Pediatric Head and Neck Tumors

Reza Rahbar · Carlos Rodriguez-Galindo
John G. Meara · Edward R. Smith
Antonio R. Perez-Atayde
Editors

Pediatric Head and Neck Tumors

A-Z Guide to Presentation and Multimodality Management

Springer

Editors
Reza Rahbar DMD, MD
Department of Otolaryngology
Harvard Medical School Boston Children's Hospital
300 Longwood Avenue - LO367
Boston, MA, USA

John G. Meara
Harvard Medical School Boston Children's Hospital
Department of Plastic and Oral Surgery
300 Longwood Avenue Enders 114
Boston, MA, USA

Antonio R. Perez-Atayde
Harvard Medical School Boston Children's Hospital
Department of Pathology
300 Longwood Avenue
Boston, MA, USA

Carlos Rodriguez-Galindo
Dana-Farber/Boston Children's Cancer and Blood Disorders Center
Harvard Medical School
450 Brookline Avenue D-3133
Boston, MA, USA

Edward R. Smith
Harvard Medical School Boston Children's Hospital
300 Longwood Avenue
Boston, MA, USA

ISBN 978-1-4939-4151-3 ISBN 978-1-4614-8755-5 (eBook)
DOI 10.1007/978-1-4614-8755-5
Springer New York Heidelberg Dordrecht London

Printed on acid-free paper

Springer is part of Springer Science+Business Media (www.springer.com)

Preface

Treatment of children with head and neck tumors exemplifies the complex multidisciplinary care that defines modern pediatric practice. From benign to malignant conditions, each tumor and each patient requires a dedicated team of specialists that understand the disease and define the best course of action, applying the most effective treatments that maximize cure options with minimal adverse effects. Accomplishing these goals requires seamless integration of many disciplines, including pathology, diagnostic and interventional radiology, otorhinolaryngology, skull base, plastic and ocular surgery, and pediatric and radiation oncology.

The Head and Neck Tumors Program at Boston Children's Hospital and Dana-Farber Cancer Institute was formed to provide a well-integrated team approach to children with those complex and often devastating diseases. In this book, we have invited a team of experts from our program to share their knowledge in the diagnosis and management of the tumors that we encounter in our practice. We would like this book to be an A to Z practical guide that provides concise reviews and treatment recommendations for the different tumors.

This work represents the efforts of many. We would like to thank all our colleagues who have so generously shared their expertise and their time, and the editors who have so patiently helped us in this process. Most of all, we are grateful to our patients and their families, whose courage and determination inspire us to continue to work, to learn, and to advance our knowledge in the treatment of these disorders.

Boston, MA, USA — Reza Rahbar, MD
Boston, MA, USA — Carlos Rodriguez-Galindo, MD
Boston, MA, USA — John G. Meara, MD, DMD, MBA
Boston, MA, USA — Edward R. Smith, MD
Boston, MA, USA — Antonio R. Perez-Atayde, MD, PhD

Contents

Contributors

Natasha M. Archer Department of Pediatric Hematology-Oncology, Dana-Farber/Boston Children's Cancer and Blood Disorders Center, Roxbury, MA, USA

Lissa C. Baird Department of Neurosurgery, Oregon Health & Science University, Portland, OR, USA

Jacob R. Brodsky Department of Otolaryngology and Communication Enhancement, Boston Children's Hospital, Harvard Medical School, Boston, MA, USA

Rafael A. Couto Department of Plastic and Oral Surgery, Boston Children's Hospital, Harvard Medical School, Boston, MA, USA

Michael J. Cunningham Department of Otolaryngology and Communication Enhancement, Boston Children's Hospital, Harvard Medical School, Boston, MA, USA

Alfredo A. Dela Rosa Department of Oral and Maxillofacial Surgery, University of the Pacific, School of Dentistry, San Francisco, CA, USA

A. Lindsay Frazier Department of Pediatric Oncology, Dana-Farber Cancer Institute, Boston, MA, USA

Catherine M. Gordon Department of Adolescent Medicine, Hasbro Children's Hospital, Providence, RI, USA

Adam L. Green Pediatric Oncology, Dana-Farber Cancer Institute, Boston, MA, USA

Lillian M. Guenther Department of Medicine, Boston Children's Hospital, Harvard Medical School, Boston, MA, USA

Stephen A. Huang Department of Medicine, Boston Children's Hospital, Harvard Medical School, Boston, MA, USA

Katherine A. Janeway Department of Pediatric Oncology, Boston Children's Hospital, Harvard Medical School, Boston, MA, USA

Dwight T. Jones Department of Otolaryngology - Head and Neck Surgery, University of Nebraska College of Medicine, Omaha, NE, USA

Vikramjit S. Kanwar Pediatric Hematology-Oncology, Albany Medical Center, Albany, NY, USA

Stephen Kieran Department of Otolaryngology, Boston Children's Hospital, Harvard Medical School, Boston, MA, USA

Sang Yoon Kim Department of Oral and Maxillofacial Surgery, INOVA Fairfax Hospital, Vienna, VA, USA

Ilkka Kivekäs Department of Otolaryngology and Communication Enhancement, Boston Children's Hospital, Harvard Medical School Boston, MA, USA

Department of Otorhinolaryngology, Tampere University Hospital and the University of Tampere, Tampere, Finland

Brian Labow Department of Plastic and Oral Surgery, Boston Children's Hospital, Harvard Medical School, Boston, MA, USA

Paul Lennon Department of Otolaryngology and Communication Enhancement, Boston Children's Hospital, Harvard Medical School, Boston, MA, USA

Jennifer W. Mack Dana-Farber Cancer Institute, Boston, MA, USA

Department of Pediatric Hematology/Oncology, Boston Children's Hospital, Harvard Medical School, Boston, MA, USA

Karen J. Marcus Pediatric Radiation Oncology, Dana Farber/Boston Children's Cancer and Blood Disorders Center, Brigham and Women's Hospital, Harvard Medical School, Boston, MA, USA

Trevor McGill Department of Otolaryngology and Communication Enhancement, Boston Children's Hospital, Harvard Medical School, Boston, MA, USA

Brendan McNeish Boston Children's Hospital, Harvard Medical School, Boston, MA, USA

John G. Meara Department of Plastic and Oral Surgery, Boston Children's Hospital, Harvard Medical School, Boston, MA, USA

Biren P. Modi Department of Surgery, Boston Children's Hospital, Harvard Medical School, Boston, MA, USA

Allison O'Neill Department of Pediatric Oncology, Harvard Medical School, Dana-Farber/ Boston Children's Hospital Cancer and Blood Disorders Center, Boston, MA, USA

Darren B. Orbach Department of Radiology, Boston Children's Hospital, Harvard Medical School, Boston, MA, USA

Interventional & Neurointerventional Radiology, Department of Radiology, Boston Children's Hospital, Harvard Medical School, Boston, MA, USA

Padua Jr. Department of Radiology, Boston Children's Hospital, Harvard Medical School, Boston, MA, USA

Horacio M. Padua Department of Radiology, Boston Children's Hospital, Harvard Medical School, Boston, MA, USA

Bonnie L. Padwa Department of Plastic and Oral Surgery, Boston Children's Hospital, Harvard Medical School, Boston, MA, USA

Antonio R. Perez-Atayde Department of Pathology, Boston Children's Hospital, Harvard Medical School, Boston, MA, USA

Dennis Poe Department of Otolaryngology and Communication Enhancement, Boston Children's Hospital, Harvard Medical School, Boston, MA, USA

Sanjay P. Prabhu Department of Radiology, Boston Children's Hospital, Harvard Medical School, Boston, MA, USA

Mark Proctor Boston Children's Hospital, Harvard Medical School, Boston, MA, USA

Melissa S. Putman Department of Endocrinology, Boston Children's Hospital, Harvard Medical School, Boston, MA, USA

Reza Rahbar Department of Otolaryngology and Communication Enhancement, Boston Children's Hospital, Harvard Medical School, Boston, MA, USA

Carlos Rodriguez-Galindo Department of Pediatric Oncology, Dana-Farber/Boston Children's Hospital Cancer and Blood Disorders Center, Harvard Medical School, Boston, MA, USA

R. Michael Scott Boston Children's Hospital, Harvard Medical School, Boston, MA, USA

Raja Shaikh Department of Interventional Radiology, Boston Children's Hospital, Harvard Medical School, Boston, MA, USA

Robert C. Shamberger Department of Surgery, Boston Children's Hospital, Harvard Medical School, Boston, MA, USA

Suzanne Shusterman Department of Pediatric Hematology-Oncology, Dana-Farber/Boston Children's Cancer and Blood Disorders Center, Boston, MA, USA

Edward R. Smith Department of Neurosurgery, Boston Children's Hospital, Harvard Medical School, Boston, MA, USA

Lisa M. Stafford College of Nanoscale Engineering, Albany, NY, USA

Amir Taghinia Department of Plastic and Oral Surgery, Boston Children's Hospital, Harvard Medical School, Boston, MA, USA

Behroze Adi Vachha Department of Radiology, Beth Israel Deaconess Medical Center, Harvard Medical School, Boston, MA, USA

Deborah Vanderveen Boston Children's Hospital, Harvard Medical School, Boston, MA, USA

Christian J. Vercler Department of Plastic and Oral Surgery, Boston Children's Hospital, Harvard Medical School, Boston, MA, USA

Section of Plastic Surgery, University of Michigan, Ann Arbor, MI, USA

Frank W. Virgin Department of Otolaryngology Head and Neck Surgery, Monroe Carell Jr. Children's Hospital at Vanderbilt, Nashville, TN, USA

Mark S. Volk Department of Otolaryngology and Communication Enhancement, Boston Children's Hospital, Harvard Medical School, Boston, MA, USA

Lynda Vrooman Boston Children's Hospital, Harvard Medical School, Boston, MA, USA

Benjamin C. Warf Department of Neurosurgery, Boston Children's Hospital, Harvard Medical School, Boston, MA, USA

Karen Watters Boston Children's Hospital, Harvard Medical School, Boston, MA, USA

Department of Otolaryngology and Communication Enhancement, Boston Children's Hospital, Harvard Medical School, Boston, MA, USA

Christopher Weldon Department of Surgery, Boston Children's Hospital, Harvard Medical School, Boston, MA, USA

Kenneth R. Whittemore, Jr. Department of Otolaryngology and Communication Enhancement, Boston Children's Hospital, Harvard Medical School, Boston, MA, USA

Part I

Evaluation and Management

Imaging

1

Behroze Adi Vachha and Sanjay P. Prabhu

Introduction

Head and neck masses are relatively common in children. Unlike adults, where the majority of neck lesions encountered are malignant, neck masses in children are usually (>90%) benign. Neck masses may be a result of a variety of congenital, infective, inflammatory, traumatic, lymphovascular, and neoplastic etiologies [1, 2].

Imaging assessment of neck masses is tailored based on the child's symptoms and findings on clinical exam. Goal of imaging should be to generate a limited list of differential diagnoses or in some cases, specify a single definitive diagnosis while keeping the ionizing radiation exposure as low as reasonably achievable (the ALARA principle).

If a lesion is thought to be neoplastic, further imaging is aimed at characterizing tumors and providing a more refined differential diagnosis, assessing the extent of the lesion, detecting involvement of adjacent structures and determining metastatic spread if the tumor is malignant, all of which are essential for appropriate treatment planning as well as to determine the prognosis of malignant tumors. Imaging is also used to guide needle biopsy and to follow response to therapy. It is important to note that while imaging can narrow the differential diagnosis of pediatric head and neck masses, biopsy and/or excision may still be required for definitive therapy.

Head and neck tumors are less common with only 5% of pediatric primary malignancies arising in the head and neck region [3]. Imaging plays an important role in the differentiation of the more benign entities from malignancies. Early diagnosis is critical as many pediatric head and neck malignancies are readily treatable and often curable by current medical and surgical management when detected early.

In this chapter we outline the various imaging techniques used to assess head and neck neoplasms (benign and malignant) in the pediatric population and review the imaging findings of most common pediatric benign and malignant tumors.

Overview of Imaging Techniques

A tailored multimodality imaging approach utilizing varying combinations of ultrasound (US), computed tomography (CT), magnetic resonance imaging (MRI), and radionuclide studies is useful in characterizing pediatric neck tumors and allows for appropriate management.

Ultrasound (US)

US is often the initial imaging modality of choice in the evaluation of palpable extracranial head and neck tumors and assessment of superficial glandular structures such as the thyroid and salivary glands in children [2].

Advantages of US in children include smaller neck size and relative lack of subcutaneous fat in children results in better sonographic penetration and resolution [4]. US plays an important role in distinguishing solid from cystic lesions and differentiating nodal from non-nodal masses [5]. In contrast to CT and MRI, US provides real-time, rapid noninvasive imaging at a lower cost and does not involve ionizing radiation exposure. It is portable and can be performed at the bedside without the need to sedate the child.

Drawbacks of US include the dependency on operator skill and experience and inherent lower spatial resolution and tissue contrast than cross-sectional imaging modalities. Optimizing US technique can help improve image quality and aid diagnosis.

S. P. Prabhu (✉)
Department of Radiology, Boston Children's Hospital, Harvard Medical School, Boston, MA, USA
e-mail: sanjay.prabhu@childrens.harvard.edu

B. A. Vachha
Department of Radiology, Beth Israel Deaconess Medical Center, Harvard Medical School, Boston, MA, USA

R. Rahbar et al. (eds.), *Pediatric Head and Neck Tumors*,
DOI 10.1007/978-1-4614-8755-5_1, © Springer Science+Business Media New York 2014

Ideally, the patient is scanned in a supine position with the neck slightly hyperextended to optimize field of view. Using high frequency linear array transducers (7–12 MHz) to evaluate superficial neck structures, small footprint high frequency small part transducers in infants and curved or sector transducers (6–8 MHz) to provide improved resolution of deeper structures in the neck are among the methods to optimize US of the neck in children [3, 4]. Color Doppler examinations and spectral tracings should be used to evaluate presence of and pattern of vascular flow within the mass [5].

Computed Tomography (CT)

Advantages of CT include its ready availability in emergent settings and ability to detect osseous changes caused by the mass such as remodeling or erosion and intralesional calcification better than MRI and US. Multidetector CT (MDCT) scanners allow for rapid scan acquisition without compromising image quality. This is especially useful in critically ill children who cannot reliably suspend respiration. Also, fast scan times decrease the potential for motion degradation and may obviate the need for sedation. Volumetric 3-D reconstruction of lesions after MDCT acquisition can be used to plan surgical approaches and assess tumor response following treatment.

Main limitation of CT in pediatric populations includes risks of ionizing radiation exposure associated with CT, particularly the potential carcinogenic effects [4, 6–8]. Technical options are now included in newer CT scanners in an effort to reduce the dose from CT exams. These include x-ray beam filtration and collimation, tube current modulation tailored to patient size and indication, peak kilovoltage optimization, improved detector efficiency, and noise reduction algorithms [9, 10]. Adhering to the ALARA concept entails applying strategies that reduce radiation exposure to the child without compromising diagnostic accuracy and alternative methods of imaging like MRI and US should be explored in all cases [11]. CT has lower tissue contrast resolution compared to MRI.

Certain technical issues need to be considered to ensure that the maximum information is gained from the CT scan. For CT of the soft tissues of the neck, the child is usually placed in the supine position with the neck slightly extended to exclude the orbits. Most studies can be performed with the child breathing quietly. Region scanned usually extends from the skull base to the top of the aortic arch. Intravenous contrast should be administered if there are no contraindications to the use of contrast for better delineation of masses from adjacent structures and to determine tumor enhancement patterns. For contrast-enhanced studies, split bolus techniques (wherein half the contrast is administered and images are then obtained after 3-min pause during the administration of the second half of the contrast bolus) provide better lesion and vascular enhancement without the need for multiple phases of scanning, which increase the radiation dose [5]. Multiplanar reconstructions are generated from the initial data set to avoid repeated scans.

Magnetic Resonance Imaging (MRI)

MRI is the ideal modality of choice for investigating neck masses due to its superior soft tissue resolution and avoidance of ionizing radiation. Contrast-enhanced MRI better defines lesion extent and margins and it can detect perineural spread of tumor and intracranial extension. Although CT provides better illustration of subtle cortical erosion, bone infiltration and cartilage invasion by soft tissue lesions is detected earlier and defined better by MRI.

The main disadvantage of MRI in children is that the many sequences require the child to lie still for a substantially longer amount of time than that needed for a CT and therefore, sedation of younger children is often required to reduce motion artifacts. Artifacts after surgical reconstruction with metallic hardware limit visualization on MRI due to susceptibility artifact, particularly on images employing fat saturation and echoplanar imaging.

MRI technique and sequence selection should be optimized based on the age of the child, the location and type of neck mass being investigated. Patients older than age 6 are placed in the supine position with the neck slightly extended and the study is performed with the child breathing quietly. Infants may be fed prior to the exam and swaddled to minimize motion artifact ("feed and wrap"). Slightly older pediatric patients (less than 6 years) often require sedation to optimize image acquisition [4].

Indication-based protocols should be employed to ensure that the diagnosis is determined with the least number of sequences and within the shortest time possible. This approach helps minimize duration of sedation and avoids the risk of patient motion in younger patients being scanned without sedation. Most head and neck protocols include multiplanar T1, fat-suppressed T2 or STIR images, a flow-sensitive gradient echo sequence, and contrast-enhanced multiplanar fat-suppressed T1-weighted sequences. Sagittal imaging may be considered for lesions around the temporomandibular joint, tongue base, nasopharyngeal, and airway lesions [12].

Diffusion-weighted imaging (DWI) has shown some value in characterization of head and neck mass lesions in children. As a rule of thumb, malignant pediatric tumors have lower apparent diffusion coefficient (ADC) than that of benign solid and cystic lesions, likely reflecting increased lesion cellularity [13]. For example, rhabdomyosarcomas (RMSs)have the lowest ADC values and mucoepidermoid carcinomas have higher ADC values than sarcomas [13].

Additional studies are required to assess the value of DWI in initial diagnosis and evaluation of response-following therapy of pediatric head and neck neoplasms.

Radionuclide Studies (Positron Emission Tomography (PET) and PET-CT)

Unlike in adults, the role of PET in management of all pediatric solid tumors is less well-defined. However, ^{18}F fluorodeoxyglucose PET (FDG-PET) and FDG-PET-CT are important tools in the noninvasive evaluation, initial staging, and continued monitoring of children with certain types of malignancies (e.g., lymphomas and some sarcomas) [3, 14, 15].

Key advantage of FDG-PET-CT over MRI or CT is the ability to distinguish viable recurrent or residual tumor from post-therapeutic changes [14].

PET and PET-CT has the risks of ionizing radiation. Further, accurate anatomic coregistration of PET and CT images requires that the child remains still throughout the procedure. As these exams can be lengthy, younger patients often require sedation or, occasionally, general anesthesia to avoid misregistration [14, 15].

Physiologic variations in FDG distribution in children include higher uptake of FDG in thymus, adenoids, and tonsils, within metabolically active brown adipose tissue, bone marrow, and spleen [16, 17]. Uptake in the bone marrow and spleen may falsely suggest metastatic disease [14, 18, 19]. Additionally, intense FDG activity in brown adipose tissue can potentially mask cervical, supraclavicular, and axillary pathology in pediatric patients [15].

Despite these limitations, PET-CT holds promise as an alternative response of assessing tumor response to therapy.

Differential Diagnosis

The following section deals with tumors, but it is important to note that infective, inflammatory, and lymphovascular lesions are relatively more common in a child and should be considered in the differential diagnosis of head and neck masses.

Specific Tumor Types

As clinical and pathological aspects of individual tumors are dealt with elsewhere in this book, the following discussion focuses on imaging characteristics of the more common head and neck benign and malignant tumors seen in the pediatric age group.

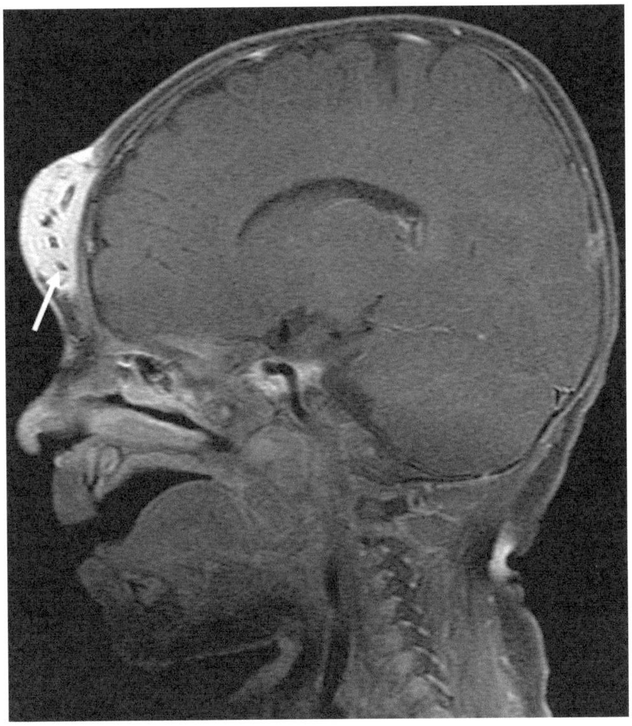

Fig. 1.1 Hemangioma. Post contrast sagittal fat-suppressed T1W image in a 6 month-old male demonstrates a large midline subcutaneous hemangioma over the forehead, characterized by marked enhancement and prominent signal void indicating presence of blood vessels (*arrow*)

Benign Tumors

Hemangioma

Hemangioma is the most common vascular tumor and arises in infants. They proliferate rapidly during the first year of life and involute over the next few years.

During the proliferative phase, US and color Doppler examinations demonstrate a soft tissue mass with prominent vessels and arterial and venous waveforms. Peak venous velocities are not as high as seen in a true arteriovenous malformation (AVM). During the involutional stage, increasing fibrofatty tissue is seen within the lesion.

Contrast-enhanced CT (CECT) demonstrates a soft tissue lobulated mass with diffuse contrast-enhancement and prominent vessels in and adjacent to the mass (Fig. 1.1).

On MRI, the lesion appears isointense to muscle during the proliferative phase and demonstrates fatty replacement during the involutional phase on T1-weighted sequences. It is mildly hyperintense to muscle on T2-weighted images. Fat saturated T1-weighted contrast-enhanced sequences demonstrate intense contrast enhancement with serpiginous flow voids in and adjacent to the mass.

Note should be made of associated abnormalities in the brain and chest in view of the known association of **p**osterior fossa malformations, **h**emangiomas, **a**rterial anomalies, **c**oarctation of the aorta and **c**ardiac defects, **e**ye abnormalities,

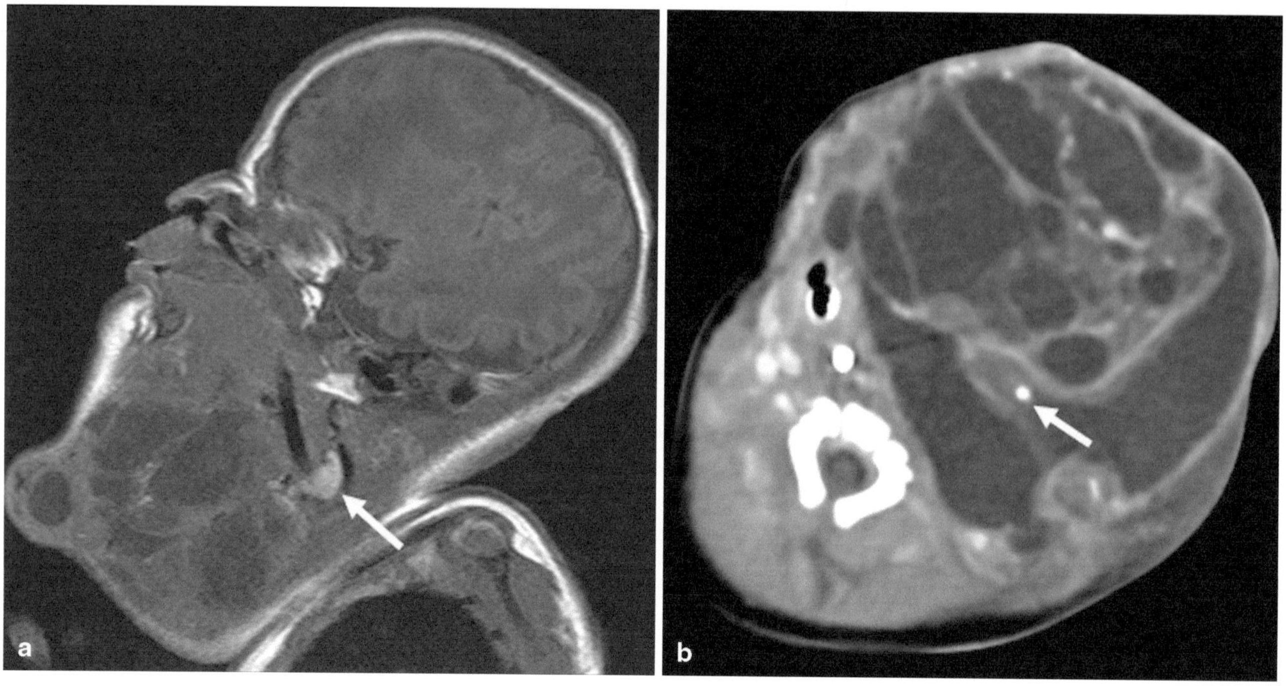

Fig. 1.2 Teratoma. **a** Sagittal T1W image shows a large mixed solid and cystic cervicofacial mass in a newborn infant. Note the hyperintense structure in the neck is the right lobe of the thyroid (*arrow*). The mass involved the left lobe of the thyroid. **b** Axial CECT shows scattered calfications within the lesion (*arrow*)

sternal malformations, and supraumbilical raphe (PHACES syndrome).

Differential diagnoses of hemangiomas include slow flow vascular malformations (venous and lymphatic malformations), arteriovenous malformations, plexiform neurofibroma, and sarcoma.

Teratoma

Teratomas are the commonest congenital head and neck tumors. Some cervicofacial teratomas are being increasingly diagnosed on antenatal US and/or MRI. These lesions present as large cervical masses can cause fatal airway compression at birth.

US demonstrates a predominantly solid or mixed cystic/solid structure.

Calcifications are virtually pathognomonic of teratoma but are seen in only half the cases and are better delineated by CT. CT demonstrates a heterogenous mass with areas of fat attenuation and calcification.

MRI signal intensities are variable and depend on the internal composition of the lesion. Presence of fat can be confirmed by using fat-saturated images (Fig. 1.2).

Differential diagnoses of cystic teratomas include lymphatic malformations and rarely infantile myofibromatosis. A useful imaging differentiating feature is that involvement of the thyroid gland by an infrahyoid congenital mass is almost pathognomonic of a teratoma (considered by some authors to be arising from the thyroid) [20].

Nerve Sheath Tumors

Plexiform neurofibromas are benign peripheral nerve sheath tumors, virtually diagnostic of neurofibromatosis Type 1. Extracranial head and neck plexiform neurofibromas arise most commonly from the trigeminal nerve at the orbital apex [21]. These lesions present as multiple masses or as fusiform enlargement of the peripheral nerves produce a “bag-of-worms” appearance [22]. On MRI, these lesions are typically hyperintense on T2-weighted images and hypointense on T1-weighted images (Fig. 1.3). Deeper lesions are typically nodular and superficial lesions have a more diffuse, infiltrating appearance involving the subcutaneous tissues and the skin.

Juvenile Nasopharyngeal Angiofibroma (JNA)

Imaging (either CT or MRI) usually confirms the diagnosis of JNA and in almost all cases, should help avoid biopsy. CT and MRI are utilized for presurgical planning of JNAs. MRI enables assessment of soft tissue extent and CT to determine the presence of skull base erosion.

Ideal imaging protocols for preoperative planning and staging include a maxillofacial CT with multiplanar reformats, maxillofacial MRI with T1-weighted fat-saturated contrast-enhanced sequences and catheter angiography of the external and internal carotid arteries (ECA and ICA, respectively) to identify feeding vessels. MR angiogram (MRA) may be performed to help evaluate the need for, and when needed, help plan catheter angiography for presurgical embolization.

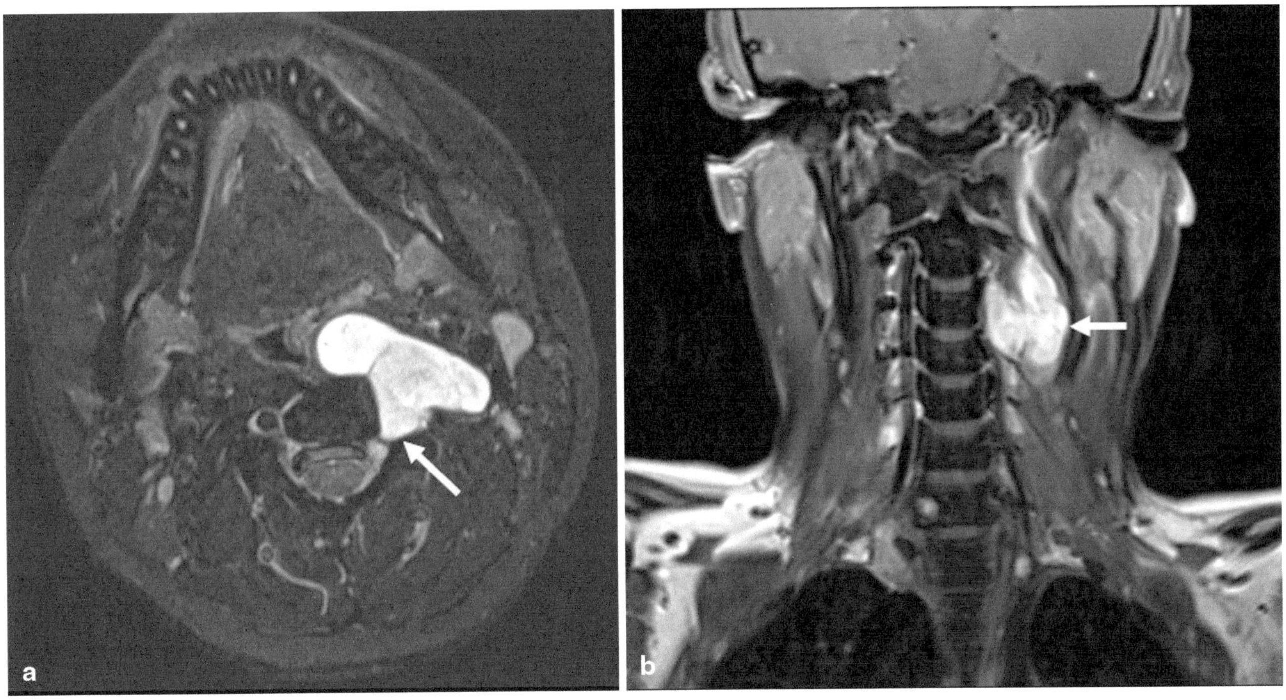

Fig. 1.3 Neurofibroma. **a** Axial fast spin echo inversion recovery (FSEIR) image shows a well-circumscribed lobulated T2 hyperintense lesion arising from the left C3-4 neural foramen in a 16 year-old male with neurofibromatosis Type 1 (*arrow*). **b** The lesion enhances avidly following contrast as seen on the coronal T1W fat-saturated images (*arrow*)

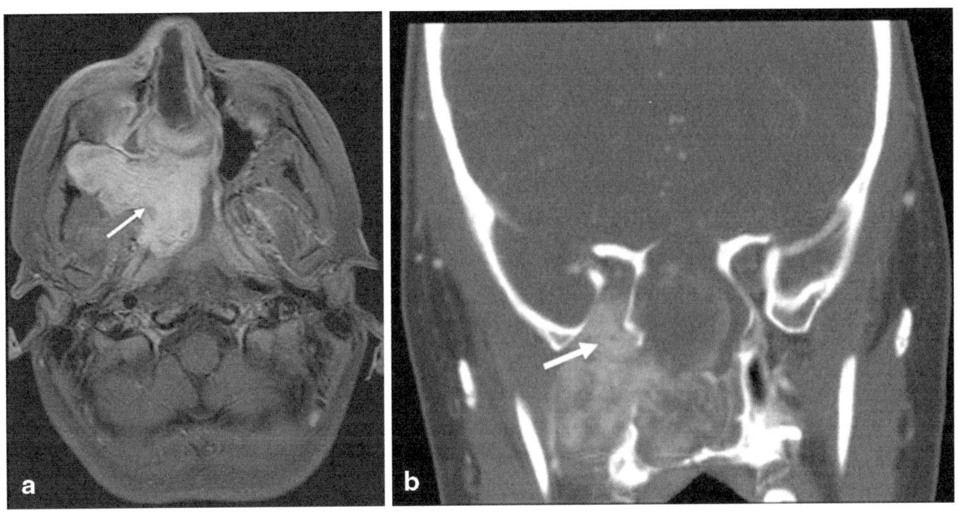

Fig. 1.4 JNA. **a** Axial fat-suppressed post contrast T1W image shows a intensely enhancing nasopharyngeal mass, eroding the sphenoid and ethmoid sinuses, expanding the pteryogopalatine fossa, and extending through the pterygomaxillary fissure into the infratemporal fossa (*arrow*) in a 12-year-old male presenting with epistaxis. **b** Coronal reformat of contrast-enhanced CT shows extension of the mass into the foramen rotundum and inferior orbital fissure (*arrow*) and extensive osseus destruction

CT usually reveals a diffusely enhancing soft tissue mass arising at the sphenopalatine foramen and extending from the posterior nasal cavity into the nasal cavity, nasopharynx, and pterygopalatine fossa (Fig. 1.4). Widening of the ipsilateral nasal cavity and pterygopalatine fossa and bowing of posterior wall of the maxillary sinus anteriorly is noted.

On MRI, a heterogeneous mass with intermediate signal is seen on T1- and T2-weighted sequences. Serpentine flow voids are typically seen within the tumor with intense enhancement post contrast administration. Coronal T1-weighted images are required to look for cavernous sinus, sphenoid sinus, and skull base extension.

Catheter angiography demonstrates a capillary blush fed by feeding vessels (usually ascending pharyngeal or internal maxillary arteries) from the ECA or occasionally, in the case of skull base or cavernous sinus extension, from the ICA.

Differential diagnoses include antrochoanal polyp, RMS, and hemangioma.

Langerhans Cell Histiocytosis (LCH)

LCH is typically characterized on CT by an enhancing soft tissue mass associated with bony involvement, which classically involves "punched out" lytic lesions. However, bony lesions may also present with irregular sclerotic margins or fragments of bone associated with smaller or no appreciable soft tissue component.

On MRI, LCH lesions show ill-defined borders, which are iso- to hypointense on T1-weighted and iso- to hyperintense on T2-weighted sequences with homogenous enhancement. The demonstration of enhancing masses on MRI helps distinguish LCH occurring in the temporal bone from other erosive processes of the temporal bone [5].

Differential diagnoses include acquired cholesteatoma, cholesterol granuloma, acute mastoiditis, and RMS.

Malignant Tumors

The most common pediatric head and neck malignancies include lymphomas, RMSs, thyroid malignancies, nasopharyngeal carcinomas (NPCs), salivary gland malignancies, neuroblastomas, and malignant teratomas.

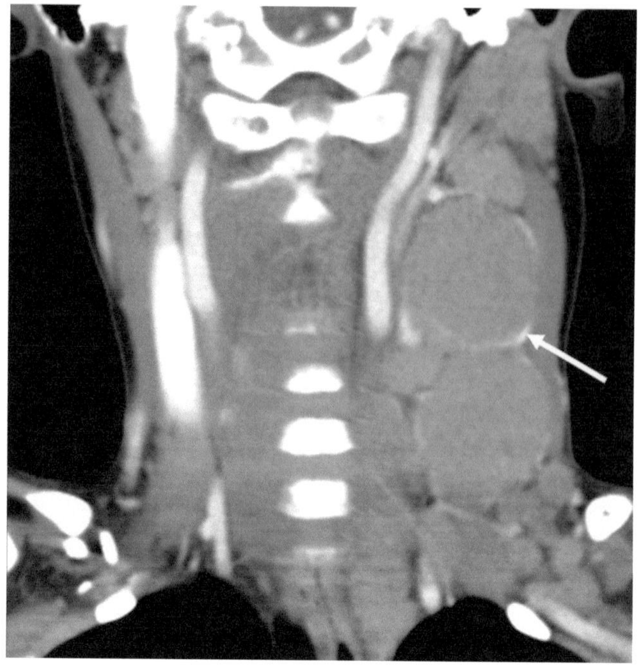

Fig. 1.5 HL. Coronal reformat of CECT shows large rounded cervical chain lymph nodes with peripheral enhancement (*arrow*)

Hodgkin Lymphoma (HL) and Non-Hodgkin Lymphomas (NHL)

US may be used to assess superficial cervical lymph nodes. Sonographic features of malignancy include increased size, loss of the normal oval shape with a more round shape, and loss of the normal echogenic hilum [4, 5]. Doppler US may demonstrate displacement of vessels, subcapsular vessels or aberrant vessels, or avascular foci.

CECT is the imaging modality of choice in assessing the disease and extent of extranodal spread, particularly involvement of lungs. CECT should include the neck chest, abdomen, and pelvis for accurate staging and may be coregistered with PET scans. Oral contrast is administered prior to the scan to help evaluate abdominal disease burden optimally.

Variable enhancement of lymph nodes may be noted (Fig. 1.5). Lymph nodes measuring less than 1 cm in short axis diameter are usually considered normal by size criteria. Central hypodensity may indicate nodal necrosis. If there is lack of fat stranding and less intense enhancement, consider lymphoma instead of infectious lymphadenitis [5]. Burkitt's lymphoma may be seen on CT as a soft tissue mass with bony involvement of the mandible and "floating teeth" [5].

MRI demonstrates enlarged, round nodes which are isointense to hypointense to muscle on T1-weighted sequences, mildly hyperintense on T2-weighted sequences, and with less avid enhancement than reactive lymph nodes following the administration of gadolinium.

FDG-PET has been shown to be superior to Gallium 67 scans in staging, evaluating tumor response to therapy and determining tumor relapse [23].

Rhabdomyosarcoma (RMS)

RMSs are typically bone-destroying and "bone-pushing" tumors. CT best depicts this osseous change. Both CT and MRI demonstrate a soft tissue mass with variable enhancement. RMS is iso- to hypointense to muscle on T1-weighted sequences and hyperintense to muscle on T2-weighted sequences with moderate-to-intense enhancement following contrast administration (Fig. 1.6) Fat-suppressed T1-weighted images are helpful for the detection of orbital masses and parameningeal tumors. MRI also helps delineate intracranial extension of parameningeal RMSs.

Follow-up imaging using the same imaging modality should be performed no earlier than 6 weeks post therapy to avoid confusion between post-therapeutic change and residual disease. Enhancement of the tumor bed after 6 weeks after therapy is considered suspicious for recurrent or residual tumor [4].

The differential diagnosis on imaging varies according to the location of the tumor and includes lymphoma, nasopharyngeal carcinoma, metastatic neuroblastoma, JNA, and LCH.

Thyroid Malignancies

Approximately 2 % of all thyroid cancers occur in children and adolescents. When a solitary thyroid nodule is identified in children and adolescents, approximately 20 % of the lesions represent malignancy compared with 5 % in adults [24]. Following initial measurement of serum thyroid-stimulating hormone (TSH), calcitonin (for diagnosis of medullary thyroid carcinoma), a neck US is the imaging modality of

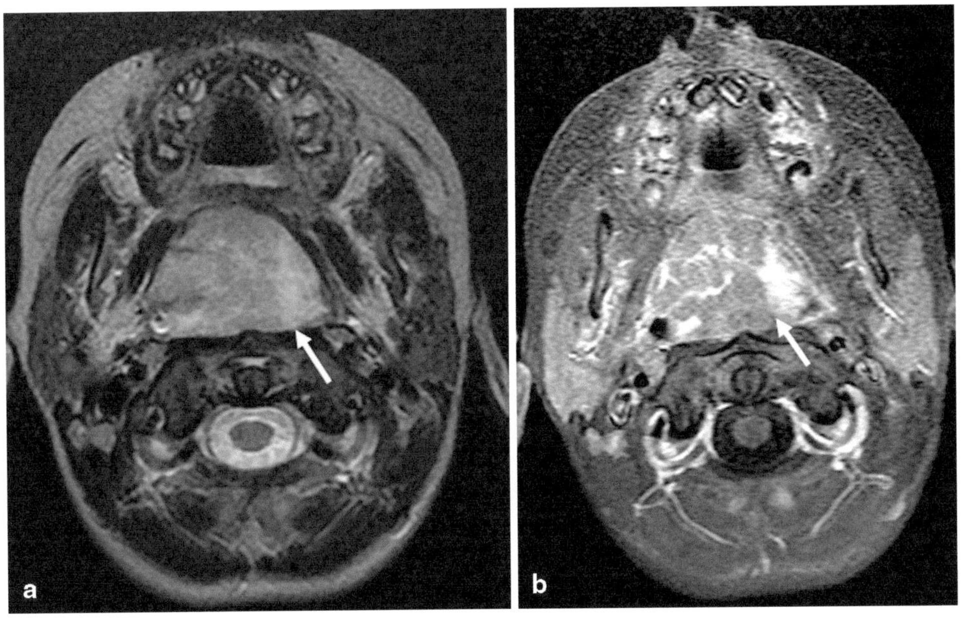

Fig. 1.6 Nasopharyngeal RMS. **a** Axial T2W image shows a large well-defined slightly T2-hypointense mass in the nasopharynx in a 28-month-old male (*arrow*). **b** Axial fat-suppressed post contrast T1W image shows the mass enhances heterogenously (*arrow*)

choice. Sonographic features suggestive of malignancy include ill-defined margins, microcalcifications, and variable echogenicity. Fine needle aspiration (FNA), which may be performed with or without US guidance may be useful for distinguishing benign and malignant nodules, but data are limited in children.

Metastases to regional cervical lymph nodes are most common in papillary thyroid carcinoma and occur in up to 90% of children affected by this type of thyroid malignancy [25].

Nasopharyngeal Carcinoma (NPC)

NPC is rare in pediatric populations and accounts for about 5% of pediatric head and neck malignancies. Children have greater bulk disease at presentation with relatively higher involvement of cranial nerves, lymph nodes, and skull base [4, 5].

NPC is characteristically seen on imaging studies as an asymmetric mass arising in the Fossa of Rosenmuller. CECT demonstrates a homogenously enhancing soft tissue mass centered in the lateral pharyngeal recess of the nasopharynx commonly associated with cervical adenopathy and skull base erosion.

On MRI, the mass is iso- to hypointense to muscle on T1-weighted sequences and hyperintense on T2-weighted sequences with homogenous enhancement following contrast administration (Fig. 1.7). Coronal contrast-enhanced T1-weighted images best depict intracranial extension of the tumor through skull base foramina. PET-CT shows FDG avid nodes.

Cervical lymph node involvement is present in 80–90% of patients at presentation, 50% of which are bilateral. As opposed to NPC in adults, necrosis within metastatic lymph nodes is uncommon in children.

Differential diagnosis based on location includes lymphoma, benign-mixed tumor, minor salivary gland malignancy, and lymphoid hyperplasia.

Salivary Gland Tumors

Although primary tumors of the salivary glands are uncommon in children, the ratio of malignant tumors to benign lesions is slightly higher in children than in adults. Tumors most commonly arise in the parotid glands. The commonest primary malignancy is mucoepidermoid carcinoma. The salivary glands may also be involved as an extra nodal site in NHL.

US, CT, and MRI are used for the evaluation of salivary gland lesions. US helps assess the size of the gland, distinguish diffuse from focal disease, and assess vascularity within the lesion and the adjacent structures, and also differentiate cystic from solid lesions. Fine-needle aspiration may be performed under US guidance.

CT is the imaging test of choice if an inflammatory mass is considered more likely and is helpful to assess for presence of calcification. MRI helps define the margins of a salivary gland mass better than CT.

Benign salivary gland tumors have a well-defined outline and do not enhance avidly on post contrast images. Calcifications within a mass on CT are highly suggestive of a benign-mixed tumor (pleomorphic adenomas). Large tumors are often lobulated. Warthin tumors are seen as well-encapsulated, homogenous cystic, or solid lesions on MRI, often in the tail of the parotid gland.

Mucoepidermoid carcinoma is the commonest malignant tumor of the salivary gland in children. CT and MRI appearances of these tumors vary with tumor grade. Lower-grade lesions resemble a pleomorphic adenoma, whereas higher-

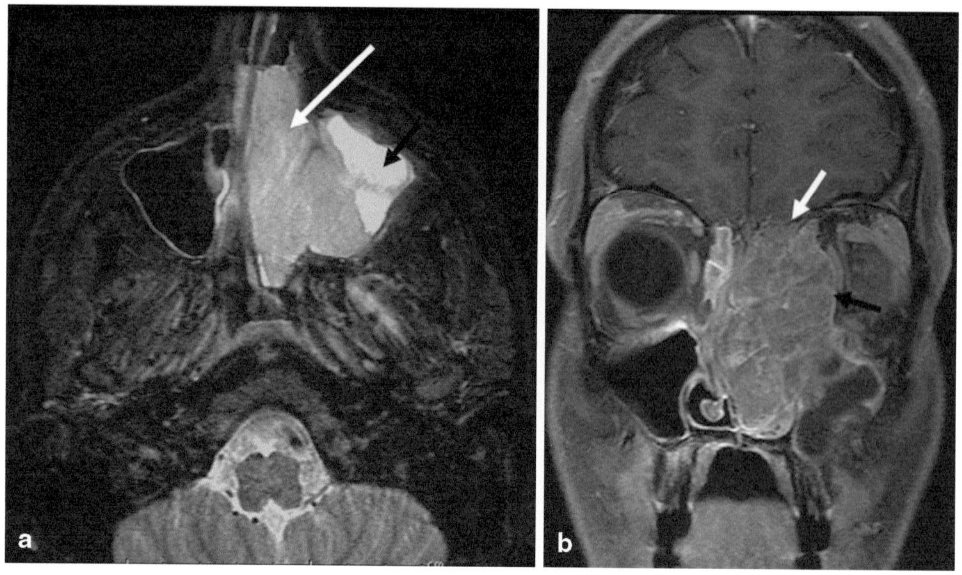

Fig. 1.7 NPC. **a** Axial FSEIR image shows sinonasal mass (*arrow*) centered along the medial left maxillary antrum and ethmoids, with low to intermediate T2 signal intensity in a 15-year-old male. Note the T2-hyperintense trapped secretions in the lateral aspect of the left maxillary sinus (*black arrow*). **b** Fat-suppressed post contrast coronal T1W image shows heterogeneous enhancement and parameningeal intracranial extension (*arrow*) through the left cribriform pate and ethmoid and also into the left orbit (*black arrow*)

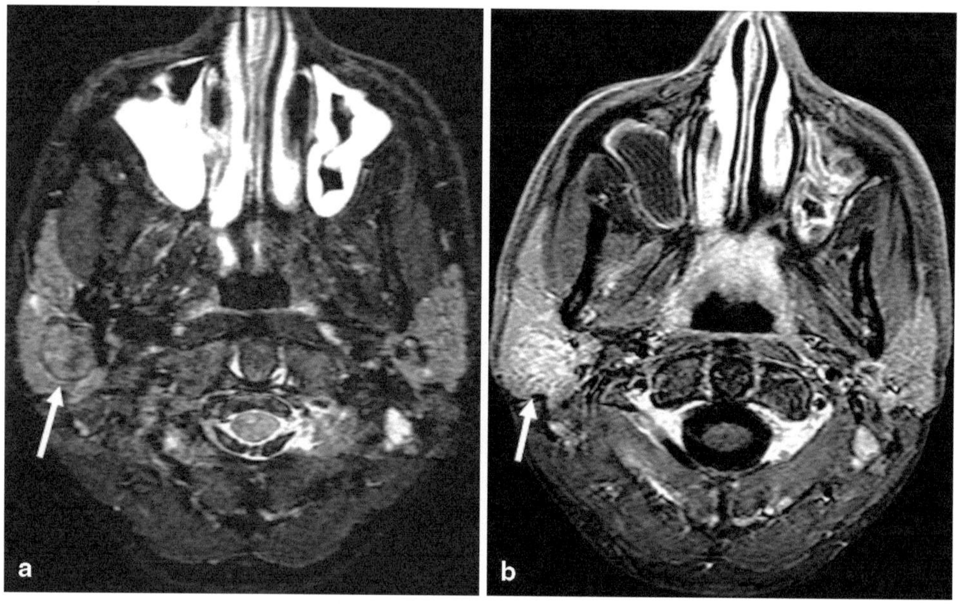

Fig. 1.8 Mucoepidermoid carcinoma. **a** Axial FSEIR image shows a well-defined heterogeneous mass (*arrow*) in the superficial and deep aspects of the right parotid gland. **b** Avid enhancement of the lesion is seen on axial fat-suppressed post contrast T1W image (*arrow*)

grade lesions have ill-defined, infiltrating margins and are more homogenous with variable enhancement (Fig. 1.8).

Neuroblastoma

Primary pediatric head and neck neuroblastomas are rare, with metastatic disease being the more common mode of involvement in this anatomic region.

Calcification may be seen on CT, but is less common in cervical neuroblastomas compared to abdominal neuroblastomas [4, 5]. Heterogeneous enhancement of the soft tissue mass is noted with CECT. Expansion of the diploic space due to marrow involvement and periosteal reaction is often seen (Fig. 1.9).

On MRI, the mass demonstrates hyperintense signal on T2-weighted images and shows heterogenous enhancement following the administration of gadolinium. Metaiodobenzylguanidine (MIBG) scans are used to assess bone and marrow involvement and in monitoring response to therapy [4].

Metastasis

Metastases in the head and neck occur more commonly to the osseous skeleton in children. These are present on CT as lytic and permeative lesions often with periosteal reaction and associated soft tissue masses. Cervical lymph nodes are variably involved. Neuroblastoma is the most common primary in children less than 2 years of age. Leukemic infiltrates are commoner in older children. Metastasis from sarcomas and other tumors is present as solitary or multiple masses. On MRI, these lesions are hypointense on T2-weighted images with avid enhancement on post contrast images.

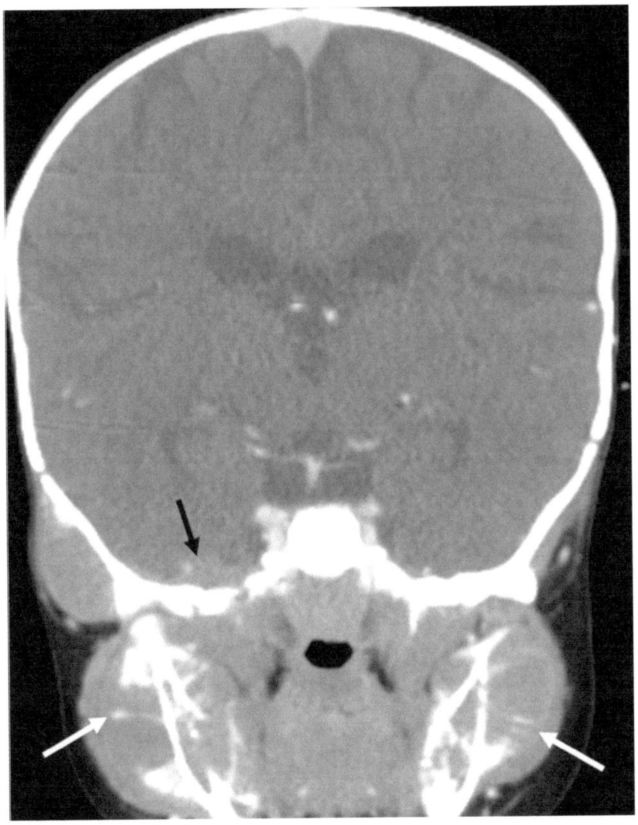

Fig. 1.9 Neuroblastoma. Coronal reformat CECT demonstrates multiple soft tissue masses around the face and neck with spiculated periosteal reaction in a 11-month-old female with increasing facial swelling and bilateral periorbital swelling and anemia (*arrows*). Note the intracranial involvement (*black arrow*)

Conclusion

The role of imaging has become increasingly important in providing maximum diagnostic information in preoperative/medical treatment planning and prognosis, and later in monitoring efficacy of therapy and detecting tumor recurrence. A carefully tailored multimodality imaging approach combined with careful history and clinical examination can help formulate a fairly accurate diagnosis and help direct appropriate patient management.

References

1. Turkington JR, Paterson A, Sweeney LE, Thornbury GD. Neck masses in children. Br J Radiol. 2005 Jan;78(925):75 85.
2. Friedman ER, John SD. Imaging of pediatric neck masses. Radiol Clin North Am. 2011 Jul;49(4):617–32, v.
3. Lloyd C, McHugh K. The role of radiology in head and neck tumours in children. Cancer Imaging. 2010;10:49–61.
4. Fefferman NR, Milla S. Ultrasound imaging of the neck in children. Ultrasound Clin. 2009;4(4):553–69.
5. Robson CD. Imaging of head and neck neoplasms in children. Pediatr Radiol. 2010 Apr;40(4):499–509.
6. Lauer MS. Elements of danger—the case of medical imaging. N Engl J Med. 2009 Aug 27;361(9):841–3.
7. Amis ES Jr, Butler PF. ACR white paper on radiation dose in medicine: three years later. J Am Coll Radiol. 2010 Nov;7(11):865–70.
8. Amis ES Jr, Butler PF, Applegate KE, et al. American college of radiology white paper on radiation dose in medicine. J Am Coll Radiol. 2007 May;4(5):272–84.
9. Mayo-Smith W. Protocol design. Image Wisely. 2010. p. 1–3.
10. Strauss KJ, Goske MJ, Kaste SC, et al. Image gently: ten steps you can take to optimize image quality and lower CT dose for pediatric patients. AJR Am J Roentgenol. 2010 Apr;194(4):868–73.
11. American College of Radiology. ACR-ASNR-SPR Practice guideline for the performance of computed tomography (CT) of the extracranial head and neck in adults and children. 2011.
12. American College of Radiology. ACR-ASNR Practice guideline for the perfomance of magnetic resonance imaging (MRI) of the head and neck. 2007.
13. Abdel Razek AA, Gaballa G, Elhawarey G, Megahed AS, Hafez M, Nada N. Characterization of pediatric head and neck masses with diffusion-weighted MR imaging. Eur Radiol. 2009 Jan;19(1):201–8.
14. Jadvar H, Connolly LP, Fahey FH, Shulkin BL. PET and PET/CT in pediatric oncology. Semin Nucl Med. 2007 Sep;37(5):316–31.
15. McCarville MB. PET-CT imaging in pediatric oncology. Cancer Imaging. 2009;9:35–43.
16. Patel PM, Alibazoglu H, Ali A, Fordham E, LaMonica G. Normal thymic uptake of FDG on PET imaging. Clin Nucl Med. 1996 Oct;21(10):772–5.
17. Weinblatt ME, Zanzi I, Belakhlef A, Babchyck B, Kochen J. False-positive FDG-PET imaging of the thymus of a child with Hodgkin's disease. J Nucl Med. 1997 Jun;38(6):888–90.
18. Hollinger EF, Alibazoglu H, Ali A, Green A, Lamonica G. Hematopoietic cytokine-mediated FDG uptake simulates the appearance of diffuse metastatic disease on whole-body PET imaging. Clin Nucl Med. 1998 Feb;23(2):93–8.
19. Sugawara Y, Fisher SJ, Zasadny KR, Kison PV, Baker LH, Wahl RL. Preclinical and clinical studies of bone marrow uptake of fluorine-1-fluorodeoxyglucose with or without granulocyte colony-stimulating factor during chemotherapy. J Clin Oncol. 1998 Jan;16(1):173–80.
20. Riedlinger WF, Lack EE, Robson CD, Rahbar R, Nose V. Primary thyroid teratomas in children: a report of 11 cases with a proposal of criteria for their diagnosis. Am J Surg Pathol. 2005 May;29(5):700–6.
21. Khanna G, Sato Y, Smith RJ, Bauman NM, Nerad J. Causes of facial swelling in pediatric patients: correlation of clinical and radiologic findings. Radiographics. 2006 Jan–Feb;26(1):157–71.
22. Lin J, Martel W. Cross-sectional imaging of peripheral nerve sheath tumors: characteristic signs on CT, MR imaging, and sonography. AJR Am J Roentgenol. 2001 Jan;176(1):75–82.
23. Hudson MM, Krasin MJ, Kaste SC. PET imaging in pediatric Hodgkin's lymphoma. Pediatr Radiol. 2004 Mar;34(3):190–8.
24. Dinauer CA, Breuer C, Rivkees SA. Differentiated thyroid cancer in children: diagnosis and management. Curr Opin Oncol. 2008 Jan;20(1):59–65.
25. Dähnert W. Radiology review manual. 7th ed. Philadelphia: Wolters Kluwer/Lippincott Williams Wilkins. 2011.

Reconstructive Surgery

2

Brian Labow and Amir Taghinia

Introduction

This chapter deals with the broad subject of reconstructive surgery in the management of pediatric head and neck tumors. The nature of the subject mandates a somewhat different format in that a wide array of tumor types and anatomic locations are considered. As such, an overview of the thought processes and management principles that guide the reconstructive surgeon will be outlined. Preoperative planning, intraoperative management, and specialized areas for reconstruction will be emphasized. Some details for specific defects and commonly used flaps and techniques will also be presented.

A few important caveats should also be stated at the outset. Many of the tumor types and resultant defects found in pediatric head and neck oncology are rare, and in some cases represent unique situations. As such, reconstructive treatment recommendations are rarely evidence-based and depend more on principles and experience rather than established protocols or algorithms. The literature supporting a given reconstructive modality is often quite limited, especially in pediatric patients and prospective well-controlled studies are lacking. The authors recognize that there is always more than one reconstructive option and that the patient's, parents', and surgeon's familiarity and comfort with the risk and rewards of various approaches may also play a role in determining the type of reconstruction method that is selected. As such, the material presented below should be viewed as a guide rather than a series of definitive treatment recommendations.

Preoperative Planning: General Considerations

Successful reconstruction of the pediatric head and neck invariably begins with careful preparation [1]. The reconstructive surgeon should be engaged as soon as it is determined that some form of reconstruction may be needed. Ideally, this should occur well in advance of tumor extirpation. This allows for a complete understanding of the diagnosis, adjuvant treatments and prognosis, as well as interdisciplinary communication by all treatment teams, including radiology. In particular, the reconstructive surgeon should be aware of what anatomic structures are definitely, likely, or possibly involved. Will immediate reconstruction be required? How will surgical margins be assessed? How likely is tumor involvement at the margins and will this mandate reexcision? What is the likelihood of local recurrence and subsequent resection? These questions should be openly discussed as the answers to these questions may influence the type and timing of reconstruction.

Adjuvant therapy and its timing should also be discussed. Radiation can significantly affect the choice of reconstructive procedure. When administered prior to resection and reconstruction, radiation can cause local tissues to be edematous and microcirculation poor [1, 2]. In this setting, local tissue rearrangement or local flaps may have a higher rate of failure. Conversely, radiation after reconstruction can produce long-lasting deleterious changes that may lead the reconstructive surgeon to defer certain elements of the reconstruction until later in childhood to avoid the direct effect of radiation on the reconstructed element in question (Fig. 2.1). In some instances, neoadjuvant chemotherapy may severely lower the ability of the patient to tolerate prolonged reconstructive procedures such as free-tissue transfers and necessitate less invasive procedures. In other cases, delays in wound healing from reconstructive complications can dangerously delay postoperative chemotherapy. In these instances, less complex reconstructive choices may be necessary initially to increase the likelihood of early, uncomplicated wound closure.

Once the reconstructive surgeon fully understands the anatomic requirements and other treatment modalities to be employed in management of the tumor, a series of reconstructive options should be generated. In some instances there may be one clear "first option", in other instances there

B. Labow (✉) · A. Taghinia
Department of Plastic and Oral Surgery, Boston Children's Hospital, Harvard Medical School, Boston, MA, USA
e-mail: brian.labow@childrens.harvard.edu

R. Rahbar et al. (eds.), *Pediatric Head and Neck Tumors*,
DOI 10.1007/978-1-4614-8755-5_2, © Springer Science+Business Media New York 2014

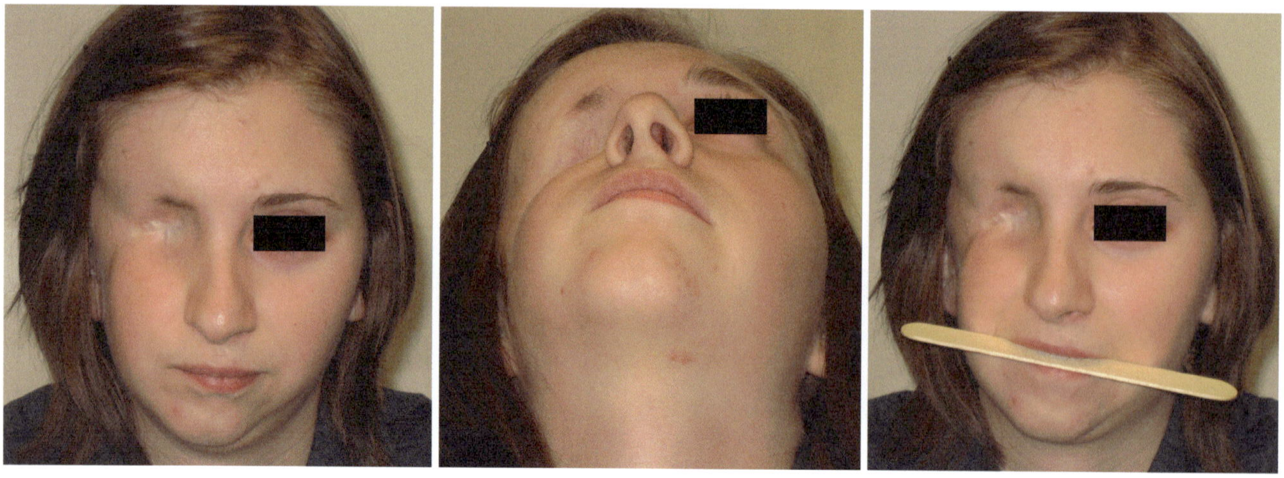

Fig. 2.1 Radiation effect. This adolescent patient underwent orbital extenteration for a rhabdomyosarcoma at the age of 4. She had free tissue transfer elsewhere followed by radiation. This case demonstrates the dramatic ill effects of radiation therapy on the growing maxillofacial skeleton. The mandible, maxilla, and orbit are substantially underdeveloped on the affected side

may be two or three equivocal options. Regardless, it is necessary to have at least one alternative procedure going into the operating room. This "lifeboat" may be deployed when intraoperative conditions change (e.g., unrecognized tumor progression, patient instability) or if the primary reconstruction modality is unsuccessful (e.g., partial or complete flap loss). When the reconstructive surgeon meets the patient and family, the rationale for the various the options should be fully discussed along with the advantages and disadvantages inherent to all reconstruction choices.

Equally important to interprovider consultation, preoperative planning must involve the parents and, when appropriate, the patient as well. The family will be overwhelmed by the diagnosis and there is often a sense of urgency to proceed as quickly as possible. The family may have been told that some form of "plastic surgery" or "reconstruction" will be required prior to the consultation with the reconstructive surgeon. A fine line must be walked between giving the family hope and inadvertently leading the family to have unrealistic expectations for the reconstruction. In addition to defining the defect and the reconstruction needs of the patient, the preferred treatment option(s) will be outlined. These may change based on anatomic considerations following physical examination or psychosocial considerations. For example, scarring from previous surgery may preclude specific donor sites for tissue or recipient vessels in case a microvascular procedure is required. Fortunately, unlike adult head and neck cancer patients, the effects of tobacco, diabetes, and other chronic comorbidities are rarely encountered. However, psychosocial considerations especially in adolescent patients, must be accounted for. It is important for the reconstructive surgeon to assess the family's and patient's understanding and tolerance for the reconstructive procedure being considered. In some cases, a simpler reconstruction with a less than ideal aesthetic outcome may be preferred if the surgical risks, recovery time, or postoperative restrictions are unacceptable to the patient or family.

All donor sites or potential donor sites for tissue, areas of scarring, and secondary deformities should be disclosed along with expectations for functional and aesthetic limitations at both the donor and recipient sites following surgery. Furthermore, depending on the age of the child, special attention should be given to the effects of growth on both of these locations. In many instances, additional procedures later in childhood will be required to address growth differences in the area of reconstruction. When this can be anticipated, the family should be made fully aware of a secondary procedure. In some instances, optimal reconstruction may require a series of staged procedures over time. Each patient and family should be viewed as unique with specific anatomic, psychological and social considerations. Care by the reconstructive team should be viewed as individualized, long-term, and may even exceed that of all other care team members.

Intraoperative Considerations

Timing and Sequence

A two-team approach is often helpful to minimize patient anesthesia and surgeon fatigue. In these situations, the free tissue flap is raised simultaneously with the extirpative operation. Clear communication between the oncologic and reconstructive teams is vital in these cases, especially when a skin flap is required. With poor communication between the teams, it is not uncommon to raise a flap that is too small for the defect. Certainly, the safest approach is to wait until the defect is complete. In our experience, however, most cases are amenable to a two-team approach.

Anesthesia

If combined with cancer ablative operations, head and neck reconstructive procedures are often lengthy. An experienced anesthesia team is crucial for optimizing care and minimizing complications.

Airway In cases that involve the oropharynx, a nasal ray endotracheal tube is obligatory. The tube can be secured to the caudal septum with a heavy silk stitch. To avoid alar rim skin necrosis, the entire tubing apparatus should be brought inferiorly and secured to the patient's foam-padded forehead with tape. A straight accordion tube extender is often useful to lengthen the circuit and avoid kinks. The tubing closer to the anesthesia machine can also be secured to the back of the headrest for additional security. Once this process is complete, the surgeon should check the integrity of this construct by turning the head in either direction.

Positioning The positioning of the patient will depend to some extent on the reconstructive plan. In the case of pedicled flaps and most free tissue flaps, supine positioning is adequate. If a large defect is anticipated and a latissimus flap is considered for reconstruction, it may be prudent to harvest the muscle flap first in a lateral decubitus position, then partially close the donor site and turn the patient supine for the extirpative operation.

Tubes and Lines Hemodynamic instability is rare during resection and reconstruction of most pediatric head and neck tumors. The main exception to this is in large vascular malformations, especially arteriovenous malformations. As such, invasive monitoring is typically limited to an arterial line and at least one and usually two peripheral intravenous lines. If postoperative chemotherapy or frequent blood sampling is anticipated postoperatively, a central venous catheter may be placed at the outset of the procedure. In patients coming to the operating room with a previously placed port-a-cath™ or long-term indwelling central venous catheter, special care must be taken to ensure appropriate handling and interrogation of these sites if they are to be used. The use of such devices should be cleared with the oncology team, parents, and the surgical team caring for the line. A nasogastric or orogastric tube is usually needed—initially for decompressing the stomach and potentially following surgery for nutrition.

Medication A broad-spectrum antibiotic that covers oral/nasal flora is routine and should be continued in the perioperative period. Other medications to consider for postoperative comfort are antiemetics and pain medications. The surgeon should communicate early with the anesthesiologist about the use of vasopressors. Too often, a wide-open arterial anastomosis has been redone only to find that the agent responsible for the pale flap was the vasopressor. Fluid, colloid, or blood product administration should be the first line of treatment in these cases.

Technical Considerations

Several important technical considerations are related to the actual execution of the operation merit discussion. Careful attention to these issues separates the good outcomes from the potential disaster cases.

Oral Cavity Separation One of the most difficult complications of oropharyngeal reconstruction is the dreaded fistula [3–12]. Fistulas may develop between the oropharynx and the nasal cavity or the skin. Typically, they occur at the flap and native mucosa juncture. To minimize the risk of fistulas, one should consider the causative factors: poor healing and inadequate seal. Poor healing may result from ischemia, infection, or a suboptimal environment (such as bathing in saliva or a radiated tissue bed). Ischemia can be controlled by bringing healthy, well-vascularized tissue to the defect and by resecting all poorly perfused tissues. Inadequate seal is almost always a result of poor surgical planning or execution. The most problematic areas for obtaining a tight seal are at the gingiva, the palate, and posterior mouth. Patients with intraoral tumor involvement, radiation, or poor oral hygiene may present with mucosa that is friable. The right approach is to remove all of the friable and suboptimal tissue from the area so that a tight seal can be created with the newly transferred flap and the surrounding tissues.

Brain–Mucosa Separation When reconstructing defects that involve the cranial base, it is critical to obtain a good seal to separate the brain from the mucosa [13]. Tumor extirpation operations that involve the cranial base typically leave a large soft tissue defect. Obliteration of the resulting dead space is paramount to avoid cerebrospinal fluid leakage and infection. It is not uncommon to have to utilize a muscle flap in addition to a fasciocutaneous flap in these cases—the former for obliteration of the dead space and the latter for mucosal reconstruction.

Microsurgery The importance of adequate vessels for microvascular anastomosis cannot be overstated—the larger the vessels, the higher the likelihood of success. Source vessels found in the neck have reliable anatomy and flow. These vessels may be too distant for more cephalic defects such as the scalp or orbit; in which case, the facial or superficial temporal vessels may be substituted [14]. In head and neck reconstruction, one rarely encounters difficulty in finding a suitable artery. However, finding an appropriate vein can sometimes be challenging. Good communication between the extirpative team and the reconstructive team from the outset of the procedure may allow for the identification and preservation of useful recipient vessels later in the procedure. In situations where the area is heavily scarred or has been previously radiated, one should consider (a) vein grafting to the opposite side or (b) use of the ipsilateral cephalic vein. It is rarely worth the risk to use less than optimal vessels in a zone compromised by scarring or radiation, to avoid the additional effort of vein grafting, using the contralateral side or the ipsilateral cephalic vein. We have found the cephalic vein quite useful in difficult outflow situations. A long segment can be harvested from the ipsilateral arm using multiple stab incisions. Minimal morbidity, anatomic consistency, and long length make this vein a perfect "bail out" strategy in difficult situations. There is ongoing debate in the literature about immediate versus delayed use of arteriovenous loops. The most recent literature suggests that staging of arteriovenous loops is not necessary [15].

Flaps

In this section, we will outline common flaps that are utilized for head and neck reconstruction. These flaps have consistent anatomy, low donor site morbidity, and long, reliable pedicles that allow a wide reach in the head and neck—they are the workhorse flaps of head and neck reconstruction [16].

Radial Forearm Flap [17, 18] This flap provides thin, reliably perfused tissue based on a long pedicle for reconstruction of small to moderate sized defects. The anatomy is consistent, the flap is easy to harvest, and outcomes have been excellent [6, 7, 11, 12, 16, 19–21]. It can be harvested as a fasciocutaneous flap or an adipofascial flap. Inclusion of the medial or lateral antebrachial cutaneous nerve creates a neurosensory flap that may be useful, to restore sensation to areas such as the palate. For small flaps, the donor site can be closed linearly. For larger flaps, a skin graft is required. The healing of this skin graft can be problematic if the paratenon over the flexor carpi radialis tendon is stripped [21–24]. Prior to harvesting this flap, one must perform an Allen's test to confirm integrity of the superficial palmar arch.

Anterolateral Thigh Flap Based on the descending branch of the lateral femoral circumflex artery, this versatile flap provides a substantial surface area of skin for reconstruction of large defects in the head and neck [16, 25–30]. The anatomy of the flap and pedicle are reliable and consistent. A large amount of skin and subcutaneous fat can be harvested with the flap and the donor site morbidity is minimal [31]. In some cases, the vascular pedicle courses along the fascial interface between the rectus femoris and the vastus lateralis muscles. However, in most cases, the vascular pedicle is intramuscular, thus making the dissection more tedious. In larger patients, its relatively remote location from the head and neck, as well as its anterior location makes it amenable to a two-team approach.

Rectus Abdominis (Myo or Myocutaneous) This flap is used in a variety of anatomic locations and in head and neck reconstruction can provide cutaneous coverage or fill large cavities (Figs. 2.2–2.7) [6, 8, 13, 32]. The flap is harvested from the lower abdomen, preferably through a low transverse incision when only muscle is required or with an ellipse of skin and fat contiguous with the underlying muscle when coverage or lining is needed. The blood supply to the flap is via the inferior epigastric system. The pedicle is typically large, long, and easy to dissect. Depending on the amount of fascia taken with the muscle, the abdominal defect can be prepared directly or with a small mesh patch. Attention must be paid to proper closure as bulges or hernias may result. Abdominal wall function and trunk support is not impacted as long as the contralateral rectus muscle is functional. When placed low enough, the donor site scar is fairly inconspicuous.

Fibula Flap (Osseous or Osseofasciocutaneous) This is another workhorse of head and neck reconstruction, especially in cases where bone is needed (Figs. 2.8–2.10) [3, 6, 16, 33–35]. The fibula flap relies on the peroneal vascular pedicle for blood flow. Dissection of this flap requires thorough anatomical knowledge of the leg and its neurovascular structures—so as to recover a healthy flap and to avoid injury to normal structures. Dissection of the skin flap along with the bone (osseofasciocutaneous flap) can be a bit more cumbersome given that there is a very thin fascia separating these structures, and the number and caliber of perforators within this fascia can be few and small, respectively. However, the long leash of the fascia provides significant versatility in positioning the skin appropriately to fit the given defect.

Summary

Reconstructive surgery is an integral part of treatment for children with head and neck tumors. Inclusion of the reconstructive surgeon at the outset of treatment improves the likelihood of an optimal outcome by facilitating interdisciplinary

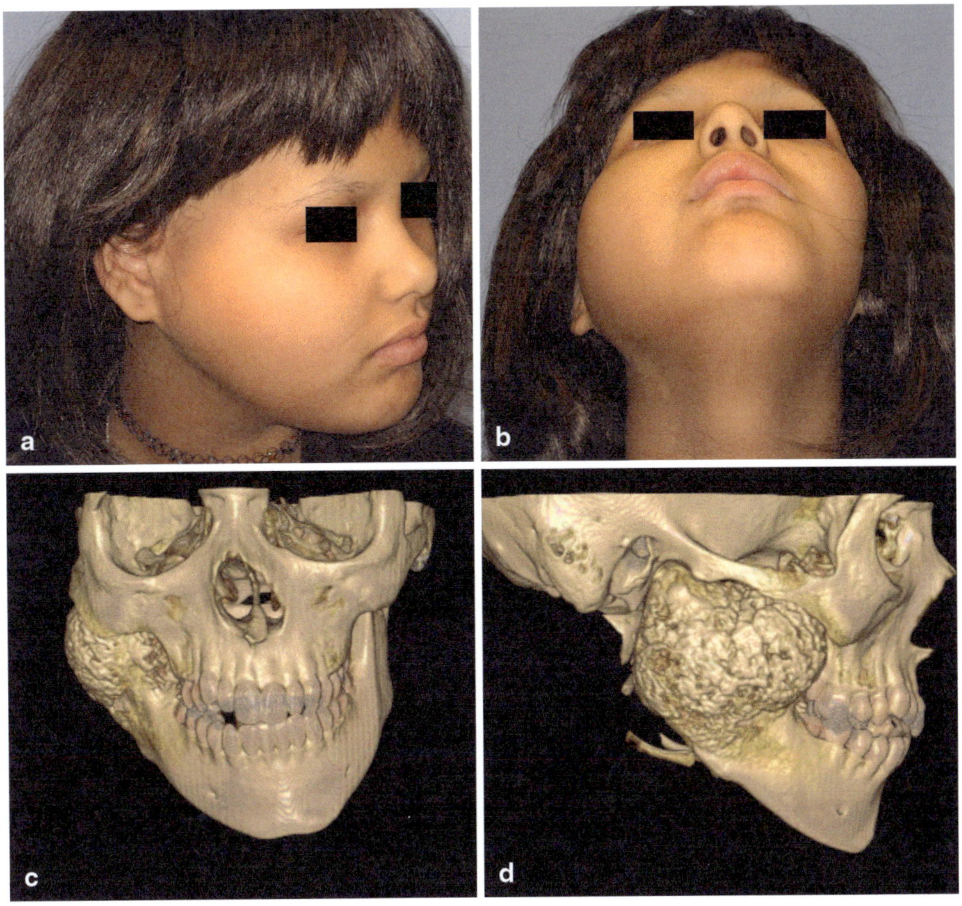

Fig. 2.2 Ten-year-old girl following neoadjuvant chemotherapy and radiation for a high grade osteogenic sarcoma of the right mandibular body (**a, b**). The 3D maxillofacial CT scans (**c, d**) demonstrate the large tumor extending up to and involving the adjacent skull base on the affected side

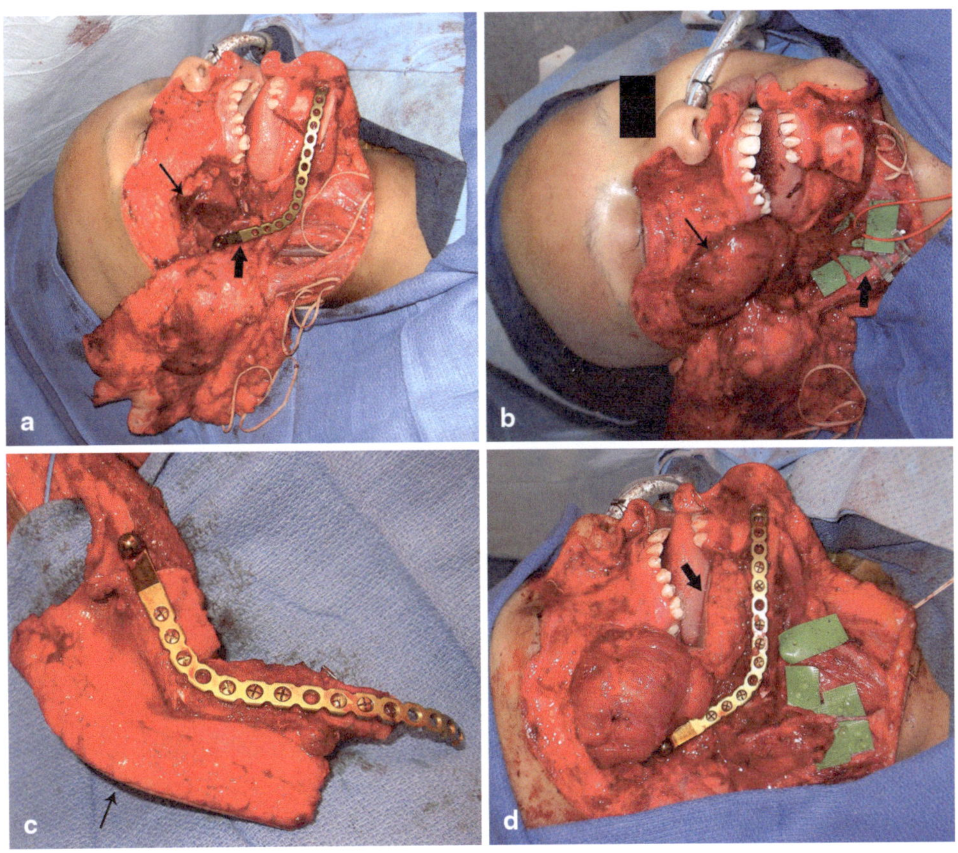

Fig. 2.3 **a** Following extirpation of this tumor via an extended Weber–Ferguson approach, loss of soft tissue and bone has created a large void adjacent to the infratemporal fossa (*thin, black arrow*). A mandibular reconstruction plate has been placed to demonstrate the absent right hemimandible (*thick, black arrow*). **b** A rectus abdominis muscle flap has been inset into the large skull base defect (*thin, black arrow*) and microvascular coaptations have been performed (*thick, black arrow*). **c** An osseofasciocutaneous fibula flap has been contoured and fixed to a mandibular reconstruction plate bent preoperatively to match the contralateral side (*thin, black arrow*). The skin paddle and soft tissue are shown inferiorly (*short, black arrow*). **d** Both flaps have now been inset. The closure of the oral lining has been completed prior to skin closure to allow for a meticulous two-layer closure under direct visualization (*thick, black arrow*)

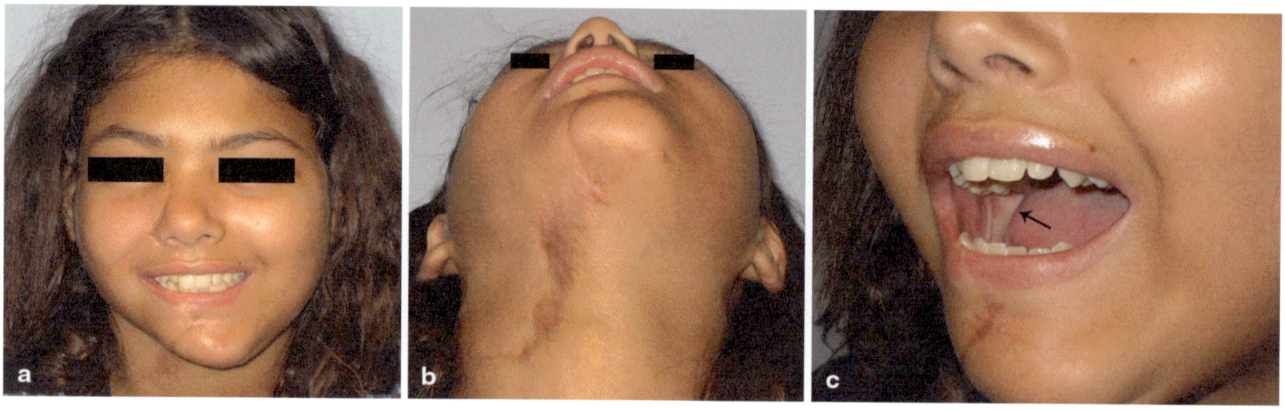

Fig. 2.4 Three years postoperatively. **a** The anteriorposterior (AP) view demonstrates some chin asymmetry secondary to differential right and left mandibular growth and soft-tissue loss on the right side. **b** Submental view demonstrating widened scarring where secondary local tissue rearrangement was required because of native skin flap loss. **c** Some degree of temporomandibular joint (TMJ) stiffness with maximal interincisal opening of 23 mm. The cutaneous portion of the flap (*thin, black arrow*) is well-healed to the adjacent pink oral mucosa

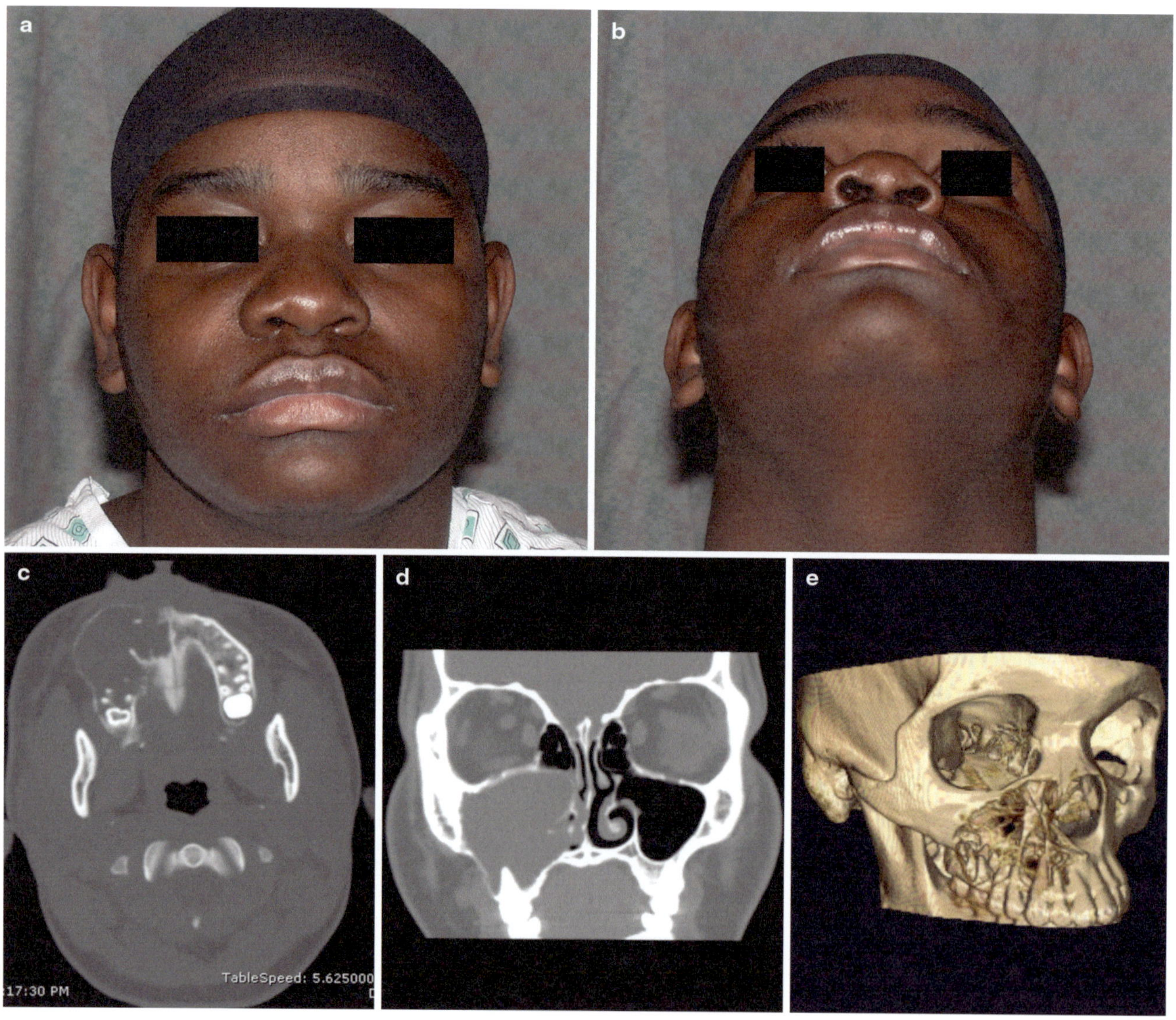

Fig. 2.5 Seventeen-year-old male who presented with swelling on the right side of his face (**a, b**). An axial (**c**) and coronal (**d**) computed tomogram demonstrate an expansile mass obliterating the right maxillary sinus. The 3D CT (**e**) view demonstrates the extent of the lesion and marked thinning of the maxillary bone. A transgingival biopsy revealed an odontogenic myxoma

Fig. 2.6 **a** The specimen following an entirely transoral resection. **b** The resultant voluminous defect extending up to and including the orbital floor. **c** Titanium mesh plates have been placed to support the globe and a rectus myocutaneous flap was used to fill the sinus and separate the sinus and oral cavity from hardware (not shown). **d** Following closure

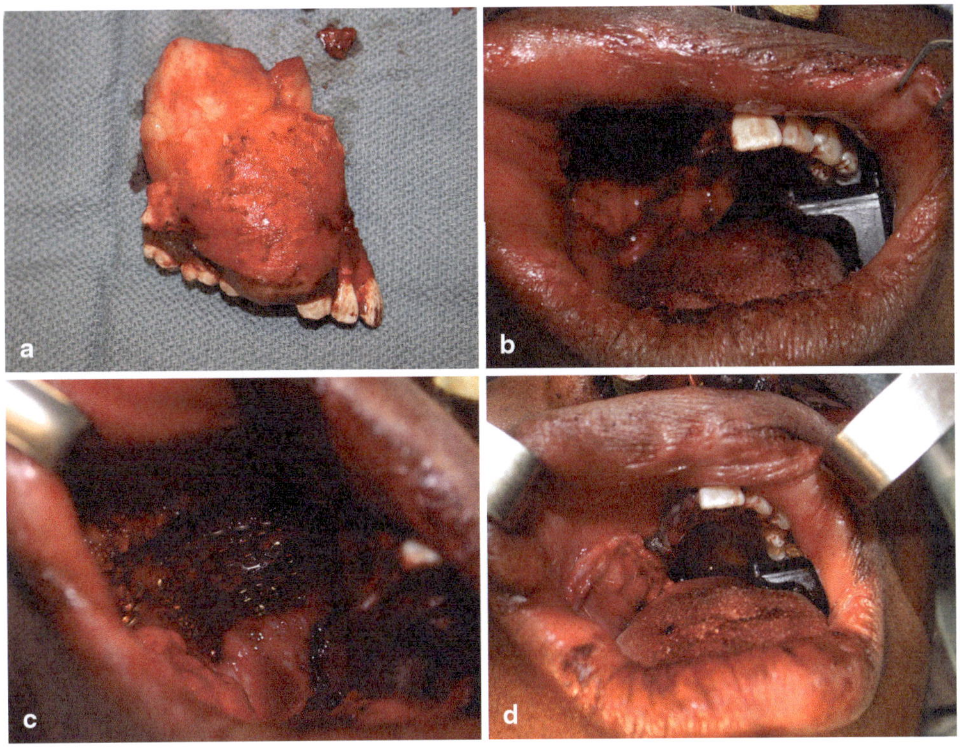

Fig. 2.7 One year after surgery with a partial denture in place (**a**). Some flattening of the right cheek and mild enophthalmos are appreciated on the submental view (**b**) but were not clinically significant

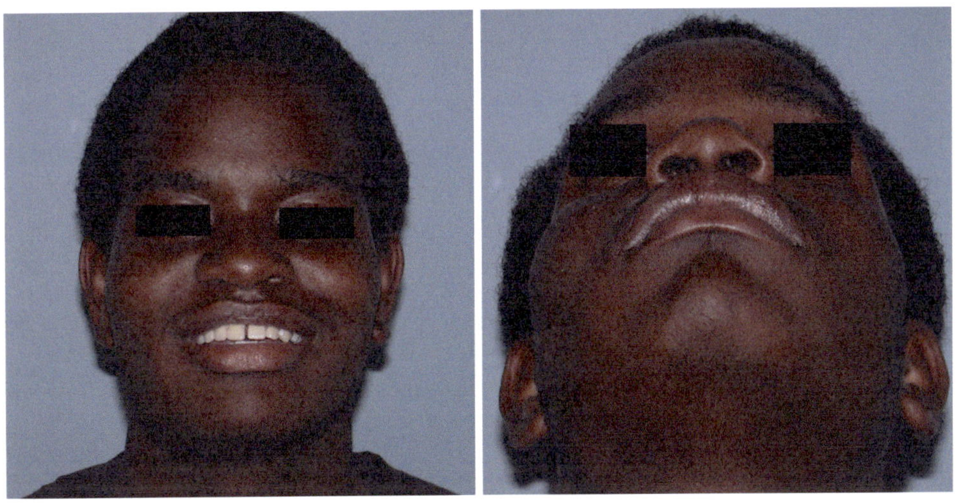

communication and integrating the reconstructive treatment into a long-term care plan. Specifically, the anatomic requirements of the reconstruction can be articulated by the extirpative team, and the rationale for, and timing of adjuvant therapy can be worked out. Preoperative consultation by the reconstructive team provides the opportunity to assess the unique patient factors (e.g., comorbidities, available donor sites, family support) that help determine the most appropriate type of reconstruction. Intraoperative coordination between surgical teams and anesthesia is also vitally important. Patient positioning, type and location of lines and tubes, and simultaneous versus staggered surgery between extirpative and reconstructive teams should be agreed upon. Although many local, regional, and distant flaps exist, a select group of workhouse flaps are commonly used. Special attention should be paid to sealing potentially problematic areas such as the oral cavity, sinuses, or cranium. The reconstructive process in the pediatric patient does not end at discharge but often extends over years. The effects of growth and time often mandate revisions as the child ages and this possibility should be fully disclosed to families at the initial consultation. Although successfully treating the patient's

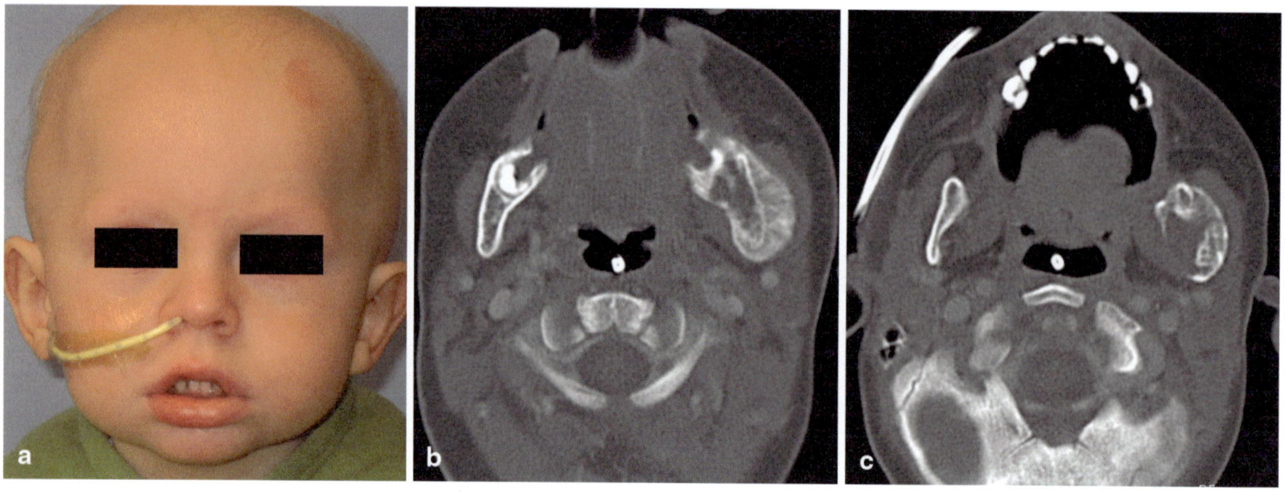

Fig. 2.8 Two-year-old boy after neoadjuvant chemotherapy for a Ewing sarcoma of the left mandible (**a**). Axial computer tomograms of the tumor involving the left mandibular body prior to (**b**) and following chemotherapy (**c**). Because of the proximity of the tumor to the oral lining, it was felt that autogenous reconstruction rather than a temporary reconstruction plate would be required

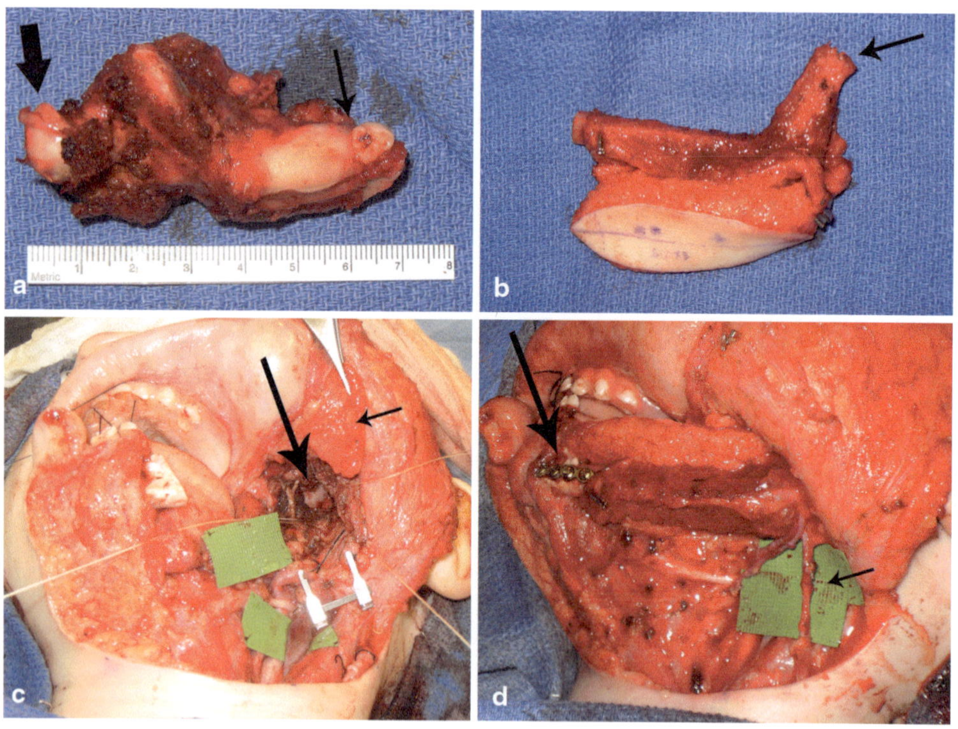

Fig. 2.9 **a** The specimen following extirpation. The condyle (*thick, black arrow*) and the oral lining and dentition (*thin, black arrow*) are seen. **b** Osseofasciocutaneous fibula flap has been harvested and contoured. The new condyle has been contoured and covered with vascularized muscle and periosteum to diminish chances of ankylosis (*black arrow*). The single osteotomy at the angle of the construct was fixed with a resorbable plate to facilitate future distraction (not shown). **c** Reconstruction of the temporomandibular joint was accomplished using vascularized buccal fat pad (*short, black arrow*) and resorbable suspension sutures to hold the new condyle in position. The glenoid fossa seen at the depths of the incision (*long, black arrow*) was not involved. **d** The mandibular construct has been inset with the distal fixation at the left parasymphysis visible (*long, black arrow*). Microvascular anastomoses between the peroneal artery and its two venae comitantes and the facial artery, facial vein, and an external jugular vein are shown (*short, black arrow*)

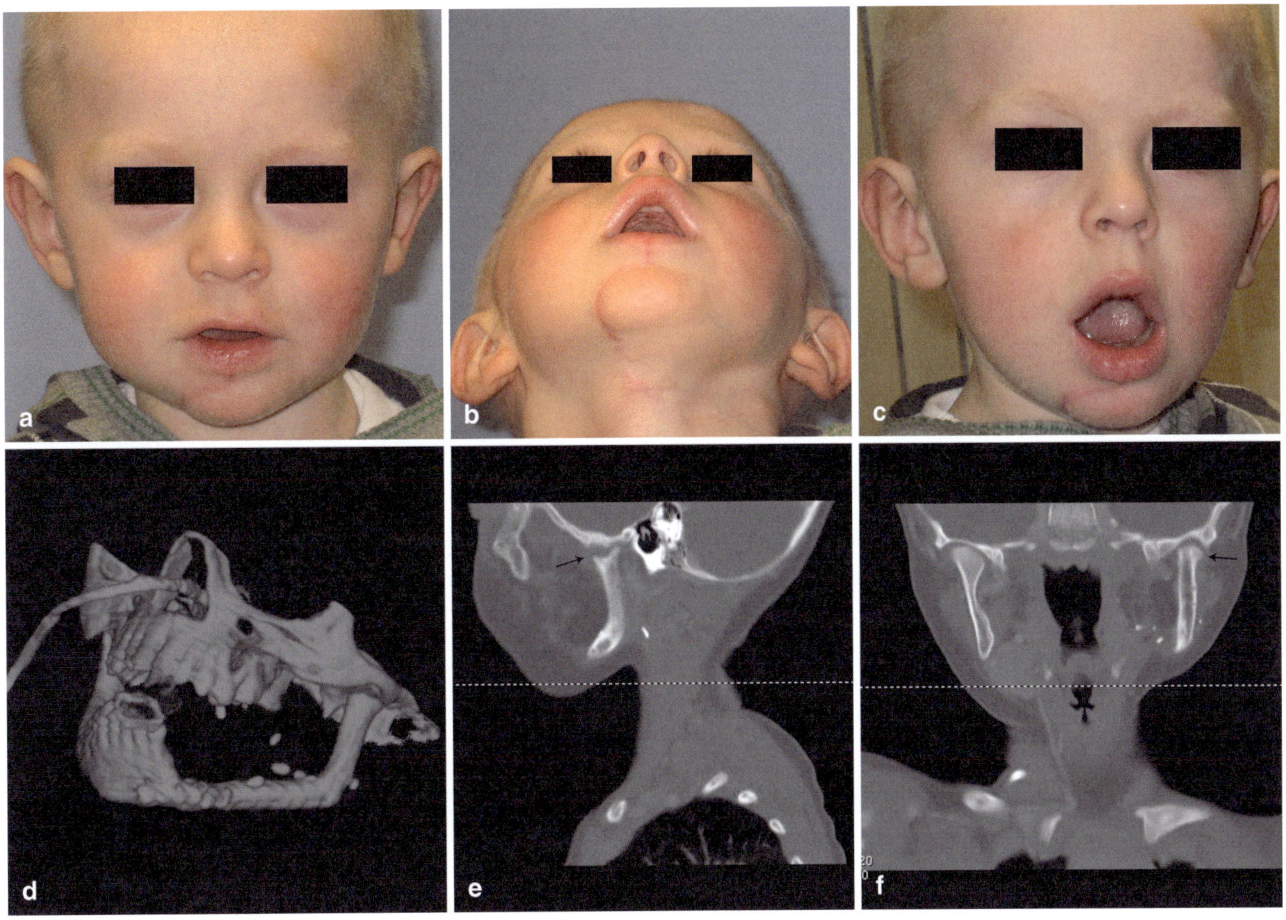

Fig. 2.10 Seven months postoperatively. The AP and submental views demonstrate healing incisions and good symmetry (**a, b**). There were no limitations in mouth opening noted on examination or by the parents (**c**). Postoperative 3D computed tomogram demonstrating the mandibular construct (**d**). Sagittal (**e**) and coronal (**f**) computed tomograms demonstrate the reconstructed condyle well-seated in the glenoid fossa with adequate joint space between condyle and glenoid seen (*long, black arrows*)

tumor remains the primary goal of therapy, the quality of the life that has been saved will be improved by a well-planned and well-executed reconstruction.

References

1. Markowitz BL, Calcaterra TC. Preoperative assessment and surgical planning for patients undergoing immediate composite reconstruction of oromandibular defects. Clin Plast Surg. 1994; Jan;21(1):9–14.
2. Duncan MJ, Manktelow RT, Zuker RM, Rosen IB. Mandibular reconstruction in the radiated patient: the role of osteocutaneous free tissue transfers. Plast Reconstr Surg. 1985 Dec;76(6):829–40.
3. Cordeiro PG, Disa JJ, Hidalgo DA, Hu QY. Reconstruction of the mandible with osseous free flaps: a 10-year experience with 150 consecutive patients. Plast Reconstr Surg. 1999 Oct;104(5):1314–20.
4. Cordeiro PG, Hidalgo DA. Soft tissue coverage of mandibular reconstruction plates. Head Neck. 1994 Mar–Apr;16(2):112–5.
5. David DJ, Tan E, Katsaros J, Sheen R. Mandibular reconstruction with vascularized iliac crest: a 10-year experience. Plast Reconstr Surg. 1988 Nov;82(5):792–803.
6. Hidalgo DA, Disa JJ, Cordeiro PG, Hu QY. A review of 716 consecutive free flaps for oncologic surgical defects: refinement in donor-site selection and technique. Plast Reconstr Surg. 1998 Sep;102(3):722–32 (discussion 733–24).
7. Hidalgo DA, Pusic AL. Free-flap mandibular reconstruction: a 10-year follow-up study. Plast Reconstr Surg. 2002 Aug;110(2):438–49 (discussion 450–31).
8. Kroll SS, Baldwin BJ. Head and neck reconstruction with the rectus abdominis free flap. Clin Plast Surg. 1994 Jan;21(1):97–105.
9. Kroll SS, Goepfert H, Jones M, Guillamondegui O, Schusterman M. Analysis of complications in 168 pectoralis major myocutaneous flaps used for head and neck reconstruction. Ann Plast Surg. 1990 Aug;25(2):93–7.
10. Panje W. Immediate reconstruction of the oral cavity. In: Thawley S, Panje W, editors. Comprehensive management of head and neck tumors. Vol I. Philadelphia: Saunders; 1987. p. 563.
11. Schusterman MA, Miller MJ, Reece GP, Kroll SS, Marchi M, Goepfert H. A single center's experience with 308 free flaps for repair of head and neck cancer defects. Plast Reconstr Surg. 1994 Mar;93(3):472–8 (discussion 479–80).
12. Urken ML, Weinberg H, Buchbinder D, et al. Microvascular free flaps in head and neck reconstruction. Report of 200 cases and review of complications. Arch Otolaryngol Head Neck Surg. 1994 Jun;120(6):633–40.

13. Carty MJ, Ferraro N, Upton J. Reconstruction of pediatric cranial base defects: a review of a single microsurgeon's 30-year experience. J Craniofac Surg. 2009 Mar;20(Suppl 1):639–45.
14. Hansen SL, Foster RD, Dosanjh AS, Mathes SJ, Hoffman WY, Leon P. Superficial temporal artery and vein as recipient vessels for facial and scalp microsurgical reconstruction. Plast Reconstr Surg. 2007 Dec;120(7):1879–84.
15. Oswald TM, Stover SA, Gerzenstein J, et al. Immediate and delayed use of arteriovenous fistulae in microsurgical flap procedures: a clinical series and review of published cases. Ann Plast Surg. 2007 Jan;58(1):61–3.
16. Lutz BS, Wei FC. Microsurgical workhorse flaps in head and neck reconstruction. Clin Plast Surg. 2005 Jul;32(3):421–30, vii.
17. Song R, Gao Y, Song Y, Yu Y. The forearm flap. Clin Plast Surg. 1982 Jan;9(1):21–6.
18. Yang G, Gao Y, Chan B. Forearm free skin transplantation. Nat Med J China. 1981;61:139.
19. Soutar DS, Scheker LR, Tanner NS, McGregor IA. The radial forearm flap: a versatile method for intra-oral reconstruction. Br J Plast Surg. 1983 Jan;36(1):1–8.
20. Urken ML, Weinberg H, Vickery C, Biller HF. The neurofasciocutaneous radial forearm flap in head and neck reconstruction: a preliminary report. Laryngoscope. 1990 Feb;100(2 Pt 1):161–73.
21. Evans GR, Schusterman MA, Kroll SS, et al. The radial forearm free flap for head and neck reconstruction: a review. Am J Surg. 1994 Nov;168(5):446–50.
22. Bardsley AF, Soutar DS, Elliot D, Batchelor AG. Reducing morbidity in the radial forearm flap donor site. Plast Reconstr Surg. 1990 Aug;86(2):287–92 (discussion 293–84).
23. Chang SC, Miller G, Halbert CF, Yang KH, Chao WC, Wei FC. Limiting donor site morbidity by suprafascial dissection of the radial forearm flap. Microsurgery. 1996;17(3):136–40.
24. Lutz BS, Wei FC, Chang SC, Yang KH, Chen IH. Donor site morbidity after suprafascial elevation of the radial forearm flap: a prospective study in 95 consecutive cases. Plast Reconstr Surg. 1999 Jan;103(1):132–7.
25. Ali RS, Bluebond-Langner R, Rodriguez ED, Cheng MH. The versatility of the anterolateral thigh flap. Plast Reconstr Surg. 2009 Dec;124(6 Suppl):e395–407.
26. Kua EH, Wong CH, Ng SW, Tan KC. The island pedicled anterolateral thigh (pALT) flap via the lateral subcutaneous tunnel for recurrent ischial ulcers. J Plast Reconstr Aesthet Surg. 2011 Jan;64(1):e21–3.
27. Kuo YR, Yeh MC, Shih HS, et al. Versatility of the anterolateral thigh flap with vascularized fascia lata for reconstruction of complex soft-tissue defects: clinical experience and functional assessment of the donor site. Plast Reconstr Surg. 2009 Jul;124(1):171–80.
28. Moiyadi AV, Ghazwan QA, Pai PS, Kelkar G, Nair D, Yadav PS. Free anterolateral thigh flap for reconstruction of complex craniofacial defects after resection of tumors of the fronto-orbitomaxillary complex. J Craniofac Surg. 2012 May 4;12(14):2378–90.
29. Park CW, Miles BA. The expanding role of the anterolateral thigh free flap in head and neck reconstruction. Curr Opin Otolaryngol Head Neck Surg. 2011 Aug;19(4):263–8.
30. Wong CH, Wei FC. Anterolateral thigh flap. Head Neck. 2010 Apr;32(4):529–40.
31. Casey WJ 3rd, Rebecca AM, Smith AA, Craft RO, Hayden RE, Buchel EW. Vastus lateralis motor nerve can adversely affect anterolateral thigh flap harvest. Plast Reconstr Surg. 2007 Jul;120(1):196–201.
32. Kroll SS, Reece GP, Miller MJ, Schusterman MA. Comparison of the rectus abdominis free flap with the pectoralis major myocutaneous flap for reconstructions in the head and neck. Am J Surg. 1992 Dec;164(6):615–8.
33. Anthony JP, Ritter EF, Young DM, Singer MI. Enhancing fibula free flap skin island reliability and versatility for mandibular reconstruction. Ann Plast Surg. 1993 Aug;31(2):106–11.
34. Hidalgo DA. Fibula free flap: a new method of mandible reconstruction. Plast Reconstr Surg. 1989 Jul;84(1):71–9.
35. Hidalgo DA. Fibula free flap mandibular reconstruction. Clin Plast Surg. 1994 Jan;21(1):25–35.

Chemotherapy

3

Carlos Rodriguez-Galindo

Introduction

Treatment of pediatric head and neck tumors requires a multimodal approach, with integration of surgical specialties, radiation therapy, pediatric oncology, and supportive care. For benign and low-grade tumors, local control with surgery is the treatment of choice, and conservative approaches that minimize disfiguration and protect function are the cornerstone of their management. However, high-grade malignancies require a more aggressive approach in order to guarantee complete local control; moreover, most pediatric cancer patients are considered to have micrometastatic disease at the time of diagnosis. For those reasons, chemotherapy is a key element in the management of pediatric head and neck malignancies.

Principles of Chemotherapy

While advances are being made in identifying specific actionable pathways that would be susceptible of molecular targeted agents, standard treatment for most pediatric cancers continues to be based on conventional, nonselective agents. Since the early years of pediatric cancer treatment, it has been recognized that combination of different agents is superior to the use of individual agents. Chemotherapeutic drugs may thus provide an additive (sum of efficacy) or a synergistic (enhanced effect beyond the sum of the parts) effect, and combinations that can achieve the maximum synergistic effect with the least toxicity are favored. The standard of care for most cancers includes multiagent regimens where drugs are delivered at maximum tolerated doses. Combinations, doses, and schedules considered standard of care are evidence based and the result of years of clinical trial development to define best treatments. Biological, pathological, and clinical characterization may lead to risk stratification for many pediatric malignancies, whereby the agents and doses used and the duration of therapy are adapted to risk [1].

Based on timing of administration of chemotherapy in relation to local control, three phases are identified (Table 3.1):

a. *Neoadjuvant chemotherapy*—In this setting, chemotherapy is administered at the time of diagnosis, prior to local control, in patients in whom surgical resection is not considered feasible, or could only be completed with a radical, usually mutilating or disfiguring approach. This is a common occurrence in head and neck malignancies, where tumor location usually limits surgical options, and chemotherapy could facilitate resection and minimize side effects. Most pediatric malignancies are very chemosensitive and thus a good response is usually expected to occur and lead to better local control.
b. *Concurrent chemotherapy*—Administration of chemotherapy in conjunction with radiation therapy may result in a synergistic effect, improve local control rates, and in some cases facilitate second-look surgery. Chemoradiotherapy of the head and neck leads to significant toxicity of the oral and pharyngeal mucosas and thus patients undergoing this treatment approach need to be carefully monitored and supportive care maximized.
c. *Adjuvant chemotherapy*—In this setting, chemotherapy is given after local control (surgery, radiation, or both), and it is mostly intended for the control of the systemic disease. Adjuvant chemotherapy may result in reactivation of mucositis in patients that have recently completed radiation therapy, particularly if doxorubicin is used.

Types of Chemotherapeutic Agents

Standard chemotherapeutic agents are divided into four broad categories based on their mechanism of action: antimetabolites, alkylating agents, topoisomerase inhibitors, and tubulin-

C. Rodriguez-Galindo (✉)
Department of Pediatric Oncology, Harvard Medical School, Dana-Farber/Boston Children's Hospital Cancer and Blood Disorders Center, Boston, MA, USA
e-mail: carlos_rodriguez-galindo@dfci.harvard.edu

R. Rahbar et al. (eds.), *Pediatric Head and Neck Tumors*,
DOI 10.1007/978-1-4614-8755-5_3, © Springer Science+Business Media New York 2014

Table 3.1 Pediatric head and neck cancers and chemotherapy delivery

Chemotherapy phase		
Neoadjuvant	Concurrent chemoradiation	Adjuvant
Neuroblastoma	Nasopharyngeal carcinoma	Neuroblastoma
Rhabdomyosarcoma	Ewing sarcoma	Rhabdomyosarcoma
Soft tissue sarcomas	Soft tissue sarcomas	Soft tissue sarcomas
Osteosarcoma	Rhabdomyosarcoma	Ewing sarcoma
Ewing sarcoma		Retinoblastoma
Nasopharyngeal carcinoma		Melanoma
Retinoblastoma		

binding drugs. In addition, advances in our understanding of cancer biology have led to the development of new classes of agents such as monoclonal antibodies, differentiating agents, and tyrosine kinase inhibitors (Table 3.2) [1].

The mechanism of action for most agents is through their interference with the synthesis or function of DNA and RNA at different levels:

a. *Antimetabolites:* These drugs are analogs of nucleoside precursors or folates and act by either depleting precursors or being incorporated into DNA or RNA. This class of agents is inhibitory only during the S phase of the cell cycle; for this reason, their effect is maximized when given in continuous infusion (such as methotrexate in acute leukemias and lymphomas or osteosarcoma or 5-fluorouracil in nasopharyngeal carcinoma) or in protracted schedules of daily administration (such as cytarabine or 5-mercaptopurine in acute leukemias).
b. *Alkylating agents:* This class of drugs damages DNA by forming covalent bonds to nucleobases and cross-linking between DNA strands. Different from antimetabolites, they are less dependent on the cell cycle and their effect is less schedule dependent. Most commonly used alkylating agents in pediatric head and neck cancers are the nitrogen mustards cyclophosphamide and ifosfamide, which are most commonly used in sarcomas, and the platinum agents cisplatin and carboplatin, which are more commonly used in embryonal cancers such as neuroblastoma and retinoblastoma.
c. *Topoisomerase inhibitors:* The topoisomerases are key enzymes in DNA topology; they create and religate single- (topoisomerase I) or double-stranded (topoisomerase II) breaks in the DNA that facilitate uncoiling and strand passage. Inhibitors of those enzymes result in DNA breaks. The most commonly used topoisomerase I inhibitors are topotecan and irinotecan; these agents have a maximum effect when given in protracted schedules over 5 days. Topotecan is used mostly in the frontline management of high-risk neuroblastoma, whereas irinotecan is used in high-risk or relapsed Ewing sarcoma and rhabdomyosarcoma. Topoisomerase II inhibitors are a larger category, with antitumor antibiotics such as doxorubicin, bleomycin, and dactinomycin, and epipodophyllotoxins, such as etoposide. This class of agents is used across the spectrum of pediatric malignancies.
d. *Tubulin binders:* Tubulin is the precursor of microtubules, high-dynamic proteins that are key in the formation of the

Table 3.2 Anticancer drugs used in pediatric oncology

Class	Drug
Antimetabolites	*Antifolates* Methotrexate
	Purine analogs 6-mercaptopurine Thioguanine Fludarabine
	Pyrimidine analogs Cytarabine 5-Fluorouracil
Alkylating agents	*Nitrogen mustards* Melphalan Cyclophosphamide Ifosfamide
	Platinum agents Cisplatin Carboplatin
	Busulfan
	Temozolomide
	Procarbazine
	Dacarbazine
Topoisomerase inhibitors	*Topoisomerase I inhibitors* Topotecan Irinotecan
	Topoisomerase II inhibitors Doxorubicin Daunomycin Idarubicin Mitoxantrone Bleomycin Dactinomycin
Tubulin binders	*Vinca alkaloids* Vincristine Vinblastine Vinorelbine
	Taxanes Paclitaxel Docetaxel
Miscellaneous	Prednisone
	Dexamethasone
	Asparaginase
Monoclonal antibodies	Anti GD-2
	Anti IGF-1R
	Anti-CTLA-4
Differentiating agents	All-trans-retinoic acid
	Cis-retinoic acid
Tyrosine kinase inhibitors	Imatinib
	Sunitinib
	Sorafenib
	Crizotinib

mitotic spindle. They are also involved in the movement of organelles within the cell and have effects on cell support and shape. The vinca alkaloids (vincristine, vinblastine, vinorelbine) inhibit tubulin by blocking microtubule polymerization; this class of agents is commonly used in pediatric cancers, usually in combination with alkylators. The taxanes (paclitaxel, docetaxel) inhibit depolymerization of the microtubules. Taxanes are less commonly used in pediatric cancer, although paclitaxel and docetaxel are used in second-line regimens for germ cell tumors and nasopharyngeal carcinoma, respectively.

e. *Monoclonal Antibodies:* This new class of agents is acquiring an increasingly important role in the treatment of some childhood malignancies. The rationale for the development of this approach is the identification of selective antigens in the surface of malignant cells that could be targets for antibody therapy. Three monoclonal antibodies may be of relevance in head and neck malignancies in children: anti-GD2, anti-IGF1R, and anti-CTLA4. Monoclonal antibodies against the tumor-associated disialoganglioside GD2, which is expressed in neuroblastoma, have been shown to increase survival in patients with high-risk neuroblastoma and are now incorporated in the frontline treatment for this group of patients [2]. Anti-IGF1R monoclonal antibodies have shown efficacy in relapsed Ewing sarcoma and their use in combination with standard chemotherapeutic agents in the frontline of patients with high-risk Ewing sarcoma and rhabdomyosarcoma is currently being evaluated [3]. Ipilimumab, an antibody against cytotoxic, T-lymphocyte-associated antigen 4 (CTLA4), has shown to prolong survival in patients with advanced melanoma [4], and it is currently being investigated in children with this malignancy.

f. *Molecularly targeted agents:* Advances in our understanding of cancer biology have resulted in the development of more selective agents designed to inhibit or activate specific pathways. Relevant agents with documented efficacy in pediatric head and neck cancer include kinase inhibitors such as crizotinib (anaplastic large cell lymphoma, neuroblastoma, and inflammatory myofibroblastic tumor) [5], sorafenib (thyroid carcinoma) [6], and vemurafenib (malignant melanoma and thyroid carcinoma) [7], and differentiating agents such as cis-retinoic acid (neuroblastoma) [2].

Pharmacokinetics of Chemotherapeutic Agents

The dose, schedule, and route of administration of antineoplastic agents are dependent on the unique pharmacokinetics of each drug, including drug absorption, distribution, metabolism, and excretion [1].

a. *Absorption:* Very few antineoplastic agents are administered orally to children; however, oral treatment is a key component in the management of acute lymphoblastic leukemia (ALL), where oral methotrexate and 6-MP form the backbone of maintenance therapy. Limitations to absorption include degradation in the gastrointestinal lumen, inability be transported across the mucosa, and metabolism in the intestinal epithelium or liver.

b. *Distribution:* Once the drug enters the systemic circulation by absorption of intravenous administration, it is transferred and distributed into the interstitial and intracellular fluids, including tumors. Each organ and tissue receives different amounts of drug; this distribution is dependent on vascular permeability, regional and systemic blood flow, rate of binding to plasma proteins, ability of the drug to bind tissue, and lipid solubility.

c. *Metabolism:* Drug metabolism entails the biochemical modification of the antineoplastic agents through specialized enzymatic systems. Metabolism is the most important determinant of variability in the pharmacokinetics of anticancer drugs; it is susceptible to constitutional variations in the levels and activity of drug-metabolizing enzymes as well as interactions with other agents. Drug-metabolizing enzymes are divided into two major groups. Phase I reactions introduce or expose a functional group on the drug, usually by oxidation, hydrolysis, reduction, or demethylation; this usually diminishes the drug's activity, although for some agents such as cyclophosphamide and ifosfamide, phase I reactions activate the drug. The CYP (cytochrome P450) superfamily of enzymes catalyze oxidation and demethylation for a large number of drugs. They have very broad and overlapping substrate specificity; CYP genes are genetically polymorphic and this may result in significant patient variability in drug metabolism. CYP enzymes are also susceptible to inhibition or induction by other drugs, thus resulting in risk of interactions that could potentially alter the effect of the anticancer agent [8]. Phase II conjugation reactions covalently link a conjugate such as glucuronic acid or glutathione to the drug; the conjugated drugs are very polar and are excreted very rapidly.

d. *Elimination:* Anticancer agents are eliminated by renal or biliary excretion, or by biotransformation or spontaneous decomposition to an inactive metabolite. Systemic exposure to the agent and its metabolites will depend on the elimination rate. Alterations in liver or renal function, which commonly occur in children with cancer, may have a significant impact in drug clearance. The routes of elimination of the most common agents used in pediatric head and neck cancers are summarized in Table 3.3.

Table 3.3 Drug elimination of antineoplastic agents commonly used in the treatment of childhood head and neck cancers

Drug	Elimination
Antimetabolites	
Methotrexate	Renal excretion
6-MP	Hepatic biotransformation
5-FU	Biotransformation
Alkylating agents	
Cyclophosphamide and Ifosfamide	Hepatic biotransformation
Cisplatin	Renal excretion, decomposition
Carboplatin	Renal excretion, decomposition
Topoisomerase Inhibitors	
Anhracyclines	Hepatic biotransformation, biliary excretion
Dactinomycin	Renal and biliary excretion
Etoposide	Biotransformation, renal excretion
Topotecan	Renal excretion
Irinotecan	Biotransformation, biliary excretion
Tubulin binders	
Vinca alkaloids	Hepatic biotransformation, biliary excretion
Taxanes	Hepatic biotransformation

Table 3.4 Organ and tissue-specific side effects of anticancer drugs commonly used in the treatment of head and neck cancers in children

Toxicity	Drug
Ototoxicity	Cisplatin
Mucositis	Anthracyclines, 5-FU
Cardiotoxicity	Anthracyclines
Hepatotoxicity	Methotrexate
Nephrotoxicity	Cisplatin, ifosfamide
Hemorrhagic cystitis	Cyclophosphamide, ifosfamide
Neurotoxicity	Methotrexate, vinca alkaloids, cisplatin

Toxicity of Chemotherapeutic Agents

Actively dividing normal cells are susceptible to the effects of anticancer drugs; those effects can be acute and reversible, or delayed (long-term) and irreversible.

a. *Acute Toxicities:* There are a number of acute side effects that are common to most class of drugs, and usually reversible, such as nausea and vomiting, mucositis, alopecia, and myelosuppression. However, certain agents are associated with organ and tissue-specific side effects (Table 3.4). *Myelosuppression* is almost universal, and all cell lines are affected. While transfusions of blood products can ameliorate anemia and thrombocytopenia, white blood cells are not typically transfused, and patients must endure variable periods of severe neutropenia. The administration of growth factors such as filgrastim (granulocyte-colony-stimulating factor, G-CSF) may shorten the duration of the neutropenia through the stimulation of the proliferation of bone marrow progenitors. G-CSF is given daily, starting 24–72 h after completion of chemotherapy and until neutropenia is resolved. A pegylated form of G-CSF is also available and can be given as a single dose. *Hemorrhagic cystitis* is caused by exposure of the urothelium to the active metabolites of cyclophosphamide and ifosfamide. This phenomenon may be minimized by aggressive hydration and diuresis to dilute the toxic metabolites and limit their time in contact with the bladder wall, and by the concomitant administration of mesna-mercaptoethane sulfonate, a scavenging agent that rapidly inactivates these metabolites in the urine. *Nephrotoxicity* may occur with several agents, thus the need to closely monitor the renal function and the electrolyte balance in patients receiving chemotherapy. Ifosfamide may cause a proximal tubulopathy that resembles Fanconi syndrome. Cisplatin may result in significant alteration of the glomerular filtration rate and tubular function; administration of aggressive hydration with hypertonic saline and osmotic diuresis with mannitol is important to prevent severe cisplatin-related renal dysfunction. Administration of high doses of methotrexate as in the treatment of ALL or osteosarcoma may also result in nephrotoxicity due to the precipitation of methotrexate and its metabolites in acidic urine; for this reason, methotrexate is typically administered with aggressive hydration and urine alkalinization. *Cardiac toxicity* is a well-known effect of doxorubicin and other anthracyclines. While acute toxicity may occur in the form of conduction abnormalities, the most common presentation is as delayed cardiomyopathy. This effect appears to be dependent on the cumulative dose of the agent administered over time, and may be ameliorated with the administration of dexrazoxane. Several agents used in the management of head and neck cancers may result in *neurologic toxicity*. Peripheral neuropathy is a common event with vinca alkaloids; this form of toxicity usually presents with loss of deep tendon reflexes, neuritic pain, foot drop, severe constipation, or vocal cord dysfunction. Cisplatin can also cause peripheral neuropathy, which usually presents in the form of symmetric paresthesias. High-dose methotrexate is associated with the development of neurotoxicity, which usually presents as an acute form, with lethargy, disorientation or seizures, or subacutely, typically as a transient stroke-like syndrome.

b. *Long-term toxicities:* Unfortunately, the administration of antineoplastic agents is associated with a wide array of long-term adverse effects. The risk of some of these long-term toxicities is augmented by the concomitant use of radiation therapy to the head and neck. The most relevant long-term toxicities include cardiotoxicity (anthracyclines), hearing loss (cisplatin), gonadal toxicity (alkylating agents), neurotoxicity (methotrexate, vinca alkaloids), renal toxicity (ifosfamide and cisplatin), and second malignant neoplasms (alkylating agents and topoisomerase II inhibitors). For this reason, it is extremely important that survivors of childhood cancer receive comprehensive, multidisciplinary care in specialized survivorship programs [9].

Overview of Most Common Anticancer Drugs Used in the Treatment of Children with Head and Neck Cancers

Vincristine

Standard dosage	Patients aged < 12 months: 0.05 mg/kg intravenously; patients aged ≥ 12 months: 1.5 mg/m^2 intravenously day 1 (maximum dose 2 mg)
Contraindications	Hypersensitivity to vincristine or any component; patients with demyelinating form of Charcot-Marie-Tooth syndrome
Main drug interactions	Cytochrome P450 isoenzyme CYP3A3/4 and CYP3A5-7 substrate; isoenzyme CYP2D6 inhibitor. Concurrent administration with itraconazole may result in worse neuromuscular side effects; voriconazole may increase plasma levels of vincristine.
Main side effects	Dose-limiting toxicity is neurotoxicity. This can be characterized by constipation and/or paralytic ileus, ptosis, vocal cord paralysis, jaw pain, abdominal pain, peripheral neuropathies, loss of deep tendon reflexes, and "foot drop."
Special points	Vincristine is a vesicant and may cause severe tissue damage if extravasation occurs.
Indications	Neuroblastoma, retinoblastoma, rhabdomyosarcoma, Ewing sarcoma, hematologic malignancies

Carboplatin

Standard dosage	Usual dose is 560 mg/m^2 intravenously on day 1 (18.6 mg/kg for patients aged < 12 months).
Contraindications	Hypersensitivity to carboplatin or cisplatin
Main drug interactions	Aminoglycosides (increased ototoxicity and nephrotoxicity); nephrotoxic drugs (increased renal toxicity); decreases phenytoin serum levels
Main side effects	Bone marrow suppression with prominent thrombocytopenia. Nausea and vomiting of moderate severity, ototoxicity, peripheral neuropathies, and reversible renal toxicity are also common.
Special points	In case of decrease in renal function, carboplatin can be administered using clearance-adjusted dosing with an area under the curve (AUC) of 6–8.
Indications	Retinoblastoma, neuroblastoma, germ cell tumors

Cisplatin

Standard dosage	Usual dose rage is 20–60 mg/m^2/d for 2–5 days, depending on disease and regimen.
Contraindications	Hypersensitivity to cisplatin or platinum-containing compounds; preexisting renal or hearing impairment
Main drug interactions	Plasma levels of anticonvulsant agents may become subtherapeutic during cisplatin therapy.
Main side effects	Severe nausea and emesis, often delayed. Bone marrow suppression with prominent thrombocytopenia. Hearing loss (high frequency). Nephrotoxicity. Peripheral neuropathy
Special points	Monitoring of glomerular filtration rate prior to initiation of therapy and during treatment is recommended. Patients also should undergo frequent hearing evaluations during and after completion of therapy.
Indications	Metastatic retinoblastoma, neuroblastoma, osteosarcoma, nasopharyngeal carcinoma

Etoposide (VP-16)

Standard dosage	Usual dose is 100 mg/m^2/d (3.3 mg/kg/d if < 12 months) intravenously for 3–5 days.
Contraindications	Hypersensitivity to etoposide or any component; pregnancy
Main drug interactions	Cytochrome P450 isoenzyme CYP3A3/4 substrate. Cyclosporine may increase the plasma levels of etoposide.
Main side effects	Myelosuppression. Hypotension can occur with rapid infusions. Etoposide injection contains

	benzyl alcohol, which may cause allergic reactions in susceptible individuals.
Special points	Etoposide has been associated with the development of secondary leukemias.
Indications	Retinoblastoma, neuroblastoma, rhabdomyosarcoma, Ewing sarcoma, germ cell tumors, osteosarcoma

Doxorubicin

Standard dosage	Usual dose is 45–60 mg/m^2 (1.5–2 mg/kg for <12 months). Doxorubicin can be given as a bolus, short infusion, or as a continuous infusion for 24–48 h.
Contraindications	Hypersensitivity to doxorubicin or any component; severe congestive heart failure or cardiomyopathy; patients who have received a total dose of 550 mg/m^2 of doxorubicin or 400 mg/m^2 in patients with previous or concomitant treatment with anthracyclines, cyclophosphamide, or irradiation of the cardiac region.
Main drug interactions	Cytochrome P450 isoenzyme CYP3A3/4 substrate; isoenzyme CYP2D6 inhibitor. Doxorubicin decreases carbamazepine, digoxin, and phenytoin levels; phenobarbital increases elimination of doxorubicin.
Main side effects	Myelosuppression and cardiotoxicity. Acute toxicity may take the form of arrhythmias, heart block, or pericarditis and may be fatal. Chronic cardiotoxicity is related to total cumulative dose and is characterized by heart failure. In general, total lifetime dosages of 450–550 mg/m^2 should not be exceeded.
Special points	Severe tissue damage and necrosis can occur upon extravasation. Radiation recall reactions can occur and may be severe. Administration of dexrazoxane prior to each dose of doxorubicin may ameliorate the risk of cardiotoxicity.
Indications	Neuroblastoma, osteosarcoma, Ewing sarcoma, soft tissue sarcomas, hematologic malignancies

Cyclophosphamide and Ifosfamide

Standard dosage	Usual dose of cyclophosphamide is as single dose of 1.2 g/m^2, or in fractionated doses of 250–500 mg/m^2/d for 5 days.Usual dose of ifosfamide is 1.8 g/m^2/d for 5 days.
Contraindications	Hypersensitivity to cyclophosphamide or ifosfamide, or any component
Main drug interactions	Cytochrome P450 isoenzyme CYP2B6, CYP2D6, and CYP3A3/4 substrate. Allopurinol (increases myelotoxicity); phenobarbital, phenytoin, and chloral hydrate may increase conversion of cyclophosphamide and ifosfamide to their active metabolites. Phenothiazines and imipramine may inhibit the metabolism of cyclophosphamide; cyclophosphamide may prolong the neuromuscular-blocking activity of succinylcholine.
Main side effects	Bone marrow suppression and cardiac toxicity. Hemorrhagic cystitis may occur and necessitates withholding therapy.
Special points	Hyperhydration and administration of mesna are recommended to prevent hemorrhagic cystitis.
Indications	Neuroblastoma, osteosarcoma, Ewing sarcoma, rhabdomyosarcoma, soft-tissue sarcomas, hematologic malignancies

Methotrexate

Standard dosage	Usual dose is 1–3 g/m^2 as 24-h infusion for hematologic malignancies, and 12 g/m^2 as 4-h infusion in osteosarcoma.
Contraindications	Severe liver or renal dysfunction. Hypersensitivity to methotrexate
Main drug interactions	Nonsteroidal anti-inflammatory drugs should not be administered prior to or concomitantly with high doses of methotrexate as they can result in impaired renal clearance. Methotrexate is partially bound to serum albumin, and toxicity may be increased because of displacement by certain drugs, such as salicylates, phenytoin, and sulfonamides. Renal tubular

	transport is diminished by probenecid. Penicillins may reduce renal clearance of methotrexate. Vitamin preparations containing folic acid or its derivatives may decrease the effect of methotrexate. Trimethroprim/sulfamethoxazole may increase bone marrow suppression through decreased tubular secretion and antifolate effect.
Main side effects	Renal toxicity, hepatotoxicity. Acute and subacute (stroke-like) encephalitis
Special points	High-dose methotrexate administration requires close monitoring of methotrexate clearance, aggressive hydration and urinary alkalinization, and rescue with folinic acid. Patients with effusions (peritoneal, pleural, subdural) may have delayed clearance.
Indications	Osteosarcoma, hematologic malignancies
Irinotecan	
Standard dosage	Irinotecan is administered in fractionated schedules. The most common schedule is 50 mg/m^2/d intravenously for 5 days. A regimen of 20 mg/m^2/d for 5 days in 2 consecutive weeks has also been used.
Contraindications	Hypersensitivity of irinotecan or its excipients
Main drug interactions	Irinotecan is a CYP3A4 substrate. Strong CYP3A4 inducers should not be administered for at least 2 weeks prior to initiation of irinotecan therapy. Strong CYP3A4 inhibitors should be discontinued at least 1 week prior to starting irinotecan therapy.
Main side effects	Bone marrow suppression is usually mild. Main side effect is diarrhea, which can present as an early, transient form (rare) due to a cholinergic reaction, or most commonly as a late diarrhea occurring more than 24 h after administration of irinotecan.
Special points	Early-onset diarrhea may be treated and prevented with subcutaneous atropine. Late-onset diarrhea may be prevented with selective intestinal decontamination, usually with cefixime or cefpodoxime, starting 2–5 days prior to initiation of the cycle and continuing until 1–2 days after the last dose of irinotecan.
Indications	Rhabdomyosarcoma, Ewing sarcoma
Topotecan	
Standard dosage	Topotecan is administered in fractionated schedules. Usual dose is 0.75–1.5 mg/m^2/d, given intravenously for 5 days.
Contraindications	Hypersensitivity to topotecan. Severe renal dysfunction
Main drug interactions	There are no drug interactions related to P450 enzymes.
Main side effects	Moderate to severe myelosuppression is common. Cutaneous reactions and fever are also common.
Special points	In case of renal dysfunction, topotecan can be administered using targeted systemic exposure methods that require pharmacokinetic evaluation. Skin reactions are not a contraindication to subsequent topotecan administration.
Indications	Neuroblastoma, Ewing sarcoma
5-Fluorouracil	
Standard dosage	Usual dose in nasopharyngeal carcinoma is 1 g/m^2/d for 4–5 days as continuous intravenous infusion.
Contraindications	Known hypersensitivity to 5-fluorouracil
Main drug interactions	Leucovorin calcium may enhance the toxicity of fluorouracil.
Main side effects	Moderate myelosuppression, mucositis and diarrhea, photosensitivity, acute cerebellar syndrome
Special points	5-fluorouracil is typically given only during the neoadjuvant (induction) phase in the treatment of nasopharyngeal carcinoma. Its concomitant administration with radiation therapy may cause severe mucositis.
Indications	Nasopharyngeal carcinoma

References

1. Widemann BC, Adamson PC. Fundamentals of cancer chemotherapy. In: Carroll WL, Finlay JL, editors. Cancer in children and adolescents. Boston: Jones and Bartlett; 2010. pp. 95–112.
2. Yu AL, Gilman AL, Ozkaynak MF, et al. Anti-GD2 antibody with GM-CSF, interleukin-2, and isotretinoin for neuroblastoma. N Engl J Med. 2010;363:1324–34.
3. Pappo AS, Patel SR, Crowley J, et al. R1507, a monoclonal antibody to the insulin-like growth factor 1 receptor, in patients with recurrent or refractory Ewing sarcoma family of tumors: results of a phase II sarcoma alliance for research through collaboration study. J Clin Oncol. 2011;29:4541–7.
4. Hodi FS, O'Day SJ, McDermott DF, et al. Improved survival with ipilimumab in patients with metastatic melanoma. N Engl J Med. 2010;363:711–23.
5. Carpenter EL, Mosse YP. Targeting ALK in neuroblastoma-preclinical and clinical advancements. Nat Rev Clin Oncol. 2012;9:391–9.
6. Gild ML, Bullock M, Robinson BG, Clifton-Bligh R. Multikinase inhibitors: a new option for the treatment of thyroid cancer. Nat Rev Endocrinol. 2011;7:617–24.
7. Bollag G, Tsai J, Zhang J, et al. Vemurafenib: the first drug approved for BRAF-mutant cancer. Nat Rev Drug Discov. 2012;11:873–86.
8. Haidar C, Jeha S. Drug interactions in childhood cancer. Lancet Oncol. 2011;12:92–9.
9. Kremer LCM, Mulder RL, Oeffinger KC, et al. A worldwide collaboration to harmonize guidelines for the long-term follow-up of childhood and young adult cancer survivors: a report from the international late effects of Childhood Cancer Guideline Harmonization Group. Pediatr Blood Cancer. 2013;60:543–9.

4 Radiotherapy

Karen J. Marcus

Radiation therapy uses ionizing radiation to destroy tumor cells. Radiation oncology is the clinical discipline that uses radiation therapy as a treatment modality in the management of malignancies, often together with chemotherapy and surgery. Malignant cells as well as normal cells are damaged by ionizing radiation. Ionizing radiations inflict damage on cells through direct effects on DNA and indirect effects on cells such as initiation of apoptotic pathways and production of free radicals through ionization of water. Some cells are able to repair the damage from ionizing radiation but some cell types are unable to do so. The biological basis of radiation therapy relies on the difference in response to ionizing radiation between malignant cells and cells of the surrounding normal tissues. Malignant cells are usually killed by ionizing radiation. However, some tumors can sustain higher amounts of damage before being eradicated. In addition, the toxicity to the surrounding normal tissues limits the total doses which can be delivered safely. The ionizing radiation is delivered to a precisely defined tumor volume with sparing of the surrounding normal tissues.

The biological effects of ionizing radiation begin within cells immediately upon exposure, resulting in the direct effects of DNA damage as well as multiple indirect effects produced by the ionization of water with the resulting free hydroxyl radicals. The direct DNA damage is dose dependent and includes lethal double-strand breaks of sublethal single-strand breaks, cross-links, and base damage. The sublethal damage can be repaired by specific genetic mechanisms such as strand break repair, mismatch repair, nucleotide excision repair, and base excision repair. The sublethal damage repair is generally complete within 4–5 h [1]. This repair of sublethal damage is the basis of fractionation in radiotherapy. Cells that progress to mitosis with unrepaired damage will usually undergo cell death during mitosis or will do so in subsequent cell divisions [2].

Radiosensitivity depends upon both intrinsic and extrinsic characteristics. Intrinsic factors include the phase of the cell cycle at the time of exposure, the activation of apoptotic pathways, the ability to repair DNA damage, and the accumulation of genetic mutations in tumor suppressor genes. The extrinsic factors relate to the tissue microenvironment such as oxygenation, nutrient and blood supply. There are underlying genetic conditions which render the host more susceptible to radiation exposure. Such genetic conditions result in greater radiosensitivity and genomic instability and are associated with cancer predisposition. Some examples of these predisposition syndromes include ataxia-telangiectasia, the Li-Fraumeni syndrome, heritable retinoblastoma, and the Nijmegan break syndrome [3–5].

The most commonly used form of therapeutic radiation is external beam irradiation and the most common type of external beam is photon beam. Photons are electromagnetic radiations which include X rays and gamma rays. X-rays are produced electrically. X-rays of low energy (5–140 kV) are used for diagnostic imaging. X-rays of higher energy (6–25 MV) are used for radiation therapy. High-energy photons are produced by linear accelerators. Electrons are accelerated which then bombard a target that stops the electron beam instantaneously, resulting in x-rays or bremsstrahlung which are then collimated to produce the therapeutic photon beam. The photon beam energy is absorbed in tissue in an exponential fashion. The rate of absorption and the depth of penetration depend upon the energy of the photon beam. Electron beams are also used in radiation therapy and have similar biological effects but are absorbed superficially. Protons are charged particles of high-energy, generated in a cyclotron. Protons are biologically similar to photons; however, the physical distribution provides significant advantages over photons. Protons enter the tissue at 20–30 % of their maximum dose. As the proton comes to rest at depth in the tissue, it releases 100 % of dose potential (the Bragg peak) after which point there is no further penetration or exit dose.

K. J. Marcus (✉)
Pediatric Radiation Oncology, Dana Farber/Boston Children's Cancer and Blood Disorders Center, Brigham and Women's Hospital, Harvard Medical School, Boston, MA, USA
e-mail: kmarcus@lroc.harvard.edu

R. Rahbar et al. (eds.), *Pediatric Head and Neck Tumors*,
DOI 10.1007/978-1-4614-8755-5_4, © Springer Science+Business Media New York 2014

This lack of exit dose provides a major advantage in radiation therapy and there is increasing use in pediatric radiotherapy treatments. There are other heavy particle irradiation beams including carbon ions and neutrons which are not in use for standard treatment of pediatric tumors and will not be discussed further.

Radiotherapy treatments evolved during the twentieth century, establishing the use of fractionated treatment delivery to maximize tumor destruction and minimize damage to the surrounding normal tissue. The international measure of radiation is the Gray (Gy). This is defined as the amount of radiation depositing 1 J of energy in 1 kg of tissue. This is equivalent to 100 rad which was the earlier term for absorbed dose where 1 rad is equal to 1 centigray (cGy) or 0.01 Gy. During this period, tolerances to normal tissues were established. The relationship between dose and time is determined by the total dose, the number of fractions required, the dose per fraction, and the overall timing to deliver these treatments. This relationship influences the biological effects. The tissue tolerances established were based on specific fraction sizes, total doses and overall timing. Formulae have been developed that relate these variables which are used when fractionation schemes are modified.

Radiotherapy is often used to treat tumors which are unable to be removed surgically. Rhabdomyosarcomas (RMS) in parameningeal locations, for example, can often not be removed surgically, and radiotherapy has been used to treat these. In some cases, when the likelihood of the tumor recurring in the area it arose is very high, radiotherapy is added. The most frequently used type of radiotherapy in cancer management is external beam therapy.

The indications for radiotherapy in the management of tumors of the head and neck in children are dependent upon the diagnosis as well as other factors. These factors include the age of the child, the stage or extent of disease and in some tumor types, the resectability. The reader is referred to the individual chapters for the specific indications for radiotherapy in the management of the many tumor types covered in this book. This chapter will review some general principles of radiotherapy, the technologies available, and the common tumors of the head and neck in children for which radiotherapy is most often indicated. The acute and long-term effects of radiotherapy will also be discussed.

Normal Tissue Responses to Radiotherapy

The effects of radiotherapy on normal tissue are divided into acute reactions, subacute reactions, and late effects. The acute effects are defined as those occurring during the course of treatment; subacute effects are those occurring within 3–9 months of treatment. Late effects are those occurring after one year following treatment. There are a variety of factors which affect the toxicities of radiotherapy. Treatment parameters which are associated with radiation therapy effects are the total dose, the dose per fraction, the fractionation schedule, and the overall time of treatment delivery. The host factors include underlying genetic predisposition to radiation damage, age, oxygenation of tissue being treated, and nutritional status. Other factors which influence radiotherapy effects include concurrent chemotherapy.

Normal tissue reactions are divided into early responding and late responding tissue depending upon the proliferating rate of the cells in the tissue. Early or acutely responding tissues manifest injury during the course of treatment as these tissues are rapidly proliferating. Skin, mucosa, and hematopoietic tissues are acutely responding. Acute effects are expected during treatment and are influenced by the dose per fraction, the dose rate and by concurrent chemotherapy. Acute reactions do not correlate with the development of late effects.

Transient cutaneous reaction of erythema can occur immediately after exposure to radiation. Sialadenitis can develop within hours of an initial treatment, resulting in painful swelling of the parotid glands if in the field. Acute toxicities of nausea, vomiting, and fatigue also occur within days of starting treatment but vary in severity and occurrence depending upon the area treated and the integral dose. The integral dose is the product of the volume exposed and the dose per fraction. These effects can also vary by age of the patient and underlying comorbidities.

Skin reactions such as hyperpigmentation and more severe reactions of dry desquamation occur approximately three weeks into a course of treatment. Hair loss begins at approximately the third week when the scalp is treated. Most severe skin reactions with development of moist desquamation are seen with higher doses and when chemotherapy, such as actinomycin D, are given concurrently.

The reactions of the mucosa occur when tumors in the head and neck are treated. These are seen beginning in the second to third week of treatment in the oral cavity, oropharynx, hypopharynx, and esophagus. These reactions are enhanced by concurrent administration of chemotherapy such as cisplatin, methotrexate, and actinomycin D. The mucosal reactions can be severe in the treatment of head and neck malignancies depending upon the dose required and the administration of concurrent chemotherapy. Topical agents and systemic pain medications are often needed. Intercurrent candidal infections should be ruled out and treated as these can occur during a course of treatment when the mucosa is damaged and will result in severe pain. Patients undergoing irradiation to the head and neck should be considered for placement of a feeding tube such a G-tube prior to starting treatment to maintain nutrition.

Subacute and late effects involve organs and tissues with slower proliferation rates. Damage to these are manifest later but can be severe or fatal. Examples of tissues and organs which demonstrate subacute and late toxicities include the kidneys, lung, spinal cord, brain, small intestine, liver, and heart [6, 7]. For these vital organs, normal tissue tolerance doses have been established in adults. The same normal tissue tolerance doses have been used in children; however, these limits are used with caution due to concerns for potentially increased sensitivity to radiotherapy in children.

Radiotherapy Techniques

Modern radiotherapy machines are linear accelerators, producing photon beams that are in the high-energy (megavoltage) range. This high energy allows the beam to penetrate tissues and treat deep-seated tumors. The dose to the skin is lower than with the early orthovoltage treatment machines. Advanced imaging with CT and MRI has been incorporated into radiotherapy treatment planning. Radiotherapy treatment fields are now designed using multiple beams to conform to the tumor shape and expose less normal tissue to ionizing radiation. This is called 3-D conformal radiation therapy. Radiotherapy treatment planning first involves the definition of the gross target volume (GTV). The GTV includes the tumor extent at diagnosis or in some situations of the postoperative tumor bed. The area surrounding the GTV which may contain microscopic extension is called the clinical target volume (CTV). The CTV includes areas of suspected or subclinical disease as well as the gross tumor volume. The CTV is an anatomical-clinical concept. The CTV may include draining lymph nodes if clinically indicated. After defining the GTV and the CTV, there is a further geometric expansion made to ensure adequate dosimetric coverage of the CTV which accounts for day-to-day variations in patient set-up or any potential movement during the actual treatment delivery. This is the planning target volume (PTV). In addition to the target volume, the identification and contouring of critical organs within the treatment volume is a mandatory part of the planning process. Earlier experiments on animals as well as outcome of patients have led to a definition of tolerance doses for normal structures. The tolerance doses and limits used for children are similar to those in adults.

Intensity-Modulated Radiation Therapy

Intensity-modulated radiation therapy (IMRT) is a more highly specialized form of conformal radiotherapy. This technology makes use of an even greater number of small fields with tiny leaves or collimators which can block parts of the treatment field. The result is that high-dose irradiation can be delivered to the tumor whilst sparing the surrounding normal tissues. Because IMRT requires highly accurate delineation of the tumor and the normal organs and structures, immobilization of the patient is critical. In addition, image guidance can be employed to follow organ and/or tumor motion during treatment. Using IMRT dose painting, different structures can be treated to different doses and the doses to critical structures can also be limited to specified doses (Fig. 4.1) With the use of IMRT, doses to many critical structures can be limited, thereby minimizing the significant late toxicity to swallowing and speech (Table 4.1).

Particle Beams

Charged particle beams such as protons and electrons are also ionizing radiation beams that are used in cancer treatments. The range of the particle in the body is determined by the energy of the beam of incoming particles which are accelerated. Protons as well as heavier ion beams deposit more energy as they go deeper into the body up to a sharp maximum at the end of their range. Near the end of the range of the particle, the residual energy is lost over a very short distance. This results in a steep rise in the absorbed dose, known as the Bragg peak. Beyond the Bragg peak, there is a rapid fall-off of dose to zero. Although the Bragg peak can be very narrow, it can be spread out to cover a longer distance. The distribution of radiation dose in the body of proton beam is characterized by a lower dose in the normal tissue proximal to the tumor, a high- and uniform-dose region across the tumor, and zero dose beyond the tumor. This is in contrast to photon radiation where the ionizing radiation energy passes on through the normal tissue beyond the tumor. The lack of exit dose of protons make proton beam preferable for many situations where a tumor is adjacent to a critical structure such as the spinal cord, which cannot tolerate high doses of ionizing radiation, or in the treatment of children, where avoiding normal tissues will significantly decrease the long-term side effects.

Proton beam for the treatment of head and neck malignancies in children can eliminate the exit dose into the brain, spare or limit the dose to the optic chiasm, salivary glands, and cochlea (Figs. 4.2 and 4.3). Presently, there are only a limited number of proton beam facilities, although more are in development. Nevertheless, this important technological advance has significant advantages in the treatment of children.

Other particle beams such as carbon ions show similar physical advantages to protons. Carbon ions have advantages over protons in that they may be more effective against some more slow growing tumors. However, carbon ion beams are not yet used commonly in the treatment of pediatric tumors.

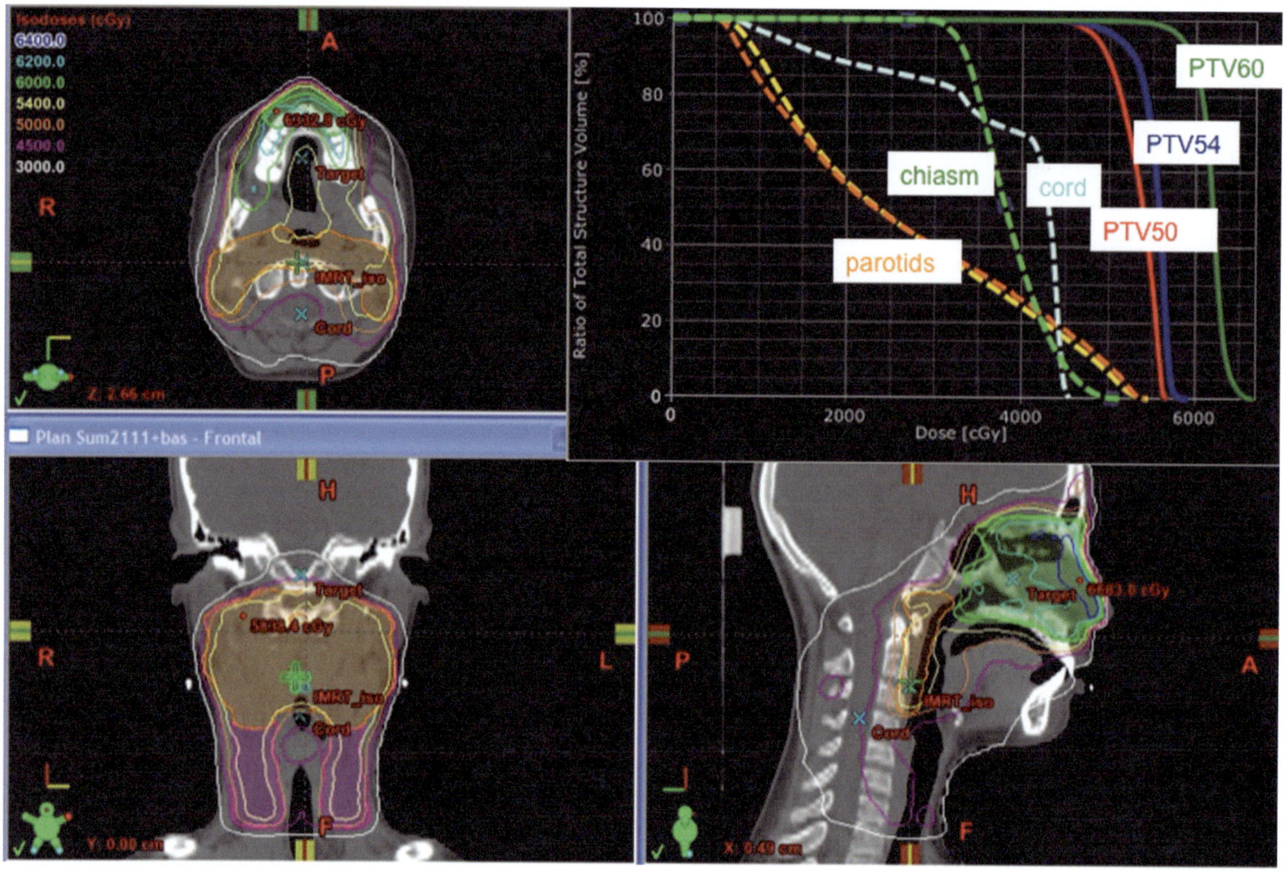

Fig. 4.1 Intensity-modulated radiation therapy (IMRT) plan for a patient with a nasopharyngeal tumor. *Upper right panel:* dose volume histogram with doses to specific critical structures (chiasm, parotid gland, spinal cord) and differentially dosed volumes

Table 4.1 IMRT dose constraints

Structure	True structure constraint	PRV constraint
Brainstem	54 Gy max. dose	No more than 1 % > 60 Gy
Spinal cord	45 Gy max. dose	No more than 1 % > 50 Gy
Optic nerves, chiasm	50 Gy max. dose	54 Gy max. dose
Mandible, TM joints	70 Gy, if not attainable, then no more than 1 cc to exceed 75 Gy	
Brachial plexus	66 Gy max. dose	
Oral cavity (excluding PTV)	Mean dose < 40 Gy	
Each cochlea (GOAL, not hard constraint)	No more than 5 % get 55 Gy or more	
Eyes	Max. dose < 50 Gy	
Lens	Max. dose < 25 Gy	
Glottic larynx	Mean dose < 45 Gy	
Esophagus/postcricoid	Mean dose < 45 Gy	
Parotids (note: submandibular and sublingual glands dose reduced as much as possible)	Mean dose in at least 1 gland < 26 Gy and/or 20 cc < 20 Gy and/or 50 % < 30 Gy	

PRV planning organ at risk volume: margin surrounding critical structure to ensure that dose is not exceeded

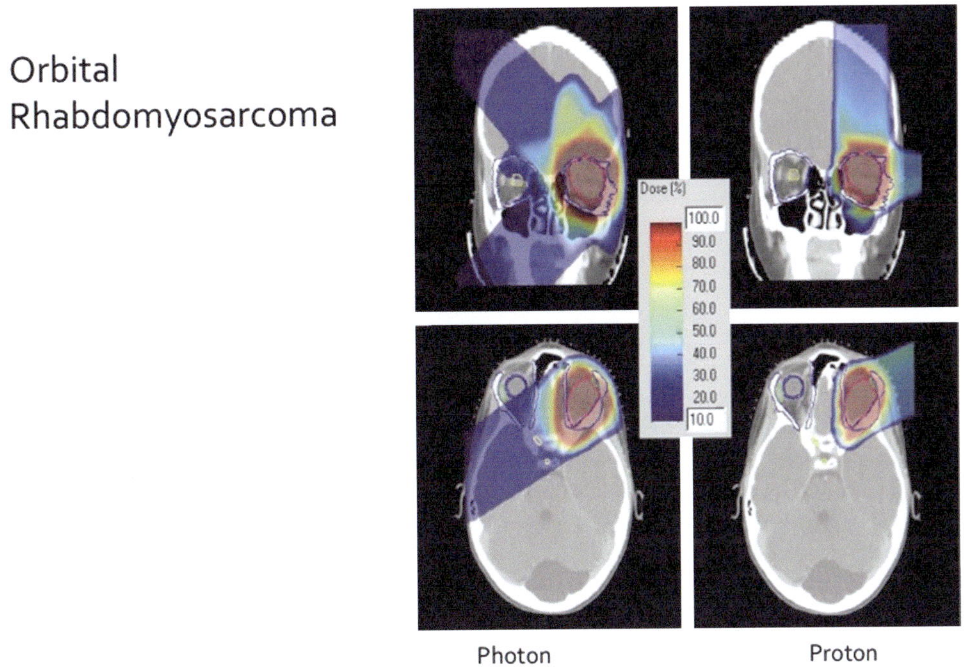

Fig. 4.2 Photon beam and proton beam radiotherapy plans for treatment of an orbital rhabdomyosarcoma (RMS) in a child. Lack of exit dose from proton beam plan is evident in the color wash [8]. (Reprinted with permission from Elsevier)

Specific Examples: Rhabdomyosarcoma and Nasopharyngeal Carcinoma

The indications for radiotherapy, the fields, doses, and timing of radiotherapy due vary depending upon the diagnosis. Several specific examples of two common pediatric tumors of the head and neck are presented in this section. Radiotherapy is used in the treatment of many children with RMS occurring in the head and neck. Radiotherapy is currently recommended for children with RMS whose tumors are inadequately resected as well as for all children whose tumor has alveolar histology [9]. The field design treats the initial tumor with a margin of 1.5–2 cm. Draining lymph nodes are not included unless clinically suspicious or pathologically proven to contain disease. Biopsy confirmation is indicated if nodes are clinically suspicious. The dose of radiotherapy for gross residual disease (group III) is 50.4 Gy in all sites except the orbit, where the dose is limited to 45 Gy. The doses for microscopic disease are 36 Gy for node negative microscopic disease and 41.4 Gy when nodes are positive.

Rhabdomyosarcomas in the head and neck region are considered either to be parameningeal if they involve the paranasal sinuses, nasal cavity, nasopharynx, middle ear,

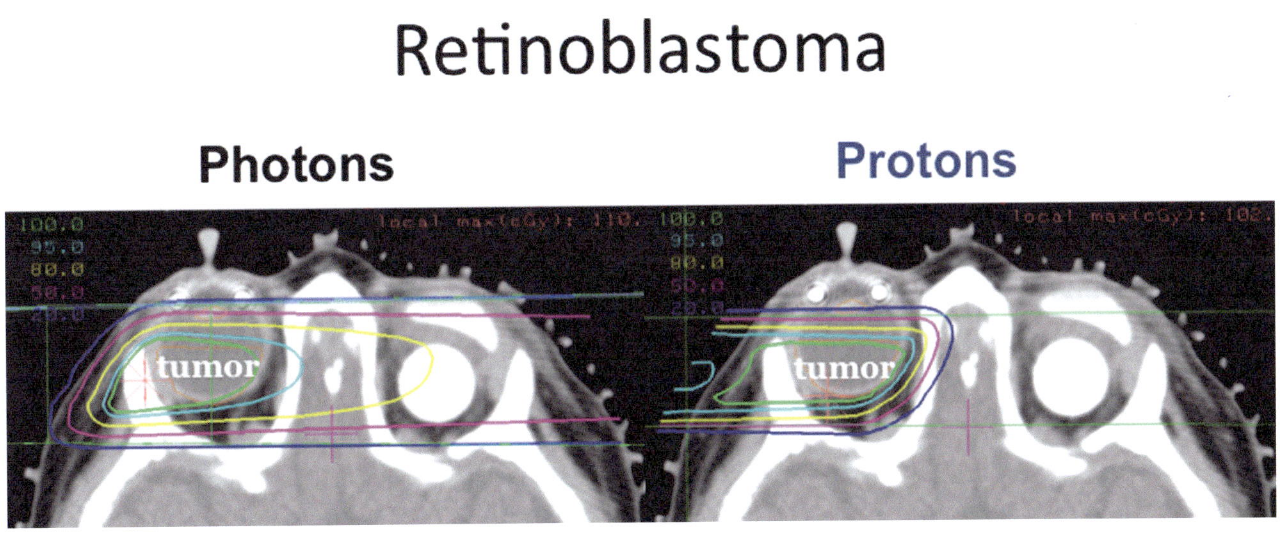

Fig. 4.3 Photon beam (*left panel*) and proton beam (*right panel*) plans for irradiation of a retinoblastoma in a child with bilateral disease who has undergone an enucleation. The proton beam plan is able to avoid irradiation of the contralateral eye; courtesy Judith Adams and Shannon MacDonald

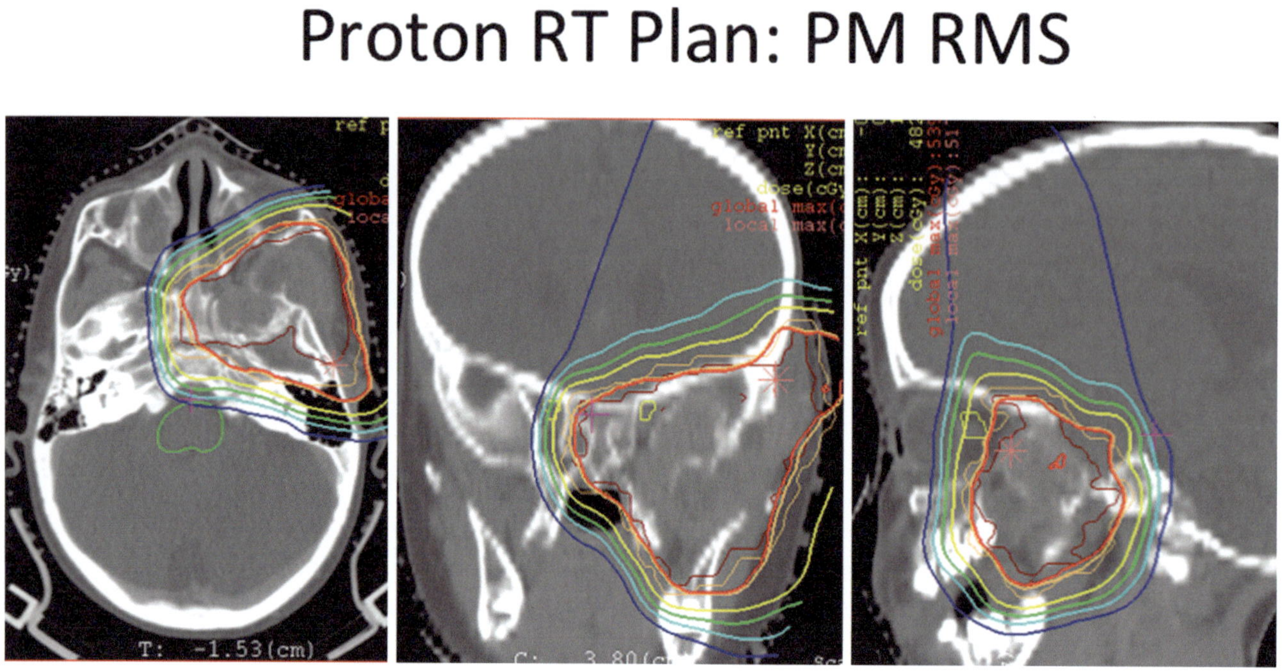

Fig. 4.4 Proton beam plan for treatment of parameningeal rhabdomyosarcoma (PM-RMS) minimizes exposure of normal tissues; courtesy Torunn Yock

infratemporal/pterygopalatine fossa, and parapharyngeal region. Those tumors arising in the orbit, scalp, oropharynx, hypopharynx, oral cavity, neck, thyroid, parotid, and larynx are all deemed head/neck nonparameningeal. The distinction is of major prognostic significance. Parameningeal sites are deemed unfavorable, whereas nonparameningeal are favorable. Both parameningeal and nonparameningeal tumors are often unresectable and therefore radiotherapy remains an important modality in the management.

Techniques for the radiotherapy have evolved from older 2-D approaches to highly conformal 3-D techniques, intensity-modulated radiotherapy, and proton beam therapy. The goals are to improve local control and to minimize late toxicity. Proton beam plan for a parameningeal rhabdomyosarcoma (PM-RMS) limits dose to the surrounding brain (Fig. 4.4).

Nasopharyngeal carcinoma is another example of a tumor arising in a location which is generally not resectable based on anatomic constraints. Nevertheless, radiotherapy treatment planning and delivery is complex due to the sensitivity of normal tissues and to the pathways of spread that are included in the treatment volume. This is true for adults as well as children. The treatment volume includes the nasopharynx, the posterior nasal cavity, the posterior ethmoid sinus, the entire sphenoid sinus, the base of skull, the posterior one-third of the maxillary sinus, the foramen ovale, the oropharyngeal wall to the mid-tonsillar fossa, the retropharyngeal nodes, and the bilateral cervical and supraclavicular lymph nodes. The treatment volume is modified based on the tumor extent. The doses of radiotherapy are 50–72 Gy in children over 10 and 5–10% lower in young children. The use of highly conformal techniques such as IMRT in the treatment of the nasopharynx is of significant benefit both in local control and diminishing short and long-term toxicities [10].

Late Effects of Radiotherapy

The long-term consequences of irradiation to the head and neck are related to normal tissues treated, the doses, and the age of the child. The salivary glands, the thyroid, and the pituitary gland might be affected. Permanent xerostomia can result from the doses of radiotherapy necessary to treat some malignancies. Although not life-threatening, xerostomia has a significant impact on quality of life. Hormonal deficiencies are the late effect of thyroid and pituitary gland irradiation [11].

In children, there are late effects of radiotherapy delivered to the head and neck not observed in adults which result in significant morbidity and even mortality. Radiotherapy in the management of retinoblastoma, for example, usually entails treating an infant, resulting in significant craniofacial bone abnormalities as the child grows. Other significant late toxicities resulting from irradiation to the head and neck area in a child are neurocognitive and neurodevelopmental effects. Focal necrosis of brain tissue can occur following doses in excess of 60 Gy. Narrowing of blood vessels in the brain can result in late vascular damage. Irradiation of the suprasellar area, as in the treatment of craniopharyngioma or optic chiasmatic tumors, can cause narrowing of one of the six major blood vessels comprising the circle of Willis [12]. The result of such narrowing causes small collateral blood vessels to develop 3–4 years following irradiation. This is a recognized syndrome known as moyamoya syndrome. Children with moyamoya are at significantly increased risk of stroke. Children treated at young ages are at greater risk of developing moyamoya, as are patients with NF-1. Another postradiation vascular late effect is the development of benign cavernomas [13]. These cavernomas can be large and, although benign, are at risk for hemorrhage.

The neurocognitive late effects of radiotherapy are well known and documented. These effects are related to the age of the child, the dose of radiotherapy, and volume of brain irradiated [14]. Irradiation of the whole brain or of those areas involved in learning and memory, particularly in young children (under 5 years), results in difficulties in attention, memory, and knowledge acquisition.

Hearing loss can result from the ototoxic effects of radiotherapy on the cochlea. Doses of at least 35 Gy can cause some degree of hearing loss. Radiation-related ototoxicity is a late consequence and generally occurs several years following treatment but can occur even later. It is irreversible. Hearing loss from combined treatment with ototoxic chemotherapy such as cisplatin can occur at lower doses of radiotherapy and can occur several years following treatment.

One of the most devastating late consequences of radiotherapy is the development of a second malignancy. A second malignancy related to prior radiotherapy is one that is of a different histology from the originally treated tumor, occurs within the previous radiotherapy field, and develops after a latency period of several years. The risk of developing a second malignancy from radiotherapy is a life-long risk. In the Children's Cancer Survivor Study cohort of 14,358 survivors, the 30-year-cumulative incidence of second malignant neoplasm was 9.3 %. On multivariable analysis, radiotherapy, age at diagnosis, family history of cancer, and primary childhood cancer diagnosis were significant [15].

References

1. Powell S, McMillan TJ. DNA damage and repair following treatment with ionizing radiation. Radiother Oncol. 1990;19(2):95–108.
2. Prise KM, Schettino G, Folkard M, et al. New insights on cell death from radiation exposure. Lancet Oncol. 2005;6(7):520–8.
3. Painter RB, Young BR. Radiosensitivity in ataxia-telangiectasia: a new explanation. Proc Natl Acad Sci U S A. 1980;77(12):7315–7.
4. Taylor AM, Harnden DG, Arlett CF, et al. Ataxia telangiectasia: a human mutation with abnormal radiation sensitivity. Nature. 1975;258(5534):427–9.
5. Demuth I, Digweed M. The clinical manifestation of a defective response to DNA double-strand breaks as exemplified by Nijmegen breakage syndrome. Oncogene. 2007;26(56):7792–8.
6. Rubin P, Casarette GW. Clinical radiation pathology. Philadelphia: Saunders, 1968.
7. Miller AR, Martenson JA, Nelson H, et al. The incidence and clinical consequences of treatment-related bowel injury. Int J Radiat Oncol Biol Phys. 1999;43(4):817–25.
8. Yock T, Schneider R, Friedmann A, Adams J, Fullerton B, Tarbell N. Proton radiotherapy for orbital rhabdomyosarcoma: clinical outcome and a dosimetric comparison with photons. Int J Radiat Oncol Biol Phys. 2005;63(4):1161–8.
9. Wolden SL, Anderson JR, Crist WM, et al. Indications for radiotherapy and chemotherapy after complete resection in rhabdomyosarcoma: a report from the Intergroup Rhabdomyosarcoma Studies I to III. J Clin Oncol. 1999;17(11):3468–75.
10. Wolden SL, Chen WC, Pfister DG, et al. Intensity-modulated radiation therapy (IMRT) for nasopharynx cancer: update of the Memorial Sloan-Kettering experience. Int J Radiat Oncol Biol Phys. 2006;64(1):57–62.
11. Hancock SL, McDougall IR, Constine LS. Thyroid abnormalities after therapeutic external radiation. Int J Radiat Oncol Biol Phys. 1995;31(5):1165–70.
12. Ullrich NJ, Robertson R, Kinnamon DD, et al. Moyamoya following cranial irradiation for primary brain tumors in children. Neurology. 2007;68(12):932–8.
13. Lew SM, Morgan JN, Psaty E, et al. Cumulative incidence of radiation-induced cavernomas in long-term survivors of medulloblastoma. J Neurosurg. 2006;104(2 Suppl):103–7.
14. Mulhern RK, Merchant TE, Gajjar A, et al. Late neurocognitive sequelae in survivors of brain tumours in childhood. Lancet Oncol. 2004;5(7):399–408.
15. Meadows AT, Friedman DL, Neglia JP, et al. Second neoplasms in survivors of childhood cancer: findings from the Childhood Cancer Survivor Study cohort. J Clin Oncol. 2009;27(14):2356–62.

5 Interventional Radiology

Raja Shaikh, Darren B. Orbach and Horatio M. Padua Jr.

Introduction

Pediatric interventional radiology (IR) is an emerging specialty. When considering "tumors" broadly, to include non-neoplastic growths, pediatric interventional radiologists are centrally involved in all aspects of diagnosis, treatment, and symptom management. With regard to neoplastic disease, oncology-related pediatric IR procedures have traditionally been limited to diagnosis, management of complications, and procedures designed as auxiliaries to open surgery. Newer landmarks in pediatric therapeutic oncological interventions are under active development, but standards remain to be established. Although many broad principles in adult and pediatric interventions are the same, some specialized topics related to procedures in children deserve discussion, as enumerated below in this introductory section.

Informed Consent Since most pediatric patients of less than 18 years of age have legal guardians or parents, a detailed preprocedural discussion is necessary to educate them of the possible complications, sometimes remaining present throughout life. Many adolescent patients are able to participate actively in the decision-making process.

Sedation and Anesthesia Almost all children require general anesthesia or higher levels of sedation to minimize motion, tolerate pain better, and allow positioning during the procedure. Deep sedation or general anesthesia can provide some postprocedure amnesia unlike adults who can tolerate most procedures under mild sedation and local anesthesia.

R. Shaikh (✉)
Department of Interventional Radiology, Boston Children's Hospital, Harvard Medical School, Boston, MA, USA
e-mail: Raja.Shaikh@childrens.harvard.edu

D. B. Orbach · H. M. Padua Jr.
Department of Radiology, Boston Children's Hospital, Harvard Medical School, Boston, MA, USA

Equipment Most available devices are designed for use in adults. Hence, bench modifications of devices developed for adults are often performed to match the smaller body habitus of children.

Contrast and Radiation Limiting the contrast and radiation dose is essential in children. Carefully monitored volume of diluted nonionic contrast should be used to minimize renal toxicity. The risk of dialysis after receiving contrast significantly increases in patients with estimated GFR <30 ml/min/1.73 [1]. Given the small caliber of the vessels, extravasation of contrast or medication can occur during percutaneous access and may result in discomfort and compartment syndrome. Due to these limitations, goals must be accomplished using less contrast than might be employed in an adult.

Likewise, maximal efforts are directed to limit the radiation dose, as the cumulative effects of radiation are of major concern in children. Most interventional radiologists practicing in adult populations concern themselves largely with the deterministic effects of radiation, related to dose and time of exposure at time of procedure. These effects are usually manifest as damage to bone marrow, gastrointestinal mucosa, or skin. It is, however, the stochastic effects, those effects which are related to any exposure to any ionizing radiation, regardless of time or dose that are far more concerning in the pediatric population than the adult [2].There is no minimum threshold radiation dose for stochastic effects to occur, and stochastic exposure (primarily related to DNA damage) may not manifest itself for decades. It is specifically in young children, with many years of life to manifest the stochastic damage that these issues are of greatest concern. Additionally, many oncology patients are exposed to high-dose external beam radiation as part of their treatment protocol, adding to the risk. The "as low as reasonably achievable" (ALARA) concept of radiation exposure is ubiquitous in radiology, but is held to much higher standard in pediatric diagnostic imaging and pediatric IR, with risk of radiation exposure always weighed against the benefits of a given image-guided

R. Rahbar et al. (eds.), *Pediatric Head and Neck Tumors*,
DOI 10.1007/978-1-4614-8755-5_5, © Springer Science+Business Media New York 2014

procedure, and every attempt made to the lowest possible radiation dose. Aggressive dose reduction methods including limiting fluoroscopy time, low-dose pulse fluoroscopy, aggressive coning and filtering applied to the smallest possible region of interest [2], and maximal utilization of imaging modalities which are nonionizing, such as ultrasound or magnetic resonance imaging (MRI). These are or should be standards of care routinely practiced in centers with large pediatric practices.

Physiologic Responses Physiologic responses to intervention can be different in a child versus an adult. For example, vasospasm is commonly seen in children, making simple access or further intravascular manipulation more challenging. Gentle massages around the vessel, warming the room temperature, the judicious use of vasodilators for spasm resolution are some options. Children react to fluid imbalances and medications more quickly. Therefore, a close monitoring of fluid balance and drug dosages based on weight or body surface area is mandatory; vigilant care on the part of specialized pediatric nurses and a pediatric anesthesia team are invaluable.

Disease Spectrum The differential diagnosis for a given head or neck tumor varies widely, depending on the patient's age. Conditions like vascular anomalies and congenital defects typically present early in life, and may require extended years of multi-session treatment spanning into adulthood. Degenerative diseases like atherosclerosis are practically nonexistent in the pediatric population.

Vascular Interventions

Introduction

Generally, endovascular interventions can be divided into two categories: (1) enlarging vascular channels (for example, balloon angioplasty of stenotic blood vessels) and (2) blocking vascular lumens (i.e., sclerotherapy and embolization). Most vascular intervention, either pediatric or adult, is concentrated on the latter category, with the goal of reducing blood flow to a given lesion to either make the pathologic target ischemic, to potentiate directly injected therapies, or to reduce the volume or flow through a vascular malformation.

We will focus the discussion on image-guided sclerotherapy and embolization, as this is by far the most common vascular intervention performed on pediatric head and neck tumors and malformations. We will discuss these procedures in the context of the more common diagnoses referred to us for these procedures.

Vascular Malformations and Vascular Tumors of the Head and Neck

These lesions can be categorized functionally as high-flow versus low-flow lesions.

High-Flow Lesions

These lesions have intrinsic arterio-venous shunting. They appear reddish, warm, firm, and pulsatile, with signs of skin ischemia, ulceration, and/or hemorrhage. Distribution of these lesions is classically seen in the cheek (31 %) (Fig. 5.1a), followed by the ear (16 %) and nose (11 %) [1]. The symptoms are typically related to regional involvement such as macrotia (ear lesions), life threatening bleeding with dental procedures (mandibular or maxillary lesion), and bleeding with chewing (tongue lesions) in addition to the pain, bruit, or thrill that accompany high-flow vascular malformations anywhere in the body. The lesions often enlarge in response to hormonal changes (e.g., puberty or pregnancy) or trauma.

MRI provides the best spatial resolution for soft tissue, with computed tomography (CT) better delineating any osseous abnormality, when the lesion is in close association with the bone. Catheter angiography remains the gold standard in terms of providing the highest spatial resolution, as well as critical insight into the flow dynamics (Fig. 5.1b, c), though catheter-based procedures are usually performed as part of the therapeutic approach, rather than purely for diagnosis. High-flow vascular malformations are usually complex lesions where the therapeutic goal is symptom control, preservation of vital functions (e.g., vision, hearing, or mastication), or aesthetic restoration, rather than cure, although for focal lesions, a combination of single or multistage preoperative embolization followed by surgical resection can sometimes be curative [1, 3, 4].

Endovascular embolization is directed towards occlusion of the nidus and initial segment of the venous outflow. This can either be performed transarterially or by percutaneous direct access of the nidus or the draining vein. Preoperative embolization provides a dry surgical field and minimizes perioperative blood loss. Gelfoam powder, polyvinyl particles, or embospheres can be used for temporary preoperative embolization. For nonoperative candidates, embolization with permanent liquid agents capable of permeating the AVM nidus, such as absolute ethanol, n-Butyl Cyano Acrylate (glue), or Onyx, may be used (Fig. 5.1d–f).

Endovascular embolization can be highly effective in cases of arterio-venous fistulas, both for preoperative adjunctive treatment and as a stand-alone cure. In contrast, for focal AVMs with multiple, small feeders, nidal embolization followed by surgical resection is the usual treatment [5].

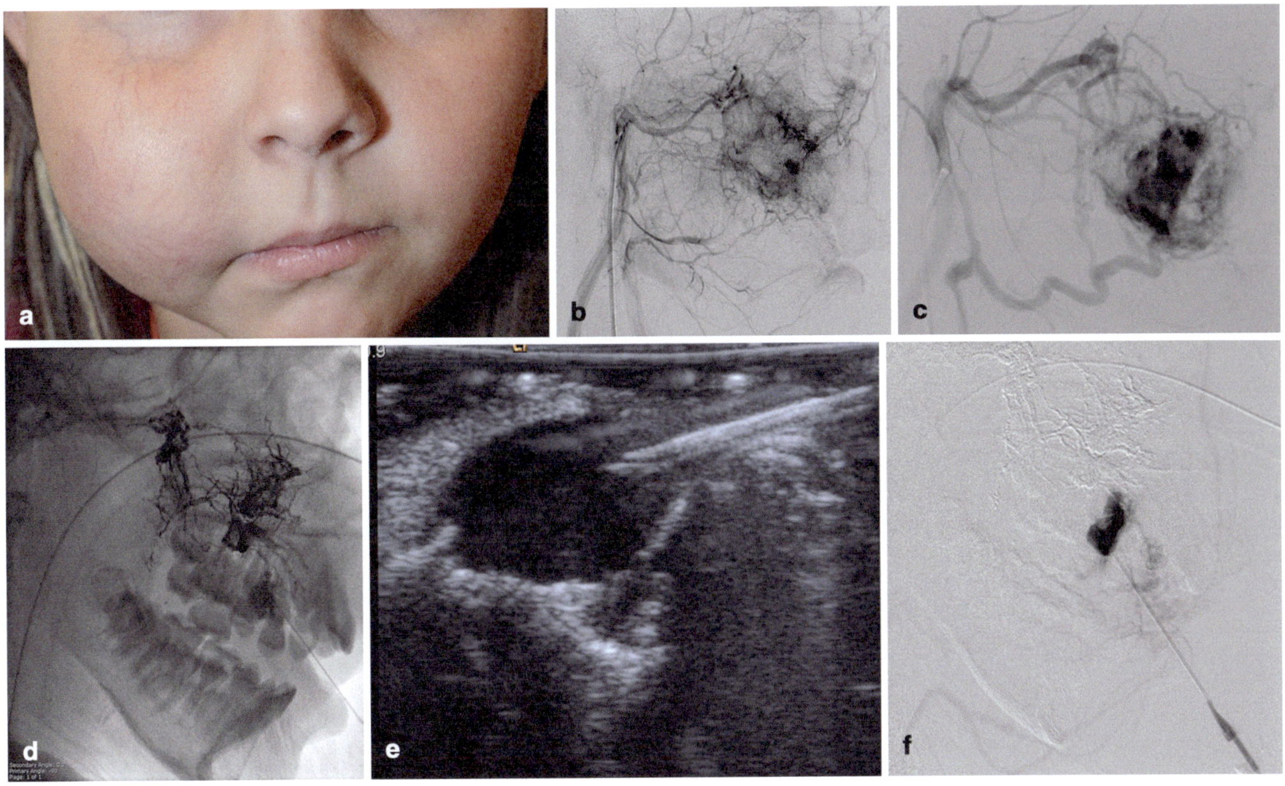

Fig. 5.1 Arteriovenous malformation (AVM): **a** Pulsatile mass of the right cheek. **b** Arterial and **c** venous phases of right external carotid angiogram demonstrating high-flow AVM with large draining veins. **d** Unsubtracted lateral fluoroscopic image demonstrating opacified Onyx embolic agent within the feeding vessels. **e** Ultrasound image of percutaneous needle access of abnormal vein. **f** Fluoroscopic image with subtraction of contrast injection of the abnormal vein

Low-Flow Malformations

These lesions are broadly classified as capillary, venous, or lymphatic malformations.

Capillary Malformations (CM) These are flat, well demarcated, lesions showing ectatic blood vessels in the dermis associated with reduction in innervation, occurring most commonly in the trigeminal V1 distribution [6, 7]. They can be seen in association with syndromes like Sturge–Weber syndrome, Klippel–Trenaunay syndrome, Parkes Weber syndrome, macrocephaly-capillary malformation syndrome, and capillary malformation-arteriovenous malformation syndrome (CM-AVM). The standard treatment is pulsed-dye laser, although only 15–20 % of lesions clear completely [8].

Venous Malformations (VMs) These represent congenital anomalies, irregular endothelial-lined channels, with thin walls deficient in smooth muscle. They typically have a bluish purplish hue, and are soft and compressible. 40 % of these lesions are found in head, neck, and extremities [9]. Episodic focal thrombosis and occurrence of phleboliths may result in swelling and pain. Larger lesions on the face can cause facial asymmetry. Trauma or hormonal changes can induce enlargement of VM, and they can extend deeper intrafascially and cause mass effect in small anatomical spaces like the orbit and oral cavity. Syndromes like glomuvenous malformation, cutaneomucosal venous malformation, and blue rubber bleb nevus syndrome have VMs as part of their manifestation [10, 11]. VMs most characteristically enhance avidly but in a patchy, heterogeneous pattern on contrast enhanced MRI. Phleboliths are typically seen as hypointense defects on MRI or as calcified foci on CT scan images (Fig. 5.2d) [12].

Lymphatic Malformations (LM) These can be either macrocystic, microcystic, or of combined types. They are soft, noncompressible, translucent masses with overlying normal or bluish skin, often with superficial dry or weeping cutaneous vesicles. Macrocystic LMs have a predilection for the head and neck region. Sudden enlargement following infection or intralesional hemorrhage and spontaneous involution are common. Syndromes associated with LM include Klippel–Trenaunay, Turner, Noonan, and trisomies 13 and 18, and others [9]. On imaging, LMs show variably sized cysts in the macrocystic type, showing debris within or fluid–fluid levels with heterogeneous signal, due to repeated hemorrhages (Fig. 5.2a). Only the septae of macrocysts enhance. Microcystic disease on ultrasound is seen as an echogenic ill-defined mass with tiny, poorly visible cysts. On contrast

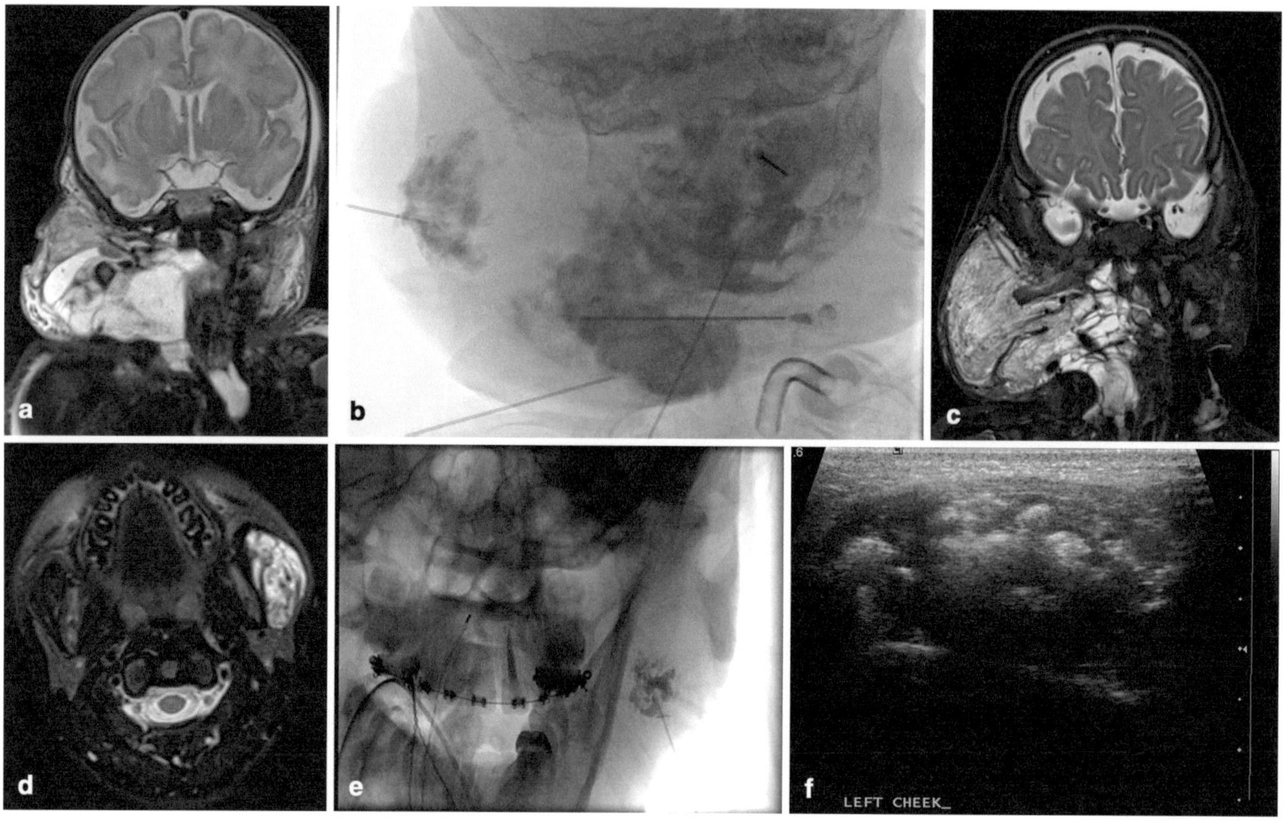

Fig. 5.2 Low-flow lesions: **a** Coronal T2-weighted MRI of newborn with large multicystic cervicofacial mass, consistent with macrocystic lymphatic malformation. **b** Anteroposterior (AP) fluoroscopic image of the neck during percutaneous sclerotherapy of multiple macrocysts. **c** Postsclerotherapy MRI demonstrating reduction of the macrocystic component and persistent microcystic disease. **d** Axial inversion-recovery MRI demonstrating VM of the left cheek. **e** AP fluoroscopic image during percutaneous sclerotherapy of the VM. **f** Ultrasound imaging of the VM after sclerotherapy injection. The echogenicity is secondary to air from foaming of the sclerosing agent

MRI, microcystic lesions may or may not enhance, with the likelihood of enhancement increased in the setting of inflammation or infection.

Treatment of Low-Flow Malformations: Percutaneous Sclerotherapy Most interventional-radiology-guided therapy of low-flow vascular malformations involves percutaneous sclerotherapy. Sclerotherapy is injection of a pharmacological agent that induces endothelial damage, elicits an avid inflammatory response, and finally leads to thrombosis (in VMs) and fibrosis. Image guidance, especially ultrasound in children, is most commonly used to gain access into the abnormal vascular channels. Digital subtraction angiograms using fluoroscopy prior to the actual injection of the sclerosant is performed to evaluate the position of the needle tip, the communications between the different components of the malformation, and the local vascular anatomy, including the hemodynamics of the venous drainage. Fluoroscopy can also help with estimation of the volume of sclerosant needed.

The sclerosant is usually reconstituted with a contrast agent, either water soluble, lipophilic (such as ethiodol), or negative contrast (air or carbon dioxide) to allow fluoroscopic and ultrasound monitoring of the injection [12] (Fig. 5.2b, e, f). Vigilantly watching for any extravasations during injection is mandatory, to prevent tissue or nerve damage. Applying direct pressure over venous drainage pathways during injection, using a tourniquet, or using double needle technique, which provides a low-pressure exit valve, can stop drainage to critical outflow veins. Escape of sclerosant into the venous drainage could potentially result in ophthalmic, cavernous, or intracranial venous thrombosis in head and neck lesions.

We most commonly use 3 % sodium tetradecyl sulfate (STS), a detergent, as the sclerosant Foaming the solution prior to injection has been reported to increase efficacy, perhaps by maximizing the surface area contact between the agent and the lesional endothelium. Ethanol, the most potent sclerosant, and one we make regular but judicious use of as well, unfortunately, has the highest rate of reported serious complications such as skin necrosis, nerve damage, central nervous system depression, acute pulmonary hypertension, thromboembolism, disseminated intravascular coagulation (DIC), hyperthermia, cardiac arrhythmias, and cardiovascular collapse and death [13]. However, STS and related detergents can cause serious adverse effects as well. Platinum coils or liquid embolics may serve as adjuncts to sclerotherapy in larger lesions, primarily to close prominent or recurrent venous channels. These agents are particularly effective in achieving preoperative short-term occlusion [12]. Bleomycin, an antibiotic with cytotoxic properties, can be of particular use in patients with intra-orbital and airway lesions, because of significantly less posttreatment edema than is seen with other agents [14]. Presclerotherapy steroids are imperative in orbital and airway malformations, for reducing postprocedural edema, which could result in increased intraocular pressure or airway compression. Sclerosants cause immediate local hemolysis and subsequent hemoglobinuria, though lesions in the head and neck are rarely large enough for the hemolysis to cause systemic problems. Generous hydration (doubling of the maintenance intravenous fluid for 4 h post procedure), monitoring of urinary output, and urinary alkalization with sodium bicarbonate intravenous fluid is recommended [12].

Localized VMs have the best responses to sclerotherapy. Diffuse malformations are less likely to have a complete response, and the treatment should, therefore, be targeted at the most symptomatic portions. For all but the smallest lesions, sclerotherapy is often repeated. Among the LMs, the macroystic variety typically responds well to sclerotherapy, whereas microcystic lesions are technically difficult to treat and show a poor response (Fig. 5.2c). Sclerosants reported for use in treating macrocystic LMs include ethanol, doxycycline, bleomycin, Ethibloc, and OK-432. Our first-line agent is most commonly doxycycline at a concentration of 10 mg/ml. For large cysts, a pigtail catheter aspiration of the contents and volume measurement is made, followed by injection and drainage of the cyst with the sclerosant. The sclerosant is allowed to dwell in the cyst for 2–3 h and then drained out. The procedure is repeated sequentially on days 2 and 3, through the indwelling catheters. It is important to disrupt the internal septations to increase the contact of the sclerosants within different compartments. Cyst involution can be assessed approximately 6 weeks after the procedure. For microcystic LM, sclerotherapy using bleomycin or OK-432 is often used. Other techniques using in-column electrocoagulation, carbon dioxide laser excision and radiofrequency ablation (RFA) have also been described [14–16]. The overall complication rate for sclerotherapy to treat VMs is 12 % [13]. Peripheral neuropathy is seen in approximately 1 %, but can be avoided if care is taken not to cause extravasation during injection; when it occurs, neuropathy is usually transient. Skin blistering and, in rare occurences, skin necrosis with permanent scarring can occur, particularly when the lesion has a more superficial component. For lesions involving the tongue, buccal surfaces, soft palate, or airway, marked postprocedural edema can cause transient dysphagia and breathing difficulties. Many such patients have a tracheostomy placed before commencing the procedure. Other lesser adverse effects include muscle atrophy and contracture if the sclerosant infiltrates the tissues [12].

Juvenile Naso-Pharyngeal Angiofibroma (JNA)

JNA is a benign vascular tumor composed of a rich vascular network within a fibrous stroma [17]. It most commonly arises in the posterolateral nasopharynx of prepubertal and adolescent males (Fig. 5.3a). JNA can behave aggressively and tend to bleed frequently. They can expand commonly beyond the nasopharynx into the cranium, nose, and paranasal sinuses [17, 18]. Profuse intraoperative bleeding leading to incomplete resection and tumor recurrence can occur, and preoperatively transarterial tumor embolization can greatly facilitate resection. JNAs are primarily fed from distal internal maxillary artery branches (Fig. 5.3b), and may recruit arterial supply from any nearby ipsilateral or contralateral vessel, requiring bilateral internal and external carotid arteriography for elucidation. Anastomosis between branches of the external and internal carotid artery and vascular spasm has to be considered when planning superselective embolization. Silastic spheres, Gelfoam, dura mater, and polyvinyl alcohol (PVA) particles (Fig. 5.3c) have been used to embolize the tumor bed and the feeding vessels [19], with PVA particles often preferred, as they are efficient and cost effective. Nontarget embolization of particles to the ophthalmic artery, the internal carotid, or vertebral arteries via anastomosis or reflux of particles injected in the external carotid artery may cause retinal or brain ischemic deficits, and thus preembolization and intraprocedural angiography must be scrupulously studied.

Glomus Tumors

Paragangliomas, also called glomus tumors, are highly vascularized tumors of neural crest origin that are derived from chemoreceptor organs in the walls of blood vessels or specific nerves in the head and neck area. They can develop in the middle ear (glomus tympanicum), the jugular foramen of the skull base (glomus jugulare), or other head and neck areas (glomus caroticum, glomus vagale). They are usually benign but locally destructive [20–23]. Preoperative embolization for devascularization greatly reduces the perioperative blood loss by a factor of 2–3, with reduction of need of transfusion in the postoperative period to less than 50 % [24]. However, extreme caution is warranted during embolization of these lesions. In particular, during embolization of carotid body tumors, particles can escape into the internal carotid artery and result in stroke, especially if particles $< 150\ \mu m$ in size are used. As in the case of JNA, vigilant angiographic search for anastomosis between the intra- and extracranial circulation is imperative. Collaterals between the vertebral artery and the C1, C2, and C3 musculoskeletal branches are

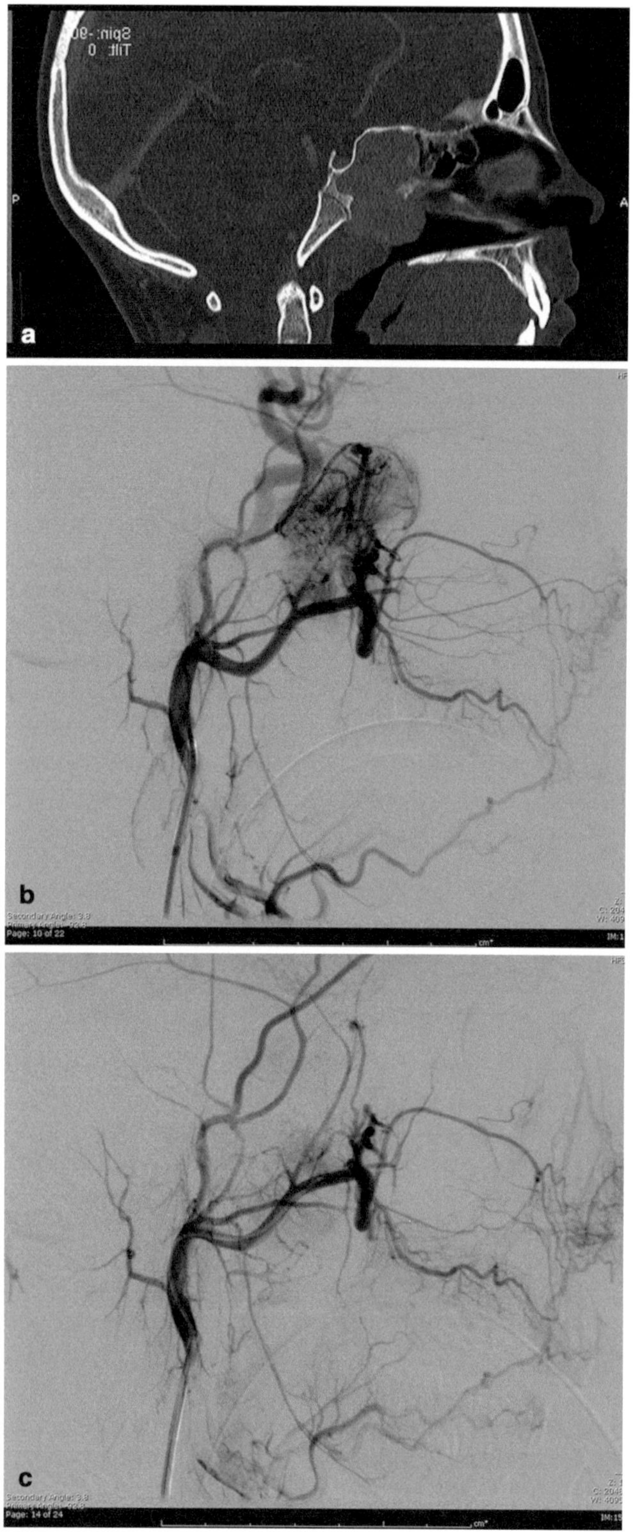

Fig. 5.3 Juvenile nasopharyngeal angiofibroma (JNA): **a** Sagittal CT-reconstructed image of the head demonstrates large enhancing nasopharyngeal mass. **b** Selective internal maxillary artery injection demonstrating hypervascular nasopharyngeal mass. **c** After selective embolization with PVA particles, there is near-complete cessation of flow to the mass with preservation of the normal circulation

common. Lower cranial nerves, such as the facial nerve or hypoglossal nerve can undergo ischemia if the vaso nervorum is inadvertently embolized. When embolizing glomus tumors, preprocedural administration of an alfa-blocking agent is often necessary to reduce catecholaminergic activity. Not infrequently, complete arterial devascularization of the tumor bed is not achieved, and several groups have recently described direct puncture and the slow injection of acrylic glue to allow for permeation of the vascular tumor bed while avoiding its passage to the venous side or its reflux into normal arterial territory [25].

Nonvascular Interventions

Introduction

Image-guided procedures that do not involve endovascular access are more common than vascular procedures in most pediatric centers. In the case of pediatric head and neck tumors, these procedures can be divided into two categories: (1) obtaining tissue for diagnosis and (2) primary treatment of tumors or tumor-like conditions using minimally invasive, image-guided methods. The following are some of the more common examples in our practice.

Percutaneous Needle Biopsy

Almost any neck mass can initially be biopsied using percutaneous needle biopsy with ultrasound guidance. Automated or semi-automated cutting needles in the range of sizes between 14-gauge and 20-gauge are available. Ultrasound guidance is usually the choice modality, given its real-time capability. Most biopsy needles are sonographically visible, and precise real-time targeting of most masses is possible, even in locations adjacent to vital structures (Fig. 5.4a–c). Risks include bleeding, infection, and injury to the structures around the target, though these risks are small when compared to surgical approaches for biopsy in the neck. Other guidance modalities can be used for targeting, including CT and MRI (Fig. 5.4d–f); these almost invariably require general anesthesia. As mentioned above, radiation exposure in CT is a concern in the pediatric population.

The most commonly biopsied structures in the neck include lymph nodes, the thyroid and the parathyroid glands, as well as soft tissue and bony masses. Accessing the deep spaces of the head and neck can be challenging and potentially hazardous. Previously operated or irradiated tissues in the neck can pose radiographic diagnostic dilemmas and can be difficult to access when situated deep to the vascular, neural, and bony structures. Blind needle biopsies have a low yield and are potentially dangerous [26]. Challenging areas

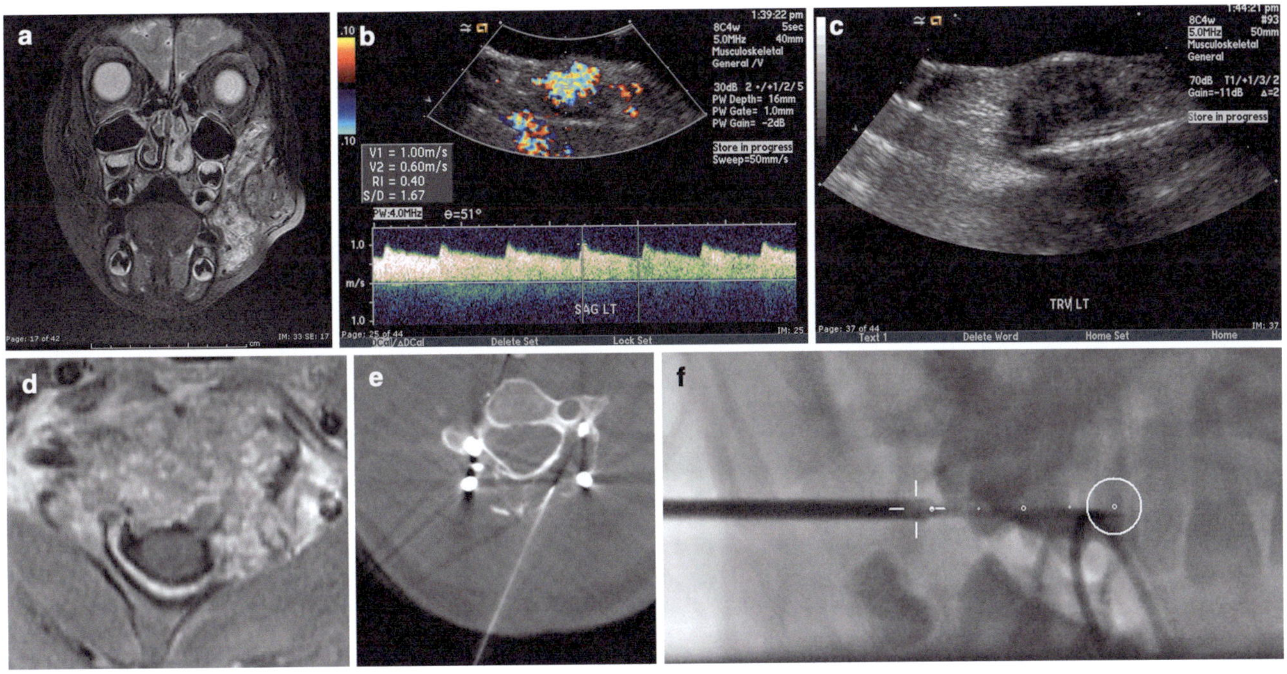

Fig. 5.4 Percutaneous image-guided needle biopsy: **a** Coronal T2 MRI of the head demonstrating large, heterogenous mass of the left face. **b** Ultrasound of the mass demonstrating moderate to high vascularity **c** Ultrasound-guided percutaneous needle biopsy with the needle (*white line*) targeting the less vascular portion of the lesion. The lesion was diagnosed as hamartoma. **d** Axial MRI of C2 with gadolinium demonstrating heterogenous mass involving the body and posterior elements with mass effect on the spinal canal. **e** CT- and **f** iGuide fluoroscopy-guided percutaneous needle biopsy of the lesion obtained tissue demonstrating the lesion to be aneurysmal bone cyst

for access include the infratemporal fossa, pterygopalatine fossa, pterygomaxillary fossa, parapharyngeal spaces, intraorbital, skull base, paralarngeotracheal and paraesophageal spaces, the retropharyngeal, parotid, thyroid, and paraspinous regions. But with cross-sectional imaging guidance, most lesions even in these areas can be sampled by core needle biopsy or fine needle aspiration (FNA). Lesions that can be visualized transorally, such as some parapharyngeal space lesions, can be approached through a transoral needle biopsy, with reported accuracy rates of 78–86% [27–29]. Depending on different locations of the abnormality, various percutaneous approaches have been described such as the retromandibular, paramaxillary, submastoid, subzygomatic, transoral, posterior, posterolateral, and anterolateral approaches [30].

Bony lesions can be particularly challenging. Benign bone tumors commonly seen in the head and neck include bony "hemangiomas" (more accurately, VMs of bone), osteomas, dermoid and epidermoid tumors, and eosinophilic granulomas. Malignant tumors include sarcomas, chondromas, and metastatic lesions. Obtaining a sample from the soft tissue mass, bone mass, and its interface is most helpful. FNA can be obtained using a 20–22-gauge needle placed co-axially via an 18–19-gauge needle. An 11- or 13-gauge needle will permit the coaxial passage of a trephine Ackermann needle (15 and 16 gauge, respectively) to complete the bone biopsy. Smaller coaxial systems such as the Bonopty system are also available. MRI or fluorodeoxyglucose positron emission tomography (FDG PET) can be used to target viable segments of the tumor.

Radiofrequency Ablation

Radiofrequency ablation (RFA) involves localized delivery of electromagnetic energy, usually via a small needle probe, to induce thermal agitation resulting in induction of cytotoxic levels of heat in the surrounding target tissue to cause coagulation necrosis. RFA probes are usually placed percutaneously using image guidance, making the procedure common in IR. As mentioned above, RFA is often used in treatment of microcystic LM [15, 16]. In the context of outside vascular malformations, RFA is most commonly used to treat osteoid osteoma.

Osteoid osteoma (OO) is a benign bone tumor mainly seen in 10–30-year old male patients [31–33]. The cervical spine, followed by the lumbar spine are the most common levels of axial involvement [34]. Classic presenting symptoms include moderate to severe pain occurring mainly at night, typically relieved by nonsteroidal anti-inflammatory medication. The characteristic radiographic pattern is a nidus under 1 cm in diameter that is cortically based, within the bone.

Percutaneous RFA for OO is usually performed under CT guidance or fluoroscopy with Dyna CT capability, for optimal resolution of the bony lesion and needle trajectory,

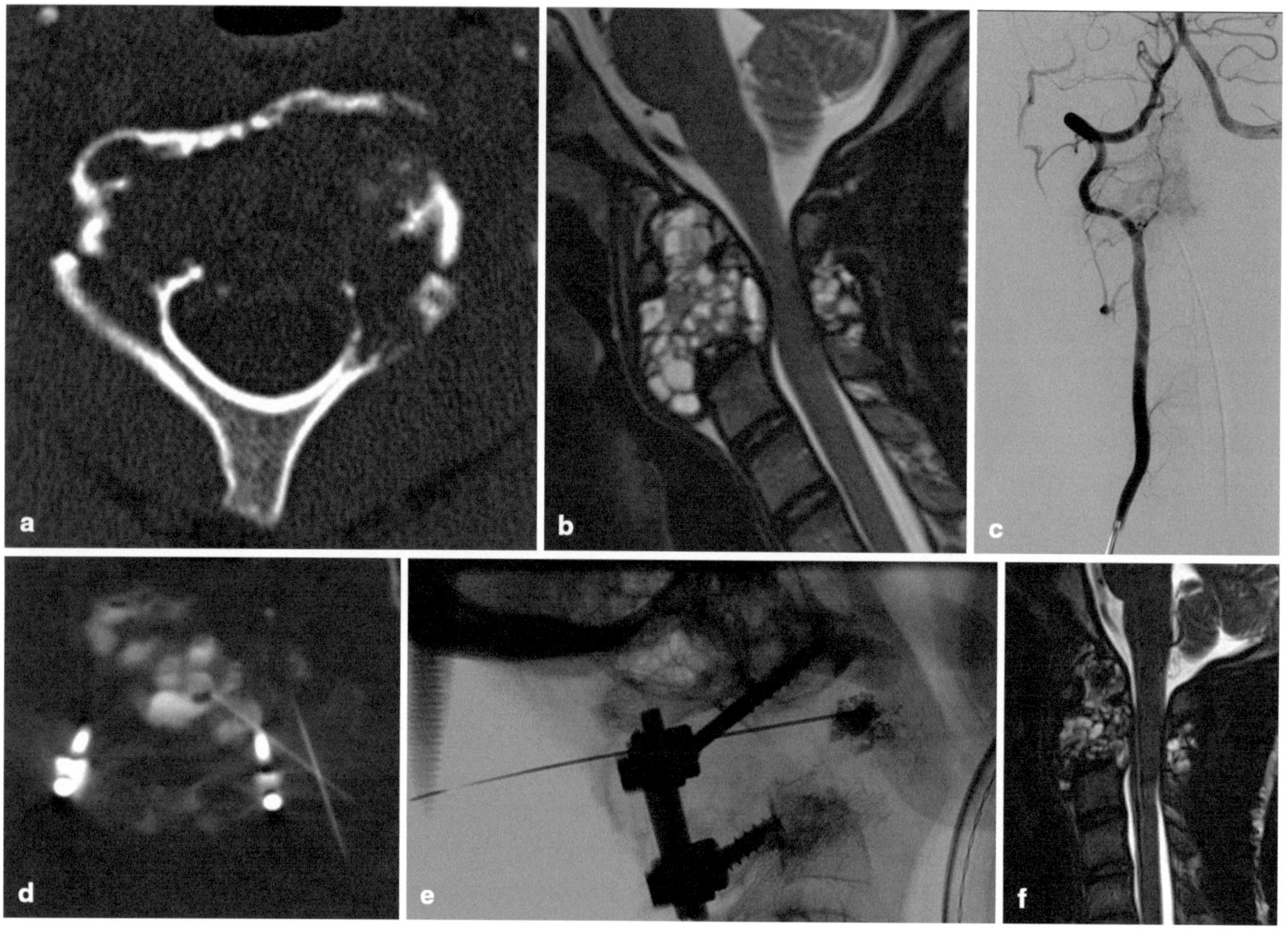

Fig. 5.5 Aneurysmal bone cyst of C2: **a** Axial CT demonstrating large expansile, lytic mass involving most of the body of C2. **b** Sagittal T2-weighted MRI demonstrating the multicystic nature of the lesion with some mass effect on the anterior spinal canal. **c** Right verterbral artery arteriogram demonstrating a small amount of vascularity. **d** dynaCT and **e** fluoroscopic-guided percutaneous sclerotherapy was performed on the lesion. **f** Follow-up MRI 4 weeks after procedure demonstrates interval improvement in the degree of mass effect on the spinal canal. There is also lower signal in the mass consistent with interval development of fibrous tissue post sclerotherapy.

with needle biopsy usually obtained at the same time. Proper placement of the grounding pads, in full contact with the skin without any air pockets, is necessary to avoid burns [35]. The target temperature is typically 90 °C. Under aseptic precautions, a small skin incision is made and an 11- or 13-gauge co-axial needle is passed under image guidance to the edge of the nidus. A 17-gauge, monopolar radiofrequency (RF) probe with a 7-mm or 1-cm active tip is placed through the coaxial needle and positioned with the active tip centered on the nidus. The coaxial needle is pulled back as far as possible on the probe to separate the coaxial needle from the active tip to avoid conduction of RF along the coaxial needle that may cause skin burns. The generator timer is set for a 6-min burn cycle and the energy is gradually increased over 1–2 min until the temperature at the probe tip registers 90 °C. Larger diameter nidus lesions may require multiple targets. Nearly all OO patients are pain-free by 2 weeks. In patients with inadequate clinical improvement, a review of procedural images to ascertain satisfactory position of the RF probe may be needed, as may a revising of the diagnosis of OO. The primary success rate for treatment of spinal OO has been cited as 76 % with a final success rate as high as 97 % [36].

Percutaneous Sclerotherapy for Aneurysmal Bone Cysts (ABC)

Sclerotherapy has been compared with gross resection for the management of ABC outside the head and neck [37]. In the head and neck, ABCs can occur in the cervical spine and result in pain, restricted neck movements and, critically, instability of the spine (Fig. 5.5a). These can be percutaneously accessed from posterior or postero-lateral approaches using cone beam CT (Fig. 5.5d) and ultrasound imaging to direct the needle into the cystic areas. Needle preference can range from 18-gauge spinal needles to 23-gauge Chiba needles, depending upon the ease of penetration through the bony cortex. Thinner needles reduce the possibility of reflux along the entry tract. If the outer cortex is difficult to penetrate, an18-gauge spinal needle is used coaxially with a

23-gauge inner needle that can be used to penetrate further into the cystic portion of the lesion. Different agents can be used for sclerotherapy, most commonly STS or doxycycline alone or in combination. Contrast injection into the cyst is performed first, to delineate the intralesional communication and the drainage pattern (Fig. 5.5e); particularly important in the neck, where drainage into veins that either drain or are in contiguity with the spinal and deep intracranial venous system is common. Extravasation into the spinal canal may result from insult to the bony margins by the expansile lesion or if the needle is partially located in the epidural space during injection. As cervical ABCs often present with significant baseline mass effect on the spinal cord (Fig. 5.5b), intraspinal injection, potentially increasing the mass effect, is of great concern, and intravenous steroids are liberally used in this setting. Moreover, we admit our patients to the intensive care unit (ICU) overnight following the procedure for careful neurologic assessment; patients understand that urgent decompression may be necessary in the setting of postprocedural edema. Another area of concern during sclerotherapy of cervical spinal ABCs is the inadvertent injury to the vertebral artery, potentially resulting in intra-arterial injection of sclerosant towards the brainstem [38] or causing vessel dissection and possible thrombosis and embolic infarct. Cervical CT angiography prior to the procedure helps to delineate the exact course and caliber of the vertebral artery in relation to the bony lesion (Fig. 5.5c). Baseline and postprocedure neurological examination are imperative. Response to treatment is evaluated by resolution of symptoms and follow-up cross-sectional imaging to look for interval fibrosis and osseous formation (Fig. 5.5f).

Conclusion

In sum, interventional radiologists are broadly involved in the management of patients with head and neck tumors, from diagnosis, to definitive treatment, treatments auxiliary to open surgery, and amelioration of symptoms. As novel, image-guided treatment approaches continue to develop, this close partnership between other specialists treating head and neck lesions and interventional radiologists will only grow and deepen.

References

1. Kohout MP, Hansen M, Pribaz JJ, et al. Arteriovenous malformations of the head and neck: natural history and management. Plast Reconstr Surg. 1998;102:643–54.
2. Miller DL, Balter S, Schueler BA, Wagner LK, et al. Clinical radiation management for fluoroscopically guided interventional procedures. Radiology. 2010;257:321–32.
3. Kim BS, Lee SK, terBrugge KG. Endovascular treatment of congenital arteriovenous fistulae of the internal maxillary artery. Neuroradiology. 2003;45:445–50.
4. Turowski B, Zanella FE. Interventional neuroradiology of the head and neck. Neuroimaging Clin N Am. 2003;13:619–45.
5. Wu IC, Orbach DB. Neurointerventional management of high-flow vascular malformations of the head and neck. Neuroimaging Clin N Am. 2009;19:219–40.
6. Tallman B, Tan OT, Morelli JG, et al. Location of portwine stains and the likelihood of ophthalmic and/or central nervous system complications. Pediatrics. 1991;87:323–7.
7. Hennedige AA, Quaba AA, Al-Nakib K. Sturge-Weber syndrome and dermatomal facial port-wine stains: incidence, association with glaucoma, and pulsed tunable dye laser treatment effectiveness. Plast Reconstr Surg. 2008;121:1173–80.
8. Katugampola GA, Lanigan SW. Five years' experience of treating port wine stains with the flashlamp- pumped pulsed dye laser. Br J Dermatol. 1997;137:750–4.
9. Dubois J, Garel L. Imaging and therapeutic approach of hemangiomas and vascular malformations in the pediatric age group. Pediatr Radiol. 1999;29:879–93.
10. Boon LM, Mulliken JB, Enjolras O, et al. Glomuvenous malformation (glomangioma) and venous malformation: distinct clinicopathologic and genetic entities. Arch Dermatol. 2004;140:971–6.
11. Garzon MC, Huang JT, Enjolras O, et al. Vascular malformations. Part II: associated syndromes. J Am Acad Dermatol. 2007;56:541–64.
12. Choi DJ, Alomari AI, Chaudry G, Orbach DB. Neurointerventional management of low-flow vascular malformations of the head and neck. Neuroimaging Clin N Am. 2009;19(2):199–218.
13. Burrows PE, Mason KP. Percutaneous treatment of low flow vascular malformations. J Vasc Interv Radiol. 2004;15:431–45.
14. Muir T, Kirsten M, Fourie P, et al. Intralesional bleomycin injection (IBI) treatment for haemangiomas and congenital vascular malformations. Pediatr Surg Int. 2004;19:766–73.
15. Grimmer JF, Mulliken JB, Burrows PE, et al. Radiofrequency ablation of microcystic lymphatic malformation in the oral cavity. Arch Otolaryngol Head Neck Surg. 2006:1251–6.
16. Kim SW, Kauvanough K, Orbach DB, Alomari AI, et al. Long-term outcome of radiofrequency ablation for intraoral microcystic lymphatic malformation. Arch Otolaryngol Head Neck Surg. 2011;137:1247–50.
17. Huang RY, Damrose EJ, Blackwell KE, et al. Extranasopharyngeal angiofibroma. Int J Pediatr Otorhinolaryngol. 2000;54:59–64.
18. Specter JG. Management of juvenile angiofibroma. Laryngoscope. 1988;98:1016–26.
19. Koç C, Ozdem C, Arıkan OK, Beriat K. Clinical value of pre-operative polyvinyl alcohol embolization in juvenile nasopharyngeal angiofibroma. Turk Arch Otolaryngol. 2001;39:267–72.
20. Erickson D, Kudva YC, Ebersold MJ, et al. Benign paragangliomas: clinical presentation and treatment outcomes in 236 patients. J Clin Endocrinol Metab. 2001;86:5210–16.
21. Bishop GB Jr, Urist MM, el Gammal T, et al. Paragangliomas of the neck. Arch Surg. 1992;127:1441–5.
22. Van Den Berg G, Rodesch G, Lasjaunias P. Management of paragangliomas: clinical and angiographic aspects. Intervent Neuroradiol. 2002;8:127–34.
23. Somasundar P, Krouse R, Hostetter R, et al. Paragangliomas: a decade of clinical experience. J Surg Oncol. 2000;74:286–90.
24. LaRouere MJ, Zappia JJ, et al. Embolization of Glomus Jugulare Tumors. Skull base surgery. 1994;4:21–5.
25. Abud DG, Mounayer C, Benndorf G, Piotin M, Spelle L, Moret J. Intratumoral injection of cyanoacrylate glue in head and neck paragangliomas. Am J Neuroradiol. 2004;25:1457–62.

26. DelGaudio JM, Dillard DG, Albritton FD, et al. Computed Tomography–Guided Needle Biopsy of head and neck lesions. Arch Otolaryngol Head Neck Surg. 2000;126:366–70.
27. Das DK, Gulati A, Bhatt NC, Mandal AK, et al. Fine needle aspiration cytology of oral and pharyngeal lesions: a study of 45 cases. Acta Cytol. 1993;37:333–42.
28. Mondal A, Raychoudhur BK. Peroral fine needle aspiration cytology of parapharyngeal lesions. Acta Cytol. 1993;37:694–8.
29. Castelli M, Gattuso P, Reyes C, Solans EP. Fine needle aspiration biopsy of intraoral and pharyngeal lesions. Acta Cytol. 1993;37:448–50.
30. Gupta S, Henningsen J, Wallace M, Madoff D, et al. Percutaneous biopsy of head and neck lesions with CT guidance: various approaches and relevant anatomic and technical considerations. RadioGraphics. 2007;27:371–90.
31. Cernesal P. Benign tumor of bone. In: Canale ST, editor. Campbell's operative orthopaedics. Philadelphia: Mosby; 2003. S 801–3.
32. Freeman BL. Scoliosis and kyphosis. In: Canale ST, editor. Campbell's operative orthopaedics. Philadelphia: Mosby; 2003. S 1921–3.
33. Choen MD, Harrington TM, Ginsburg WW. Osteoid osteoma: 95 cases and review of literature. Semin Arthritis Rheum. 1983;12:265–80.
34. Linville DA. Other disorders of spine. In: Canale ST, editor. Campbell's operative orthopaedics. Philadelphia: Mosby; 2003. S 2106–7.
35. Owen RP, Silver CE, Ravikumar TS, et al. Techniques for radiofrequency ablation of head and neck tumors. Arch Otolaryngol Head Neck Surg. 2004;130:52–6.
36. Vanderschueren GM, Obermann WR, Dijkstra SP, et al. Radiofrequency ablation of spinal osteoid osteoma: clinical outcome. Spine. 2009;34:901–4.
37. Varshney MK, Rastogi S, Khan SA, Trikha V. Is sclerotherapy better than intralesional excision for treating aneurysmal bone cysts? Clin Orthop Relat Res. 2010;468:1649–59.
38. Turowski B, Schellhammer F, Herdmann J, et al. Fatal ethibloc embolization of vertebrobasilar system following percutaneous injection into aneurysmal bone cyst of the second cervical vertebra. Am J Neuroradiol. 2005;26(7):1883–4.

Sentinel Lymph Node Biopsy

6

Christopher Weldon

Introduction

The role of a sentinel lymph node biopsy (SLNB) in the management of head and neck tumors is dependent on two factors: (1) the propensity for the known malignancy to spread to and through the lymphatic system from local to regional lymph node basins, especially in the absence of enlarged or suspected pathologic lymph nodes (LN) by physical exam and/or radiographic studies, and (2) the need to confirm that the tumor in question has spread to the most proximal, 'upstream' lymph node draining basin for staging information and determination of the best therapeutic option. The technique of SLNB has been employed in a variety of malignancies since its inception almost 4 decades ago with a great deal of success. It is now a vital component of staging tumors as varied as melanoma [1], breast cancer [2], and certain sarcomas [3], in addition to squamous cell head and neck tumors [4]. In children's cancers, prospective, randomized, controlled trials documenting its utility and prognostic success are lacking. However, if results on the same cancers afflicting adults are extrapolated to children and if we review the data available for its utility in children is reviewed, then specific pediatric applications can be identified.

Key Points

- SLNB is a safe and effective operative technique performed in the outpatient setting that is utilized to document the presence of occult lymph node metastases from specific head and neck malignancies (melanoma; various sarcomas [rhabdomyosarcoma, epithelioid sarcoma, synovial cell sarcoma]) afflicting children.
- The technique relies upon both preoperative (via lymphatic mapping by lymphoscintigraphy utilizing technetium 99m sulfur colloid) and intraoperative detection (via administration of blue dye [isosulfan blue]) by visual documentation of a discolored lymph node and/or detection of the radiolabelled tracer (technetium 99m sulfur colloid) by using a handheld gamma probe of the occult, first 'upstream' lymph node(s) with subsequent removal for pathological evaluation. One or several lymph nodes can be harvested and sent for pathologic determination depending on intraoperative results.

Objectives

An in depth review of the specific cancers and specific data tracing its utility as a technique is beyond the scope of this work. However, pediatric tumors in which this technique demonstrated utility in the accurate staging and management include melanoma [5], other melanocytic lesions [6], rhabdo- and some nonrhabdomyomatous soft-tissue sarcomas (epithelioid, synovial cell, clear cell, alveolar soft part, fibrosarcoma), and breast cancer [7].

Presentation

Patients will present in a variety of ways at diagnosis, and the symptoms will be related to the specific tumor type, in addition to the size and location of the tumor or organ of origin, especially when one considers the anatomic area that houses the tumor with resultant functional loss. Furthermore, for the dermatological-based cancers (melanoma), there is often no presenting symptom save the presence of the skin lesion and possible changes in the size, border, color, thickness, or general appearance of the lesion. The patient will generally require an initial history and physical exam documenting any loss of function, in addition to the anatomical boundaries and characteristics of the involved mass or

C. Weldon (✉)
Department of Surgery, Boston Children's Hospital, Harvard Medical School, Boston, MA, USA
e-mail: christopher.weldon@childrens.harvard.edu

R. Rahbar et al. (eds.), *Pediatric Head and Neck Tumors*,
DOI 10.1007/978-1-4614-8755-5_6, © Springer Science+Business Media New York 2014

lesion. A dedicated evaluation of *all possible* draining lymph node basins should be undertaken both at the initial evaluation and all subsequent visits. These investigations will begin with a physical exam, but they will also include radiographic (ultrasound [US], computed tomograms [CT], or magnetic resonance [MR]) and nuclear medicine (positron emission scanning [PET]) studies. Though it would be common to assume that cervical lymph node chains are the only likely lymphatic metastatic sites of head and neck lesions (especially melanomas), this may not always be the case. Hence, it is imperative that preoperative lymphatic mapping be performed to determine the precise draining basin(s), especially for those lesions or masses at the base of the neck. The axillae, inguinal regions, and intrathoracic locations have been known to provide drainage for some melanomas discovered in the head and neck.

Diagnosis and Evaluation

Physical Examination

- *ALL* possible draining lymph node basins should be evaluated by an in-depth physical exam upon presentation of a child with a head and neck malignancy. These would include anterior and posterior cervical locations, in addition to supraclavicular, axillary, and inguinal regions. One should attempt to palpate for any enlarged masses that could represent clinically evident lymphadenopathy. A careful palpation of the skin and subcutaneous tissue between the lesion or primary tumor and the possible draining lymph node basins should be performed to ensure that skip metastases are not present. Furthermore, with some bulkier tumors (sarcomas), there may be concomitant infectious processes secondary to the obstruction of the sinuses or the like that may be the etiology for any observed palpable or radiographic lymphadenopathy. Therefore, the clinician must perform a thorough head and neck exam to document other signs and symptoms consistent with the presence of an active infection that might be responsible for any observed lymphadenopathy.

Laboratory Data

- Preoperative tests documenting adequate normal clotting function, hemogram, and platelets are required. Other specific laboratory evaluations will be tumor specific.

Imaging Evaluation

- Complete staging studies should be performed, but these will vary according to the tumor type involved. In most instances, axial imaging studies (MR or CT) of the involved anatomic area will be required, and other studies documenting involvement of the brain, lungs, bone marrow, or other organs will be tumor specific. PET scanning may also prove useful depending on the disease types. Caution must be raised, however, with the recommendation of utilizing CT and PET scans in pediatric patients secondary to the risk of associated malignancies from exposure to ionizing radiation [8]. For adequate radiographic staging of the immediate draining lymph node basins, either MR or CT would be appropriate. Discussions should be held with the radiologist in advance of the studies to ensure that all necessary sequences are secured in order to evaluate the desired lymph node regions. If concerns arise regarding the presence of a radiographically positive lymph node(s) once the above studies are obtained, then a dedicated US of the area can often be helpful to ensure the accuracy of the axial imaging. Finally, nuclear medicine studies (PET) either alone or in conjunction with the axial studies may be performed to possibly add further clarity and accuracy [9].

Pathology

The pathological evaluation of the sentinel lymph node (SLN) removed at surgery will rely on a direct discussion with the pathologist and the surgeon in the operating room. All LNs removed should be documented as to their color (darkest to lightest 'blue' color if dye is used) and/or gamma counts recorded intraoperatively and then given directly to the pathology team for appropriate handling and processing. The precise conduct of the histopathological processing and evaluation of the LNs is beyond the scope of this work, but utilizing a pathology service well versed in evaluating these specimens and tumor types is critical [10].

Treatment

Surgical therapy

- The SLNB procedure can be married to the initial diagnostic biopsy procedure or performed remotely from it. Combining procedures under one anesthetic is certainly more advantageous, but often the precise diagnoses requiring appropriate staging with an SLNB are not necessarily suspected in advance, nor has the patient been evaluated for suitability of the procedure.
- In the patient with both clinically and radiographically negative lymph node basins in the setting of a cancer that has a predisposition to spread to regional LNs, an outpatient procedure consisting of same-day preoperative lymphoscintigraphy utilizing injections of technetium

99m sulfur colloid injected intradermally or peritumorally (depending on the type and location of the tumor involved) will be performed. Precise determination of the draining node(s) is then confirmed prior to proceeding to the operating room. Counts can be determined in the nuclear medicine suite preoperatively, and the exact location of the LN can be marked externally on the skin.

- After the lymphoscintigraphy procedure, the patient is taken to the operating room and prepared for surgery. Immediately prior to prepping the skin, if 1 % isosulfan blue dye is being used in conjunction with the sulfur colloid, it is injected peritumorally as well, utilizing a tuberculin syringe, 30-gauge needle, and 0.5 cc per injection site (total of four, radially around the primary tumor site).
- Once prepared, the site directly over the marked LN is opened and the area thoroughly explored for all positive LNs by both color (blue) and by increased counts (generally greater than 10-fold over general background of the wound). All LNs are removed and sent for pathological analysis, each individually marked. Generally, there may be one of several LNs removed.
- Once all concerning LNs are identified and removed, the wound is closed and sterile dressings applied.

Complications

- Standard complications include bleeding, infection, scarring and cosmesis concerns, numbness or pain at the wound site, hematoma/seroma/lymphocele formation, injury to any anatomic structure in the area during the course of the dissection, and an inability to find the involved SLN. Precise discussion of the accuracy of the technique is tumor specific and beyond the scope of this work, but there is little doubt that for melanoma, breast and rhabdomyosarcoma, it is both a useful and appropriate staging technique [7]. Additionally, application of this technique in certain nonrhabdomyomatous sarcomas may also be warranted [7].
- Though adverse allergic reactions have been reported with the use of dye, [7, 11], these are rare and should not necessarily negate utilization of this technique.

Outcomes

Data from large, multicenter, randomized trials do not exist for the use of SLNB in the pediatric population. In fact, most results documenting its utility and success stem from results published from adult series on the similar/same cancers. The majority of data available on the use of SLNB in pediatric patients is from single institutions with varied diagnoses over relatively long periods of time. Kayton et al. [7] from the *Memorial Sloan–Kettering Cancer Center* (MSKCC) evaluated their use of the technique in 30 patients over ten years. In all patients, they found the SLN in all cases, and lymphoscintigraphy identified the SLN in 97 % (30/31) preoperatively. There were no complications, and SLNs were positive in 1/9 patients with rhabdomyosarcoma and 2/5 with breast cancer. There were no recurrences over a median follow-up of 48 months.

In pediatric melanoma, Mu et al. [5] queried the SEER database regarding the use and results from SLNB in children and young adults with melanoma. Children (<20 years old) were more likely to have a positive SLNB considering all other factors than young adults (20–24 years old), especially in the cohort with a lesion measuring between 1–2 mm thick. In fact, these patients were six times more likely to have a positive SLNB than their young adult (20–24 year-old) counterparts. Furthermore, these patients were also more likely to die of their disease corroborating earlier date from Australia [12].

References

1. Lee CCF, Ollila D, Moschos S. Historical review of melanoma treatment and outcomes. Clin Dermatol. 2013;31(2):141–7.
2. Kumar APR, Gadgil PV, Jatoi I. Sentinel lymph node biopsy in primary breast cancer: window to management of the axilla. World J Surg. 2012;36(7):1453–9.
3. Andreou D, Tunn PU. Sentinel node biopsy in soft tissue sarcoma. Recent Results Cancer Res. 2009;179:25–36.
4. Thompson CFSJM, Lawson G, Grogan T, Elashoff D, Mendelsohn AH. Diagnostic value of sentinel lymph node biopsy in head and neck cancer: a meta-analysis. Eur Arch Otorhinolaryngol. 2013;270:2115–22.
5. Mu ELJ, Strouse JJ. Comparison of the use and results of sentinel lymph node biopsy in children and young adults with melanoma. Cancer. 2012;118(10):2700–7.
6. Mills OLMS, Zager JS, Sondak VK, Messina JL. Sentinel node biopsy in atypical melanocytic neoplasms in childhood: a single institution experience in 24 patients. J Cutan Pathol. 2012;39(9):331–6.
7. Kayton MLDR, Busam K, Cody HS III, Athanasian EA, Coit D, La Quaglia MP. Experience with 31 sentinel lymph node biopsies for sarcomas and carcinomas in pediatric patients. Cancer. 2008;112(9):2052–9.
8. Shah DJSR, Wilson DJ. Radiation-induced cancer: a modern view. Br J Radiol. 2012;85(1020):e1166–73.
9. Krause BJSS, Souvatzoglou M. FDG PET and PET/CT. Recent Results Cancer Res. 2013;187:351–69.
10. Mathew R, Messina JL. Recent advances in pathologic evaluation and reporting of melanoma. Semin Oncol. 2012;39(2):184–91.
11. Montgomery LLTA, Van Zee KJ, Fey J, Heerdt AS, Gemignani M, Port E, Petrek J, Cody HS III, Borgen PI. Isosulfan blue dye reactions during sentinel lymph node mapping for breast cancer. Anesth Analg. 2002;95(2):385–8.
12. Howman-Giles RSH, Scolyer RA, Murali R, Wilmott J, McCarthy SW, Uren RF, Thompson JF. Sentinel lymph node biopsy in pediatric and adolescent cutaneous melanoma patients. Ann Surg Oncol. 2010;17(1):138–43.

Part II

Disease Specific

Arteriovenous Malformations: Extracranial

7

Rafael A. Couto and Arin K. Greene

Introduction

An arteriovenous malformation (AVM) is a fast-flow vascular anomaly characterized by the shunting of blood from the arterial to venous circulation. Shunting reduces capillary oxygen delivery to tissues, causing ischemia. AVMs can produce deformity, ulceration, bleeding, congestive heart failure, and/or destruction of vital structures (see Fig. 7.1a). Treatment consists of embolization and/or resection. Certain AVMs are part of inherited syndromes (see Fig. 7.1b, c): (1) capillary malformation-arteriovenous malformation (CM-AVM), (2) hereditary hemorrhagic telangiectasia (HHT), and (3) PTEN-associated vascular anomaly (PTEN-AVA).

Key Points

- The most common site of extracranial AVM is the head/neck, followed by the limbs, viscera, and trunk [1].
- AVM worsens over time, and can be classified according to the Schobinger staging system (see Table 7.1) [2, 3].
- Despite the high likelihood of recurrence, embolization, and/or resection can palliate an AVM by reducing its size and alleviating pain and bleeding.
- AVM should be treated in a vascular anomalies center by a multidisciplinary team.

Biology and Epidemiology

AVM results from abnormal vascular development during embryogenesis. Lack of a capillary bed causes shunting of blood directly from the arterial to venous circulation through a fistula (direct connection of an artery to a vein) or nidus (abnormal channels bridging the feeding artery to the draining veins) [4]. Although the presence of AVM may be problematic, expansion of the lesion is the main cause of morbidity [3].

Pathophysiology

- Increasing tissue mass requires neovascularization to support its expansion through angiogenesis (growth of new blood vessels from pre-existing vasculature) [5, 6] or vasculogenesis (de novo formation of new vasculature) [7–9]. Vasculogenesis, rather than angiogenesis, may contribute to the expansion of AVM [10].
- Although neovascularization may be a primary stimulus for AVM growth, it might be secondary to ischemia. Ischemia, a potent stimulator of neovascularization, causes enlargement of AVM after proximal arterial ligation or trauma [2, 11, 12]. Alternatively, increased blood flow from arteriovenous shunting may promote vascular endothelial growth factor (VEGF) production and endothelial proliferation [13, 14].
- Both males and females have a two-fold risk of progression in puberty; increased circulating hormones during this period may promote AVM expansion [3].

Molecular/Genetic Pathology

- CM-AVM is an autosomal dominant condition that results from a loss-of-function mutation in *RASA1*, which encodes p120RasGAP. This protein inhibits RAS p21 control of cellular proliferation, survival, and differentiation [15].
- HHT is due to an alteration in endoglin and activin receptor-like kinase 1 (ALK-1) which affect transforming growth factor-beta (TGF-β) signaling [16, 17].
- PTEN-AVA is an autosomal dominant disease caused by a mutation in *PTEN* (phosphatase and tensin homologue)

A. K. Greene (✉) · R. A. Couto
Department of Plastic and Oral Surgery, Boston Children's Hospital, Harvard Medical School, Boston, MA, USA
e-mail: arin.greene@childrens.harvard.edu

R. Rahbar et al. (eds.), *Pediatric Head and Neck Tumors*,
DOI 10.1007/978-1-4614-8755-5_7,

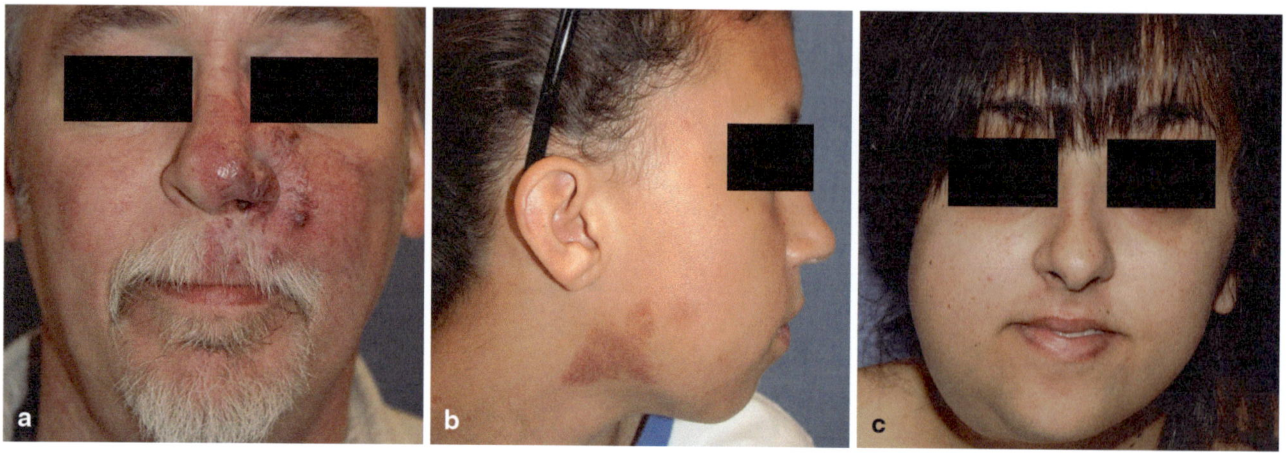

Fig. 7.1 Types of AVM. **a** Fifty-one-year-old male patient with a Stage II AVM of the left cheek, nose, and orbit, causing epistaxis. **b** Nine-year-old female patient with capillary CM-AVM (positive for RASA-1 mutation) and fast-flow stains of the right cheek and neck. **c** Twenty-one-year-old female patient with PTEN-AVA (positive for PTEN mutation) with an enlarging right cheek and submandibular lesion

Table 7.1 Schobinger staging of AVM

Stage	Clinical Findings
I (Quiescence)	Warm, pink-blue, shunting on Doppler
II (Expansion)	Enlargement, pulsation, thrill, bruit, tortuous veins
III (Destruction)	Dystrophic skin changes, ulceration, bleeding, pain
IV (Decompensation)	Cardiac failure

[18]. The gene encodes a tumor suppressor lipid phosphatase that mediates cell cycle arrest and apoptosis [19]. Patients with PTEN mutations have PTEN hamartoma tumor syndrome (PHTS) [18].

Incidence and Prevalence

- AVMs comprise 14.3 % of vascular malformations treated in a vascular anomalies center [20].
- The prevalence of CM-AVM is estimated to be 1 in 100,000 Caucasians [15].

Age Distribution

- Although present at birth, AVM may not become clinically evident until childhood or adolescence [3].
- Approximately three-fourths of patients with AVM require treatment in childhood or adolescence; the remaining individuals do not need intervention until adulthood [3].

Sex Predilection

- Males and females are affected equally.

Risk Factors

- The offspring of patients with CM-AVM or PTEN-AVA have a 50 % risk of inheriting the mutated gene; however, phenotypic heterogeneity is common within families [15, 18, 21].
- Progesterone-only oral contraceptives are recommended because estrogen has greater proangiogenic activity than progesterone [1, 22–25].
- Pregnant women with Stage I lesions do not have an increased rate of progression, compared to non-pregnant women [3]. However, pregnancy in women with Stage II-IV AVM has not been studied, and thus pregnancy may exacerbate the malformation.

Relationships to Other Disease States, Syndromes

- Parkes Weber syndrome (PWS) is a diffuse AVM of an extremity with an overlying capillary malformation (CM) [26]. The extremity is overgrown and the lower limb is most commonly affected [26]. Patients are at risk for leg length discrepancy and congestive heart failure [26].

Presentation

Arteriovenous Malformation

- Lesions appear pink-red, are warm, have a palpable thrill or bruit, and may be mistaken for a CM or hemangioma [1].
- Hand-held Doppler shows fast flow.

Capillary Malformation-Arteriovenous Malformation

- Although the CM is rarely problematic, 30 % have associated AVMs that can cause major morbidity: PWS (12 %), extracerebral AVM (11 %), or intracerebral AVM (7 %) [21].
- An individual may have as many as 53 CMs, ranging in size from 1 to 15 cm, although 6 % of patients have a solitary lesion [21].
- An association between CM-AVM and spinal arteriovenous lesions exists [27].
- Five percent of patients have benign or malignant tumors, most commonly involving the nervous system (neurofibroma, optic glioma, vestibular schwannoma) [21].
- Patients with PWS should be followed by a cardiologist to monitor signs of congestive heart failure. Orthopedic evaluation is necessary to rule out a leg length discrepancy [21].

PTEN-Associated Vascular Anomaly

- Patients with PTEN mutations have PHTS. Approximately one-half (54 %) of patients have a unique fast-flow vascular anomaly with arteriovenous shunting [18].
- Patients may have multiple PTEN-AVAs (57 %), and 85 % are intramuscular [18].
- Patients with PHTS are followed for the presence of tumors, particularly, endocrine and gastrointestinal malignancies [1, 18].

Symptoms

- Arteriovenous shunting causes ischemia, which can lead to pain, ulceration, bleeding, and congestive heart failure.
- AVM also may cause deformity, destruction of tissues, and obstruction of vital structures.
- High-pressure shunting of blood can cause venous hemorrhage and rupture of arteries in weakened areas, such as aneurysms.
- Arterial bleeding most commonly occurs at skin or mucosal surfaces from erosion into a superficial component of the lesion.

Differential Diagnosis

Capillary malformation (CM)
Congenital hemangioma (CH)
Infantile hemangioma (IH)
Kaposiform hemangioendothelioma (KHE)
Lymphatic malformation (LM)
Pyogenic granuloma (PG)
Venous malformation (VM)

Diagnosis and Evaluation

Physical Examination

Arteriovenous Malformation

Ninety percent of AVMs are diagnosed by history and physical examination [28, 29].

Findings

- Lesions are usually warm, pink-red, and have a palpable thrill or bruit.
- Unlike IH, AVM expands after infancy.
- Hand-held Doppler examination showing fast flow excludes slow-flow vascular anomalies (e.g., CM, LM, VM).

Capillary Malformation-Arteriovenous Malformation

Diagnosis is made by history and physical examination. A patient presenting with multiple CMs, especially with a family history of similar lesions, should be evaluated for possible AVMs. Patients are counseled about the autosomal dominant inheritance pattern.

Findings

- Atypical CMs that are small, multifocal, round, pinkish-red, and surrounded by a pale halo (50 %) [15, 21].
- Unlike sporadic CM, Doppler examination in CM-AVM often shows fast flow.
- An overgrown extremity with a CM suggests PWS [26].

PTEN-Associated Vascular Anomaly

Suspicion of a PTEN-AVA usually is initiated after reviewing the magnetic resonance imaging (MRI) or angiographic study of a patient thought to have an AVM. Vascular anomalies with fast-flow lesions consistent with a PTEN-AVA are evaluated for possible PHTS. PTEN-AVA is an autosomal dominant condition; patients are counseled about the risk of transmitting the gene to their offspring.

Findings

- Unlike typical AVM, PTEN-AVA can be multifocal, associated with ectopic fat tissue, and have disproportionate, segmental dilation of the draining veins [4, 18].
- Patients with PHTS have macrocephaly (>97th percentile), and all males have penile freckling [18].
- PHTS is associated with mental retardation/autism (19 %), thyroid lesions (31 %), or gastrointestinal polyps (30 %) [18].

Laboratory Data

- *RASA1* gene testing confirms the diagnosis of CM-AVM. However, not all patients with CM-AVM clinically will have a *RASA1* mutation, suggesting that unknown mutations in *RASA1* or other genes may result in the same phenotype [21].
- *PTEN* gene testing is confirmative; however, a germline mutation is not found in 9% of families clinically diagnosed with PHTS [30].

Imaging Evaluation

Arteriovenous Malformation

Ultrasonography (US)	Exhibits a hypervascular lesion with arteriovenous shunting and no significant parenchymal mass. Color Doppler shows feeding arteries and large draining veins.
Computed Tomography (CT)	May be indicated if the lesion involves the bone.
Magnetic Resonance Imaging (MRI)	Demonstrates dilated feeding arteries and draining veins, enhancement, and flow voids [4]. MRI is usually indicated to: (1) confirm the diagnosis, (2) determine the extent of the lesion, and (3) plan treatment. MRI with contrast and fat suppression, as well as T2-weighted sequences, is necessary to adequately asses the anomaly [1, 4].
Angiography	Displays tortuous, dilated, arteries with arteriovenous shunting and enlarged draining veins [4]. The nidus manifests as dysplastic, tortuous, small vessels, with ill-defined larger contiguous vascular spaces. Angiography is indicated when: (1) the diagnosis is unclear after US and MRI, (2) embolization or resection is planned.

Capillary Malformation-Arteriovenous Malformation

Imaging features for CM-AVM are similar to non-syndromic AVMs. Patients with CM-AVM are at risk for intracranial and spinal fast-flow lesions; MRI of the brain and/or spine should be considered [31]. Because extracranial AVM has not been found to involve the viscera, exploratory imaging of other anatomical areas is not necessary [21].

PTEN-Associated Vascular Anomaly

Unlike typical AVM, PTEN-AVA can be multifocal, associated with ectopic adipose tissue, and have disproportionate, segmental dilation of the draining veins [4, 18]. Intramuscular lesions replace the architecture with disorganized fat, in contrast to non-syndromic muscular AVMs [18].

Pathology

Arteriovenous Malformation

AVM generally shows large, tortuous arteries, as well as dilated, thick-walled veins [32]. In the early stage, veins have a hypertrophic muscular layer. As the lesion progresses, smooth muscle is replaced by collagen, and the vessel becomes fibrotic (see Fig. 7.2) [32].

Capillary Malformation-Arteriovenous Malformation

CM-AVM shares most of the histopathological features that are found in non-syndromic AVM.

PTEN-Associated Vascular Anomaly

Similar to non-syndromic AVM, PTEN-AVA shows tortuous arteries with transmural muscular hyperplasia and clusters of abnormal veins with variable smooth muscle [18]. However, skeletal muscle infiltration with adipose tissue, fibrous bands, and lymphoid aggregates is unique to PTEN-AVA.

Treatment

Pharmacological therapy does not exist for AVM. Problematic lesions are embolized and/or resected. The goal of treatment usually is to control the lesion; cure is rare. Interventions focus on alleviating symptoms (e.g., bleeding, pain, ulceration), preserving vital functions (e.g., vision, mastication), and for improving a deformity. Asymptomatic AVMs should be observed unless they can be managed with minimal morbidity; embolization or subtotal resection of an asymptomatic malformation may provoke it to enlarge and become problematic. Therapy is determined by the (1) size and location of the lesion, (2) patient's age, and (3) Schobinger stage. Resection of a non-problematic Stage I AVM offers the best chance for long-term control. However, intervention must be individualized based on the deformity that would result from excision and reconstruction [1, 3]. For example, a large Stage I AVM in a non-anatomically important location (e.g., trunk, proximal extremity) may be resected without significant morbidity, before it progresses to a higher stage when excision is more complicated and the recurrence rate is greater [1, 3]. Similarly, a small, well-localized AVM in a more difficult location (e.g., face, hand) may be removed for

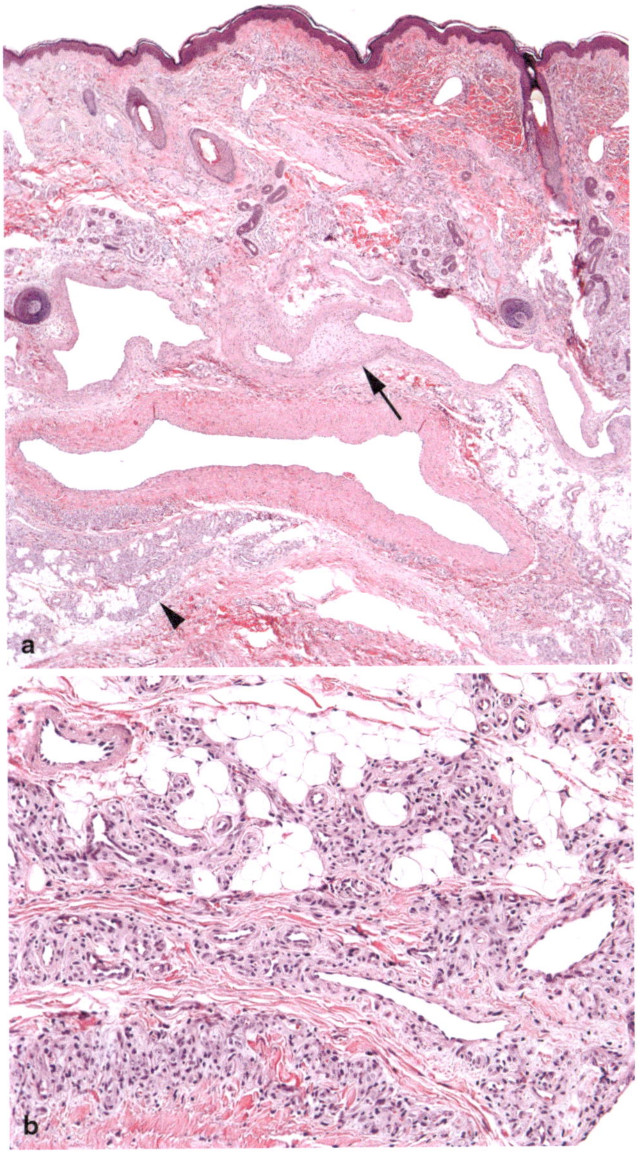

Fig. 7.2 Arteriovenous malformation, scalp. **a** Malformed large arteries and veins occupy superficial and deep dermis as well as subcutaneous tissue. A venous channel with high flow, hypertensive changes, is indicated by arrow. Arrowhead on the bottom left indicates small vessel component. **b** Small vessel component of AVM in subcutaneous tissue at higher magnification is characterized by groups of small channels in close proximity to each other and lined by plump endothelium

possible "cure" before it expands and complete extirpation is no longer possible [1, 3].

In contrast, a large, asymptomatic lesion located in an anatomically sensitive region (e.g., face) is best observed; especially in a young child not ready for a major procedure [1, 3]. Resection may cause a worse deformity and the malformation can recur. Some children (17.4 %) do not experience morbidity from their AVM until adulthood [3].

Intervention for Stage II AVMs is similar to Stage I lesions. However, the threshold for treatment is lower if an enlarging malformation is causing a worsening deformity or if functional problems are expected [1, 3]. Treatment for Stage III and IV AVMs is necessary to control pain, bleeding, ulceration, or congestive heart failure [1, 3].

Non-Operative Management

For superficial AVMs, patients should apply hydrated petroleum to prevent desiccation and subsequent ulceration [1]. Compression garments for extremity lesions may reduce pain and swelling, but can also worsen symptoms [1]. If bleeding occurs it is readily controlled by compression; further intervention is rarely necessary [1].

Embolization

Delivery of an inert substance, through an arterial catheter, occludes blood flow and/or fills vascular spaces. Fibrosis may further reduce arteriovenous shunting and shrink the lesion. Even if significant volume reduction is not obtained after embolization, symptoms are reduced [1]. Embolizing the arterial inflow to the nidus is contraindicated because recannalization occurs, and the lesion becomes inaccessible for future embolization [4]. Patients and families are counseled that the AVM is likely to re-expand; additional embolizations may be required in the future.

Liquid (n-butyl cyanoacrylate [n-BCA], Onyx, ethanol) or solid (polyvinyl alcohol particles [PVA], coils) may be used for embolization [4]. The choice of agent depends on whether embolization is utilized as a primary treatment or as a pre-operative adjunct to excision [1, 4]. For primary treatment, permanent liquid agents capable of permeating the nidus (ethanol, n-BCA, Onyx) are used. Our institution prefers Onyx, an ethylene-vinyl alcohol copolymer (EV3 Neurovascular, Irvine, CA) that precipitates on the surface after contact with blood [1, 4, 33]. It maintains a non-adhesive liquid core that allows multiple injections of different compartments. For pre-operative embolization, temporary occlusive substances (gelfoam powder, PVA, embospheres) are used. Delivery of different particle sizes permits the initial occlusion of small, distal vessels followed by blockage of more proximal branches with larger emboli. Our institution is now using Onyx for pre-operative embolization [1, 4, 33].

Patients are typically observed overnight in the hospital. If swelling is a concern, dexamethasone can be administered peri-operatively [1, 4, 33]. If airway or orbital lesions are embolized, post-treatment swelling may require close monitoring. Embolization of deep extremity lesions are at risk for compartment syndrome. Ulceration is the most common complication of embolization, especially in superficial lesions [1, 4, 33]. Wounds are allowed to heal secondarily with local wound care.

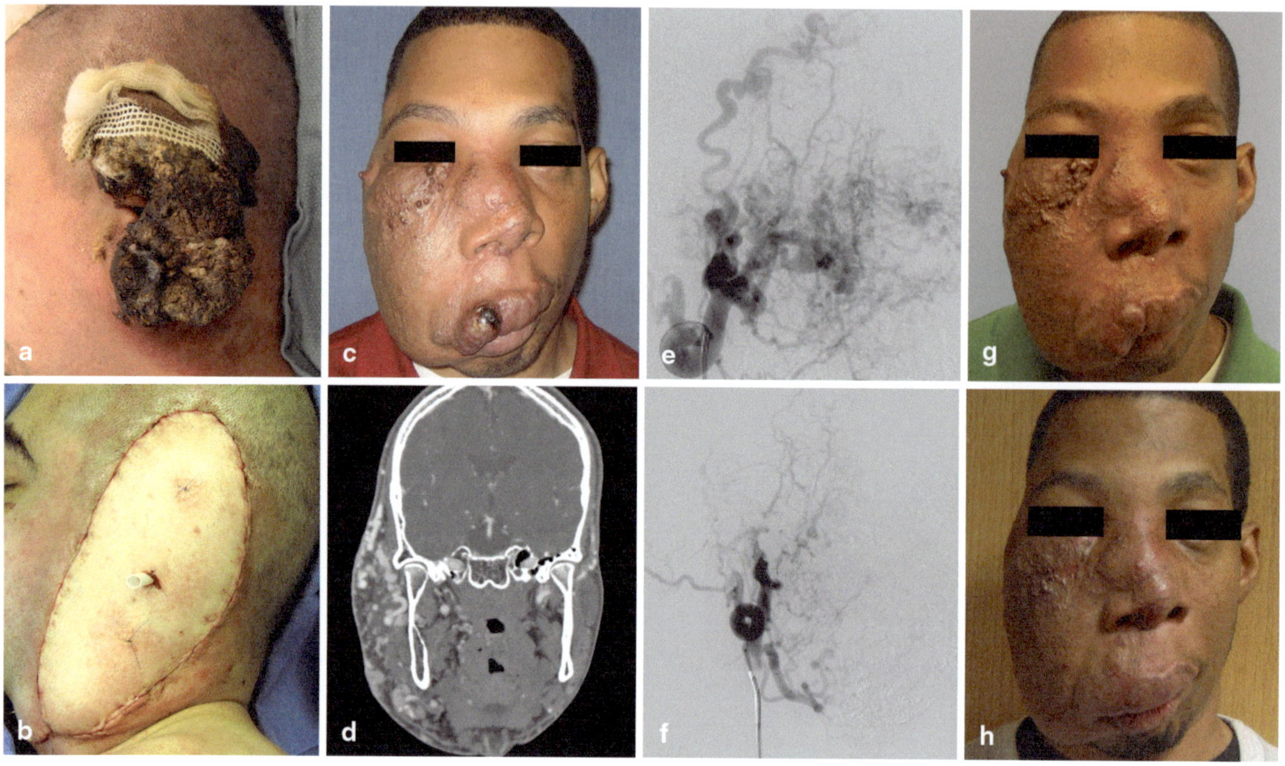

Fig. 7.3 Operative management of AVM. **a** Twenty-two-year-old male patient with a Stage III auricular AVM causing pain, bleeding, and infection. **b** Following embolization and wide resection, a free latissimus dorsi myocutaneous flap was used to close the defect. **c** Twenty-five-year-old male patient with a Stage III AVM causing a significant deformity, bleeding, pain, and ulceration. Because the lesion involved all structures of the face (including orbit, maxilla, mandible), radical resection would cause a greater deformity than the AVM. Embolization and subtotal resection of the ulcerated, bleeding lip and cheek lesions were performed. **d** Coronal computed tomography angiogram illustrates prominent, diffuse vascular anomaly with soft tissue enlargement. **e** Angiogram showing diffuse nidus. **f** Nonopacification of most of the AVM nidus after embolization. **g** Healed lip ulceration and resolution of bleeding following six embolizations. **h** Improved appearance after subtotal resection of the upper lip and cheek. Reprinted from Clinics in Plastic Surgery, 38/1, Greene AK, Orbach DB, Management of Arteriovenous Malformations, 100–101, 2011, with permission from Elsevier

Sclerotherapy

Transcutaneous injection of a substance into the malformation causes endothelial destruction and thrombosis. Subsequent fibrosis decreases the size of the lesion and improves symptoms. Sclerotherapy is reserved for an AVM that cannot be accessed transarterially, or for a well-localized lesion [1, 4]. Sclerosant use in a high-flow lesion is at risk for escaping into the systemic circulation [1, 4]. Sodium tetradecyl sulfate (STS) and absolute ethanol are the preferred scleroscents at our institution [1, 4]. Ethanol is more effective than STS, but has a higher complication rate; it should be used carefully in proximity to important structures (e.g., facial nerve) [1, 4].

Resection

Excision of an AVM has a lower recurrence rate than embolization, and is considered for localized lesions to correct a focal deformity (e.g., bleeding or ulcerated areas, labial hypertrophy) (see Fig. 7.3) [1]. Wide extirpation and reconstruction of a large, diffuse AVM should be performed with caution because (1) cure is rare and the recurrence rate is high, (2) the resulting deformity is often worse than the appearance of the malformation, and (3) resection can cause significant blood loss and iatrogenic injury [3].

Pre-operative embolization facilitates resection by reducing the size of the lesion and minimizing blood loss. Excision should be carried out 24–72 hours after embolization, before recannalization restores blood flow, especially if particulate agents, such as PVA, are used [3]. Infusing an epinephrine-containing local anesthetic throughout the operative field reduces blood loss. Small, well-localized AVMs or those that cannot be accessed for embolization may be treated by resection alone.

Surgical margins are best determined by assessing the amount of bleeding from the wound edges [2]. Most defects can be reconstructed by advancing local skin flaps. Skin grafting ulcerated areas has a high failure rate because the underlying tissue is ischemic; excision with regional flap transfer may be required [1]. Free-flap reconstruction permits wide resection and primary closure of complicated defects but does not improve long-term control [2, 3, 12, 34].

Outcome

Embolization

Embolization does not remove the AVM; almost all lesions will eventually expand after treatment. Although studies suggest that multiple embolizations do not lower the rate of recurrence, newer embolic agents (e.g., Onyx) may offer more lasting results [3]. Stage I AVM has a lower recurrence rate than higher-staged lesions. Most recurrences occur within the first year after embolization and 98.0 % re-expand within 5 years; although this may reflect results obtained with older embolic agents [1, 3]. The recurrence rate after embolization in PTEN-AVA lesions seems to be higher than non-syndromic AVMs [1]. Despite the high recurrence rate, embolization can effectively palliate an AVM.

Resection

Despite subtotal and presumed "complete" extirpation, most AVMs recur [3]. Recurrences typically occur within the first year after intervention, and 86.6 % re-expand within 5 years [3]. It is our experience that PTEN-AVA has a higher recurrence rate compared to non-syndromic AVM, possibly because the loss of the tumor suppressor protein favors a more proliferative environment [1]. Patients not displaying recurrence 5 years following intervention are more likely to have long-term control [3]. However, 5.2 % will experience re-expansion more than 10 years post-operatively [3]. Patients and families are told that AVM is likely to recur following resection, and further intervention may be needed in the future.

References

1. Greene AK, Orbach DB. Management of arteriovenous malformations. Clin Plast Surg. 2011;38(1):95–106.
2. Kohout MP, Hansen M, Pribaz JJ, et al. Arteriovenous malformations of the head and neck: natural history and management. Plast Reconstr Surg. 1998;102:643–54.
3. Liu AS, Mulliken JB, Zurakowski D, et al. Extracranial arteriovenous malformations: natural progression and recurrence after treatment. Plast Reconstr Surg. 2010;125:1185–94.
4. Wu IC, Orbach DB. Neurointerventional management of high-flow vascular malformations of the head and neck. Neuroimag Clin N Am. 2009;19:219–40.
5. Folkman J. Tumor angiogenesis: therapeutic implications. N Engl J Med. 1971;285:1182–86.
6. Folkman J. Is tissue mass regulated by vascular endothelial cells? Prostate as the first evidence. Endocrinology. 1998;139:441–2.
7. Asahara T, Murohara T, Sullivan A, et al. Isolation of putative progenitor endothelial cells for angiogenesis. Science. 1997;275:964–67.
8. Takahashi T, Kalka C, Masuda H, et al. Ischemia- and cytokine-induced mobilization of bone marrow-derived endothelial progenitor cells for neovascularization. Nat Med. 1999;5:434–8.
9. Tepper OM, Capla JM, Galiano RD, et al. Adult vasculogenesis occurs through in situ recruitment, proliferation, and tubulization of circulating bone marrow-derived cells. Blood. 2005;105:1068–77.
10. Lu L, Bischoff J, Mulliken JB, et al. Increased endothelial progenitor cells and vasculogenic factors in higher-staged arteriovenous malformations. Plast Reconstr Surg. 2011;128(4):260e–9e.
11. Young AE, Mulliken JB. Arteriovenous Malformations. In: Mulliken JB, Young AE, editors. Vascular birthmarks: hemangiomas and malformations. Philadelphia: Saunders;1988. p. 228–45.
12. Wu JK, Bisdorff A, Gelbert F, et al. Auricular arteriovenous malformation: evaluation, management, and outcome. Plast Reconstr Surg. 2005;115:985–95.
13. Masuda H, Zhuang YJ, Singh TM, et al. Adaptive remodeling of internal elastic lamina and endothelial lining during flow-induced arterial enlargement. Arterioscler Thromb Vasc Biol. 1999;19:2298–307.
14. Karunanyaka A, Tu J, Watling A, et al. Endothelial molecular changes in a rodent model of arteriovenous malformation. J Neurosurg. 2008;109:1165–72.
15. Eerola I, Boon LM, Mulliken JB, et al. Capillary malformation-arteriovenous malformation: a new clinical and genetic disorder caused by RASA1 mutations. Am J Hum Genet. 2003;73:1240–9.
16. Urness LD, Sorensen LK, Li DY. Arteriovenous malformations in mice lacking activin receptor-like kinase-1. Nat Genet. 2000;26:328–31.
17. Thomas B, Eyries M, Montagne K, et al. Altered endothelial gene expression associated with hereditary haemorrhagic telangiectasia. Eur J Clin Invest. 2007;37:580–8.
18. Tan WH, Baris HN, Burrows PE, et al. The spectrum of vascular anomalies in patients with PTEN mutations: implications for diagnosis and management. J Med Genet. 2007;44:594–602.
19. Sansal I, Sellers WR. The biology and clinical relevance of the PTEN tumor suppressor pathway. J Clin Oncol. 2004;22:2954–63.
20. Greene AK, Liu AS, Mulliken JB, et al. Vascular anomalies in 5621 patients: guidelines for referral. J Peditr Surg. 2011;46(9):1784–9.
21. Revencu N, Boon LM, Vikkula M. From germline towards somatic mutations in the pathophysiology of vascular anomalies. Hum Mol Genet. 2009;18:65–75.
22. Johanisson E, Oberholzer M, Swahn ML, et al. Vascular changes in the human endometrium following the administration of the progesterone antagonist RU 486. Contraception. 1989;39:103–17.
23. Hyder SM, Huang JC, Nawaz Z, et al. Regulation of vascular endothelial growth factor expression by estrogens and progestins. Environ Health Perspect. 2000;108(Suppl 5):785–90.
24. Heryanto B, Rogers PA. Regulation of endometrial endothelial cell proliferation by oestrogen and progesterone in the ovariectomized mouse. Reproduction. 2002;123:107–13.
25. Kayisli UA, Luk J, Guzeloglu-Kayisili O, et al. Regulation of angiogenic activity of human endometrial endothelial cells in culture by ovarian steroids. J Clin Endocrinol Metab. 2004;89:5794–802.
26. Mulliken JB, Fishman SJ, Burrows PE. Vascular anomalies. Curr Probl Surg. 2000;37:517–84.
27. Thiex R, Mulliken JB, Revencu N, et al. A novel association between RASA1 mutations and spinal arteriovenous anomalies. Am J Neuroradiol. 2010;31(4):775–9.

28. Mulliken JB, Glowacki J. Hemangiomas and vascular malformations in infants and children: a classification based on endothelial characteristics. Plast Reconstr Surg. 1982;69:412–22.
29. Finn MC, Glowacki J, Mulliken JB. Congenital vascular lesions: clinical application of a new classification. J Pediatr Surg. 1983;18:894–900.
30. Marsh DJ, Coulon V, Lunetta KL, et al. Mutation spectrum and genotype-phenotype analyses in Cowden disease and Bannayan-Zonana syndrome, two hamartoma syndromes with germline PTEN mutation. Hum Mol Genet. 1998;7:507–15.
31. Limaye N, Boon LM, Vikkula M. From germline towards somatic mutations in the pathophysiology of vascular anomalies. Hum Mol Genet. 2009;18:65–75.
32. Gupta A, Kozakewich H. Histopathology of vascular anomalies. Clin Plast Surg. 2011;38(1):31–44.
33. Thiex R, Wu I, Mulliken JB, et al. Safety and clinical efficacy of onyx for embolization extracranial head and neck vascular anomalies. Am J Neuroradiol. 2011;32:1082–6.
34. Upton J, Coombs CJ, Mulliken JB, et al. Vascular malformations of the upper limb: a review of 270 patients. J Hand Surg Am. 1999;24:1019–35.

Arteriovenous Malformations: Intracranial

8

Brendan McNeish and Edward R. Smith

Introduction

Arteriovenous malformations (AVMs) are among the most important vascular anomalies in the nervous system of children; they are relatively common and usually require treatment. They consist of direct arterial-to-venous connections without intervening capillaries and occur in the cerebral hemispheres, brainstem, and spinal cord [1]. AVMs can present with hemorrhage, seizure, headache, progressive ischemia ("steal"), or can be found incidentally. Treatment is predicated on obliteration of the lesion, which can be achieved by surgery, radiation, embolization, or a combination of therapies.

Key Points

- AVMs are the most common symptomatic intracranial vascular abnormality [2]. In a large autopsy series, the overall frequency of detection for AVMs was 1.4 % [3].
- Hemorrhagic events from an AVM in childhood have been associated with a 25 % mortality rate [4].
- Computed tomography angiography (CTA) has increasingly been employed as an initial study for children presenting with nontraumatic intracranial hemorrhage to the emergency department, followed by magnetic resonance imaging (MRI) and catheter-based digital subtraction angiography (DSA) if AVM is found [5].
- Treatment for pediatric AVM should be performed at experienced centers with multidisciplinary teams able to offer all modalities of therapy (surgery, embolization, and radiation) whenever possible.

E. R. Smith (✉)
Department of Neurosurgery, Boston Children's Hospital, Harvard Medical School, Boston, MA, USA
e-mail: edward.smith@childrens.harvard.edu

B. McNeish
Boston Children's Hospital, Harvard Medical School, Boston, MA, USA

R. Rahbar et al. (eds.), *Pediatric Head and Neck Tumors*,
DOI 10.1007/978-1-4614-8755-5_8, © Springer Science+Business Media New York 2014

Biology and Epidemiology

AVMs consist of direct arterial-to-venous connections without intervening capillaries; they occur in the cerebral hemispheres, brainstem, and spinal cord. Functional neural tissue does not reside within the lesion [1].

Pathophysiology

- The mechanism of expansion of AVM has been debated. One possibility is "mechanical" dilatation as the result of increased flow through poorly differentiated vessels and recruitment of collateral arterial feeders. Ischemia and surrounding microhemorrhages with resultant gliosis may promote enlargement of the AVM by destruction of the surrounding parenchyma.
- Expansion of an AVM may also result from sprouting of new blood vessels from preexisting branches, i.e., angiogenesis—a complex process regulated by a wide range of proteins, including metalloproteinases and related growth factors such as vascular endothelial growth factor (VEGF) [6–12]. Immunochemical studies on resected cerebral AVMs have shown upregulation of VEGF, more prominently after preoperative embolization: supporting the concept that postnatal influences can affect the development and evolution of these lesions [10, 12–14].

Molecular/Genetic Pathology

- AVMs and cerebral cavernous malformation (CCMs) have been shown to express VEGF and increased levels of structural proteins in the endothelium and subendothelium and transforming growth factor alpha in endothelial and perivascular layers [8].
- The RASA1 mutation, resulting in familial AVMs and/or cutaneous capillary malformations, has been associated

with symptomatic cerebral AVMs in a small number of families [14].

- Hereditary hemorrhagic telangiectasia (HHT) is a genetic condition that predisposes affected individuals to AVMs. Transgenic mice with one deletion of *endoglin* (the gene that causes HHT) showed progressive destruction of the capillary bed related to endothelial cell nitric oxide synthetase deficiency [15].

Incidence and Prevalence

- AVM is the most common symptomatic intracranial vascular abnormality [2].
- In a large autopsy series, the overall frequency of detection for AVMs was 1.4% (46 among 3,200 brain tumor cases) [3].
- In another report, the annual incidence of symptomatic AVMs was 1.1 per 100,000 [16].
- The pediatric age group comprises 12–18% of all AVMs from major centers and the overall prevalence in children is about 0.02% of the pediatric population [17–20].

Age Distribution

- Most AVMs present in adulthood, with a mean age of presentation approximately 30–40 years old. About 20% of all symptomatic AVMs will present before 15 years of age [21].

Sex Predilection

- There is no sex predilection for pediatric AVMs.

Geographic Distribution

- AVMs are about one-seventh as common as saccular aneurysms; they may be more frequent in Asian populations [22].

Risk Factors—Environmental, Life Style

- None

Relationships to Other Disease States, Syndromes

- Thirty-five percent of cases were associated with HHT. Twenty-three percent of patients had multiple AVMs, with mean age at presentation being 35 years [16].
- The RASA1 mutation, resulting in familial AVMs and/or cutaneous capillary malformations, has been associated with symptomatic cerebral AVMs in a small number of families [14].

Presentation

Symptoms

- Hemorrhage and seizure are most common, may also include headache, focal neurologic deficits, and cognitive decline, or may be asymptomatic.
- Hemorrhage:
  - 80–85% of all pediatric AVMs present with hemorrhage. May present with seizures, headache, or focal neurologic deficits.
  - AVM hemorrhages are usually intraparenchymal (IPH) because of the location of the AVM within the substance of the brain. A nontraumatic IPH should raise concerns for the presence of an AVM or tumor.
  - The rate of major bleeding has been reported as 4.0% per year, and the mortality rate as 1.0% per year.
  - Hemorrhagic AVMs have been associated with a 25% mortality rate.
- Mass effect/ischemia:
  - Produce deficits through mass effect or from cerebral ischemia that is due to diversion of blood to the AVM from the normal cerebral circulation ("steal").

Patterns of Evolution

- The presentation of symptoms in AVM is generally acute if related to hemorrhage or seizure, often occurring within minutes to hours or chronic over months if related to steal phenomenon or headache.

Evaluation at Presentation

- *CT:* If a child presents with an IPH without a clear etiology on initial evaluation, AVM should be considered and a CTA may be helpful in the acute setting to identify the presence of dilated vessels or nidus.
- If no clear lesion is found, repeat imaging with MRI in 4–6 weeks should be performed to evaluate the hemorrhage cavity after the clot has cleared.
- Further testing is dependent on the stability of the patient. In general, MRI is helpful for three dimensional visualization of lesional anatomy, in particular for delineating the relationship between the malformation and underlying

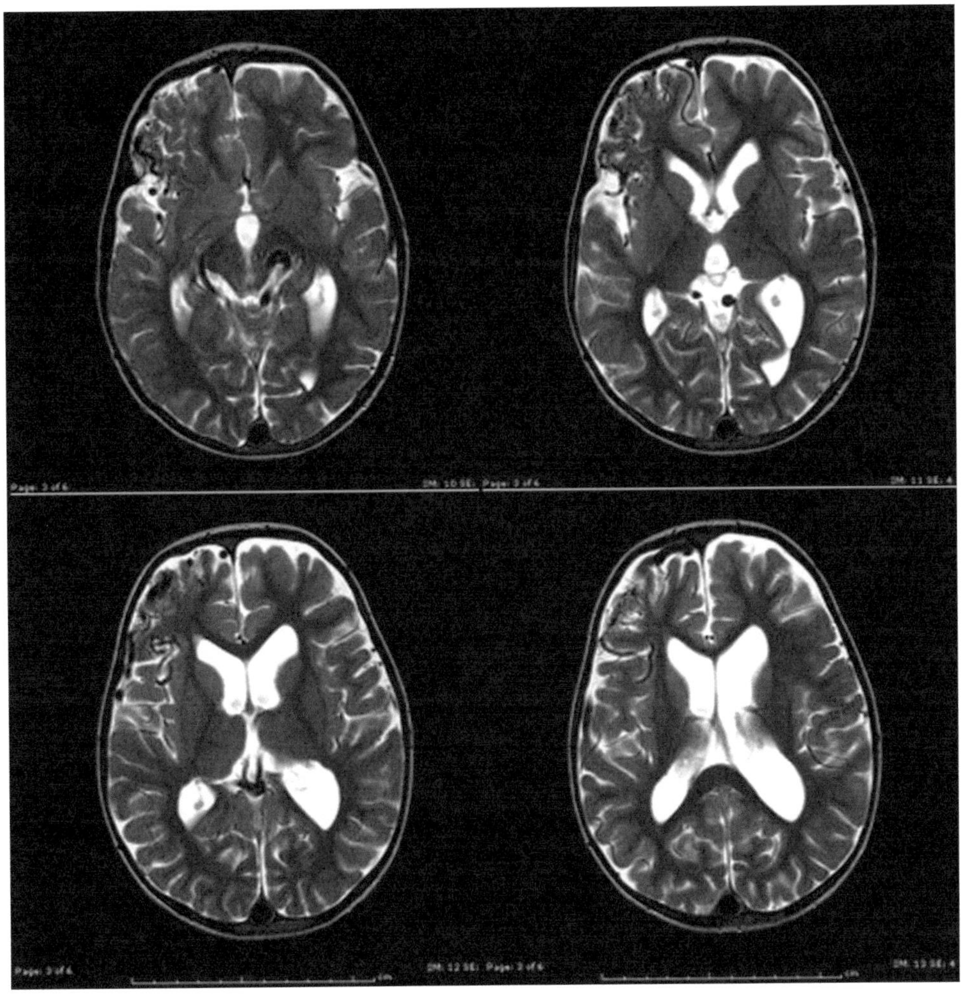

Fig. 8.1 MRI (axial T2 images) demonstrating right frontal AVM in 2-year-old child. Note dilated vessels in right frontal region, including anterior (ACA) and middle cerebral (MCA) branches, as well as dilated draining veins, both superficial and deep (esp. ultimate drainage to basal veins of Rosenthal). In addition, brain atrophy with sulcal prominence and ex vacuo ventriculomegaly are present

brain structures (Fig. 8.1). DSA is critical for defining angioarchitecture (see evaluation) (Fig. 8.2).

- Standard preoperative laboratory studies (complete blood count (CBC), clotting times prothrombin time/partial thromboplastin time (PT/PTT), type and cross (T&C) for blood bank, chemistry panel (Chem 7)).

Intervention

- Initial therapeutic maneuvers are dependent on the presentation of the child. For the healthy child or for the child who presents with chronic symptoms (seizure, developmental delay), there are often no immediate interventions necessary (with the exception of antiepileptic medication if seizures are present). The following steps are warranted for the child who presents with an intracranial hemorrhage. It is important to note that severity of presentation can vary greatly, and thus treatment must be individually tailored.

Stabilization

- Access: Large bore IV (at least 2), arterial line, bladder catheter (airway intubation if unable to protect airway), and nasogastric tube if intubated.
- Blood pressure control (labetolol or nipride) with goal of normotension for age.
- ICP intracranial pressure control—external ventricular drain if hydrocephalus (NB; avoid overdrainage of cerebrospinal fluid (CSF) to prevent rerupture, often no more than 5 cc at a time), head of bed (HOB) elevated.
- Antiepileptic medication if concern for seizure.

Preparation for Definitive Intervention, Nonemergent

- As previously discussed, nonemergent management varies greatly depending on presentation. In elective cases, preoperative labs and imaging are needed. For the patient with a hemorrhage but minimal deficits, admission to the intensive care unit for blood pressure control and preoperative imaging studies are the two important interventions. (Emergent management is detailed above.)

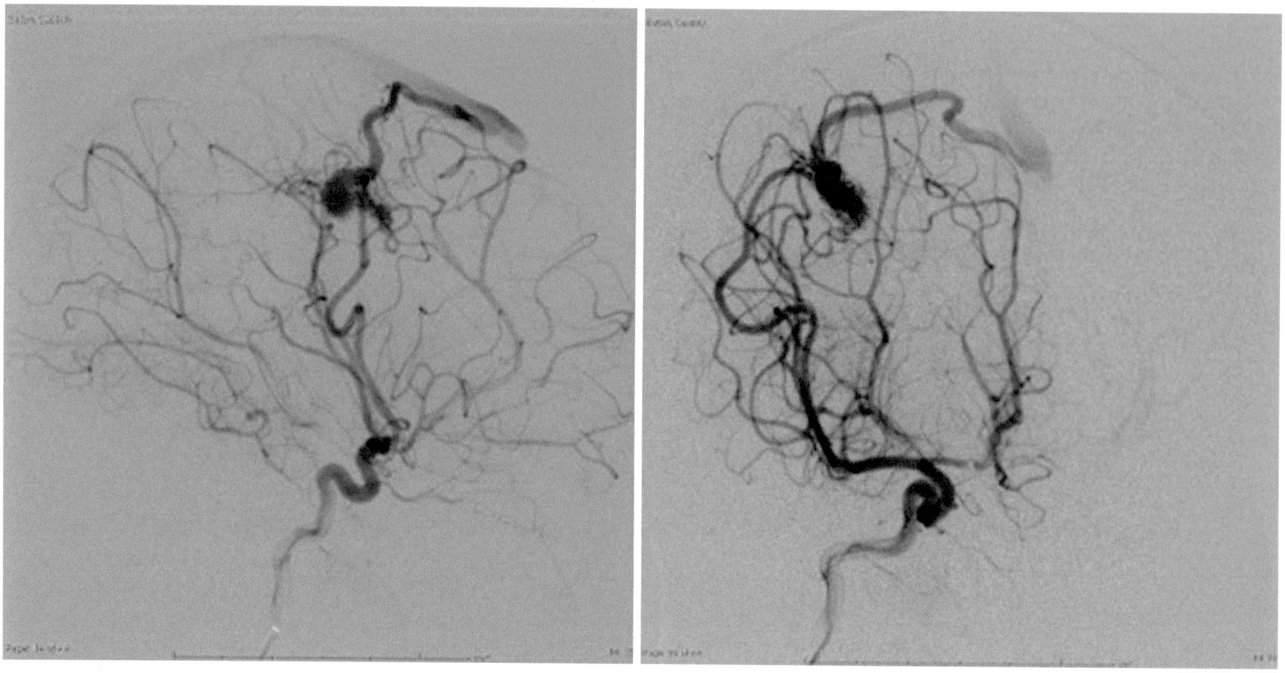

Fig. 8.2 Two projections of left internal carotid artery injection angiogram demonstrating high-flow right frontal AVM in 1-year-old child. Note dilated MCA feeding vessel and early superficial draining vein

Preparation for Definitive Intervention, Emergent

- In addition to the steps noted in the stabilization section, the operating room should be notified to prepare for surgery. Equipment should include the operating microscope, multiple suctions, bipolar electrocautery, an array of AVM/aneurysm clips, a craniotome (drill), and a retraction system.
- Anesthesia should be consulted and appropriate measures made to ensure that multiple large bore IV access is present and adequate blood products are in the room.
- It is helpful to have the microscope draped and clips prepared prior to starting the case if possible, so that quick access can be obtained should unexpected bleeding occur during opening (Fig. 8.3).

Differential Diagnosis

Many patients will be asymptomatic on examination if the lesion is found incidentally. If a spontaneous intracranial intraparenchymal/intraventricular or subarachnoid hemorrhage is found, the following differential diagnosis should be considered:

- AVM
- Brain tumor
- Aneurysm (including mycotic lesions)
- Bleeding/clotting disorder
- Venous thrombosis
- Moyamoya
- (Trauma, while not "spontaneous", should be excluded in recent history)

Diagnosis and Evaluation

Physical Examination

- Many patients will be asymptomatic on examination. However, a detailed neurologic examination and history are always important. Attention should be paid to evidence of neurologic dysfunction in the history (see list below).

Findings Suggestive of an Intracranial Lesion

- Headache in the early morning hours or awakening patient from sleep
- Vomiting
- Headache of less than 6 months duration
- Confusion or behavioral changes
- Abnormal neurologic examination findings

  (Positive correlation between number of predictors and risk of surgical lesion)

On examination, findings may be present secondary to (1) local effects (focal weakness, visual changes, etc.), (2) increased intracranial pressure (papilledema, increased head circumference, etc.), or (3) high flow (dilated scalp vessels, bruit on auscultation, cardiac failure).

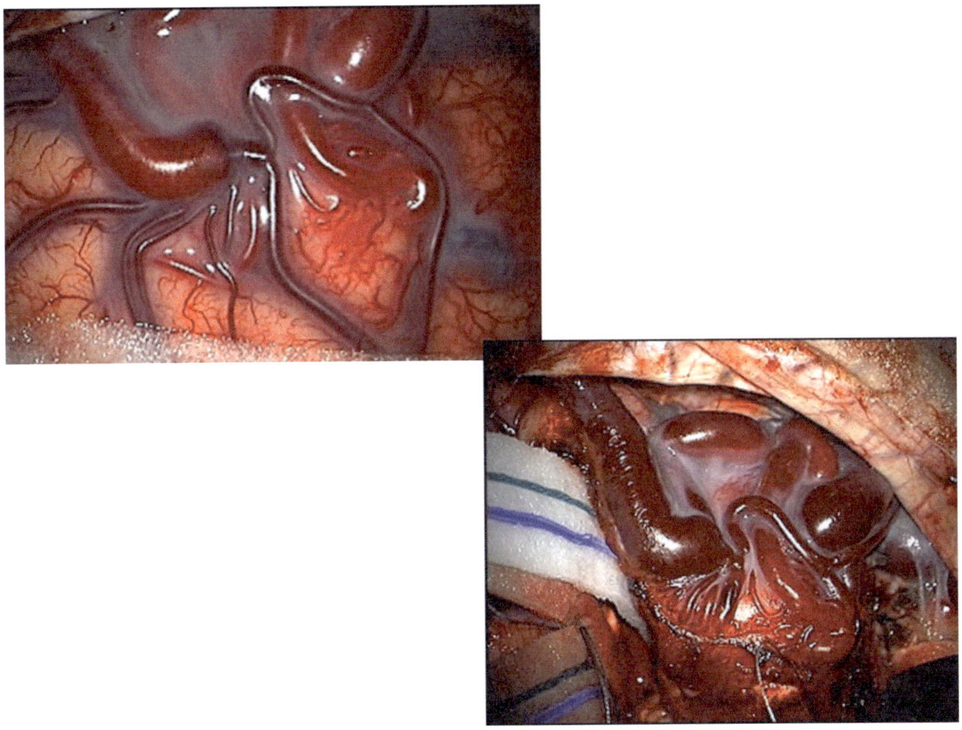

Fig. 8.3 Intraoperative images of superficial cortical AVM. Initial image shows dilate and arterialized draining vein. Subsequent image illustrates method of circumferential dissection around AVM with preservation of draining vein until final portion of case. Note reduction in caliber of draining vein and change to stagnant, deoxygenated venous blood after interruption of arterial supply

"Red Flags" on Examination or History

- Bradycardia, hypertension, decreased respirations (cushing response)
- Dilated pupil, hemparesis (uncal herniation)
- Fixed downward gaze (Parinaud's syndrome)
- Lethargy, tense open anterior fontanelle in infants
- Ataxia with nausea and vomiting
- Sudden onset of a third nerve palsy, including involvement of the pupil (appearing dilated)
- Sudden onset of severe headache

Laboratory Data

- Standard preoperative laboratory studies (CBC, clotting times (PT/PTT), T&C for blood bank, chemistry panel (Chem 7)).

Imaging Evaluation

- CT: If a child presents with a hemorrhage without a clear etiology on initial evaluation, AVM should be considered and repeat imaging in 4–6 weeks with MRI should be performed to evaluate the hemorrhage cavity after the clot has cleared.
- AVM typically appears as a heterogeneous area of mixed density with serpiginous areas of enhancement after infusion of contrast material. Cerebral atrophy may sometimes be seen on the affected side. A large malformation or an intracerebral hematoma may distort the normal intracranial anatomy.
- MRI is useful for 3D anatomy and identification of chronic ischemia, presumably a result of "steal" phenomena; AVM may be identified on MRI as bright signal of the surrounding brain on FLAIR or T2 images (Fig. 8.1).
- The typical MRI appearance is that of a latticework of signal-void spaces, highly contrasted against surrounding cerebral tissue on both T1- and T2-weighted sequences, intermixed with regions of various signal intensities corresponding to blood products in different stages of evolution, and occasionally calcium and hemosiderin [23, 24]. The serpiginous shape of vessels may be distinctive, identified as flow-voids, and relevant anatomy can be well visualized with MR angiography. Susceptibility imaging will sometimes disclose evidence of previous hemorrhage as a dark "bloom" around the nidus [25]. Chronic ischemic changes, presumably a result of "steal" phenomenon or venous hypertension, may be identified on MRI as bright signal of the surrounding brain on FLAIR or T2 images.
- Digital subtraction angiography is the definitive investigation. It establishes the nature and extent of the lesion to its blood supply and its venous drainage [26] (Fig. 8.2). Angiography entails bilateral injection of all potential arterial sources of supply to the AVM, both pial and dural (with 15 % of cerebral AVMs receiving some blood supply from ipsilateral or contralateral meningeal arteries [27]): typically at least the internal carotid arteries bilaterally, as well as the ipsilateral external carotid and vertebral

arteries. Three-dimensional angiography with computer-generated reconstruction is increasingly employed to depict lesional anatomy. The typical angiographic appearance of an AVM is that of distended, tortuous afferent, and efferent vessels connecting with a tangled vascular mass, through which the circulation time is rapid; i.e., arteriovenous shunting. Other vessels or structures are not displaced unless there is an intracerebral hematoma, which appears as an avascular mass.

- A recent analysis of 241 consecutive pediatric patients revealed a 0 % complication rate during the procedure and a 0.4 % post-procedural complication rate. Evaluation should look for:
  - High-flow vs. low-flow lesions.
  - Outflow stenoses.
  - Varices in subarachnoid or ventricular spaces.
  - Number and location of feeding vessels.
  - *Aneurysms:* Flow-related aneurysms are rarely seen in association with AVMs. Often these flow-related aneurysms will spontaneously regress following the reduction in blood flow after treatment of the AVM.
- Screening is not justified in the general population. Patients with HHT may be candidates for MRI/A studies of the CNS during childhood to screen for AVMs, as they may be present in 5–10 % of children with HHT.

Nuclear medicine tests	Not usually indicated with AVMs.
Electrodiagnostic tests	Electroencephalography (EEG) may be warranted if the concern for seizure exists.
Neuropsychological tests	Not usually indicated with AVMs, although may be helpful as baseline study in selected children to help with recovery strategies.

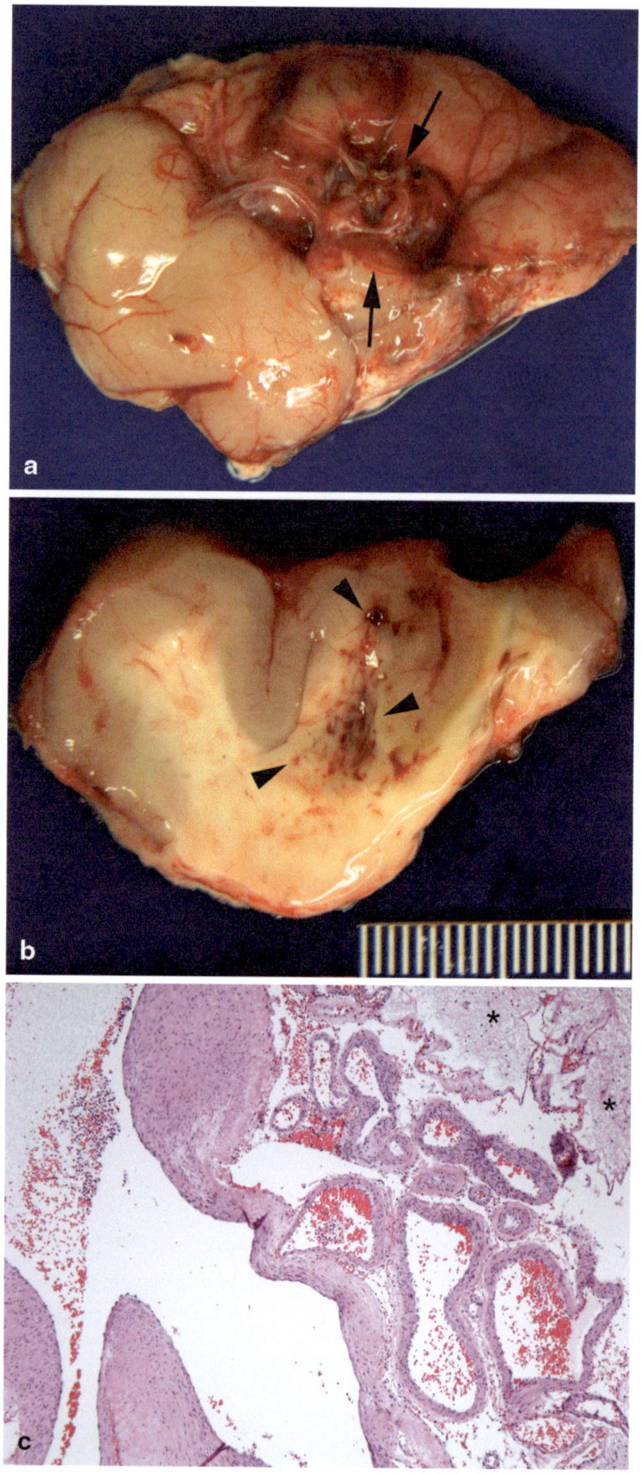

Fig. 8.4 Pathology of central nervous system arteriovenous malformation. **a** Temporal lobe with arteriovenous malformation (*between arrows*), characterized by a circumscribed cluster of large tortuous blood vessels. **b** On cut section, abnormal vessels and petechiae are observed in the white matter (*arrow heads*). **c** Large malformed arteries and veins. Large veins have hypertrophic walls with variable thickness, consistent with high-flow, hypertensive changes

Pathology

AVM consist of direct arterial-to-venous connections without intervening capillaries; they occur in the cerebral hemispheres, brainstem, and spinal cord. Functional neural tissue does not reside within the lesion (Fig. 8.4) [1].

Treatment

Goal To remove the risk of bleeding or growth.

There are no currently accepted medical therapies for the primary treatment of AVM. While adjuvant medical therapy may be helpful (antiepileptic medication for seizure, pain medication for headache, etc.), the obliteration of an AVM is currently achieved by either surgical resection or treatment with radiation.

- The treatment goal is complete removal/obliteration of the lesion. Two major modalities are used—surgery or radiation. The decision to operate on an AVM is based on several factors: (1) eloquence of cortical location (speech, motor function, and sensation), (2) pattern of venous drainage, (3) size, (4) associated aneurysms, (5) recent hemorrhage, (6) clinical deterioration, and (7) risk of complication from other modalities of therapy (such as radiation injury to the developing brain) [28, 29]. Several of these factors are combined in the Spetzler-Martin [30] grade that incorporates eloquence of location, pattern of venous drainage, and size and is considered predictive of outcome from surgical management. Spetzler-Martin grade helps to predict surgical risk. If a low grade lesion (1–3) is present, surgery should be considered. Higher-grade lesions (4 and 5) often benefit from multidisciplinary approach and might be considered for radiation therapy.

Spetzler-Martin AVM grading scale	
Size	
0–3 cm	1
>3–6 cm	2
>6 cm	3
Location	
Non-eloquent	0
Eloquent	1
Deep venous drainage	
Not present	0
Present	1

Surgical Therapy

Timing: If a child presents with symptoms of increased ICP then urgent operation may be necessary. If there are worrisome findings on angiography (high-flow lesion with intraventricular varices or aneurysms) then surgery may be planned within the same hospital stay. If not, then a delay of several weeks may help, with delayed reimaging offering better understanding of the anatomy for surgical or radiosurgical planning, as well as an easier surgical approach once the clot has resorbed.

- A primary surgical principle for AVM resection is the obliteration of feeding arteries before occlusion of draining veins, as premature closure of outflow can lead to AVM rupture with uncontrolled bleeding.
- AVMs are often wedge or cone shaped, and resection can be performed in a circumferential pattern, staying close to—but not entering—the nidus. It is helpful to try to maintain an even depth of resection around the lesion to avoid getting in a "hole" and caution must be taken to minimize retraction on draining vessels during dissection.
- Repeated inspection of the surrounding brain for swelling or bleeding can aid the surgeon in preventing complications by early identification of poorly placed retractors or clips (Fig. 8.3).
- AVM vessels may coagulate poorly and consideration should be given to clip application or gentle tamponade (if the bleeding is of small volume) if bipolar electrocautery is not working. Every attempt should be made to avoid operating within the nidus itself.

Complications

- Bleeding is the most immediate complication of surgery and risks are magnified in smaller children, who have little reserve. The loss of one-quarter of blood volume can induce shock and there may be rapid decompensation in children, which mandates careful monitoring and replacement of blood products by the operative team.
- Normal perfusion pressure breakthrough is a phenomenon that is thought to occur after resection of high-flow AVMs in which the blood previously transmitted through the AVM is redirected to smaller, normal vasculature after the AVM has been removed, with subsequent inability of the vessels to handle the increased flow. This can result in brain swelling, increased intracranial pressure, seizure, neurologic dysfunction, or hemorrhage. The problem may be minimized by staged preoperative embolization and rigorous blood pressure control postoperatively.
- Neurologic deficit can occur following AVM resection, although specific rates are hard to derive, given the wide variability in AVM size and location.
- Overall, there is low postoperative morbidity in low-grade (1–3) Spetzler-Martin lesions (ranging from 0–12 %), along with a high rate of complete obliteration (up to 100 %), suggesting that surgical resection of these lesions is warranted—especially when performed in experienced centers [29, 31–33].

Radiation Therapy

Conventional fractionated radiation is not helpful in the majority of AVMs, however, stereotactic radiosurgery offers cure rates of up to 90 % in lesions under 3 cm in size. This approach is beneficial for surgically inaccessible lesions or in patients who are high-risk surgical candidates. Shortcomings of this approach include a delay of up to 3 years for lesion obliteration and exposure to radiation in children. Radiation has increased risk in younger populations, making its application less appealing in those children under 3 years of age.

Complications

The long delay between treatment and lesion obliteration in radiosurgery for AVMs means that the child is at risk of the complication of bleeding during this interval. Patients with small (less than 3 cm diameter), deep-seated lesions (in the basal ganglia, internal capsule, and thalamus) are the best candidates for radiosurgery. A study of 42 children with lesions in these locations documented a 62 % angiographic cure rate within 2 years [34]. However, radiosurgery in these sites have shown a higher risk of rebleeding when compared to AVMs treated in other areas of the brain [35].

Young children have risk of radiation-induced damage, including injury to the surrounding developing brain and potential for development of secondary malignancies. These risks limit radiation use to older children in most cases.

Embolization

Although not traditionally used as a stand-alone treatment for AVMs other than in rare cases with a small nidus and a small number of feeding pedicles, there is a growing literature on the use of newer embolization agents (Onyx) for definitive treatment of brain AVM in adults. However, the situation in children is more complex and embolization is rarely used as a stand-alone modality, as the recurrence rate is higher, and lesion immaturity may preclude complete visualization angiographically. Regardless, embolization is a significant aid in the treatment of AVMs, reducing their blood supply and facilitating operative approaches (usually <72 h before surgery). Embolization also has a role in targeted treatment of nonoperative lesions, by occluding areas at risk of hemorrhage such as aneurysms or high-risk varices (those that are intraventricular).

Outcomes

Outcome After Surgery

- In pediatric patients with grade I–III Spetzler-Martin AVMs treated by resection [33], good recovery was achieved in 90 % and deaths occurred at a rate of 5 %. Radiographic obliteration rates were 89 %.
- Although class I or II data are lacking, the combined class III data strongly support resection as a primary treatment for patients with Spetzler-Martin grade 1 or 2 AVM. The relatively low postoperative morbidity in these lesions (ranging from 0–12 %), along with a high rate of complete obliteration (up to 100 %), suggests that delayed control, inherent to radiosurgery, might not be warranted [29, 31–33].

Outcome After Nonsurgical Treatments

- For comparison, a similar group of patients treated with radiosurgery alone had a reported 80 % efficacy of lesion obliteration at 36 months with 4 out of 53 patients having recurrent hemorrhage posttreatment [36].
- One large pediatric AVM study included 40 patients and confirmed radiographic obliteration of the AVM nidus in 35 % of the patients [37]. The cumulative posttreatment hemorrhage rate was 3.2 % per patient per year in the first year and 4.3 % per patient per year over the first 3 years [37]. These rates of obliteration, which are notably lower than that reported in the adult population, were potentially complicated by a slightly larger than average size of treated AVM in the study group. In contrast, when a group of 53 pediatric patients was stratified by AVM size (<3 cm^3, 3–10 cm^3, and >10 cm^3), in the smallest and middle group, obliteration rates of 80 % and 64.7 % were reported [36].
- Although class I and II data are lacking, the aggregate class III data strongly support the use of radiosurgery in the treatment of small (less than 3 cm diameter), deep-seated lesions in eloquent cortex. For Spetzler-Martin grade I and most grade II lesions, open resection is generally recommended over radiosurgery, unless there are specific considerations which make the patient unsuitable for resection. Radiosurgery should only be used for larger lesions (grade II–V), if the objective is complete obliteration of the AVM [38].

Outcome After Multimodal Therapies

- Multimodality therapy of AVM has been advocated by several investigators (Fig. 8.2) [29, 31, 39, 40]. Neurointerventionalists, radiation oncologists, and neurosurgeons work together to determine the best strategy for a particular patient. Using a multimodality approach, angiographic obliteration rates of 92.9 % have been reported.
- The efficacy of multimodality treatment of large, complex lesions is supported by a group of 53 children at a 3 year follow-up in whom a 58 % cure rate was noted for AVMs greater than 6 cm in diameter [41].
- In summary, the high likelihood of obliteration, coupled with low-complication rates, make a convincing argument in favor of multimodality treatment of pediatric AVMs. Although no class I or II data directly support this recommendation, the class III data are compelling and there is wisdom in pooling the skills of the concerned specialists.

Follow-up

Frequency of Office Visits

- Postoperative care will frequently consist of an office visit approximately 1 month postoperatively, then annually thereafter. Radiation therapy also involves annual visits posttreatment.

Frequency of Imaging

- In addition to the perioperative angiogram to confirm obliteration of the AVM, a MRI/A at 6 months may be helpful as a baseline study, to then be compared to subsequent annual MRI/A. Imaging is performed annually for 5 years, if feasible.
- An angiogram (DSA) is often performed at 1 year postoperatively to confirm durable cure.

AVMs and Pregnancy

- Treatment of a known AVM should be undertaken prior to pregnancy, whenever possible. There are rare situations of documented intracranial AVM in a pregnancy. Either the AVM was not addressed prior to gestation or neurological sequelae led to its discovery. Data in this small group of patients are inconclusive, particularly with regard to the rate of hemorrhage during the pregnancy [42–48]. MRI is safe for initial evaluation of the anatomy of the lesion [49]. No specific recommendations can be made if the AVM is diagnosed during pregnancy, because individual risk-benefit relationships need to be assessed. If the mother has an untreated or partially treated AVM, caesarean section should be considered [1, 40, 46, 48, 50].

References

1. Friedlander RM. Clinical practice. Arteriovenous malformations of the brain. N Engl J Med. 2007;356:2704–12.
2. Brown RD Jr, Wiebers DO, Torner JC, O'Fallon WM. Incidence and prevalence of intracranial vascular malformations in Olmsted County, Minnesota, 1965 to 1992. Neurology. 1996;46:949–52.
3. Olivecrona H, Riives J. Arteriovenous aneurysms of the brain: their diagnosis and treatment. Arch Neurol Psychiatry. 1948;59:567–603.
4. Altschuler E, Lunsford LD, Kondziolka D, et al. Radiobiologic models for radiosurgery. Neurosurg Clin N Am. 1992;3:61–77.
5. Tan CL, Li DT, Shen SB. Detection of brain vascular diseases with CT angiography. Hunan Yi Ke Da Xue Xue Bao. 2001;26:460–2. Chinese.
6. Sonstein WJ, Kader A, Michelsen WJ, Llena JF, Hirano A, Casper D. Expression of vascular endothelial growth factor in pediatric and adult cerebral arteriovenous malformations: an immunocytochemical study. J Neurosurg. 1996;85:838–45.
7. Rothbart D, Awad IA, Lee J, Kim J, Harbaugh R, Criscuolo GR. Expression of angiogenic factors and structural proteins in central nervous system vascular malformations. Neurosurgery. 1996;38:915–24; discussion 24–5.
8. Kilic T, Pamir MN, Kullu S, Eren F, Ozek MM, Black PM. Expression of structural proteins and angiogenic factors in cerebrovascular anomalies. Neurosurgery. 2000;46:1179–91; discussion 91–2.
9. Hashimoto T, Emala CW, Joshi S, et al. Abnormal pattern of Tie-2 and vascular endothelial growth factor receptor expression in human cerebral arteriovenous malformations. Neurosurgery. 2000;47:910–8; discussion 8–9.
10. Sure U, Butz N, Schlegel J, et al. Endothelial proliferation, neoangiogenesis, and potential de novo generation of cerebrovascular malformations. J Neurosurg. 2001;94:972–7.
11. Shenkar R, Elliott JP, Diener K, et al. Differential gene expression in human cerebrovascular malformations. Neurosurgery. 2003;52:465–77; discussion 77–8.
12. Gault J, Sarin H, Awadallah NA. Pathobiology of human cerebrovascular malformations: basic mechanisms and clinical relevance. Neurosurgery. 2004;55:1–17.
13. Sure U, Butz N, Siegel AM, Mennel HD, Bien S, Bertalanffy H. Treatment-induced neoangiogenesis in cerebral arteriovenous malformations. Clin Neurol Neurosurg. 2001;103:29–32.
14. Boon LM, Mulliken JB, Vikkula M. RASA1: variable phenotype with capillary and arteriovenous malformations. Curr Opin Genet Dev. 2005;15:265–9.
15. Jerkic M, Rivas-Elena JV, Prieto M, et al. Endoglin regulates nitric oxide-dependent vasodilatation. Faseb J. 2004;18:609–11.
16. Jessurun GA, Kamphuis DJ, van der Zande FH, Nossent JC. Cerebral arteriovenous malformations in The Netherlands Antilles. High prevalence of hereditary hemorrhagic telangiectasia-related single and multiple cerebral arteriovenous malformations. Clin Neurol Neurosurg. 1993;95:193–8.
17. Celli P, Ferrante L, Palma L, Cavedon G. Cerebral arteriovenous malformations in children. Clinical features and outcome of treatment in children and in adults. Surg Neurol. 1984;22:43–9.
18. Kahl W, Kessel G, Schwarz M, Voth D. Arterio-venous malformations in childhood: clinical presentation, results after operative treatment and long-term follow-up. Neurosurg Rev. 1989;12:165–71.
19. Kader A, Goodrich JT, Sonstein WJ, Stein BM, Carmel PW, Michelsen WJ. Recurrent cerebral arteriovenous malformations after negative postoperative angiograms. J Neurosurg. 1996;85:14–8.
20. D'Aliberti G, Talamonti G, Versari PP, et al. Comparison of pediatric and adult cerebral arteriovenous malformations. J Neurosurg Sci. 1997;41:331–6.
21. Di Rocco C, Tamburrini G, Rollo M. Cerebral arteriovenous malformations in children. Acta Neurochir (Wien). 2000;142:145–56; discussion 56–8.
22. Tay CH, Oon CL, Lai CS, Loong SC, Gwee AL. Intracranial arteriovenous malformations in Asians. Brain. 1971;94:61–8.
23. Leblanc R, Levesque M, Comair Y, Ethier R. Magnetic resonance imaging of cerebral arteriovenous malformations. Neurosurgery. 1987;21:15–20.
24. Smith HJ, Strother CM, Kikuchi Y, et al. MR imaging in the management of supratentorial intracranial AVMs. AJR Am J Roentgenol. 1988;150:1143–53.
25. Chappell PM, Steinberg GK, Marks MP. Clinically documented hemorrhage in cerebral arteriovenous malformations: MR characteristics. Radiology. 1992;183:719–24.
26. Pott M, Huber M, Assheuer J, Bewermeyer H. Comparison of MRI, CT and angiography in cerebral arteriovenous malformations. Bildgebung. 1992;59:98–102.
27. Newton TH, Cronqvist S. Involvement of dural arteries in intracranial arteriovenous malformations. Radiology. 1969;93:1071–8.

28. Fisher WS 3rd. Therapy of AVMs: a decision analysis. Clin Neurosurg. 1995;42:294–312.
29. Hoh BL, Chapman PH, Loeffler JS, Carter BS, Ogilvy CS. Results of multimodality treatment for 141 patients with brain arteriovenous malformations and seizures: factors associated with seizure incidence and seizure outcomes. Neurosurgery. 2002;51:303–9; discussion 9–11.
30. Spetzler RF, Martin NA. A proposed grading system for arteriovenous malformations. J Neurosurg. 1986;65:476–83.
31. Humphreys RP, Hoffman HJ, Drake JM, Rutka JT. Choices in the 1990s for the management of pediatric cerebral arteriovenous malformations. Pediatr Neurosurg. 1996;25:277–85.
32. Morgan MK, Rochford AM, Tsahtsarlis A, Little N, Faulder KC. Surgical risks associated with the management of Grade I and II brain arteriovenous malformations. Neurosurgery. 2004;54:832–7; discussion 7–9.
33. Kiris T, Sencer A, Sahinbas M, Sencer S, Imer M, Izgi N. Surgical results in pediatric Spetzler-Martin grades I-III intracranial arteriovenous malformations. Childs Nerv Syst. 2005;21:69–74; discussion 5–6.
34. Andrade-Souza YM, Zadeh G, Scora D, Tsao MN, Schwartz ML. Radiosurgery for basal ganglia, internal capsule, and thalamus arteriovenous malformation: clinical outcome. Neurosurgery. 2005;56:56–63; discussion 63–4.
35. Pollock BE, Gorman DA, Brown PD. Radiosurgery for arteriovenous malformations of the basal ganglia, thalamus, and brainstem. J Neurosurg. 2004;100:210–4.
36. Levy EI, Niranjan A, Thompson TP, et al. Radiosurgery for childhood intracranial arteriovenous malformations. Neurosurgery. 2000;47:834–41; discussion 41–2.
37. Smyth MD, Sneed PK, Ciricillo SF, et al. Stereotactic radiosurgery for pediatric intracranial arteriovenous malformations: the University of California at San Francisco experience. J Neurosurg. 2002;97:48–55.
38. Ogilvy CS, Stieg PE, Awad I, et al. Recommendations for the management of intracranial arteriovenous malformations: a statement for healthcare professionals from a special writing group of the Stroke Council, American Stroke Association. Circulation. 2001;103:2644–57.
39. Ter Brugge K, Lasjaunias P, Chiu M, Flodmark O, Chuang S, Burrows P. Pediatric surgical neuroangiography. A multicentre approach. Acta Radiol Suppl. 1986;369:692–3.
40. Lee BB, Do YS, Yakes W, Kim DI, Mattassi R, Hyon WS. Management of arteriovenous malformations: a multidisciplinary approach. J Vasc Surg. 2004;39:590–600.
41. Chang SD, Marcellus ML, Marks MP, Levy RP, Do HM, Steinberg GK. Multimodality treatment of giant intracranial arteriovenous malformations. Neurosurgery. 2003;53:1–11; discussion 11–3.
42. Horton JC, Chambers WA, Lyons SL, Adams RD, Kjellberg RN. Pregnancy and the risk of hemorrhage from cerebral arteriovenous malformations. Neurosurgery. 1990;27:867–71; discussion 71–2.
43. Lanzino G, Jensen ME, Cappelletto B, Kassell NF. Arteriovenous malformations that rupture during pregnancy: a management dilemma. Acta Neurochir (Wien). 1994;126:102–6.
44. Karlsson B, Lindquist C, Johansson A, Steiner L. Annual risk for the first hemorrhage from untreated cerebral arteriovenous malformations. Minim Invasive Neurosurg. 1997;40:40–6.
45. Yih PS, Cheong KF. Anaesthesia for caesarean section in a patient with an intracranial arteriovenous malformation. Anaesth Intensive Care. 1999;27:66–8.
46. Trivedi RA, Kirkpatrick PJ. Arteriovenous malformations of the cerebral circulation that rupture in pregnancy. J Obstet Gynaecol. 2003;23:484–9.
47. Piotin M, Mounayer C, Spelle L, Moret J. [Cerebral arteriovenous malformations and pregnancy: management of a dilemma]. J Neuroradiol. 2004;31:376–8. French.
48. English LA, Mulvey DC. Ruptured arteriovenous malformation and subarachnoid hemorrhage during emergent cesarean delivery: a case report. Aana J. 2004;72:423–6.
49. Shojaku H, Seto H, Kakishita M, Yokoyama M, Ito J. Use of MR angiography in a pregnant patient with thalamic AVM. Radiat Med. 1996;14:159–61.
50. Terao M, Kubota M, Tamakawa S, Kawada K, Ogawa H. [Anesthesia for cesarean section in a patient with intracranial A-V malformation]. Masui. 1995;44:1700–2. Japanese.

Capillary Malformations

9

Rafael A. Couto and Arin K. Greene

Introduction

Capillary malformation (CM) is the most common vascular malformation in the general population, affecting approximately 1 in 300 newborns [1]. It is a slow-flow vascular anomaly characterized by dilated venule-type channels in the superficial dermis (see Fig. 9.1). It is present at birth and the color may darken overtime [2, 3]. CM can cause psychosocial morbidity and functional problems because of soft-tissue and skeletal overgrowth [2]. CM is a component of several syndromes, such as capillary malformation-arteriovenous malformation (CM-AVM), cutis marmorata telangiectatica congenita (CMTC), macrocephaly-capillary malformation (M-CM), and Sturge-Weber syndrome (SWS) [3]. Fading capillary stains involving the forehead and/or posterior scalp/neck are common in Caucasians, and typically resolve by 2 years of age (see Fig. 9.2) [3].

Key Points

- Most CMs are small and sporadic, and do not require treatment.
- CMs may represent an underlying syndrome.
- Pulse dye laser (PDL) is the primary treatment for CMs.
- Most CMs can be managed by a single specialist, although syndromic patients or those with significant overgrowth are best managed in a vascular anomalies center by a multidisciplinary team.

A. K. Greene (✉) · R. A. Couto
Department of Plastic and Oral Surgery, Boston Children's Hospital, Harvard Medical School, Boston, MA, USA
e-mail: arin.greene@childrens.harvard.edu

Biology and Epidemiology

Pathophysiology

- The pathogenesis of CM is not understood. Stasis in dilated, thin-walled channels may cause progressive vascular ectasia and soft-tissue thickening [4, 5]. Cobblestoning may be due to a lack of neural control of blood flow [6–8], or a loss of connective tissue support of the vessel wall [4, 9].
- The mechanism of osseous overgrowth is unknown. It may be secondary to increased blood flow, the production of localized growth factors, or intraosseous CM [2].

Molecular/Genetic Pathology

- CM-AVM is an autosomal dominant condition that results from a loss-of-function mutation in *RASA1*, which encodes p120RasGAP. This protein inhibits RAS p21 control of cellular proliferation, differentiation, and survival [10].
- The etiologies of CMTC, M-CM, and SWS are unclear; they occur sporadically [3].

Incidence and Prevalence

- Fading capillary stain is present in up to 40 % of Caucasian infants [3].
- The birth prevalence of CM is approximately 0.3 % [1].
- CMs comprise 11 % of vascular malformations treated in a vascular anomalies center [11].
- The prevalence of CM-AVM is estimated to be 1 in 100,000 Caucasians [10].
- SWS occurs 1 in 50,000 live births [12–14].

R. Rahbar et al. (eds.), *Pediatric Head and Neck Tumors*,
DOI 10.1007/978-1-4614-8755-5_9,

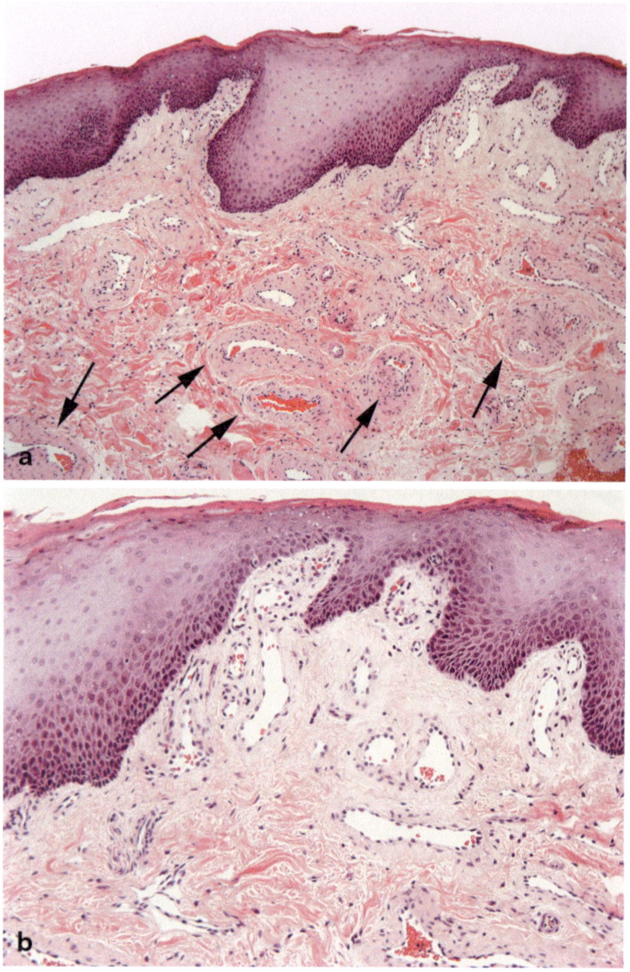

Fig. 9.1 Capillary malformation, face. **a** Hypertrophic lip with numerous ecstatic thin-walled venules on the superficial submucosa and thick-walled veins with prominent smooth muscle walls in a deeper submucosal location (*arrows*). **b** Superficial submucosal ecstatic thin-walled venules at higher magnification

Age Distribution

- CM is present at birth.

Sex Predilection

- CMs have equal gender distribution [1, 11].

Risk Factors

- The offspring of patients with CM-AVM have a 50%-risk of inheriting the condition; phenotypic heterogeneity is common [10, 15, 16].

Relationships to Other Disease States, Syndromes

- Parkes-Weber syndrome (PWS) is a diffuse arteriovenous malformation (AVM) in an overgrown extremity with an overlying CM [17].
- Klippel-Trénaunay syndrome (KTS) consists of a capillary-lymphatic-venous malformation (CLVM) of an extremity in association with soft-tissue and/or skeletal overgrowth [2].

Presentation

Fading Capillary Stain

- Vascular stain that resolves during early childhood [3].
- Popularly referred as "angel kiss" when located on the forehead and "stork bite" when on the occipital scalp/posterior neck.

Capillary Malformation

- CM is present at birth; however, the stain may not be evident because it can be hidden by the erythema of neonatal skin.
- Facial CMs are associated with hypertrophy of the lip, cheek, or forehead; the lip is most commonly affected [2].
- Fibrovascular nodules with cutaneous thickening and cobblestoning occur in 10–24% of patients with nonsyndromic CM, especially when located in the second and third trigeminal nerve distribution [18–20].
- Eighteen percent of patients develop pyogenic granulomas (PG) within the CM [2].
- Enlargement of the maxilla or mandible can cause occlusal cant (vertical maxillary overgrowth) with increased dental show and malocclusion [2].

Capillary Malformation-Arteriovenous Malformation

- The CM is typically nonproblematic; however, 30% of patients have AVMs that can cause major morbidity: PWS (12%), extracerebral AVM (11%), or intracerebral AVM (7%) [16].
- An individual may have multiple CMs; however, 6% of patients have a single lesion [16].
- Five percent of patients have benign or malignant tumors, most commonly involving the nervous system (neurofibroma, optic glioma, vestibular schwannoma) [16].

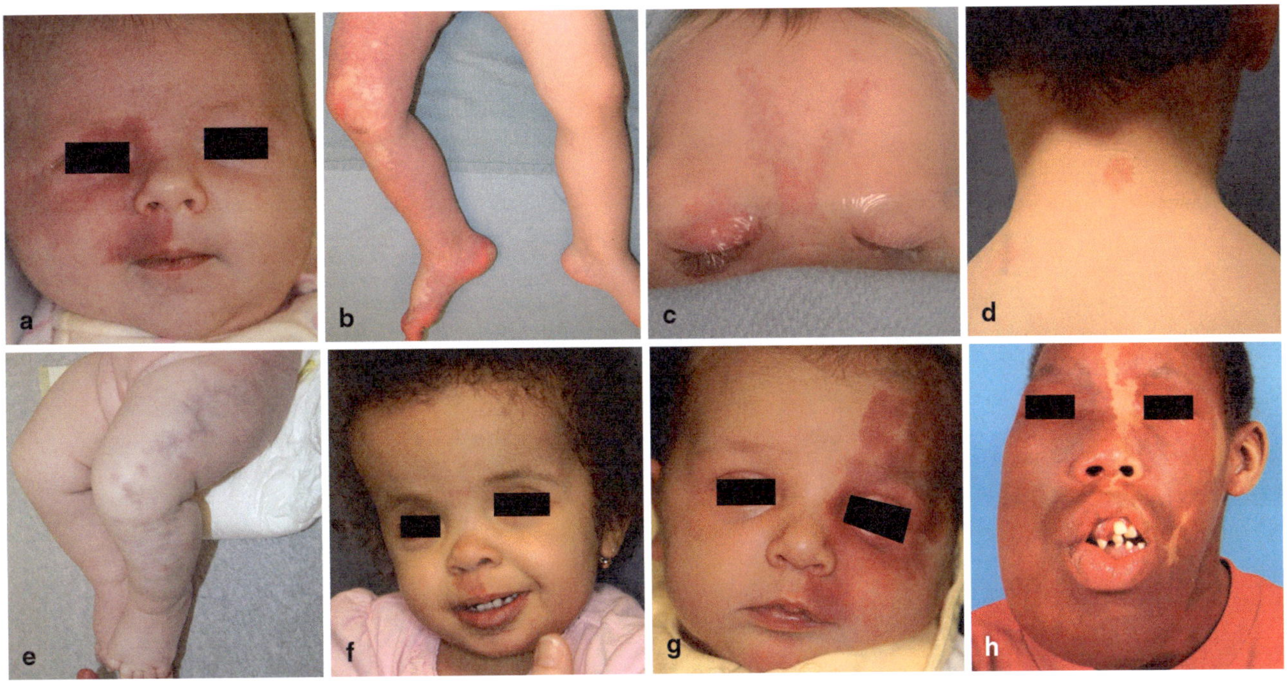

Fig. 9.2 Types of capillary malformation (CM). **a** 1-month-old girl with a sporadic CM. **b** Diffuse lower extremity CM with overgrowth in a 2-year-old boy. **c** Six-month-old boy with fading capillary stain of the forehead and right eyelid. **d** Three-year-old boy with a capillary malformation-arteriovenous malformation (CM-AVM) of the posterior neck exhibiting fast flow and a peripheral halo. **e** Three-month-old girl with cutis marmorata telangiectatica congenita (CMTC). Note the serpiginous and discolored craters of the left extremity. **f** Two-year-old girl with macrocephaly, frontal bossing, and CM of the philtrum—typical features of macrocephaly-capillary malformation (M-CM). **g** Two-week-old girl with Sturge-Weber syndrome. **h** Sixteen-year-old boy with Sturge-Weber syndrome showing soft-tissue and osseous overgrowth

Cutis Marmorata Telangiectatica Congenita

- A reticulated cutaneous stain that is unresponsive to warm temperatures, and becomes pronounced with low temperatures or crying [21].
- Usually involves the extremities; limb asymmetry is present in 33–68 % of patients [3, 21].
- Most infants show improvement during the first year of life, continuing into adolescence [22, 23].
- Atrophy, pigmentation, and ectasia of the superficial veins typically persist into adulthood.
- Associated with hypoplasia of the iliac and femoral veins [24].

Macrocephaly-Capillary Malformation

- A reticular CM, commonly on the face, associated with developmental delay and neurologic abnormalities [25].

Sturge-Weber Syndrome

- Consists of: (1) upper facial CM, (2) ocular abnormalities (e.g., glaucoma, choroidal vascular anomalies), and (3) leptomeningeal vascular malformation [26].
- Approximately 6–10 % of patients with a CM in the V1 distribution have SWS [27].
- Leptomeningeal vascular anomalies ipsilateral to the CM can cause seizures and developmental delay [26].

Differential Diagnosis for Capillary Malformations

Arteriovenous malformation (AVM)
Congenital hemangioma (CH)
Infantile hemangioma (IH)
Kaposiform hemangioendothelioma (KHE)
Lymphatic malformation (LM)
Venous malformation (VM)

Diagnosis and Evaluation

Physical Examination

Fading Capillary Stain

- Findings:
  - Macular red stain, which typically resolves by 2 years of age.
  - Usually located on the eyelids, glabella, nose, philtrum, and posterior neck; stains on the face normally fade, but those in the nuchal area may persist [3].

Capillary Malformation

- Findings:
  - CMs initially may have a bright pink, red, or violaceous color. Darkening and thickening occurs over time [2, 3].
  - Lesions are located in the extremity (43.9 %), head/neck (32.8 %), or trunk (23.3 %) [11].
  - Hand-held Doppler examination shows normal flow in CMs, while hemangiomas and arteriovenous malformations exhibit fast flow.

Capillary Malformation-Arteriovenous Malformation

- Findings:
  - Atypical CMs that are small, multifocal, and round; 50 % have a surrounding pale halo [10, 16].
  - Unlike nonsyndromic CMs, Doppler examination usually shows fast flow.
  - An enlarged extremity with an overlying CM may be PWS.

Cutis Marmorata Telangiectatica Congenita

- Findings:
  - The skin is depressed and has a purple, reticulated pattern.
  - The stain may be localized, segmental, or generalized.
  - Most frequently involves the extremities, is unilateral (65 %), and affects the lower limb (69 %) [21].

Macrocephaly-Capillary Malformation

- Findings:
  - Unlike CMTC, the cutaneous stain found in M-CM has a patchy pattern and does not ulcerate or fade [3, 28].
  - The vascular lesion is commonly located on the glabella, philtrum, or nose, but may also affect the extremities or trunk [3].

Sturge-Weber Syndrome

- Findings:
  - Facial CM with ocular abnormalities (e.g., glaucoma, choroidal vascular anomalies) and leptomeningeal vascular malformation [2, 26].
  - Refractory seizures, contralateral hemiplegia, and delayed motor and cognitive development may be observed in this condition.
  - Soft-tissue overgrowth is present in 55–70 % of patients: lip (28–64 %), cheek (14 %), and forehead (5–6 %) [2].
  - Skeletal hypertrophy affects 22–45 % of patients: mandible (6–17 %), maxilla (48–72 %), or both jaws (22–35 %) [2].
  - Patients with SWS can have extracraniofacial CM (29 %) and extremity hypertrophy (14 %) [2].

Laboratory Data

- *RASA1* gene testing confirms the diagnosis of CM-AVM. However, not all patients with CM-AVM clinically will have a *RASA1* mutation, suggesting that unknown mutations in *RASA1* or other genes may exist [16].

Imaging Evaluation

More than 90 % of CMs are diagnosed by history and physical examination; imaging is rarely necessary.

Ultrasonography (US):	Can be performed without sedation. CM-AVM may show fast flow.
Computed Tomography (CT):	May be used to assess osseous overgrowth.
Magnetic Resonance Imaging (MRI):	MRI of the brain and/or spine should be considered for patients with CM-AVM because they are at risk for intracranial and spinal fast-flow lesions [29]. MRI with gadolinium is the optimal study for SWS; patients have pial vascular enhancement, cerebral atrophy, and cortical calcifications [3].

Pathology

Histopathological diagnosis of CM is rarely necessary. In young children, the malformation shows dilated capillaries in the superficial dermis [30]. With increasing age, ectatic, venular-like vessels become more prominent in the papillary and reticular dermis [30]. Vessel size and density increase with age [4, 30]. CM-AVM shows large, tortuous arteries, and dilated, thick-walled veins (see Fig. 9.1) [30].

Treatment and Outcomes

Nonoperative Management

Drug therapy for CMs is not available. Abnormal periorbital and choroidal vascularity in patients with SWS can cause glaucoma, often leading to blindness [2]. Ophthalmologic examination should be performed every 6 months until the age of 2, and yearly thereafter [3].

Seventy-five percent of patients with SWS have seizures, which typically manifest during infancy [31]. Anticonvulsant therapy and regular neurology follow-up is necessary [31]. Neurosurgical intervention may be required for patients with severe seizures, drug therapy failures, or if antiepileptic medication is contraindicated [32].

Laser Therapy

Pulsed Dye Laser (PDL)

Originally developed for selective ablation of vascular lesions, PDL (595 nm wavelength) is the primary therapy for CM [3]. The laser penetrates 0.75–1.2 mm and thus deeper and larger vessels may not be affected. The settings used are 0.45–1.5 m/s pulse duration, 6–10 J/cm^2 fluence, and 7–10 mm spot size [3]. It is effective and has a low risk of scarring [3, 33–36]. Intervention with PDL during early childhood is recommended because: (1) superior lightening of the lesion is achieved [37, 38], (2) the risk of darkening and hypertrophy is reduced [37], and (3) psychosocial morbidity is minimized. Multiple treatments, 6 weeks apart, are often required until the CM fails to improve [3].

Approximately 15% of patients achieve 90% lightening, 65% improve 50–90%, and 20% respond poorly (see Fig. 9.2) [39]. Results are superior for smaller CMs and those treated at a younger age [37, 40]. PDL is less effective in large CMs with soft-tissue overgrowth [3]. Lesions on the head/neck region respond better than malformations located in the extremities [41–43]. Treatment response is inferior in Asian patients with facial CMs; only 14% demonstrate 50% or more lightening [44]. CMs often redarken following laser therapy [45]. Pigmentary alterations are more common in individuals with darker skin [44, 46]. Reactivation of herpes simplex virus [47], superinfection of molluscum contagiosum [48], and development of warts [49] can occur.

Long-Pulsed Nd:YAG (LP-Nd:YAG)

A laser with a wavelength of 1064 nm penetrates deeper into the dermis compared to the PDL [3]. It is the second-line therapy for CMs with large, deep vessels, and/or cutaneous thickening that do not respond to PDL [3, 50]. It has a greater risk for scarring compared to PDL [3].

Pulse Dye Laser (PDL) + Long-Pulsed Nd:YAG (LP-Nd:YAG)

This is a sequential dual wavelength system that delivers alternate pulses of 595 nm (PDL) and 1064 nm (LP-Nd:YAG) [43]. PDL converts oxy-hemoglobin to methemoglobin within the treated vessels [43]. Because methemoglobin has an absorption peak of approximately 1064 nm, the efficacy of LP-Nd:YAG is enhanced [43]. Indicated for PDL-resistant CMs [51, 52].

Alexandrite Laser

A wavelength of 755 nm, which has selectivity for deoxy- and oxy-hemoglobin, is used to treat vessels within the malformation [53]. It is effective for deep vessels within hypertrophic CMs [3]. It has a significant risk of edema, bullae, and scarring [3, 53].

Intense Pulsed Light (IPL)

A noncoherent light that allows the targeting of a broad range of vessel sizes within the malformation [54]. Although it is associated with reduced purpura and fewer complications than PDL, it is less effective [55, 56].

Photodynamic Therapy (PDT)

The topical or systemic administration of photosensitizing chromophores (e.g., hepatoporphyrin, benzoporphyrin, aminolavulinic acid) that accumulate in the endothelium of abnormal vessels within the CM. Photoreaction of these compounds produce oxygen radicals that cause endothelial injury and ablation of capillaries [3, 57]. The use of systemic photosensitizers followed by the exposure of copper vapor laser (wavelengths at 510 and 578 nm) seems effective [3, 57–59]. Topical aminolavulinic acid does not increase the efficiency of PDL in CMs [60].

Operative Management

Uncomplicated CMs usually do not require operative intervention. Surgical procedures are not typically indicated to remove the cutaneous stain, but to correct overgrowth caused by the malformation (e.g., pyogenic granuloma, fibrovascular nodules, soft-tissue/osseous hypertrophy; see Fig. 9.3). Because overgrowth is not present at birth, most patients do not require contouring until adolescence or adulthood. Patients

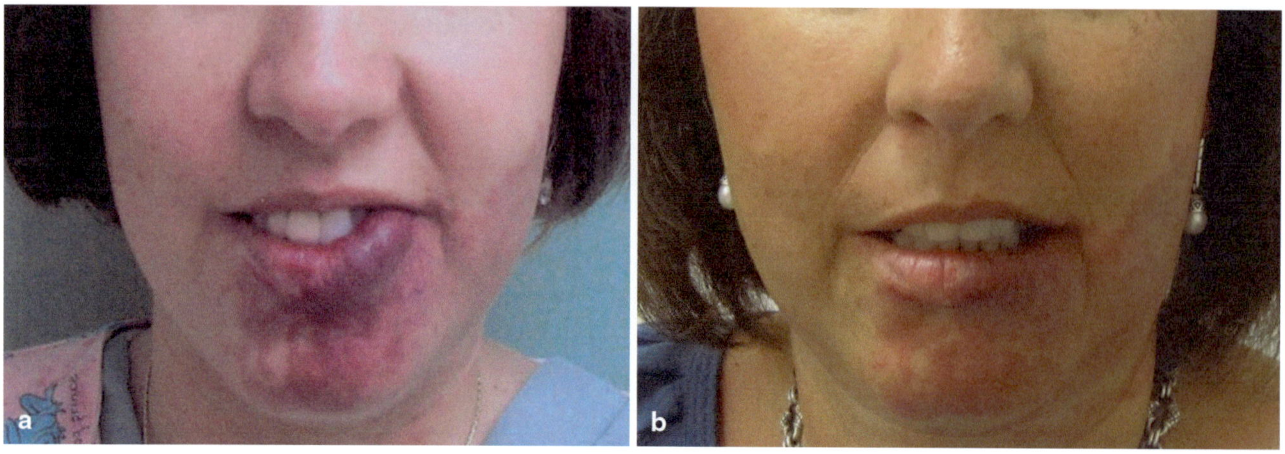

Fig. 9.3 Operative and pulse dye laser treatment of capillary malformation. **a** Forty-two-year-old woman with a capillary malformation of the lower lip and chin causing labial hypertrophy. **b** Improved contour after subtotal resection using a transverse mucosal incision. Note lightening of the chin lesion after pulse dye laser treatment

commonly undergo labial reduction (61 %), excision of localized cutaneous growth (33 %), malar reduction (11 %), palpebral debulking (11.0 %), and orthognatic correction (11 %) [2]. Severe cutaneous thickening and cobblestoning can be resected and reconstructed by linear closure, skin grafts, or local flaps. Malocclusion can be improved in adolescence with orthodontic management. If correction of occlusion cannot be achieved with orthodontics, an orthognatic procedure is considered after completion of skeletal growth. Le Fort 1 osteotomy or a bimaxillary procedure may be necessary [2]. Facial asymmetry caused by overgrowth of the zygoma, maxilla, or mandible can be improved by contour burring [2]. Trunk or extremity CM can be associated with increased subcutaneous adipose tissue. Suction-assisted lipectomy can reduce the deformity while avoiding a long incision.

References

1. Jacobs AH, Walton RG. The incidence of birthmarks in the neonate. Pediatrics. 1976;58:218–22.
2. Greene AK, Taber SF, Ball KL, et al. Sturge-Weber syndrome: soft-tissue and skeletal overgrowth. J Craniofac Surg. 2009;20 (Suppl 1):617–21.
3. Maguiness SM, Liang MG. Management of capillary malformations. Clin Plast Surg. 2011;38(1):65–73.
4. Barsky SH, Rosen S, Geer DE, et al. The nature and evolution of port-wine stains: a computer-assisted study. J Invest Dermatol. 1980;74:154–7.
5. Finley JL, Noe JM, Arndt KA, et al. Port-wine stains: morphologic variations and developmental lesions. Arch Dermatol. 1984;120:1453–5.
6. Smoller BS, Rosen S. Port-wine stain: a disease of altered neural modulation of blood vessels? Arch Dermatol. 1986;122:177–9.
7. Rydh M, Malm M, Jernbeck J, et al. Ectatic blood vessels in port wine stains lack innervation: possible role in pathogenesis. Plast Reconstr Surg. 1991;87:419–22.
8. Del Pozo J, Pazos JM, Fonseca E. Lower lip hypertrophy secondary to port-wine stain: combined surgical and carbon dioxide laser treatment. Dermatol Surg. 2004;30:211–4.
9. Sanchez-Carpintero I, Mihm MC, Mizeracki A, et al. Epithelial and mesenchymal hamartomatous changes in a mature port-wine stain: morphologic evidence for a multiple germ layer field defect. J Am Acad Dermatol. 2004;50:608–12.
10. Eerola I, Boon LM, Mulliken JB, et al. Capillary malformation-arteriovenous malformation: a new clinical and genetic disorder caused by RASA1 mutations. Am J Hum Genet. 2003;73:1240–9.
11. Greene AK, Liu As, Mulliken JB, et al. Vascular anomalies: 5621 patients: guidelines for referral. J Peadiatr Surg. 2011;46(9):1784–9.
12. Sturge WA. A case of partial epilepsy apparently due to a lesion of one of the motor centers of the brain. Trans Clin Soc London. 1879;12:112.
13. Parkes-Weber F. Right sided hemihypertrophy resulting from right-sided congenital spastic hemiplegia with a morbid condition of the left side of the brain revealed by radiogram. J Neurol Neurosurg Psychiatry. 1922;37:301–11.
14. Thomas-Sohl KA, Vaslow DF, Maria BL. Sturge Weber syndrome. J Child Neurol. 2003;30:303–10.
15. Tan WH, Baris HN, Burrows PE, et al. The spectrum of vascular anomalies in patients with PTEN mutations: implications for diagnosis and management. J Med Genet. 2007;44:594–602.
16. Revencu N, Boon LM, Vikkula M. From germline towards somatic mutations in the pathophysiology of vascular anomalies. Hum Mol Genet. 2009;18:65–75.
17. Mulliken JB, Fishman SJ, Burrows PE. Vascular anomalies. Curr Probl Surg. 2000;37:517–84.
18. Mills CM, Cooper PH, Fechner RE. Lobular capillary hemangioma: the underlying lesion of pyogenic granuloma. Am J Surg Pathol. 1980;4:471–9.
19. Klapman MH, Yao JF. Thickening and nodules in port-wine stains. J Am Acad Dermatol. 2001;44:300–2.
20. Sheehan DJ, Lesher JL. Pyogenic granulomas arising within port wine stain. Cutis. 2004;73:175–80.
21. Amitai DB, Fichman S, Merlob P, et al. Cutis marmorata telangiectatica congenita: clinical findings in 85 patients. Pediatr Dermatol. 2000;17:100–4.
22. Mulliken JB, Young A. Vascular Birthmarks: hemangiomas and malformations. Philadelphia:Saunders; 1988.

23. Devillers AC, de Waard-van der Spek FB, Oranje AP. Cutis marmorata telangiectatica congenita: clinical features in 35 cases. Arch Dermatol. 1999;135:34–8.
24. Morgan JM, Naisby GP, Carmichael AJ. Cutis marmorata telangiectatica congenita with hypoplasia of the right iliac and femoral veins. Br J Dermatol. 1997;137:119–22.
25. Moore CA, Toriello HV, Abuelo DN, et al. Macrocephaly-cutis marmorata telangiectatica congenita: a distinct disorder with developmental delay and connective tissue abnormalities. Am J Med Genet. 1997;70:67–73.
26. Comi AM. Pathophysiology of Sturge-Weber syndrome. J Child Neurol. 2003;18:509–16.
27. Tallman B, Tan OT, Morelli JG, et al. Location of port-wine stains and the likelihood of ophthalmic and/or central nervous system complications. Pediatrics. 1991;87:323–7.
28. Toriello HV, Mulliken JB. Accurately renaming macrocephaly-cutis marmorata telangiectatica congenital (M-CMTC) as macrocephaly-capillary malformation (M-CM). Am J Med Gen. 2007;143A:3009.
29. Greene AK, Orbach DB. Management of arteriovenous malformations. Clin Plast Surg. 2011;38(1):95–106.
30. Gupta A, Kozakewich H. Histopathology of vascular anomalies. Clin Plast Surg. 2011;38(1):31–44.
31. Comi AM. Sturge-Weber syndrome and epilepsy: an argument for aggressive seizure management in these patients. Expert Rev Neurother. 2007;7:951–6.
32. Bourgeois M, Crimmins DW, de Oliveira RS, et al. Surgical treatment of epilepsy in Sturge-Weber syndrome in children. J Neurosurg. 2007;106(Suppl 1):20–8.
33. Tan E, Vinciullo C. Pulsed dye laser treatment of port-wine stains: a review of patients treated in Western Australia. Med J Aust. 1996;164:333–6.
34. Wimmershoff MB, Wenig M, Hohenleutner U, et al. Treatment of port-wine stains with the flash lamp pumped dye laser. 5 years of clinical experience. Hautarzt. 2001;52(11):1011–5.
35. Lam SM, Williams EF. Practical considerations in the treatment of capillary vascular malformations, or port wine stains. Facial Plast Surg. 2004;20(1):71–6.
36. Cordisco MR. An update on lasers in children. Curr Opin Pediatr. 2009;21(4):499–504.
37. Chapas AM, Eickhorst K, Geronemus RG. Efficacy of early treatment of facial port wine stains in newborns: a review of 49 cases. Lasers Surg Med. 2007;39(7):563–8.
38. Minkis K, Geronemus RG, Hale EK. Port wine stain progression: a potential consequence of delayed and inadequate treatment? Lasers Surg Med. 2009;41(6):423–6.
39. Astner S, Anderson RR: Treating vascular lesions. Dermatol Ther. 2005;18:267–81.
40. Stier MF, Glick SA, Hirsch RJ. Laser treatment of pediatric vascular lesions: port wine stains and hemangiomas. J Am Acad Dermatol. 2008;58:261–85.
41. Tan OT, Sherwood K, Gilchrest BA. Treatment of children with port-wine stains using the flashlamp-pulsed tunable dye laser. N Engl J Med. 1989;320:416–21.
42. van der Horst CM, Koster PH, de Borgie CA, et al. Effect of the timing of treatment of port-wine stains with the flash-lamp-pumped pulsed-dye laser. N Engl J Med. 1998;338(15):1028–33.
43. Jasim ZF, Handley JM. Treatment of pulsed dye laser-resistant port wine stain birthmarks. J Am Acad Dermatol. 2007;57(4):677–82.
44. Chan HH, Chan E, Kono T, et al. The use of variable pulse width frequency doubled Nd:YAG 532 nm laser in the treatment of port-wine stain in Chinese patients. Dermatol Surg. 2000;26:657–61.
45. Huikeshoven M, Koster PH, de Borgie CA, et al. Redarkening of port-wine stains 10 years after pulsed-dye-laser treatment. N Engl J Med. 2007;356:1235–40.
46. Sommer S, Sheehan-Dare RA. Pulsed dye laser treatment of port-wine stains in pigmented skin. J Am Acad Dermatol. 2000;42:667–71.
47. Owens WW, Lang PG. Herpes simplex infection and colonization with Pseudomonas aeruginosa complicating pulsed-dye laser treatment. Arch Dermatol. 2004;140(6):760–1.
48. Strauss RM, Sheehan-Dare R. Local molluscum contagiosum infection as a side-effect of pulsed-dye laser treatment. Br J Dermatol. 2004;150(5):1047–9.
49. Chen T, Frieden IJ. Development of extensive flat warts after pulsed dye laser treatment of a port-wine stain. Dermatol Surg. 2007;33(6):734–5.
50. Yang MU, Yaroslavsky AN, Farinelli WA, et al. Long-pulsed neodymium:yttrium-aluminum-garnet laser treatment for port-wine stains. J Am Acad Dermatol. 2005;52(3 Pt 1):480–90.
51. Alster TS, Tanzi EL. Combined 595-nm and 1,064-nm laser irradiation of recalcitrant and hypertrophic port-wine stains in children and adults. Dermatol Surg. 2009;35(6):914–8.
52. Borges da Costa J, Boixeda P, Moreno C, et al. Treatment of resistant port-wine stains with a pulsed dual wavelength 595 and 1064 nm laser: a histochemical evaluation of the vessel wall destruction and selectivity. Photomed Laser Surg. 2009;27(4):599–605.
53. Izikson L, Nelson JS, Anderson RR. Treatment of hypertrophic and resistant port wine stains with a 755 nm laser: a case series of 20 patients. Lasers Surg Med. 2009;41(6):427–32.
54. Bjerring P, Christiansen K, Troilius A. Intense pulsed light source for the treatment of dye laser resistant port-wine stains. J Cosmet Laser Ther. 2003;5(1):7–13.
55. Ho WS, Ying SY, Chan PC, et al. Treatment of port wine stains with intense pulsed light: a prospective study. Dermatol Surg. 2004;30(6):887–90.
56. Faurschou A, Togsverd-Bo K, Zachariae C, et al. Pulsed dye laser vs. intense pulsed light for port-wine stains: a randomized side-by-side trial with blinded response evaluation. Br J Dermatol. 2009;160(2):359–64.
57. Yuan K, Li Q, Yu W, et al. Photodynamic therapy in treatment of port wine stain birthmarks—recent progress. Photodiagnosis Photodyn Ther. 2009;6(3–4):189–94.
58. Gu Y, Huang NY, Liang J, et al. Clinical study of 1949 cases of port wine stains treated with vascular photodynamic therapy (Gu's PDT). Ann Dermatol Venereol. 2007;134(3 Pt 1):241–4.
59. Yuan K, Li Q, Yu W, et al. Comparison of photodynamic therapy and pulsed dye laser in patients with port wine stain birthmarks: a retrospective analysis. Photodiagnosis Photodyn Ther. 2008;5(1):50–7.
60. Evans AV, Robson A, Barlow RJ, et al. Treatment of port wine stains with photodynamic therapy, using pulsed dye laser as a light source, compared with pulsed dye laser alone: a pilot study. Lasers Surg Med. 2005;36(4):266–9.

10 Carcinoma/Undifferentiated Tumor

Jennifer W. Mack

Introduction

Squamous cell carcinomas of the head and neck, including carcinomas of the lip, oral cavity, oropharynx, hypopharynx, larynx, and sinus, are common malignancies among adults, often associated with tobacco and alcohol use. However, these tumors are exceedingly rare in children. When they do occur in the pediatric age group, predisposing factors such as Fanconi anemia must be considered. Outcomes appear similar to those in adults, and the mainstay of treatment is aggressive local control, with chemotherapy reserved for special pathologic risk factors and advanced disease.

Key Points

- Squamous cell carcinomas of the head and neck are rare in children, and management, therefore, relies on established treatment strategies in adults.
- Early-stage disease can generally be treated with either surgery or radiation; choice of modality depends on resectability as well as expected functional outcome.
- For patients with advanced disease, chemotherapy improves outcomes over local control alone.
- Especially after radiation therapy, children tend to experience significant acute toxicity and late effects.

J. W. Mack (✉)
Dana-Farber Cancer Institute, Boston, MA, USA

Department of Pediatric Hematology/Oncology, Boston Children's Hospital, Harvard Medical School, Boston, MA, USA
e-mail: Jennifer_mack@dfci.harvard.edu

Biology and Epidemiology

Squamous cell carcinomas originate in the squamous epithelium that lines the mucosal surfaces of the head and neck. They are classified according to the organ of origination. Oral cavity cancer originates from the lips, anterior two-thirds of the tongue, the buccal and gingival mucosae, the floor of the mouth, and the hard palate. Oropharygeal cancer arises from the soft palate, base of tongue, and tonsils. Additional anatomic locations include the hypopharynx, the larynx, the paranasal sinuses, and the nasal cavity.

Adult squamous cell carcinomas are relatively common, accounting for about 3 % of all cancers in the USA or about 50,000 new incident cancers per year [1], and are frequently associated with smoking and alcohol use. However, these tumors are extremely rare in children. Their presence in childhood should raise the question of predisposing factors. DNA repair defects such as Fanconi anemia [2], Bloom syndrome, ataxia telangiectasia, and dyskeratosis congenita should be considered, as well as xeroderma pigmentosum [3–5]. Even children without characteristic morphologic features of Fanconi anemia should have consideration of appropriate testing, given the frequent use of radiation in treatment of head and neck tumors, and its potential toxicity in this disease [2]. In addition, Li-Fraumeni syndrome, an inherited defect of *TP53*, is associated with squamous cell carcinomas of the larynx [3, 5]. A careful family history may be suggestive, but because not all affected patients have a positive family history, genetic testing may be indicated.

Aside from genetic factors, pediatric cancer survivors, especially those with a history of prior irradiation of the head and neck, are also at risk for developing squamous cell cancers [6]. Oral carcinomas have also been noted in patients with a history of allogeneic bone marrow transplantation and oral graft-versus-host disease [7–9], in which chronic mucosal injury and repair may create a cycle not unlike that seen in adult users of tobacco.

In addition, the human papilloma virus (HPV) has been implicated in squamous cell carcinomas [10, 11], especially

R. Rahbar et al. (eds.), *Pediatric Head and Neck Tumors*,
DOI 10.1007/978-1-4614-8755-5_10, © Springer Science+Business Media New York 2014

oropharyngeal cancers originating from the tonsils and base of tongue. HPV-16 appears to be the subtype that is most commonly involved and is believed to have a role in oncogenesis [10, 11]. The incidence of HPV-associated oropharyngeal cancers is increasing [12], although increasing vaccination rates of children may halt that rise in young people. The existence of HPV infection confers a favorable prognosis and may therefore have implications for treatment [13].

Finally, midline carcinomas with the BRD-NUT translocation t(15;19) have been described in young people and tend to have a highly aggressive course (see also the chapter on nasopharyngeal carcinomas) [14, 15]. Consideration of this entity and evaluation for the translocation should take place in children with midline squamous cell carcinomas.

Presentation

Signs and symptoms of squamous cell carcinomas of the head and neck depend on the tissue of origination. However, oral lesions frequently present as a nonhealing mucosal ulcer, pain or bleeding in the mouth, or mucosal erythema or leukoplakia (Fig. 10.1a). Pharyngeal and laryngeal lesions may present as dysphagia, otalgia, or hoarseness. Nasal and sinonasal lesions commonly present as nasal obstruction, epistaxis, rhinorrhea, chronic sinusitis, or headaches. In addition, a solitary neck mass or bilateral cervical enlargement, evident because of involved regional lymph nodes, is a common presentation with each of these cancers.

Diagnosis and Evaluation

Unfortunately, because of the rarity of these tumors in children, it is not uncommon for patients to come to attention after incomplete resection of what was felt to be a benign lesion. However, such procedures can create greater challenges for local control in the future, and initial resection through tumor is associated with a poorer prognosis [16]. Therefore, whenever possible, initial nasal or oral endoscopy can offer opportunity for biopsy under direct visualization. Careful examination can also help to define the extent of disease. If necessary, the diagnosis can also be made using biopsy of involved cervical lymph nodes in the presence of an identified mucosal lesion.

Imaging studies should include visualization of the primary tumor and nodal areas, including anterior cervical, posterior cervical, and retropharyngeal nodes. Both head and neck magnetic resonance imaging (MRI), for optimal soft tissue involvement, and computed tomography (CT), for evaluation of bony structures and identification of tumor erosion into bones, are indicated. A positron emission tomography (PET) scan should be performed to evaluate for regional and distant disease, and can help to identify involved lymph nodes, although reactive lymph nodes can also be PET positive, so interpretation of results often involves clinical correlation. Finally, evaluation for distant

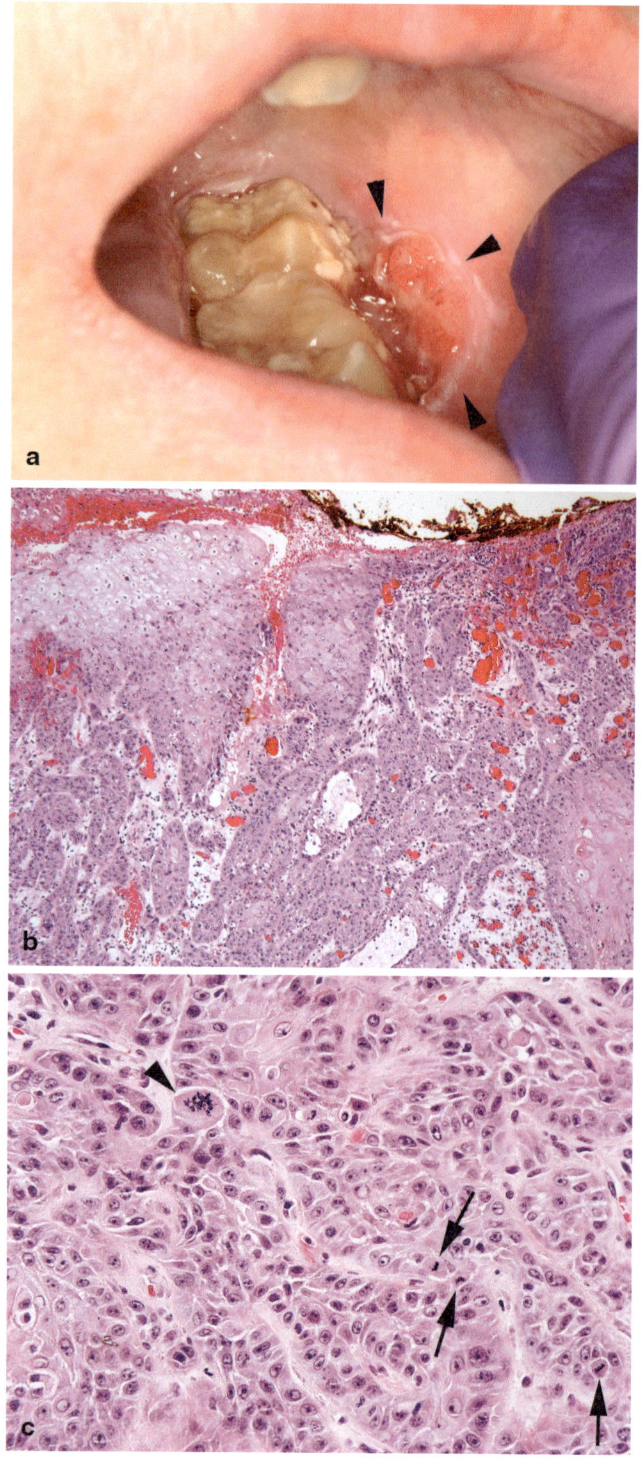

Fig. 10.1 Squamous cell carcinoma of the oral cavity. **a** Large ulceration of the gum (*between arrowheads*) with friable, necrotic surface. Posterior molars are seen to the left of the ulcer. **b** Infiltrating moderately well-differentiated squamous cell carcinoma with ulcerated surface. **c** Nests of pleomorphic, moderately differentiated squamous cells with numerous mitoses (*arrows*), some of them atypical (*arrowhead*)

disease at diagnosis should include a chest CT scan for pulmonary metastases.

Squamous cell carcinomas of the head and neck can be classified pathologically according to the Broder classification [17], which relies on differentiation:

G1 well differentiated
G2 moderately well differentiated
G3 poorly differentiated
G4 undifferentiated

Most squamous cell carcinomas are moderately or poorly differentiated (Fig. 10.1b, c); differentiation is not, however, predictive of survival [18, 19]. Pathology should also be evaluated for lymphovascular and perineural invasion as well as extracapsular lymph node spread, which are predictive of outcomes and response to therapy [20].

Staging of squamous cell carcinomas of the head and neck involves the American Joint Committe on Cancer (AJCC) staging system [21], which predicts clinical outcomes and guides therapy. Each anatomic site has a unique staging system based on the extent of the primary tumor, involvement of regional lymph nodes, and distant metastases. We provide here staging for oral cavity cancer as an illustrative example, but staging should always be based on current AJCC staging for the primary site of origin (Tables 10.1 and 10.2).

In general for squamous cell carcinomas of the head and neck, early-stage cancers are those designated as stages I and II. These tumors are small in size without deep invasion of surrounding structures, and without regional lymph node involvement or distant metastases. Advanced tumors, which are stage III and IV tumors, have significant local invasion, regional lymph nodes, and/or distant metastases. Early-stage and advanced tumors are distinct prognostically and require different treatment modalities.

Table 10.1 AJCC staging system for oral cavity squamous cell carcinoma

Value	Definition
Primary tumor (T)	
T1	Tumor 2 cm or less in greatest dimension
T2	Tumor more than 2 cm but not more than 4 cm in greatest dimension
T3	Tumor more than 4 cm in greatest dimension
T4a	Moderately advanced local disease Lip: Tumor invades through cortical bone, inferior alveolar nerve, floor of mouth, or skin of face, that is, chin or nose Oral cavity: Tumor invades adjacent structures only
T4b	Very advanced local disease Tumor invades masticator space, pterygoid plates, or skull base, and/or encases internal carotid artery
Regional lymph nodes (N)	
N0	No regional lymph node metastasis
N1	Metastasis in a single ipsilateral lymph node, 3 cm or less in greatest dimension
N2	Metastasis in a single ipsilateral lymph node, 3–6 cm in greatest dimension; or in multiple ipsilateral lymph nodes, none more than 6 cm in greatest dimension; or in bilateral or contralateral lymph nodes, none more than 6 cm in greatest dimension
N3	Metastasis in a lymph node >6 cm in greatest dimension
Distant metastasis (M)	
M0	No distant metastasis
M1	Distant metastasis

Table 10.2 Summary staging for oral cavity cancer

Stage	T stage	N stage	M stage
Stage I	T1	N0	M0
Stage II	T2	N0	M0
Stage III	T3	N0	M0
	T1-3	N1	M0
Stage IVA	T4a	N0-1	M0
	T1-4a	N2	M0
Stage IVB	T1-4a	N3	M0
	T4b	N0-3	M0
Stage IVC	Any T	Any N	M1

Treatment

Overview

Because of the rarity of these cancers in children and the consequent lack of clinical trials, treatment is largely based on adult regimens. This is supported by small series demonstrating similar outcomes in pediatric and adult patients with oral and tongue carcinomas [22, 23], although data in the pediatric setting remain quite limited. Special consideration should be taken of the consequences of aggressive surgery and radiation in children.

Approximately one-third of adult patients present with early-stage (stages I and II) squamous cell carcinomas, and aggressive local control confers excellent survival for most early-stage patients. Use of either surgery or radiation, depending on the resectability of the lesion, is usually sufficient. Treatment modality, including choice of radiation or surgery for local control, should be determined for each patient on an individual basis. Thus, careful discussion with a multidisciplinary team including otorhinolaryngology, oncology, and radiation oncology can offer optimal planning for individual patients before local control is attempted. When high-risk features are found at resection, adjuvant radiation or chemoradiation is recommended.

In contrast, patients with advanced (stage III and IV) disease usually require combined modality therapy, including aggressive local control and systemic chemotherapy, although the optimal sequence of these modalities is not known.

Early-Stage Disease

Because both surgery and radiation can offer excellent cancer control, primary considerations include whether surgical local control is possible and whether surgery or radiation will provide a better functional outcome. In the adult setting, surgery is often the modality of choice for early-stage disease at most anatomic sites. Surgery requires wide local excision [24]; positive margins require re-resection or postoperative radiotherapy. Thus, surgical resection should be attempted only for lesions that are deemed to be resectable with wide margins. For lesions that invade the skull base, for example, radiation alone should be considered, because even an aggressive resection is not expected to obviate the need for radiation. Frozen sections may be used intraoperatively to ensure adequacy of surgical margins.

Even in patients with a clinically negative neck, neck dissection should be considered [25]. Evaluation of the neck helps to determine the extent of disease for consideration of adjuvant radiation or chemoradiotherapy. Typically ipsilateral dissection is adequate in the absence of clinical concerns; however, midline lesions such as those in the palate, base of tongue, and supraglottic larynx may require bilateral dissection, given the high risk of bilateral lymphatic drainage. In addition, lesions of the anterior tongue and floor of mouth require evaluation of the submandibular glands. For oral cavity cancers, the depth of invasion predicts nodal involvement; thus, neck dissection should be considered for lesions with a depth of greater than 4 mm [26]. Any clinically involved nodes should be removed, with bilateral dissections for patients with clinically significant bilateral nodes.

Although surgery is the treatment of choice for many patients with resectable limited-stage disease, patients with laryngeal carcinoma benefit from radiation, which offers the prospect of voice preservation [27]. Similarly, radiation may provide the optimal functional outcome for patients with oropharyngeal cancers at the base of tongue or tonsils. Finally, patients with nasal or sinonasal tumors frequently require postoperative radiation, given high rates of local recurrence with resection alone, except in the smallest (T1) lesions.

For children, the balance of risks and benefits of surgery and radiation is complicated by added pediatric toxicity of radiation, which impairs bony growth for children who are not fully mature, and which confers a lifetime second tumor risk that is magnified over the long hoped-for lifetime of these young patients. The use of proton beam radiotherapy has been proposed as one way to mitigate these risks, but it is not widely available, and the extent to which it mitigates these risks is not known.

Finally, even patients with disease defined preoperatively as early stage may benefit from adjuvant therapy. Postoperative chemoradiotherapy is recommended for adult patients with extracapsular nodal spread or positive surgical margins [20]. Given the morbidity of radiation in children, surgical re-resection could be considered as an alternative strategy for positive margins if a complete resection is deemed possible. In addition, even if lesions are fully resected, histopathologic features including perineural or vascular invasion, or the presence of multiple positive lymph nodes, portend a high risk for recurrence. Thus, postoperative radiation is generally indicated for such patients [20].

Advanced Disease

For patients with advanced disease, three basic strategies have been used: up-front chemoradiotherapy; initial surgery with adjuvant radiation or chemoradiation when indicated, as recommended for early-stage disease; or induction chemotherapy followed by radiation or chemoradiation. To date, no single strategy has been defined as superior [28]; however, concurrent chemotherapy and radiation are generally recommended for most patients. Cisplatin (100 mg/m^2 every 3 weeks concurrent with radiation) offers a modest increase in disease-free survival among patients with locally advanced disease over radiation alone [29, 30]. However, results have been mixed as to whether this regimen improves overall survival, and it comes with a cost of significant toxicity, particularly oral mucositis. Other chemoradiotherapy regimens have been used, including carboplatin/5-fluorouracil [31], cisplatin/paclitaxel [32], and carboplatin/paclitaxel [33], but without clear improvements over cisplatin alone. Cetuximab, which is an IgG1 antibody against the ligand-binding domain of the epidermal growth factor receptor (EGFR), has also been used concurrent with radiation to enhance its cytotoxic effects. An early trial demonstrated survival gain over radiation alone, but without clear improvements over historical findings with cisplatin [34, 35].

Others have advocated for induction chemotherapy followed by radiotherapy or chemoradiotherapy for patients with advanced disease [36, 37]. Neoadjuvant chemotherapy has been proposed as a way to reduce distant metastases as a cause of treatment failure, but results have been mixed, and a reduction in distant recurrence has not been definitively demonstrated. In addition, patients experience significant mucosal toxicity when chemotherapy precedes head and neck radiation. However, because neoadjuvant chemotherapy can offer tumor reduction prior to local control and quick institution of therapy while surgical and radiation planning are underway, it may offer practical benefits to the care of some patients. Regimens are cisplatin based and have included cisplatin/docetaxel/5-fluorouracil [36, 37] or cisplatin/paclitaxel/5-fluorouracil [38]. Following induction chemotherapy, radiotherapy can be used alone or in conjunction with agents such as weekly cetuximab or carboplatin.

Patients with Distant Metastases

Finally, for patients with distant disease, chemotherapy can be used to attempt systemic control, although prognoses remain poor [39]. Therefore, in the adult oncology setting, treatment for metastatic disease usually begins with chemotherapy only, with radiation offered for palliative purposes if local disease is causing significant symptoms. Because of the rarity of this disease in children and the lack of full knowledge about outcomes, it may be appropriate to treat metastatic disease aggressively, with initial chemotherapy and, depending on the systemic response, consideration of aggressive local control with curative intent for those who have responded. Nonetheless, cure of systemic disease is likely to be uncommon in children, just as it is in adults, so evidence of poorly responsive disease merits reconsideration of the aggressiveness of therapy.

Supportive Care

Particularly for patients who will receive chemoradiotherapy, acute toxicity of treatment can be significant, marked by profound mucositis. For patients who present with significant weight loss or swallowing dysfunction, or for patients whose radiation plan involves a large field of mucosa with anticipated significant mucositis, prophylactic gastrostomy tube placement is recommended. Even without these risk factors, close nutritional follow-up and support may be beneficial.

In addition, assessment of speech and swallowing is indicated for patients who either present with deficits or who are expected to have deficits following local control. A careful dental examination prior to therapy also offers the opportunity to treat caries and improve hygiene in mucosal areas that may be compromised during treatment. Finally, patients who develop significant mucositis should have aggressive pain control, as mucosal healing can take weeks or even months after radiation and especially after chemoradiation.

Late Effects

Treatment can have significant long-term effects, especially for children who receive radiation. These include endocrine effects, such as hypothyroidism in children who receive neck irradiation and hypopituitarism in children who receive radiation to the skull base; xerostomia and dental caries after salivary gland radiation; impaired bony growth; swallowing dysfunction and esophageal strictures; speech impairment; and a risk for secondary malignancies in the radiation field. Thus, careful long-term follow-up is indicated for these patients.

References

1. National Cancer Institute: Cancer Statistics. 2012. http://seer.cancer.gov/statfacts/html/lungb.html. Accessed 23 Mar 2012.
2. Kutler DI, et al. High incidence of head and neck squamous cell carcinoma in patients with Fanconi anemia. Arch Otolaryngol Head Neck Surg. 2003;129(1):106–12.
3. Trizna Z, Schantz SP. Hereditary and environmental factors associated with risk and progression of head and neck cancer. Otolaryngol Clin North Am. 1992;25(5):1089–103.
4. Jefferies S, et al. The role of genetic factors in predisposition to squamous cell cancer of the head and neck. Br J Cancer. 1999;79(5–6):865–7.
5. Baez A. Genetic and environmental factors in head and neck cancer genesis. J Environ Sci Health C Environ Carcinog Ecotoxicol Rev. 2008;26(2):174–200.
6. Bassal M, et al. Risk of selected subsequent carcinomas in survivors of childhood cancer: a report from the Childhood Cancer Survivor Study. J Clin Oncol. 2006;24(3):476–83.
7. Szeto CH, et al., Squamous cell carcinoma of the tongue complicating chronic oral mucosal graft-versus-host disease after allogeneic hematopoietic stem cell transplantation. Am J Hematol. 2004;77(2):200–2.
8. Montebugnoli L, et al. Multiple squamous cell carcinomas of the oral cavity in a young patient with graft-versus-host disease following allogenic bone marrow transplantation. Int J Oral Maxillofac Surg. 2011;40(5):556–8.
9. Mawardi H, et al. Oral epithelial dysplasia and squamous cell carcinoma following allogeneic hematopoietic stem cell transplantation: clinical presentation and treatment outcomes. Bone Marrow Transplant. 2011;46(6):884–91.
10. Mork J, et al. Human papillomavirus infection as a risk factor for squamous-cell carcinoma of the head and neck. N Engl J Med. 2001;344(15):1125–31.
11. Mineta H, et al. Human papilloma virus (HPV) type 16 and 18 detected in head and neck squamous cell carcinoma. Anticancer Res. 1998;18(6B):4765–8.
12. Jemal A, et al. Annual report to the nation on the status of cancer, 1975–2009, featuring the burden and trends in human papillomavirus (HPV)-associated cancers and HPV vaccination coverage levels. J Natl Cancer Inst. 2013;105(3):175–201.
13. Licitra L, et al. High-risk human papillomavirus affects prognosis in patients with surgically treated oropharyngeal squamous cell carcinoma. J Clin Oncol. 2006;24(36):5630–6.
14. Vargas SO, et al. Upper respiratory tract carcinoma with chromosomal translocation 15;19: evidence for a distinct disease entity of young patients with a rapidly fatal course. Cancer. 2001;92(5):1195–203.
15. French CA, et al. BRD4 bromodomain gene rearrangement in aggressive carcinoma with translocation t(15;19). Am J Pathol. 2001;159(6):1987–92.
16. Scholl P, et al. Microscopic cut-through of cancer in the surgical treatment of squamous carcinoma of the tongue. Prognostic and therapeutic implications. Am J Surg. 1986;152(4):354–60.
17. Bansberg SF, Olsen KD, Gaffey TA. High-grade carcinoma of the oral cavity. Otolaryngol Head Neck Surg. 1989;100(1):41–8.
18. Bachar G, et al. Outcome of oral tongue squamous cell carcinoma in patients with and without known risk factors. Oral Oncol. 2011;47(1):45–50.
19. Janot F, et al. Prognostic value of clinicopathological parameters in head and neck squamous cell carcinoma: a prospective analysis. Br J Cancer. 1996;73(4):531–8.
20. Bernier J. et al. Defining risk levels in locally advanced head and neck cancers: a comparative analysis of concurrent postoperative radiation plus chemotherapy trials of the EORTC (#22931) and RTOG (# 9501). Head Neck. 2005;27(10):843–50.

21. Edge SB, et al., editors. AJCC Cancer Staging Manual. 7th ed. New York: Springer; 2010.
22. Morris LG, et al. Squamous cell carcinoma of the oral tongue in the pediatric age group: a matched-pair analysis of survival. Arch Otolaryngol Head Neck Surg. 2010;136(7):697–701.
23. Morris LG, Ganly I. Outcomes of oral cavity squamous cell carcinoma in pediatric patients. Oral Oncol. 2010;46(4):292–6.
24. Looser KG, Shah JP, Strong EW The significance of "positive" margins in surgically resected epidermoid carcinomas. Head Neck Surg. 1978;1(2):107–11.
25. Ferlito A, et al. Elective and therapeutic selective neck dissection. Oral Oncol. 2006;42(1):14–25.
26. Melchers LJ, et al. Tumour infiltration depth ≥ 4 mm is an indication for an elective neck dissection in pT1cN0 oral squamous cell carcinoma. Oral Oncol. 2012;48(4):337–42.
27. Forastiere AA, et al. Concurrent chemotherapy and radiotherapy for organ preservation in advanced laryngeal cancer. N Engl J Med. 2003;349(22):2091–8.
28. Haddad R, et al. Induction chemotherapy followed by concurrent chemoradiotherapy (sequential chemoradiotherapy) versus concurrent chemoradiotherapy alone in locally advanced head and neck cancer (PARADIGM): a randomised phase 3 trial. Lancet Oncol. 2013;14(3):257–64.
29. Bernier J, et al. Postoperative irradiation with or without concomitant chemotherapy for locally advanced head and neck cancer. N Engl J Med. 2004;350(19):1945–52.
30. Cooper JS, et al. Postoperative concurrent radiotherapy and chemotherapy for high-risk squamous-cell carcinoma of the head and neck. N Engl J Med. 2004;350(19):1937–44.
31. Denis F, et al. Final results of the 94–01 French Head and Neck Oncology and Radiotherapy Group randomized trial comparing radiotherapy alone with concomitant radiochemotherapy in advanced-stage oropharynx carcinoma. J Clin Oncol. 2004;22(1):69–76.
32. Garden AS, et al. Preliminary results of Radiation Therapy Oncology Group 97–03: a randomized phase ii trial of concurrent radiation and chemotherapy for advanced squamous cell carcinomas of the head and neck. J Clin Oncol. 2004;22(14):2856–64.
33. Suntharalingam M, et al. The use of carboplatin and paclitaxel with daily radiotherapy in patients with locally advanced squamous cell carcinomas of the head and neck. Int J Radiat Oncol Biol Phys. 2000;47(1):49–56.
34. Bonner JA, et al. Radiotherapy plus cetuximab for squamous-cell carcinoma of the head and neck. N Engl J Med. 2006;354(6):567–78.
35. Bonner JA, et al. Radiotherapy plus cetuximab for locoregionally advanced head and neck cancer: 5-year survival data from a phase 3 randomised trial, and relation between cetuximab-induced rash and survival. Lancet Oncol. 2010;11(1):21–8.
36. Vermorken JB, et al. Cisplatin, fluorouracil, and docetaxel in unresectable head and neck cancer. N Engl J Med. 2007;357(17):1695–704.
37. Posner MR, et al. Cisplatin and fluorouracil alone or with docetaxel in head and neck cancer. N Engl J Med. 2007;357(17):1705–15.
38. Hitt R, et al. Phase III study comparing cisplatin plus fluorouracil to paclitaxel, cisplatin, and fluorouracil induction chemotherapy followed by chemoradiotherapy in locally advanced head and neck cancer. J Clin Oncol. 2005;23(34):8636–45.
39. Fury MG, Pfister DG. Current recommendations for systemic therapy of recurrent and/or metastatic head and neck squamous cell cancer. J Natl Compr Canc Netw. 2011;9(6):681–9.

Chiari Malformation

11

Edward R. Smith, Lissa C. Baird and Benjamin C. Warf

Introduction

The term Chiari malformation has accrued multiple meanings over time. Formally, this includes various groupings of hindbrain dysmorphism, with four numbered malformations (I–IV) which describe different cerebellar configurations. It is worth noting that while types I-III all include displacement of the cerebellar tonsils through the foramen magnum, type IV is cerebellar hypoplasia and likely a completely separate process from the other three—linked only by name. For the sake of simplicity: type I is displacement of the tonsils below the plane of the foramen magnum; type II is a far more complex malformation that includes displacement of the hindbrain, IVth ventricle, and cerebellar tonsils and vermis below the foramen magnum as well as a more diffuse constellation of brain anomalies with varying degrees of severity found in association with myelomeningocele; and, type III is similar to type II but found in association with a suboccipital or high cervical encephalocele. Patients with types II and III commonly have hydrocephalus. Historically, some have linked the work of Arnold with the type II malformation (Arnold-Chiari), although his contributions were minimal relative to Chiari. In addition, some groups have described a so-called Chiari 0, in which there are symptoms of brainstem compression or foramen magnum outlet obstruction without tonsillar herniation, presumably secondary to other anatomic structures such as arachnoid bands or scar [1].

Further note should be made of the terms *syringomyelia* and *hydromyelia,* which are often used interchangeably to describe the presence of fluid (presumably cerebrospinal fluid, CSF) within the substance of the spinal cord, a finding commonly associated with cases of Chiari malformation. Technically, if the fluid cavity is lined with ependyma (i.e., and expansion of the central canal), the term hydromyelia is used, while syringomyelia is defined as a fluid space within the spinal cord that is not lined by ependyma (also called a *syrinx*).

This chapter will focus on the Chiari I malformation (CM I), as it is the most commonly encountered type. There is a great deal of controversy surrounding the diagnosis and treatment of Chiari I, including the degree of displacement required for diagnosis (with most requiring at least 5 mm of herniation below the foramen magnum, but some accepting 0–2 mm) and what constitutes a pathologic Chiari I. Some experts have called for renaming the condition to Chiari "anomaly," as it is thought to be present in about 0.75 % of the population [1–3]. Here we will review pathologic Chiari I malformations with associated treatment and outcomes.

Key Points

Chiari I malformations are defined as displacement of the cerebellar tonsils at least 5 mm below the foramen magnum (Fig. 11.1).

The vast majority of Chiari I malformations are asymptomatic and do not need intervention [3].

When symptomatic, Chiari I malformations often present with sudden-onset suboccipital headaches classically aggravated by activities that invoke a valsalva maneuver. Less commonly, patients can present with lower cranial nerve dysfunction (especially dysphagia or sleep apnea), cerebellar dysfunction (e.g., ataxia), or spinal cord dysfunction secondary to an associated hydromyelia (weakness, scoliosis).

Treatment (when necessary) is predicated on surgical decompression of the cervicomedullary junction.

E. R. Smith (✉) · B. C. Warf
Department of Neurosurgery, Boston Children's Hospital, Harvard Medical School, Boston, MA, USA
e-mail: edward.smith@childrens.harvard.edu

L. C. Baird
Department of Neurosurgery, Oregon Health & Science University, Portland, OR, USA

R. Rahbar et al. (eds.), *Pediatric Head and Neck Tumors,*
DOI 10.1007/978-1-4614-8755-5_11, © Springer Science+Business Media New York 2014

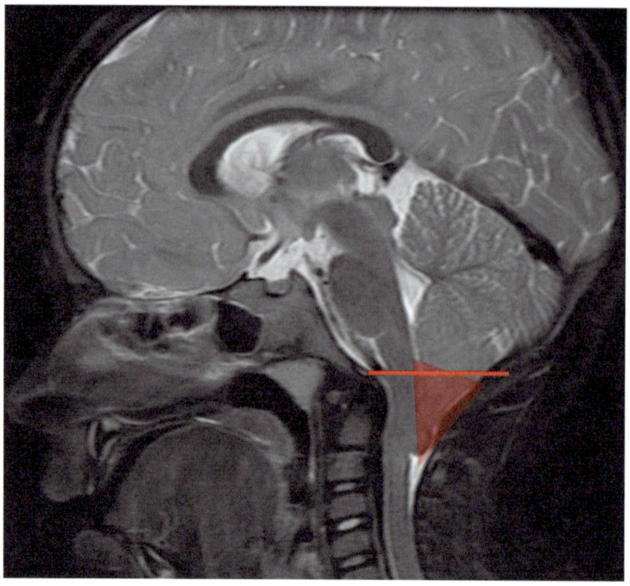

Fig. 11.1 Sagittal T2 magnetic resonance imaging (MRI) demonstrates presence of a CM I, with herniation of the cerebellar tonsils (*shaded in red*) below the foramen magnum (*red line*), compressing the cervicomedullary junction

Biology and Epidemiology

The etiology of CM I remains controversial. The majority of cases are considered to be developmental and a result of a mismatch between growth of the brain and that of the posterior fossa. Evidence comes from craniosynostosis patients and the observation of the clinical constellation of symptoms developing over time, as well as the observation that tonsillar displacement can change for better or worse over time during childhood, sometimes even resolving altogether [2, 4]. A minority of Chiari malformations can be acquired, presumably secondary to an abnormal pressure differential across the foramen magnum such as from hydrocephalus or a mass lesion from above or a lumboperitoneal shunt from below [5].

Pathophysiology

Symptoms from Chiari malformations are generally considered to be secondary to local compression or irritation. Tonsillar compression and scar-related tethering of the dura (particularly with valsalva maneuvers) irritate pain fibers in the dura, leading to headache [6].

Direct compression of the brainstem may contribute to dysfunction of local tracts and nucleui, leading to problems with swallowing, respiration, phonation, and other lower cranial nerve palsies.

Obstruction of normal CSF flow at the cervicomedullary junction has been implicated in the development of hydromyelia (or syringomyelia). This can cause chronic injury to pain and temperature fibers (which cross centrally in the spinal cord to produce a classic "suspended" sensory loss), compression of anterior horn motor neurons leading to lower motor neuron weakness (typically in the hands), compression of corticospinal tracts leading to upper motor neuron weakness with spasticity (typically in the legs), and possible scoliosis from weakness of the axial musculature [7].

Molecular/Genetic Pathology

- The majority of Chiari I malformations are thought to be sporadic, although 3 % of cases are found to be familial [8].
- There are no known genes specifically implicated in the cause of CM I, but links have been suggested to craniofacial disorders (including some craniosynostosis syndromes) and some connective tissue disorders [9, 10].
- Patients may have other findings, including Klippel-Feil, basilar invagination, or other areas of bony fusion [11].

Incidence and Prevalence

- Approximately 1/150 individuals will have some degree of tonsillar displacement potentially consistent with a CM I [1–3].
- Of all Chiari I malformations, only ~3 % are familial [8].

Age Distribution

- Mean age of presentation with symptoms = ~ 30 y/o
- Syrinx present in ~ 40 %
- Amount of tonsillar displacement correlated with symptoms:
  - Asymptomatic ~ 7 mm
  - Headache ~ 8 mm
  - Central cord symptoms ~ 10 mm
  - Brainstem compression symptoms ~ 12 mm [6, 12]

Sex Predilection

- There is a slight female preponderance at 3:2 [12].

Geographic Distribution

- None

Risk Factors—Environmental, Life Style

- None

Relationships to Other Disease States, Syndromes

- As noted above, there are several associations between Chiari I and other conditions [11]:
  - Hydrocephalus
  - Craniosynostosis
  - Endocrinopathies (growth hormone deficiency and acromegaly)
  - Hyperostosis
  - Bone mineral deficiency
  - Cutaneous disorders (neurofibromatosis type I, blue rubber bleb nevus)
  - Spinal defects (Klippel Feil, spondyloepiphyseal dysplasia)

Presentation

Symptoms/Signs

- Headache (occipital or suboccipital, tussive, worse with flexion/extension)—most common (about 2/3 of patients).
- Scoliosis was the 2nd most common reported finding in symptomatic Chiari I malformations in children [8].
- Lower cranial nerve dysfunction (hoarseness, dysphagia, dysphonia, aspiration, swallowing problems, snoring, apnea).
- Cerebellar syndrome (dysmetria, ataxia, nystagmus).
- Central cord syndrome (loss of pain and temperature sensation, weakness with lower motor nerve injury, scoliosis (often with syrinx)).
- Greater degrees of displacement often correlate with increasing severity of symptoms [6, 12].

Patterns of Evolution

- The presentation of symptoms in CM I is often chronic, over a period of months or years.

Evaluation at Presentation

- MRI is the current standard for evaluation of the cervicomedullary junction (CMJ).
- Discovery of a CM I often includes imaging of the brain to exclude mass lesions rostrally and—on occasion—MR imaging of the spine to assess for the presence and extent of syrinx.
- In some cases (such as those with a history of neck trauma), the history or imaging findings may suggest the need to assess the bony anatomy of the CMJ with other diagnostic studies, such as flexion–extension radiographs or computerized tomography.
- Standard preoperative laboratory studies (complete blood count (CBC), clotting times Prothrombin Time/Partial Thromboplastin Time (PT/PTT), type and cross (T&C) for blood bank, chemistry panel (Chem 7)) may be considered prior to planned surgery.

Differential Diagnosis

Many patients will be asymptomatic on examination if the lesion is found incidentally. The diagnosis of a CM I is relatively straightforward, with the difficulty primarily arising from the exercise of using clinical judgment to select appropriate surgical candidates. The main issue with differential diagnosis is to ascertain whether a proximate cause for the CM I exists. As such, imaging of the head and spine may be warranted to exclude intracranial mass lesions, hydrocephalus or areas of spinal CSF leak. Furthermore, careful history taking is important to determine if things such as lumbar puncture or intracranial pressure (ICP)-elevating medications (such as retinoic acid) may be contributing to the radiographic findings. Lastly, given the often subjective nature of complaints in CM I, the clinician must carefully evaluate the patient for other causes that may explain presenting symptoms.

Diagnosis and Evaluation

Physical Examination

- Many patients will be asymptomatic on examination. However, a detailed neurologic examination and history are always important. Attention should be paid to evidence of neurologic dysfunction in the history.
  - Headache—usually occipital and tussive which can often be replicated on exam, need to assess whether the pain is related to flexion or extension of the neck
  - Lower cranial nerve dysfunction—apnea (infants), snoring, dysphonia, dysphagia, trapezius weakness
  - Spinal cord dysfunction—weakness in the arms or legs (especially the hands with signs of muscle wasting), long tract signs (with hyperreflexia Babinski, "cape" sensory loss distribution), scoliosis

Laboratory Data

- Standard preoperative laboratory studies (complete blood count (CBC), clotting times (PT/PTT), type and cross (T&C) for blood bank, chemistry panel (Chem 7)).

Imaging Evaluation

MRI is the imaging modality of choice in the evaluation of CM I. If possible, studies of the brain should be obtained (either MRI or computed tomography, CT) to exclude the possibility of mass lesions or hydrocephalus as proximate, treatable causes of CM I. The use of high-resolution MRI (such as Fast Imaging Employing Steady State Acquisition (FIESTA)) may be useful in assessing for the possibility of obstruction to the outflow of the 4th ventricle. Contrast is usually not needed, although it may be helpful in assessing the location of the confluence of sinuses in the posterior fossa or the choroid in the 4th ventricle (as well as excluding other lesions such as tumor or vascular anomalies, if suspected).

In addition to the objective measurement of tonsillar herniation, there are subjective measures that can be assessed using MRI to help determine the extent of compression. These subjective findings include the presence of "peg-like" tonsils, obliteration of CSF spaces at the CMJ, the presence of a syrinx (sometimes requiring dedicated spinal imaging) and the quantification of CSF flow.

CSF flow studies have been considered as diagnostic tools when considering surgical decompression of Chiari malformation. In patients who clearly have symptoms related to their Chiari, diminished CSF flow in preoperative assessment appears to correlate well with surgical outcome. There is no good evidence, however, that CSF flow studies have any advantage over clinical impression in determining whether a Chiari malformation is symptomatic [13].

CT and plain films are generally not warranted unless there is a concern for basilar invagination, atlanto-axial instability, or other bony injury that might not be readily assessed with MRI. However, in some cases, such as reoperations (in which the extent of bony decompression may need to be seen) or in situations that might require arthrodesis (such as those children with rheumatoid arthritis), CT or flexion–extension plain films can be helpful.

Nuclear medicine tests

- Not usually warranted with CM I

Electrodiagnostic tests

- Not usually warranted with CM I

Neuropsychological tests

- Not usually indicated with CM I

Treatment

Goal To remove compression at the cervicomedullary junction, restore physiologic pulsatile CSF flow, and thereby alleviate symptoms and/or provide protection from future injury.

Surgical therapy

Surgical Indications One of the greatest challenges in CM I is appropriate selection of surgical candidates. "The Chiari malformation is, in fact, one of the few conditions for which the AANS (American Association of Neurological Surgeons) issued a position statement regarding the inappropriate use of surgery (AANS Position Statement on the Use of Cervical Decompression for Chronic Fatigue Syndrome, March 2000). When a patient presents with two common conditions, there is always going to be some degree of coincidental overlap, and surgeons must be careful not to perform surgery in patients in whom there is little chance that the Chiari malformation is symptomatic [2]."

In general, operation is indicated in patients with associated symptoms (see above) and clear radiographic evidence of disease (>5 mm herniation, +/− syrinx). For those with atypical symptoms (frontal headache, fatigue, etc.) and minimal radiographic findings, a conservative approach with a referral to pain management might be appropriate. Surgery for asymptomatic patients (including incidentally found lesions) remains controversial and has been justified on the basis that this lesion has the potential to become symptomatic or could place the patient at greater risk of spinal cord injury if left untreated, although this has not been substantiated.

One of the factors to support surgical intervention for asymptomatic Chiari includes prevention of an exacerbation after trauma. Development of symptoms related to a Chiari after a minor traumatic event has occurred, with reports indicating approximately 13 % of previously asymptomatic CM I developing symptoms after trauma (including isolated case reports of sudden death in severe cases) [14, 15].

Athletes with Chiari malformation present additional challenges in the determination of appropriate management for an incidentally found Chiari. Numerous athletes have been found to have Chiari malformation on imaging obtained after suffering a concussion, and reports of athletes with known Chiari experiencing drop attacks have been reported. The implication of these associations is unclear, and it has yet to be determined whether athletes with asymptomatic Chiari who play contact sports are at a greater risk for catastrophic injuries. A known Chiari with clear associated symptoms is often considered a contraindication to contact sports. Asymptomatic Chiari malformation may be a rela-

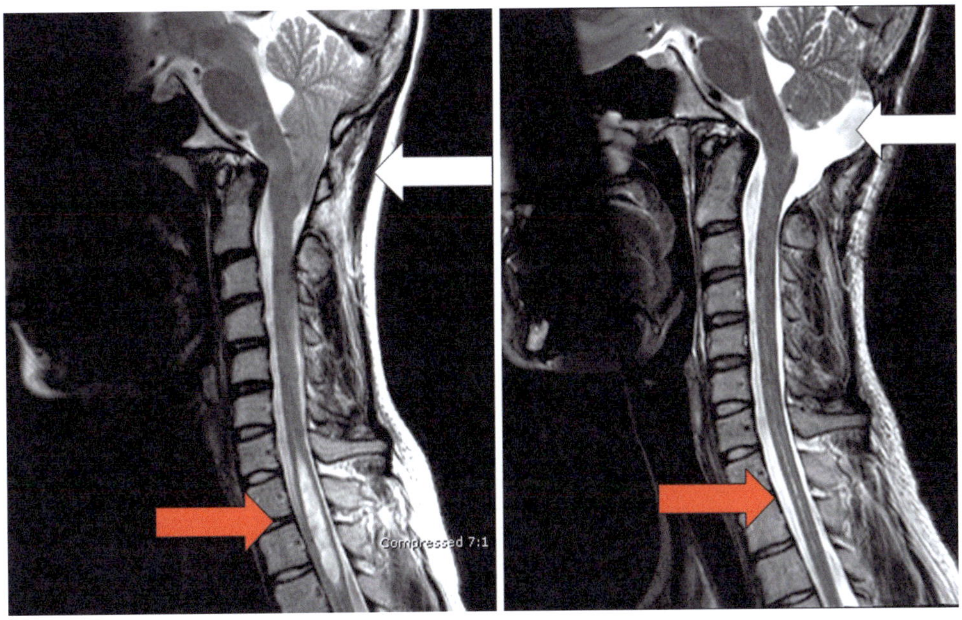

Fig. 11.2 Sagittal T2 MRI of the posterior fossa and cervical spine showing preoperative images (*left*) with an extensive CM I (*white arrow*) and cervical cord syrinx (*red arrow*), coupled with postoperative images from the same patient 6 months later (*right*), revealing decompression of the cervicomedullary junction (*white arrow*) and marked reduction in the syrinx (*red arrow*)

tive contraindication due to increased risk of injury based on anecdotal evidence. A careful discussion with the athlete and family is important. Most athletes can return to sports after undergoing a surgical Chiari decompression.

Surgical Techniques

The method of decompression is also a topic of debate. Generally, a suboccipital craniectomy is performed, often with removal of the posterior ring of C1. Controversy exists as to the utility of opening the dura and placing a dural patch, with some authors calling for the use of intraoperative ultrasound to assess the extent of decompression after bony removal and using the findings to guide the need for dural opening. Overall, 7% of pediatric neurosurgeons only perform bony decompression (without dural opening), while 36% always open the dura [16].

Relieve external pressure on the crowded foramen magnum region
- Suboccipital craniectomy, C1 laminectomy
- Open dura and place dural graft (either routinely or only after ultrasound)

Reestablish normal CSF flow out of IVth ventricle in patients with syringomyelia
- Remove scarring from IVth ventricle outflow
- Possible "shunt" from IVth ventricle to cervical subarachnoid space

Complications [16]

Overall, published complication rates for pediatric CM I operation range from 2–40% [8, 17].

- Bleeding is the most immediate complication of surgery and risks are magnified in smaller children, who have little reserve. In particular, high venous pressures and large dural sinuses in the posterior fossa increase the risk of hemorrhage.
- CSF leak can occur when dura is opened, including pseudomeningocoele.
- Chemical meningitis.
- Vertebral artery injury.
- "Cerebellar slump" is a controversial entity often ascribed to excessive decompression of the posterior fossa, resulting in sag of the tonsils and recrudescence of Chiari-related symptoms.

Outcomes

Outcome After Surgery (Fig. 11.2)

- In a recent large series, average hospital stay and "return to school" time after surgery were 3 and 12 days, respectively [8].
- In carefully selected, symptomatic patients, 60% will demonstrate durable improvement in symptoms following surgery [18].
- In patients with symptomatic syrinx, over half will experience improvement clinically within 10 months [19].
- Three percent of patients will need reoperation for recurrence (more likely with younger patients) [8].

Follow-up

Frequency of Office Visits

- Postoperative care will frequently consist of an office visit approximately one month postoperatively.
- Rare long-term issues include recurrence and craniocervical instability. While most patients can be discharged from care after routine postoperative visits, some may require long-term follow-up.

Conclusions

The management of CM I remains controversial, with debate centered on operative indications and surgical approach. Candid discussions with patients and families are useful in establishing realistic plans of action and expected outcomes.

References

1. Chern JJ, Gordon AJ, Mortazavi MM, Tubbs RS, Oakes WJ. Pediatric Chiari malformation Type 0: a 12-year institutional experience. J Neurosurg Pediatr. 2011;8:1–5.
2. Proctor MR, Scott RM, Oakes WJ, Muraszko KM. Chiari malformation. Neurosurg Focus. 2011;31:Introduction.
3. Meadows J, Kraut M, Guarnieri M, Haroun RI, Carson BS. Asymptomatic Chiari Type I malformations identified on magnetic resonance imaging. J Neurosurg. 2000;92:920–6.
4. Alden TD, Ojemann JG, Park TS. Surgical treatment of Chiari I malformation: indications and approaches. Neurosurg Focus. 2001;11:E2.
5. Payner TD, Prenger E, Berger TS, Crone KR. Acquired Chiari malformations: incidence, diagnosis, and management. Neurosurgery. 1994;34:429–34; discussion 34.
6. Arnett BC. Tonsillar ectopia and headaches. Neurol Clin. 2004;22:229–36.
7. Heiss JD, Patronas N, DeVroom HL, et al. Elucidating the pathophysiology of syringomyelia. J Neurosurg. 1999;91:553–62.
8. Tubbs RS, Beckman J, Naftel RP, et al. Institutional experience with 500 cases of surgically treated pediatric Chiari malformation Type I. J Neurosurg Pediatr. 2011;7:248–56.
9. deSouza RM, Zador Z, Frim DM. Chiari malformation type I: related conditions. Neurol Res. 2011;33:278–84.
10. Strahle J, Muraszko KM, Buchman SR, Kapurch J, Garton HJ, Maher CO. Chiari malformation associated with craniosynostosis. Neurosurg Focus. 2011;31:E2.
11. Loukas M, Shayota BJ, Oelhafen K, et al. Associated disorders of Chiari Type I malformations: a review. Neurosurg Focus. 2011;31:E3.
12. Elster AD, Chen MY. Chiari I malformations: clinical and radiologic reappraisal. Radiology. 1992;183:347–53.
13. Hofkes SK, Iskandar BJ, Turski PA, Gentry LR, McCue JB, Haughton VM. Differentiation between symptomatic Chiari I malformation and asymptomatic tonsilar ectopia by using cerebrospinal fluid flow imaging: initial estimate of imaging accuracy. Radiology. 2007;245:532–40.
14. Wan MJ, Nomura H, Tator CH. Conversion to symptomatic Chiari I malformation after minor head or neck trauma. Neurosurgery. 2008;63:748–53; discussion 53.
15. Wolf DA, Veasey SP 3rd, Wilson SK, Adame J, Korndorffer WE. Death following minor head trauma in two adult individuals with the Chiari I deformity. J Forensic Sci. 1998;43:1241–3.
16. Rocque BG, George TM, Kestle J, Iskandar BJ. Treatment practices for Chiari malformation type I with syringomyelia: results of a survey of the American Society of Pediatric Neurosurgeons. J Neurosurg Pediatr. 2011;8:430–7.
17. Parker SR, Harris P, Cummings TJ, George T, Fuchs H, Grant G. Complications following decompression of Chiari malformation Type I in children: dural graft or sealant? J Neurosurg Pediatr. 2011;8:177–83.
18. Furtado SV, Thakar S, Hegde AS. Correlation of functional outcome and natural history with clinicoradiological factors in surgically managed pediatric Chiari I malformation. Neurosurgery. 2011;68:319–27; discussion 28.
19. Attenello FJ, McGirt MJ, Gathinji M, et al. Outcome of Chiari-associated syringomyelia after hindbrain decompression in children: analysis of 49 consecutive cases. Neurosurgery. 2008;62:1307–13; discussion 13.

Cholesteatoma

12

Ilkka Kivekäs and Dennis Poe

Introduction

Cholesteatoma is a pathologic condition characterized by the presence of keratinizing squamous epithelium within the middle ear and/or mastoid cavity. The foreign epithelium layer exfoliates keratinaceous debris that accumulates as a nonvascularized cystic mass which is prone to chronic infection. The epithelial layer also induces an inflammatory response, including upregulated osteoclastic activity that can cause erosion of the ossicles and other bony structures. Cholesteatomas associated with chronic persistent infection or erosion into the labyrinth, facial nerve, or intracranial fossa are among some of the common reasons for developing serious complications of otitis media. The most common symptoms are otorrhea and hearing loss, but only occasionally otalgia. The diagnosis is based on clinical findings and imaging studies. Active treatment is exclusively surgical. Postoperative management involves following patients long-term for residual disease (incomplete surgical removal of cholesteatoma) or recurrence (development of a new cholesteatoma).

Key Points

- Clinical findings may include a tympanic membrane perforation with squamous epithelium migrating into the middle ear cavity, chronic persistent or recurrent middle ear infection with otorrhea, a retraction pocket in the tympanic membrane in which there is an accumulation of squamous debris and margins extending deeply into the middle ear or mastoid recesses, or even a white mass seen behind an otherwise intact tympanic membrane.
- The main goals of treatment are eradication of the disease and prevention of recurrence. Reconstruction of hearing is done after optimizing those first two priorities. Additionally, functional reconstruction of the anatomy may be done to create a dry, healthy, self-cleaning ear. These goals may be achieved through means such as restoration of the ear canal wall, mastoid obliteration, or cartilage reconstruction of an attic defect.
- Residual or recurrent cholesteatomas may present many years after surgery and require long-term follow-up.
- Once a cholesteatoma or retraction pocket has been removed, there may be a persistent upregulated biological tendency to form a new retraction and ultimately a new cholesteatoma. Such retraction pockets may occur despite healthy Eustachian tube function.
- There is a wide variability in the biological activity of cholesteatomas between patients. In general, pediatric cholesteatomas tend to be more aggressive in rate of growth and have higher recurrence rates than seen in adult patients.
- The incidences of cholesteatoma and complications from cholesteatoma, such as facial paralysis, suppurative labyrinthitis, and intracranial complications are markedly reduced since the introduction of antibiotic and tympanostomy tubes for the management of otitis media.

Biology and Epidemiology

There are two types of cholesteatomas in children: (1) acquired from a tympanic membrane perforation or retraction pocket (Figs. 12.1, 12.2 and 12.3) and (2) congenital which are typically recognized in childhood years (Figs. 12.4 and 12.5). It is estimated that only 1–5% of pediatric cholesteatomas are congenital [1]. Acquired cholesteatomas may

D. Poe (✉) · I. Kivekäs
Department of Otolaryngology and Communication Enhancement, Boston Children's Hospital, Harvard Medical School, Boston, MA, USA
e-mail: Dennis.Poe@childrens.harvard.edu

I. Kivekäs
Department of Otorhinolaryngology, Tampere University Hospital and the University of Tampere, Tampere, Finland
e-mail: ilkka.kivekas@fimnet.fi

R. Rahbar et al. (eds.), *Pediatric Head and Neck Tumors*,
DOI 10.1007/978-1-4614-8755-5_12, © Springer Science+Business Media New York 2014

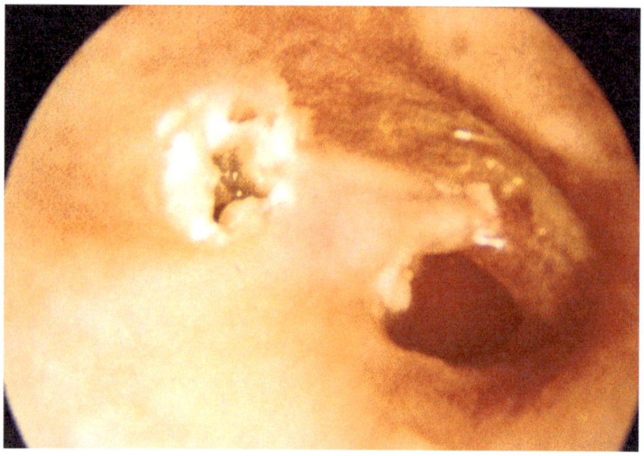

Fig. 12.1 Endoscopic view of the right ear with an attic cholesteatoma and pars tensa perforation. (Copyright held by Dennis S. Poe, MD, PhD, Boston Children's Hospital)

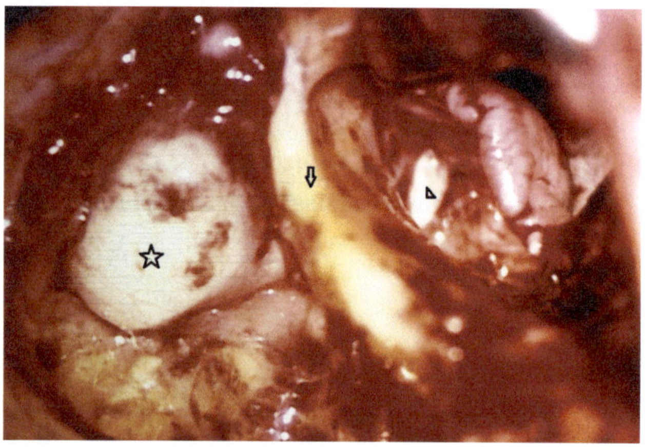

Fig. 12.2 Intraoperative microscopic view of the right ear with an attic (*triangle*) and mastoid (*star*) cholesteatoma. Posterior canal wall marked with an *arrow*. (Copyright held by Dennis S. Poe, MD, PhD, Boston Children's Hospital)

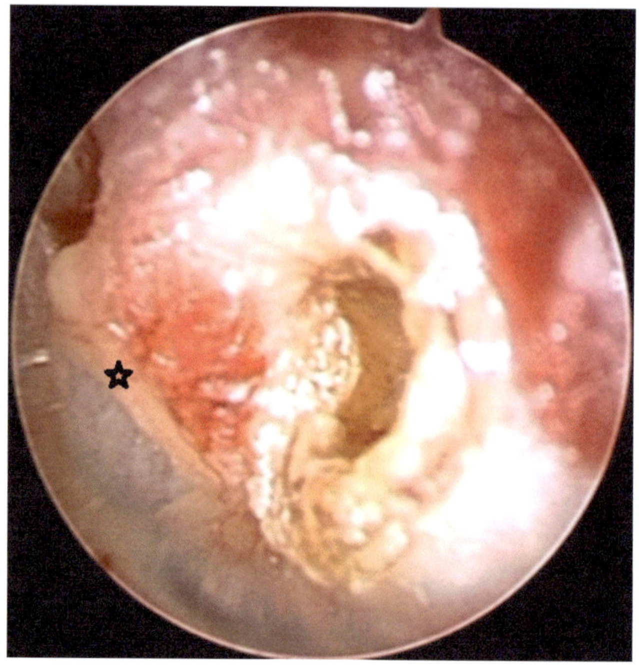

Fig. 12.3 Endoscopic view of the left ear with a posterior superior cholesteatoma and a pars flaccida retraction pocket. Malleus handle marked with a *star*. (Copyright held by Dennis S. Poe, MD, PhD, Boston Children's Hospital)

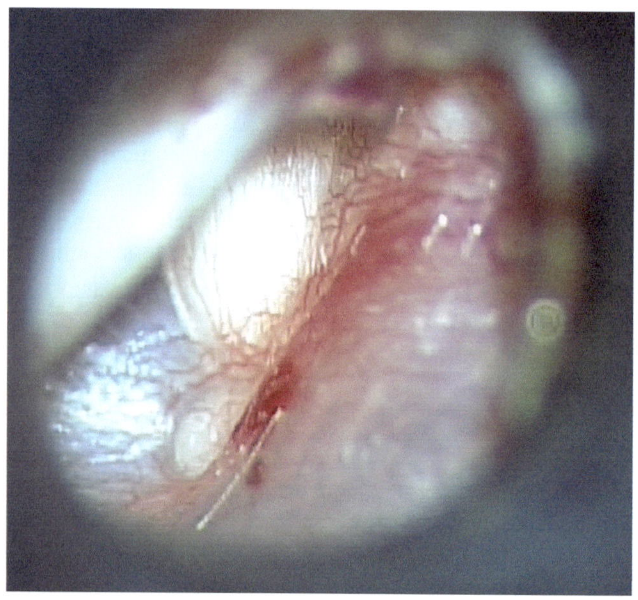

Fig. 12.4 Microscopic view of the left ear with a congenital cholesteatoma behind an intact tympanic membrane. (Copyright held by Dennis S. Poe, MD, PhD, Boston Children's Hospital)

occur in adulthood, but many represent the slow progression of squamous epithelial migration or accumulation of debris from defects in the tympanic membrane dating back to childhood.

Pathophysiology

- Eustachian tube dysfunction is probably the principal pathologic condition that leads to acquired cholesteatoma [2].
- There are three different conditions in which squamous epithelium may gain access into the middle ear: (1) tympanic membrane retraction pocket, (2) migration or displacement of squamous epithelium into the middle ear through an acute or chronic perforation in the tympanic membrane, (3) iatrogenic, e.g., through ventilation tube or after middle ear operation [3].
- The chronic inflammation associated with cholesteatoma induces squamous epithelial proliferation, migration, and bone resorption [1, 4].

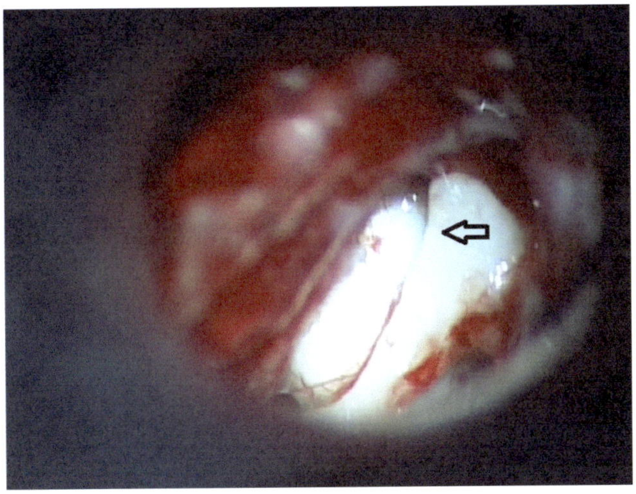

Fig. 12.5 Intraoperative microscopic view of the same (Fig. 12.4) left ear with a congenital cholesteatoma. Malleus marked with an *arrow* and cholesteatoma mass located anterior to malleus. (Copyright held by Dennis S. Poe, MD, PhD, Boston Children's Hospital)

- A cholesteatoma is defined as congenital when there is a completely intact tympanic membrane without any evidence of retraction or perforation and there is an absence of any history of significant otitis media [5].

Molecular/Genetic Pathology

- Osteoclast activity and thus bone resorption are increased because of chronic inflammation caused by cholesteatoma and presence of bacteria [6].
- Proteolytic inflammatory cytokines (metalloproteinases, MMP2, MMP9) have been shown to be increased in pediatric cholesteatoma in comparison to adults [4].
- Angiogenesis seen in the perimatrix of cholesteatoma is higher in pediatric than adult patients [4].

Incidence and Prevalence

- Pediatric prevalence is about 3/100,000 compared to 9/100,000 in adults [7].

Age Distribution

- The mean age of children with acquired cholesteatoma is 9–10 years and with congenital cholesteatoma 4–5 years [5, 8].

Sex Predilection

- Cholesteatoma is slightly more common in male patients with the incidence being about 1.4 times higher in male than in female patients [7, 8].

Risk Factors—Environmental, Life Style

- Eustachian tube dysfunction, middle ear infections, cleft palate [8], craniofacial anomalies, Turner [9] or Down [10] syndromes, or a family history of chronic middle ear infection or cholesteatoma [3].

Presentation

Symptoms

The full spectrum of chronic middle ear infection symptoms may be seen in acquired cholesteatoma:

- Foul smell otorrhea and hearing loss are the main symptoms in acquired pediatric cholesteatoma.
- Facial weakness and vestibular symptoms are marks of more extensive disease.
- Intracranial symptoms are ararity.

A congenital cholesteatoma might not have any symptoms until it reaches a size that causes conductive hearing loss or it blocks the Eustachian tube to cause otitis media. Often, it is discovered as a white mass behind an intact tympanic membrane.

Patterns of Evolution

- Most commonly, chronic retraction of the tympanic membrane results in a persistent pocket that becomes bound down by fibrous adhesion to the undersurface of the attic, superior tympanic ring, or the ossicles. This pocket may progressively enlarge and deepen or perforate, eventually generating or collecting squamous debris around the margins or within the pocket. The pocket may subsequently enlarge, erode bone, or become infected with progressive chronicity or local destruction.
- The presentation of symptoms in acquired cholesteatoma is typically similar to those of chronic middle ear infection and it is often resistant to topical and systemic treatments, with otorrhea recurring promptly after repeated treatments.

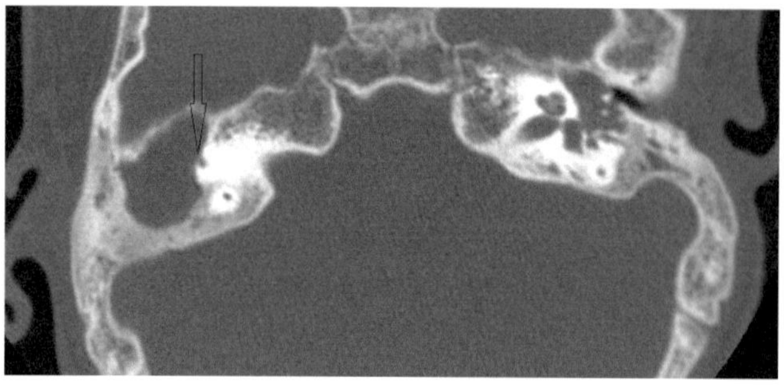

Fig. 12.6 An axial CT image of the right ear with a cholesteatoma. Extensive erosion with typical scalloping of bone is seen in the right mastoid cavity in which there is also a fistula to the anterior limb of the superior semicircular canal (ampullated end marked with a *black arrow*). (Copyright held by Dennis S. Poe, MD, PhD, Boston Children's Hospital)

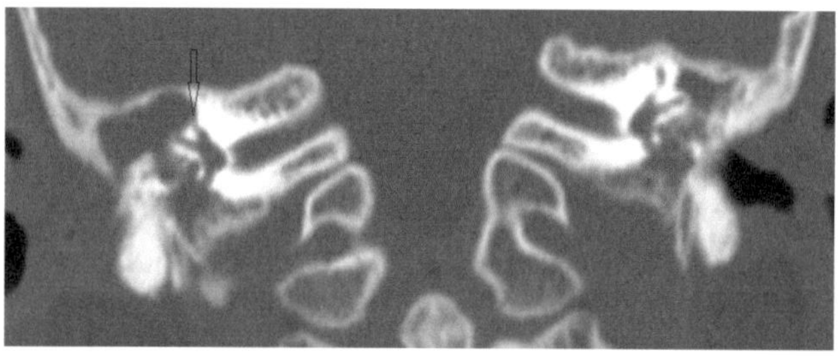

Fig. 12.7 A coronal CT image of the same patient as in Fig. 12.6. The superior semicircular canal fistula is marked with a *black arrow*. (Copyright held by Dennis S. Poe, MD, PhD, Boston Children's Hospital)

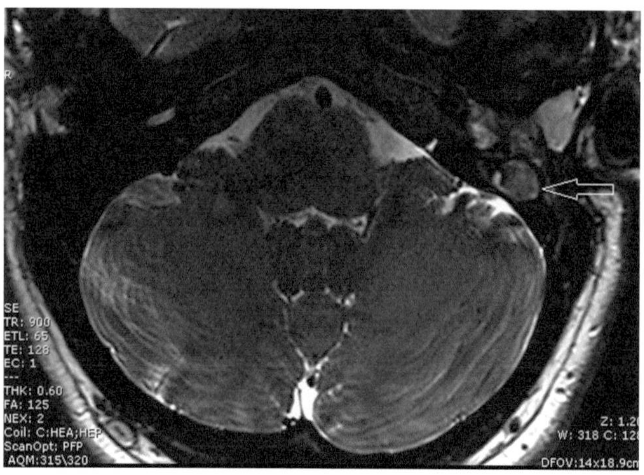

Fig. 12.8 A T2 MR image of a left ear with residual cholesteatoma adjacent to the posterior fossa dura (*white arrow*). (Copyright held by Dennis S. Poe, MD, PhD, Boston Children's Hospital)

Differential Diagnosis

Chronic middle ear infection, cholesterol cyst (granuloma).

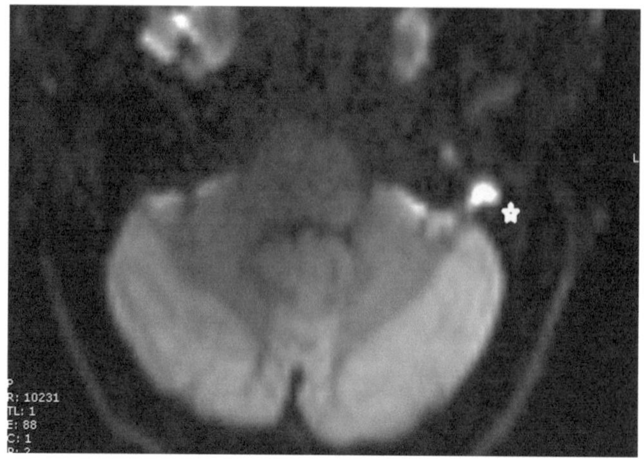

Fig. 12.9 A diffusion-weighted sequence MR image of the cholesteatoma in Fig. 12.8 showing bright signal that represents restricted diffusion. Cholesteatoma marked with a *star*. (Copyright held by Dennis S. Poe, MD, PhD, Boston Children's Hospital)

Diagnosis and Evaluation

Physical Examination

- Otomicroscopic examination may reveal a deep tympanic membrane retraction pocket, a tympanic membrane perforation with squamous epithelium migrating into the middle ear, granulation tissue, or polyps in the middle ear [2].
- Retraction pockets are typically seen in the posterior superior part of the pars tensa or in the pars flaccida.
- Hearing loss is typically conductive. Sensorineural hearing loss may be associated with more extensive, aggressive, or chronic disease.

Imaging Evaluation

- Temporal bone CT or MRI should be considered preoperatively. CT is particularly helpful for evaluating the size and pneumatization of the mastoid cavity (which helps in planning the type of mastoidectomy), assessing the extent of the cholesteatoma, revealing complications (e.g., semicircular canal fistulas or tegmen dehiscence), and detecting anatomical variants [1]. Typical findings on CT would be middle ear or mastoid cavity opacification or rounded lesions with soft tissue or fluid density and bony erosion (Figs. 12.6 and 12.7).
- MR imaging has recently become helpful using high-resolution diffusion-weighted sequences that demonstrate the relatively specific findings of restricted diffusion in the presence of cholesteatoma. It may be particularly useful for differentiating between fluid/adhesions and residual cholesteatoma in following patients after surgery (Figs. 12.8 and 12.9) [11].

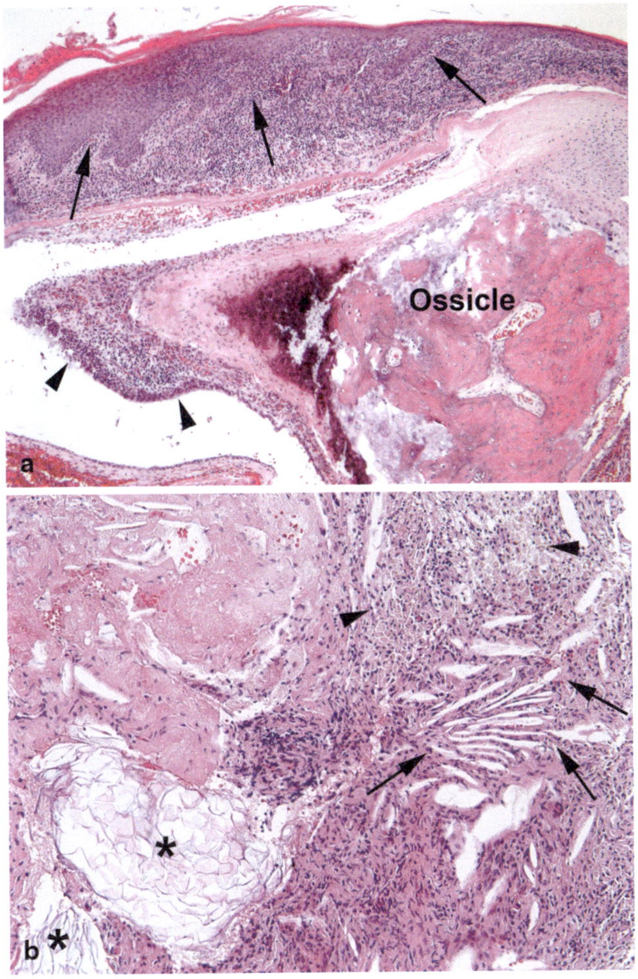

Fig. 12.10 **a** Chronically inflamed middle ear mucosa (*arrowheads*) covering an ear ossicle. Cholesteatoma consists of keratinizing squamous epithelium with marked submucosal chronic inflammation (arrows). **b** Components of cholesteatoma consisting of cholesterol crystal ghosts (*arrows*), iron- and ceroid-laden macrophages (between *arrowheads*) and clusters of keratin squames (*stars*)

Pathology

Cholesteatoma is a clinical diagnosis which is confirmed by CT imaging and at surgery. Biopsies are not needed for preoperative confirmation of diagnosis. Findings are normal appearing keratinizing squamous epithelium matrix or capsule within the middle ear or mastoid cavities and often with surrounding inflammation and bony erosion (Fig. 12.10). There is often accumulation of keratin and desquamated debris within the lumen of the epithelial capsule. Metaplastic cells are not seen.

Treatment

Medical and Preventive Intervention

- Optimizing Eustachian tube function. Identification and medical treatment of possible etiologies (adenoid hypertrophy, allergies, chronic rhinosinusitis, reflux).
- Debridement of retraction pockets to minimize the tendency to accumulate debris. This is most effective in very cooperative pediatric and adult patients.
- Operative treatment of persistent tympanic membrane retraction pockets to lyse the binding adhesions before it becomes a progressive cholesteatoma. Lysis of adhesions in younger children may permit effective regrowth of the middle fibrous layer of the tympanic membrane and fully restore its normal contours.

Surgical Considerations

The clinical picture of pediatric cholesteatoma is generally more aggressive than adult cholesteatoma; residual and recurrence are more common in the pediatric population. Small cholesteatomas may be removed through standard tympanoplasty techniques. Larger disease involving the mastoid cavity are principally operated through one of two surgical approaches: canal wall up or canal wall down approach [2]. A small mesotympanic congenital cholesteatoma may be operated through a transcanal (through the ear canal) approach.

In the canal wall up operation, the posterior wall of the external ear canal is preserved or reconstructed. It maintains the normal ear canal anatomy and provides a scaffold upon which the tympanic membrane may be reconstructed. In the canal wall down operation, the posterior wall of the external ear canal is removed to better view the cholesteatoma and its sites of origin. In the canal wall down approach, there is an option that the mastoid cavity may be obliterated in the primary operation or later.

Preparation for Definitive Intervention, Nonemergent

- The present infection should be treated as thoroughly as possible in an attempt to eradicate active infection before surgery. In addition to topical antibiotic drops or oral antibiotic therapy (if indicated), daily or periodic irrigations with white distilled vinegar and water (50:50) are often effective in controlling a chronically draining ear. Vinegar/water is usually well tolerated when there is no exposed middle ear mucosa and the mixture is flushed into the ear at 37 °C. An audiogram should be done preoperatively.

Preparation for Definitive Intervention, Emergent

- Presence of intracranial complications in an acutely ill patient but otherwise medically stable condition should be considered for emergent operation. In such cases, drainage of purulent material and management of the complications are the principal objectives. Definitive removal of cholesteatoma, especially the live matrix, will usually be deferred to a later date after which the acute infection will have been treated and subsided.
- Facial weakness, acute sensorineural hearing loss, or acute vestibular symptoms should be considered for emergent operation in the face of cholesteatoma.

Surgical Therapy

- The main goal is to eradicate the underlying cholesteatoma disease. Surrounding inflammation and granulations will usually resolve, even if some such disease remains after removal of the cholesteatoma.
- Canal wall up mastoidectomy restores the normal anatomical structures and hearing outcome is more frequently better than in canal wall down operations, at least in the initial postoperative period. The hearing results after several years approach those of canal wall down operations in many series. There is usually minimal office maintenance required subsequently.
- Canal wall down approach allows improved intraoperative exposure of the cholesteatoma, which facilitates removal and reduces the residual rate in most series compared with canal wall up.
- Recurrent and residual cholesteatoma are more common after canal wall up operations [12]. Consequently, consideration for second-look (staged) operations or imaging studies are more commonly made after canal wall up surgery.
- Ossicular chain reconstructions are often deferred for a second-look operation where potential residual or recurrent disease is anticipated or seen.
- Second-look operations are often scheduled for 4–6 months following primary surgery in younger children. Adolescents and adults are often planned for 6–12 months postoperatively.

Complications

- Complications are much more commonly caused by extensive disease rather than by surgery. Surgical complications include similar injuries as seen in other temporal bone operations: facial nerve paralysis, semicircular canal fistula or other inner ear fistula with vertigo or sensorineural hearing loss.

Outcomes

Outcome After Surgery

- Residual or recurrent disease is more common in the pediatric than in the adult population. Recurrence rates of 16–46 % have been published [12].
- Male gender, younger age than 8 years, pars flaccida type of cholesteatoma, and otitis media with effusion seem to be risk factors for recurrence and residual disease [13, 14].

Natural History of Untreated Cholesteatoma

- Temporal bone and intracranial complications were far more common in the presurgical era and continue to be seen in patients lacking adequate access to medical care.
- Chronic otorrhea, inner ear injury (hearing loss, balance problems), intracranial complications and loss of life still occur today.

Follow-up

Office Visits

- Children need more frequent office follow-up than adults because of their increased likelihood for developing recurrent or residual cholesteatoma. Pediatric patients are generally followed at least annually until adulthood.

Frequency of Imaging

- In the case of suspicion for residual disease within the middle ear or mastoid not visible clinically, imaging is typically recommended annually for at least 3 years.

References

1. Nevoux J, Lenoir M, Roger G, Denoyelle F, Ducou Le, Pointe H, Garabédian EN. Childhood cholesteatoma. Eur Ann Otorhinolaryngol Head Neck Dis. 2010 Sep;127(4):143–50.
2. Shohet JA, de Jong AL. The management of pediatric cholesteatoma. Otolaryngol Clin North Am. 2002 Aug;35(4):841–51.
3. Isaacson G. Diagnosis of pediatric cholesteatoma. Pediatrics. 2007 Sep;120(3):603–8.
4. Dornelles Cde C, da Costa SS, Meurer L, Rosito LP, da Silva AR, Alves SL. Comparison of acquired cholesteatoma between pediatric and adult patients. Eur Arch Otorhinolaryngol. 2009 Oct;266(10):1553–61.
5. Lim HW, Yoon TH, Kang WS. Congenital cholesteatoma: clinical features and growth patterns. Am J Otolaryngol. 2012 Sep–Oct;33(5):538–42.

6. Nason R, Jung JY, Chole RA. Lipopolysaccharide-induced osteoclastogenesis from mononuclear precursors: a mechanism for osteolysis in chronic otitis. J Assoc Res Otolaryngol. 2009 Jun;10(2):151–60.
7. Nelson M, Roger G, Koltai PJ, Garabedian EN, Triglia JM, Roman S, Castellon RJ, Hammel JP. Congenital cholesteatoma: classification, management, and outcome. Arch Otolaryngol Head Neck Surg. 2002 Jul;128(7):810–4.
8. Kemppainen HO, Puhakka HJ, Laippala PJ. Sipilä MM, Manninen MP, Karma PH. Epidemiology and aetiology of middle ear cholesteatoma. Acta Otolaryngol. 1999;119(5):568–72.
9. Dhooge IJ, De Vel E, Verhoye C, Lemmerling M, Vinck B. Otologic disease in turner syndrome. Otol Neurotol. 2005;26:145–50.
10. Bacciu A, Pasanisi E, Vincenti V, Giodano D, Caruso A, Lauda L, Bacciu S. Surgical treatment of middle ear cholesteatoma in children with Down syndrome. Otol Neurotol. 2005;26:1007–10.
11. Plouin-Gaudon I, Bossard D, Fuchsmann C, Ayari-Khalfallah S, Froehlich P. Diffusion-weighted MR imaging for evaluation of pediatric recurrent cholesteatomas. Int J Pediatr Otorhinolaryngol. 2010 Jan;74(1):22–6.
12. Schraff SA, Strasnick B. Pediatric cholesteatoma: a retrospective review. Int J Pediatr Otorhinolaryngol. 2006 Mar;70(3):385–93.
13. Iino Y, Imamura Y, Kojima C, Takegoshi S, Suzuki JI. Risk factors for recurrent and residual cholesteatoma in children determined by second stage operation. Int J Pediatr Otorhinolaryngol. 1998 Nov 15;46(1–2):57–65.
14. Ahn SH, Oh SH, Chang SO, Kim CS. Prognostic factors of recidivism in pediatric cholesteatoma surgery. Int J Pediatr Otorhinolaryngol. 2003 Dec;67(12):1325–30.

Craniopharyngioma

13

Edward R. Smith and R. Michael Scott

Introduction

Craniopharyngiomas are tumors usually found in the region of the infundibulum, although they can develop anywhere along an axis from the nasopharynx to the third ventricle. They comprise approximately 5–10 % of pediatric brain tumors and present with signs and symptoms referable to their location, including visual loss, hormonal disturbances, hydrocephalus, and headache. The broad spectrum of management strategies employed in the treatment of these tumors—including surgical resection, radiation, and intratumoral delivery of chemotherapeutic agents or radioisotopes—underscores the difficulty of achieving successful cures with acceptable morbidity and has fostered considerable controversy among physicians involved in the care of children with these lesions.

Key Points

- Craniopharyngiomas comprise approximately 5–10 % of pediatric brain tumors and present with signs and symptoms referable to their location, including visual loss, hormonal disturbances, hydrocephalus, and headache.
- Magnetic resonance imaging (MRI) is useful for identification of tumors and delineation of the relationship of the tumor to surrounding neurovascular structures including the carotids and their branches, optic apparatus, pituitary gland and stalk, and the hypothalamus/ventricular system. Computed tomography (CT) is important in the diagnosis and surgical planning for craniopharyngiomas due to the frequent presence of calcium in the lesions and the need to understand sinus anatomy if a transsphenoidal approach is planned.
- Patients with craniopharyngioma should undergo preoperative endocrinologic assessment and visual field testing may be useful.
- Treatment for craniopharyngioma should be performed at experienced centers with multidisciplinary teams able to offer all modalities of therapy whenever possible and long-term follow-up is essential to identify recurrence.

Biology and Epidemiology

The term craniopharyngioma was coined by Harvey Cushing in 1932 to describe a class of tumor found in the sellar region first reported by Erdheim in 1904 [1, 2]. Microscopic examination has revealed that craniopharyngiomas are comprised of two distinct subtypes, adamantinomatous and papillary, which some consider to have separate—if related—embryologic origins. (Mixed subtypes of tumor, with both adamantinomatous and papillary regions, have also been described [3–5].)

Pathophysiology

Evidence supports the premise that craniopharyngiomas originate from cells derived from the development of the adenohypophysis and tend to arise primarily from the region of the infundibulum [6, 7]. At the end of the first month of gestation, part of the oral cavity (the stomodeum) projects up toward the brain (Rathke's pouch). This tissue interfaces with the infundibulum, a downward projection of the brain. Over the next 2 weeks, the connection between the oral cavity and the brain (the pharyngohypophyseal stalk within the craniopharyngeal duct) involutes as the sphenoid bone grows and closes off the two spaces, while Rathke's pouch contributes to the development of the anterior pituitary gland [1, 6–8].

Craniopharyngiomas are thought to arise from remnants of Rathke's pouch and tissue from the craniopharyngeal duct [9, 10]. In particular, there is some evidence suggesting that

E. R. Smith (✉) · R. M. Scott
Boston Children's Hospital, Harvard Medical School, Boston, MA, USA
e-mail: edward.smith@childrens.harvard.edu

R. Rahbar et al. (eds.), *Pediatric Head and Neck Tumors*,
DOI 10.1007/978-1-4614-8755-5_13, © Springer Science+Business Media New York 2014

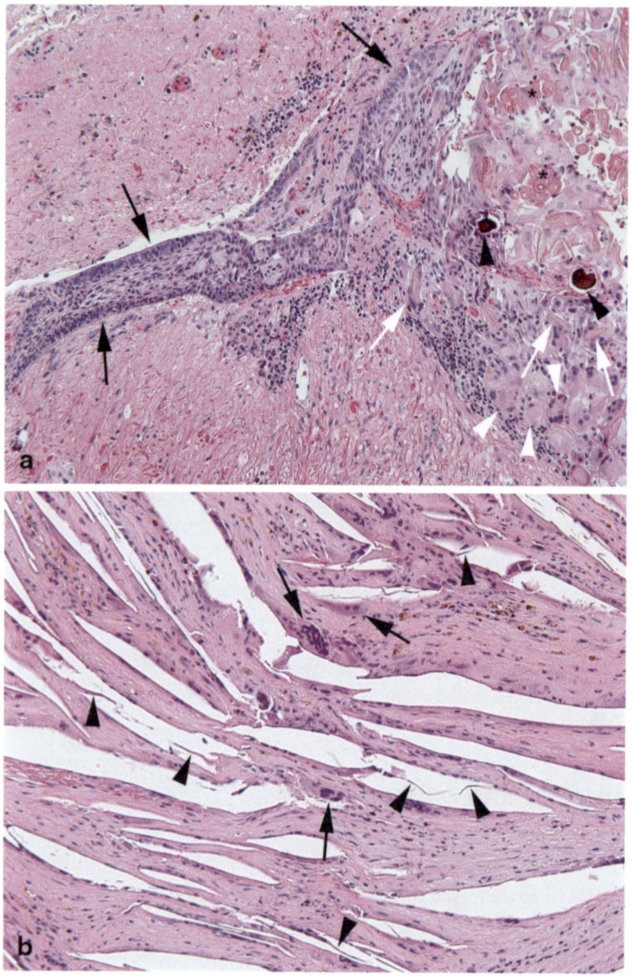

Fig. 13.1 Pathology of craniopharyngioma. **a** Adamantinomatous craniopharyngioma characterized by trabecules of stratified squamous epithelium with peripheral palisading of basaloid cells (*black arrows*). A microcystic component (on the *right*) contains degenerated squamous cells (*), keratin debris, and microcalcifications (*black arrowheads*). A solid component (on the *bottom right*), consists of foreign body multinucleated giant cells (*white arrowheads*) reactive to keratin debris and squames (*white arrows*). The lesion's periphery consists of dense fibrous tissue. **b** Another component of craniopharyngioma with extensive fibrosis, cholesterol clefts, hemosiderin deposition, multinucleated giant cell reaction (*arrows*) and squames (*arrowheads*)

adamantinomatous lesions are derived from neoplastic transformation of epithelial remnants of the craniopharyngeal duct [8, 9]. This is contrasted against the squamous papillary subtype of craniopharyngioma, which is considered to result from metaplasia of adenohypophyseal cells [8, 11].

These tumor subtypes differ pathologically in several ways. Adamantinomatous craniopharyngiomas are most common in children and share characteristics with tooth enamel forming and long-bone tumors of the skeletal system (the eponymous "adamantinomas"), including the tendency to produce calcified deposits intratumorally. The epithelial cells have a keritanized squamous layer that flakes off and degenerates into a characteristic cholesterol-rich "crankcase oil" fluid [4, 10, 11]. In contrast, the papillary subtype (also called "squamous papillary") found nearly exclusively in adults (albeit still less frequently than adamantinomatous tumors) and is characterized by stratified squamous epithelium that does not usually exhibit the calcification or cystic degeneration evident in the adamantinomatous tumors [4, 10–12] (Fig. 13.1).

Greater than 90 % of all pediatric craniopharyngiomas are adamantinomatous, with fewer than 2 % pure papillary and the remainder exhibiting mixed features [10–13].

Molecular/Genetic Pathology

Disruptions in apoptotic pathways involving beta-catenin and Wnt may contribute to neoplastic transformation of craniopharyngiomas [8].

Growth factors and angiogenic peptides have been implicated in craniopharyngioma growth and development [8]. These are relevant not only for the light that they shed on the basic mechanisms of tumorigenesis but also because they facilitate development of novel methods of tumor detection and follow-up, such as recent data suggesting that urine may be able to noninvasively detect brain tumors, specifically including craniopharyngiomas [14, 15].

Incidence and Prevalence

In the United States, approximately 340 craniopharyngiomas are diagnosed annually in the combined pediatric and adult population, of which 100 are in children between 0 and 14 years of age [16].

Craniopharyngioma has an incidence of 1.3 cases diagnosed per million person-years [16].

Age Distribution

About one-third of cases will occur in children and the remaining two-third will present in adults, with the largest peak at 5–14 years of age and a smaller one at 50–74 years of age [1, 16].

Sex Predilection

There is no sex predilection for craniopharyngioma.

Geographic Distribution

None.

Risk Factors—Environmental, Life Style

None.

Relationships to Other Disease States, Syndromes

Craniopharyngiomas represent 5–10 % of all intracranial tumors in children in many series and represent more than half of all sellar region tumors in this population [11, 16, 17].

They are the most common nonglial intracranial tumors in children [18].

Presentation

Symptoms

The most common clinical findings include sequelae of increased intracranial pressure (ICP) due to mass effect and hydrocephalus (especially headache, nausea and vomiting), visual loss and/or endocrinologic dysfunction [6, 18, 19]. These signs and symptoms are directly related to the location of the tumor and variations in the site of origin help to explain variations in presentation. Generally, cranipharyngiomas exhibit one of three growth patterns—prechiasmatic (affecting the optic nerves/chiasm), retrochiasmatic (affecting the hypothalamus, optic tracts, and drainage of cerebrospinal fluid (CSF)), and sellar (affecting hormonal function).

ICP

Nearly one-fourth of patients with craniopharyngioma have hydrocephalus at presentation [19].

Vision

Visual deterioration can be quite severe before detection by family or clinicians and may be asymmetric depending on the growth pattern of the tumor [18, 20]. (Careful documentation of visual function is critical as it may substantially influence subsequent planning for operative approaches.)

Endocrinologic Dysfunction

Similarly insidious is the development of endocrinologic dysfunction, which may remain unnoticed for long periods of time due to the often subtle onset of symptoms, such as growth delay. While deficiency of growth hormone is the most common endocrinopathy found in the setting of craniopharyngioma (followed by hypothyroidism and diabetes insipidus), abnormalities of any and all of the pituitary hormones may be manifest and careful retrospective analysis of patients reveals some form of endocrine dysfunction in 60–90 % of patients at diagnosis [18, 21].

Hypothalamic Injury

Hormonal symptoms can be compounded by effects resulting from hypothalamic injury, including temperature intolerance/dysregulation, weight gain, and behavioral disturbances.

Diagnosis and Evaluation

Physical Examination

A detailed neurologic examination and history are always important, with one-fourth of patients presenting with hydrocephalus and nearly half presenting with signs referable to increased ICP. Attention should be paid to evidence of endocrinologic or visual dysfunction in the history (see list). Growth arrest is particularly common in children with craniopharyngioma.

Findings Suggestive of an Intracranial Lesion

- Headache in the early morning hours or awakening patient from sleep
- Vomiting
- Headache of less than 6 months duration
- Confusion or behavioral changes
- Abnormal neurologic examination findings
- (Positive correlation between number of predictors and risk of surgical lesion)

On examination, findings may be present secondary to (1) local effects (focal weakness, visual changes, etc.), (2) increased ICP (papilledema, increased head circumference, etc.), or (3) high flow (dilated scalp vessels, bruit on auscultation, cardiac failure).

"Red Flags" on Examination or History

- Bradycardia, hypertension, decreased respirations (Cushing response)
- Dilated pupil, hemparesis (Uncal herniation)
- Fixed downward gaze (Parinaud's syndrome)
- Lethargy, tense open anterior fontanelle in infants
- Ataxia with nausea and vomiting
- Sudden onset of a third nerve palsy, including involvement of the pupil (appearing dilated)
- Sudden onset of severe headache

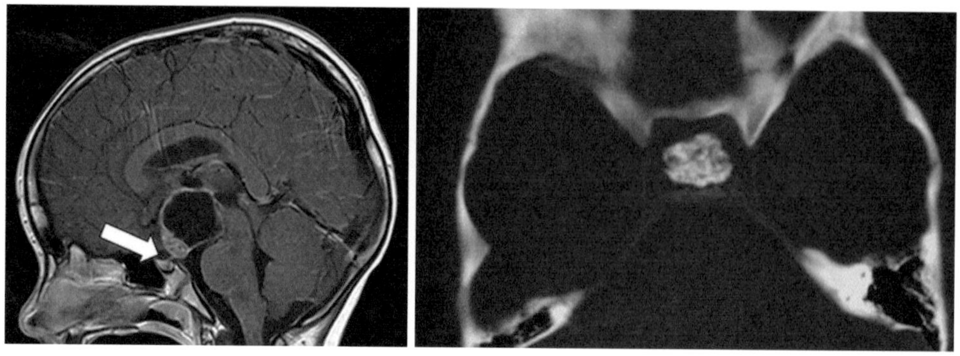

Fig. 13.2 Radiographic appearance of craniopharyngioma. The T1 sagittal enhanced image (*left*) reveals the large, cystic lesion in the suprasellar region, extending up toward the third ventricle with mixed imaging characteristics. The axial noncontrast CT study (*right*) demonstrates a solid calcified core in another tumor, a finding of substantial utility in formulating an appropriate treatment strategy

Imaging Evaluation (13.2)

MRI MRI is particularly useful for identification of tumors and delineation of the relationship of the tumor to surrounding neurovascular structures including the carotids and their branches, optic apparatus, pituitary gland and stalk, and the hypothalamus/ventricular system (Fig. 13.2). The tumor may appear heterogeneous, with cystic components bright on T1 and T2 and solid portions of the tumor exhibiting variable enhancement following administration of contrast (Fig. 13.2). Obtaining an MRI with axial, sagittal, and coronal planes with and without contrast is critical to preoperative planning and postoperative follow-up. Increasingly, magnetic resonance angiography (MRA) is helpful in delineating vascular anatomy for these same reasons.

CT CT is important in the diagnosis and surgical planning for craniopharyngiomas. A distinguishing feature of these tumors is the presence of calcium, which may be difficult to detect on MRI (Fig. 13.2). Regions of calcification are present in the majority of pediatric tumors (up to 90 %) and more than half of adult lesions [10, 17, 22]. Preoperative radiographic visualization of solid calcium deposits (when present) is invaluable to the surgeon in determining the feasibility of specific operative approaches. Moreover, CT is helpful in ascertaining the degree of pneumatization of the sphenoid, ethmoid, and frontal sinuses—relevant to transsphenoidal approaches for sellar tumors (sphenoid), drilling down the planum sphenoidale for frontal approaches (sphenoid/ethmoids), and bifrontal approaches for suprasellar tumors (frontal).

Laboratory Data

Standard preoperative laboratory studies (complete blood count (CBC), clotting times (PT/PTT), type and cross (T&C) for blood bank, chemistry panel (Chem 7)). Replacement of deficient hormones will be performed as needed, with particular attention to cortisol deficiency—patients with craniopharyngioma should be considered in need of supplemental stress dose steroids perioperatively. Replacement of corticosteroids frequently averts disaster in these cases (one can administer dexamethasone 1–4 mg/IV, although hydrocortisone 30 mg/m^2 is also effective).

Laboratory Tests for Endocrinology Evaluation

- Prolactin
- T4, THBR, TSH, Free T4
- IGF-1, IGFBP-3
- Cortisol (if not receiving steroids)
- DHEA-sulfate over age 6 years (if not receiving steroids)
- FSH, LH
- Estradiol (if female)
- Testosterone (if male)
- Electrolytes, BUN, creatinine, and serum osmolality
- Bone age (at least by the time of hospital discharge)

Other Investigations

When possible, a formal assessment of visual fields and an ophthalmologic examination should be performed prior to surgery [18, 20]. This not only establishes a baseline, but also may help to guide the surgical approach if one optic nerve is substantially impaired and the other has retained function.

Differential Diagnosis

The differential diagnosis of tumors in the hypothalamic/sellar region is large and includes congenital lesions (Rathke's cleft cyst, arachnoid cyst, dermoid/epidermoid, hypothalamic hamartoma), tumors (pituitary adenomas, germinomas/nongerminomatous germ cell tumors, lymphoma, meningiomas, schwannomas of the cranial nerves, optic gliomas), vascular lesions (aneurysm, cavernous malformation), and inflammatory conditions (neurosarcoid, lymphocytic hypophysitis) [9, 10, 23]. The characteristic calcification and cystic regions of craniopharyngiomas (especially in children) often help substantially with confirming the radiographic diagnosis.

Treatment

Goal

The primary objective of craniopharyngioma treatment is the restoration and preservation of neurologic function with minimal morbidity. There is substantial debate regarding the most effective method for achieving this goal. The difficulty in developing definitive guidelines for care stems in large part from the variability in presentation, the need for exceptionally long follow-up to assess efficacy, and the rarity of these tumors. The preferential use of specific treatments—radical surgery, subtotal resection, radiation, intracystic administration of chemotherapy—may be influenced by both published data and institutional bias. Here we present an overview of surgical techniques used in the management of craniopharyngioma—approaches that will be of use for both radical and subtotal resections.

Stabilization

- Access: Large bore IV (at least 2), arterial line, bladder catheter (airway intubation if unable to protect airway), and nasogastric tube if intubated.
- Steroid replacement if needed.
- ICP control—external ventricular drain if hydrocephalus.

Preparation for Definitive Intervention, Nonemergent

Prior to undertaking an operation, it is critical to define the goals of surgery. An important distinction is whether the objective is a complete resection or a planned subtotal debulking. This topic is controversial and data exist arguing in support of both strategies [1, 6, 18, 24–29]. The policy at our institution is to attempt a total resection at initial presentation in most cases, but exceptions are made when preoperative imaging suggests that surgical morbidity would be unacceptable [18].

Surgical Therapy

Timing

If a child presents with symptoms of increased ICP then urgent operation may be necessary, although it is often possible to temporize with an external ventricular drain and steroids. Given the complex anatomy in the location of these tumors, lengthy operations are common and performing surgery electively is preferable if possible.

A primary surgical goal is complete removal of the tumor, with the best opportunity often present at initial operation. It is important to understand that there can be several equally valid approaches that may be efficacious for a given tumor.

Approach

The growth pattern of an individual tumor can direct a surgeon to a particular approach. In general, craniopharyngiomas fall into three distinct groups: suprasellar/prechiasmatic, suprasellar/postchiasmatic, and sellar. When viewed through this lens, it can be helpful to pair the common approaches (subfrontal, pterional, subtemporal, transcallosal/transventricular, and transsphenoidal) with specific growth patterns to maximize access to the tumor.

Potential Surgical Approaches Based on Craniopharyngioma Growth Patterns

- Suprasellar
  - Primarily intraventricular—Transcallosal/transventricular
  - Prechiasmatic—Subfrontal
- Pterional
  - Postchiasmatic—Subfrontal
- Pterional
- Subtemporal
- Sellar—Transsphenoidal (microscopic/endoscopic)

Specific Approaches

Subfrontal

The subfrontal approach allows for excellent visualization of optic nerves, carotids, and lamina terminalis. This approach is useful for most craniopharyngiomas, albeit less so for isolated sellar lesions. It affords a wide range of access to the suprasellar region and can easily be combined with other approaches such as pterional, transcallosal/intraventricular, and even sellar (with drilling of the planum sphenoidale). The approach can be unilateral or bilateral, depending on the anatomy of the tumor. For retrochiasmatic and intraventricular tumors, removal of the superior orbital rim and roof improves visualization while minimizing retraction on the frontal lobes (Fig. 13.3).

Limitations of the approach include risk of anosmia with injury to the olfactory nerves, the concern of venous congestion from ligation of the superior sagittal sinus (which is usually minimal), and the extensive nature of the craniotomy, including violation of the frontal sinus with the attendant risk of CSF leak and mucocoele.

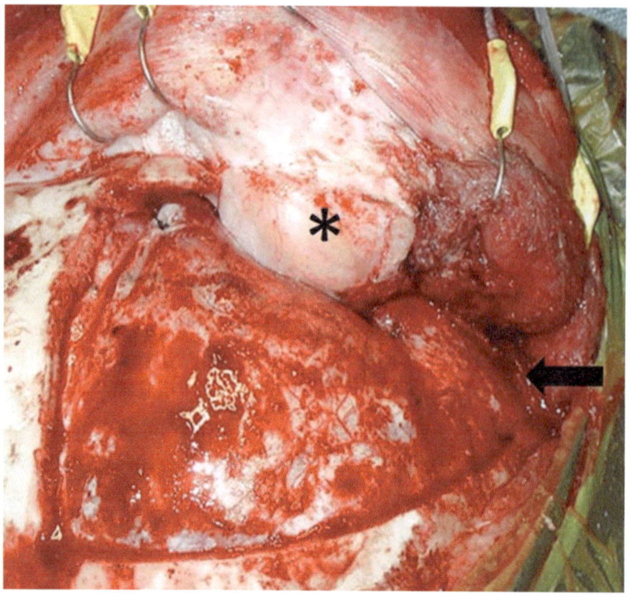

Fig. 13.3 Operative approach (extradural). A unilateral subfrontal approach is demonstrated, with removal of the orbital roof (*). In addition, the craniotomy has been extended inferiorly in order to provide an element of a pterional approach (*arrow*), highlighting the versatility of these approaches and the importance of preserving flexibility in the operating room

Pterional

The pterional approach is often used with suprasellar tumors that are both pre- and retrochiasmatic. It offers a more lateral view than the subfrontal route and can be combined with other approaches (subfrontal, subtemporal, transcallosal/transventricular) to expand access to larger masses. In addition to this versatility, it has the advantage of being familiar to many neurosurgeons. The primary limitation of the pterional approach is reduced visualization of the contralateral optico-carotid complex (Fig. 13.4).

A common preference is to perform a right-sided craniotomy (assuming this to be the nondominant hemisphere), although one will alter this based on tumor anatomy and function of the optic nerves. Should one optic nerve have markedly impaired function, it may be safer to approach from the side of the healthy nerve in order to better visualize and protect it. Depending on the size of the tumor and the preference of the surgeon, the Sylvian fissure can be opened to increase exposure at the bifurcation of the carotid.

Subtemporal

The subtemporal approach is employed primarily for access to suprasellar retrochiasmatic craniopharyngiomas that extend down toward the pons or laterally under the temporal lobe. Care must be taken to seal mastoid air cells with bone wax to prevent CSF leak postoperatively. It is important to preserve the trochlear nerve by cutting the tentorium behind the point at which they cross.

Transcallosal/Transventricular

Transcallosal/transventricular approaches are most helpful for tumors located high within the third or lateral ventricles. This route can be used independently or in combination with other approaches. The main limitation is the inability to visualize neurovascular structures near the sella. Care must be taken to avoid injury to the fornices and internal cerebral veins.

Transsphenoidal (Microscopic and Endoscopic)

The development of the transsphenoidal approach has generally been employed in the removal of sellar craniophayngiomas (Fig. 13.5). While tradionally limited to purely sellar lesions, surgeons have become increasingly capable of successfully resecting sellar lesions with suprasellar extension with the improved visualization afforded by the operating endoscope. The main advantages of the transsphenoidal approach (either microscopic or endoscopic) include decreased surgical morbidity, shorter hospital stays, and improved access to sellar tumors. However, transsphenoidal

Fig. 13.4 Intraoperative view of craniopharyngioma (pre- and postresection). The *left* image demonstrates the view of a suprasellar/retrochiasmatic cystic craniopharyngioma as seen from a right pterional approach. Note the tumor (*) in the opticocarotid triangle. The *arrow* points out the relatively limited access to the contralateral optic nerve, one shortcoming of this approach

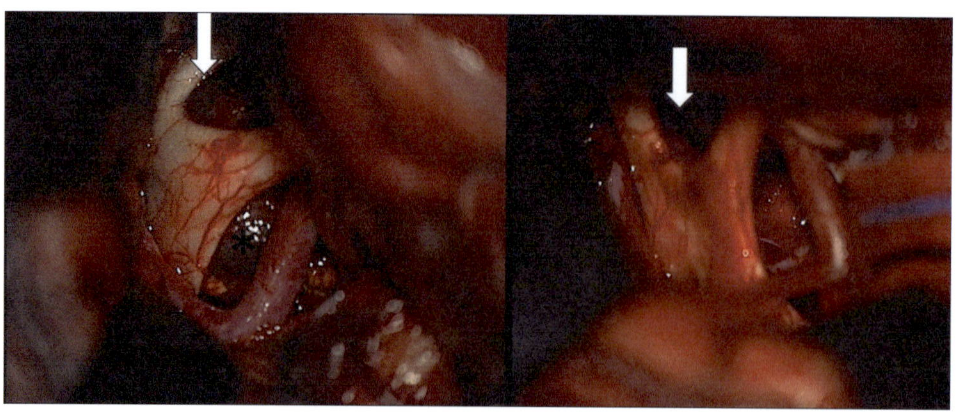

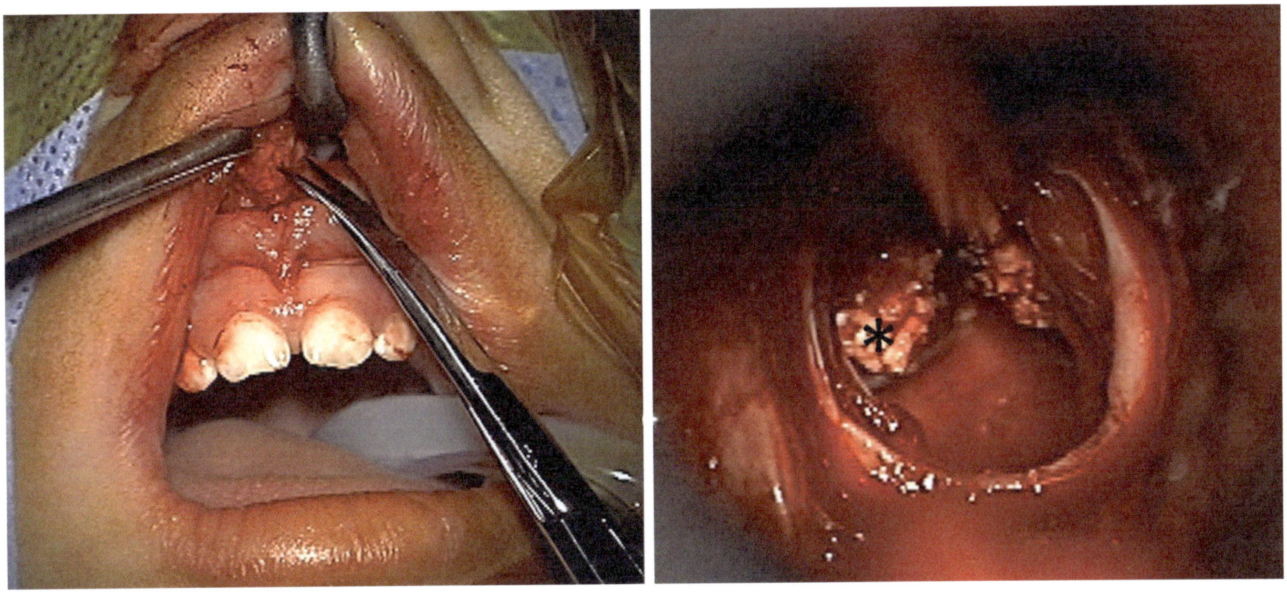

Fig. 13.5 Transsphenoidal approach (translabial/transsphenoidal). The transsphenoidal approach is most useful for sellar tumors confined to the midline. In young children or in adults with small nares, the translabial approach (*left image*) affords a wider viewing and working route. Care must be taken to leave a reasonable cuff of tissue above the gums to prevent injuring the nutrient vessels and nerves to the teeth. Once exposed, the tumor can be clearly identified (*) and removed. Maintaining the integrity of the diaphragm sella reduces the risk of a postoperative CSF leak and inspection of the operative field with an angled endoscope or dental mirror at the conclusion of the case can help to ensure a complete resection

surgery has markedly limited lateral exposure, minimal ability to control bleeding, and an increased risk of CSF leak/meningitis. Rare, but catastrophic injury can occur following injuries to the carotid arteries and their major branches. Moreover, heavily calcified lesions are difficult to remove with the access provided from this route. Low tumors, particularly ones that are primarily midline, infradiaphragmatic, and cystic are well-suited to this approach.

Complication avoidance includes careful preselection of appropriate cases, as described above. In young children, the small working spaces and nonpneumatized sphenoid do not preclude this approach, but do require consideration. With children or in adults with small nares that might inhibit the easy passage of surgical instruments, the translabial/transsphenoidal approach can be used to afford greater visualization and working access (Fig. 13.5). Image guidance, either with frameless stereotaxy and/or fluoroscopy has proved useful to maintain a safe midline approach, especially in reoperated cases. On occasion, the decision to stage a procedure and perform a craniotomy at a subsequent date to remove suprasellar portions of a tumor may be prudent.

In cases with large tumors and evidence of a widened sella on preoperative imaging, the use of a lumbar drain may be helpful to prevent CSF leak and promote healing in the immediate postoperative period. Reconstruction of the sellar floor, often with a synthetic or bony graft, is important at the conclusion of the case.

Alternative Surgical Treatments

In addition to operative approaches targeted at removing the tumor, alternative surgical strategies exist to manage the issues caused by craniophayngioma cysts and/or resultant hydrocephalus. Generally, it is our practice to attempt to treat the underlying cause of the hydrocephalus before resorting to a ventriculoperitonal shunt. In some craniopharyngiomas with large cystic components, placement of a catheter within the cyst can allow for delivery of sclerosing agents, such as bleomycin (an antibiotic that inhibits protein synthesis) or P32 (a radioisotope with limited penetration to surrounding tissues). Generally, these catheters are placed with stereotatic guidance, as accuracy is of paramount importance. Leakage of toxic agents into the subarachnoid space or normal neural parenchyma is to be avoided. Often contrast will be instilled through the catheter, and an imaging study will be done to document the absence of a leak prior to delivery of the sclerosing agent.

Immediate Postoperative Care

Following surgical resection of a craniopharyngioma, patients are usually monitored in the intensive care unit (ICU). Primary concerns center on management of hormonal replacement (especially with regards to diabetes insipidus and stress-dose corticosteroids), repeated assessment of visual function (monitoring for hemorrhage or blood-pressure-dependent changes to eyesight) and documentation of level of consciousness (watching for delayed hydrocephalus and effects of hypothalamic injury). As discussed below, postoperative imaging is useful. Continued discussion between ICU staff, nursing, and the neurosurgical team is critical to maximize the likelihood of a successful outcome.

Complications

- Endocrine dysfunction is common, with immediate concerns centered on diabetes insipidus (with proper fluid management throughout the case) and corticosteroid replacement (given risk of decompensation from acute physiologic stressors). Long-term hormone replacement is often needed.
- CSF leak can occur, particularly with the transsphenoidal approach or when the frontal sinus is compromised at craniotomy. Preparation for abdominal fat graft and/or external CSF drainage can help.
- Bleeding is a major concern, given the location of the tumor within the circle of Willis.
- Neurologic injury can be severe, including damage to the hypothalamic nuclei, optic apparatus, and—with bifrontal craniotomies—olfactory nerves.

Preoperative Complication Avoidance—General Principles

Review of the case with nursing and anesthetic staff well beforehand allows anticipation of needed medications, hormone replacement, blood products, equipment and potential emergencies. In addition to discussing the case with colleagues, a candid assessment of expected outcomes and risks of the surgery with the patient and family is vital. In the operating room, consideration of needs such as abdominal fat grafts, pericranial flaps to provide vascularized coverage of defects, and placement of ventricular or lumbar drains are best done well in advance of the initial preparation. In planning operative approaches, it is useful to allow for additional exposure (through extension of the incision and bone flap) if possible. While often not needed, the ability to improve access to the tumor intraoperatively can be invaluable.

Radiation Therapy

Both fractionated radiation and stereotactic radiosurgery can be very useful in the treatment of craniopharyngioma. Reported rates of cure vary greatly, with tumor size and length of follow-up important variables to consider. This approach is beneficial for surgically inaccessible lesions or in patients who are high-risk surgical candidates and is considered as first-line therapy in some cases. Shortcomings of this approach include a delay of up to 3 years for lesion obliteration and exposure to radiation in children. Radiation has increased risk in younger populations, making its application less appealing in those children under 3 years of age.

Complications

Young children have risk of radiation-induced damage, including injury to the surrounding developing brain and potential for development of secondary malignancies. These risks limit radiation use to older children in most cases. In addition, there seems to be an association between an arteriopathy similar to moyamoya and craniopharyngioma as well as a link between cranial radiation for brain tumor treatment and moyamoya, suggesting that there may be increased risk of moyamoya syndrome in children with craniopharyngioma treated with radiation [30].

Outcomes

Endocrine, Metabolic, and Cognitive Issues

Endocrine dysfunction is common following surgical treatment of craniopharyngiomas, with reports of diabetes insipidus occurring in greater than 80 % of patients and need for hormone replacement in more than 90 % of patients who underwent gross total resections [19, 21, 22, 26, 27, 31–33]. Equally high percentages exist for replacement of thyroid hormone, sex hormones (following puberty), and corticosteroids [33]. More than half of all surgically treated children are candidates for growth hormone replacement [33]. Obesity resulting from hypothalamic injury is present in more than half of children following resection [28, 33]. For many of these patients, these deficits are permanent. As such, long-term endocrinologic follow-up is needed, with appropriate adjustments in hormone replacement (age-specific sex hormones, dosing of growth hormone, and careful monitoring of volume status for DDAVP replacement). Critically important is the recognition of the need for stress-dose corticosteroids in the setting of physiologic challenges such as illness and injury.

Increasingly appreciated are the consequences of surgical treatment of craniopharyngioma on cognitive and emotional function. In the most severe state, akinetic mutism may render patients unable to function in society, but more subtle deficits in intelligence, emotion, and memory may add to the lifetime burden of this disease [34, 35]. Awareness of these potential problems may facilitate appropriate consultation to neuropsychology, psychiatry, and social work to provide additional support and coping mechanisms for affected patients [19, 35].

Long-Term Issues and Recurrence

Several series report average time to recurrence following operation with gross total resection is 2.5–3 years, with about 50 % of patients remaining disease-free at 5 years, although these statistics remain controversial, with some reports indicating much better long-term disease-free intervals after gross total resection [1, 13, 19, 28, 36]. However, craniopharyngioma is notable for its capacity to recur decades after seemingly successful treatment and—as such—warrants prolonged monitoring [18, 25]. Some reports note a 15–40 % recurrence of tumor at 15 years, regardless of therapy administered [1, 18, 37]. If recurrence occurs, it substantially reduces survival, even in delayed cases (10-year survival without recurrence is >99 %, while patients with recurrence have a <70 % survival at 10 years) [19].

If recurrence is detected, the risks and benefits of treatment modalities must be weighed. In younger patients there is often an impetus to attempt surgical re-resection in order to avoid long-term risks of radiation (particularly in those preschool-age children). Gross total resection at reoperation has been reported, with rates ranging from 30 to 70 % [1, 25, 28, 29]. Prior radiation therapy and increasing size of tumor are noted as risk factors limiting the success of reoperation [18, 25, 29]. The wide range of clinical and radiographic presentation of these tumors, coupled with the variety of treatments administered (surgery, radiation, instillation of sclerosing agents, etc.) limits the ability to formulate general guidelines for the management of recurrent disease. As such, many patients are evaluated on a case-by-case basis, emphasizing the importance of providing treatment at an experienced center so that the treating surgeon can more accurately assess the likelihood of success [25, 26, 29].

Follow-up

Frequency of Office Visits

Postoperative care will frequently consist of an office visit approximately 1 month postoperatively, then annually thereafter. Radiation therapy also involves annual visits post-treatment.

Frequency of Imaging

Postoperative imaging is critical to assess the extent of tumor resection and to establish a baseline for comparison to future studies, usually done within 72 h of operation. CT is also performed postoperatively to ascertain whether any calcification remains in the operative bed—a finding considered by some to indicate residual tumor. Calcified regions of tumor are sometimes unable to be safely removed and may thereby be deliberately left in place. Small flecks of calcium—if found to be the only abnormality present on postoperative imaging—are often observed, as their natural history as predictors of tumor recurrence is unclear [38].

Subsequent imaging varies, although many groups will obtain MRI studies every 3–6 months for 1–2 years, then annually thereafter. It is worthwhile noting that craniopharyngiomas have the potential to recur at very delayed dates after surgery, supporting the practice of long-term follow-up.

Conclusion

The surgical management of craniopharyngioma is challenging and best provided by neurosurgeons who routinely treat these tumors at institutions with the resources to administer the required multidisciplinary care. Preoperative assessment should include both MRI and CT for imaging, coupled with a complete endocrinologic and visual evaluation. Operative approaches should be selected based on anatomic routes of access, awareness of pre-existing deficits to preserve remaining function, and surgeon's experience. The goal of complete resection should be weighed against the risk of severe surgical morbidity and may sometimes prompt abandoning attempts of further tumor removal. Follow-up studies include immediate perioperative imaging and endocrinologic replacement as needed. Multidisciplinary care is helpful in the long-term management of these patients. Appreciation of the possibility of delayed recurrence—even decades later—should encourage continued monitoring well after the surgery has finished. Optimal management of patients affected by craniopharyngiomas remains controversial and ongoing collaborative research will hopefully guide clinicians toward increasingly effective treatments.

References

1. [Craniopharyngioma in children. 41st annual congress of the French Society of Neurosurgery. Lisbon, Portugal, 4–7 June 1991]. Neurochirurgie 1991;37(Suppl 1):1–174. French.
2. Lindholm J, Nielsen EH. Craniopharyngioma: historical notes. Pituitary. 2009;12:352–9.
3. Kleihues P, Burger PC, Scheithauer BW. The new WHO classification of brain tumours. Brain Pathol. 1993;3:255–68.
4. Louis DN, Ohgaki H, Wiestler OD, et al. The 2007 WHO classification of tumours of the central nervous system. Acta Neuropathol. 2007;114:97–109.
5. Kleihues P, Louis DN, Scheithauer BW, et al. The WHO classification of tumors of the nervous system. J Neuropathol Exp Neurol. 2002;61:215–25 (discussion 26–9).
6. Jane JA Jr, Laws ER. Craniopharyngioma. Pituitary. 2006;9:323–6.
7. Kanter AS, Sansur CA, Jane JA Jr, Laws ER Jr. Rathke's cleft cysts. Front Horm Res. 2006;34:127–57.

8. Pettorini BL, Frassanito P, Caldarelli M, Tamburrini G, Massimi L, Di Rocco C. Molecular pathogenesis of craniopharyngioma: switching from a surgical approach to a biological one. Neurosurg Focus. 2010;28:E1.
9. Donovan JL, Nesbit GM. Distinction of masses involving the sella and suprasellar space: specificity of imaging features. AJR Am J Roentgenol. 1996;167:597–603.
10. Zada G, Lin N, Ojerholm E, Ramkissoon S, Laws ER. Craniopharyngioma and other cystic epithelial lesions of the sellar region: a review of clinical, imaging, and histopathological relationships. Neurosurg Focus. 2010;28:E4.
11. Miller DC. Pathology of craniopharyngiomas: clinical import of pathological findings. Pediatr Neurosurg. 1994;21(Suppl 1):11–7.
12. Crotty TB, Scheithauer BW, Young WF Jr, et al. Papillary craniopharyngioma: a clinicopathological study of 48 cases. J Neurosurg. 1995;83:206–14.
13. Weiner HL, Wisoff JH, Rosenberg ME, et al. Craniopharyngiomas: a clinicopathological analysis of factors predictive of recurrence and functional outcome. Neurosurgery. 1994;35:1001–10 (discussion 10–1).
14. Smith ER, Manfredi M, Scott RM, Black PM, Moses MA. A recurrent craniopharyngioma illustrates the potential usefulness of urinary matrix metalloproteinases as noninvasive biomarkers: case report. Neurosurgery. 2007;60:E1148–9 (discussion E9).
15. Smith ER, Zurakowski D, Saad A, Scott RM, Moses MA. Urinary biomarkers predict brain tumor presence and response to therapy. Clin Cancer Res. 2008;14:2378–86.
16. Bunin GR, Surawicz TS, Witman PA, Preston-Martin S, Davis F, Bruner JM. The descriptive epidemiology of craniopharyngioma. J Neurosurg. 1998;89:547–51.
17. Samii M, Tatagiba M. Surgical management of craniopharyngiomas: a review. Neurol Med Chir (Tokyo). 1997;37:141–9.
18. Scott RM. Craniopharyngioma: a personal (Boston) experience. Childs Nerv Syst. 2005;21:773–7.
19. Karavitaki N, Brufani C, Warner JT, et al. Craniopharyngiomas in children and adults: systematic analysis of 121 cases with long-term follow-up. Clin Endocrinol (Oxf). 2005;62:397–409.
20. Feletti A, Marton E, Mazzucco GM, Fang S, Longatti P. Amaurosis in infancy due to craniopharyngioma: a not-exceptional but often misdiagnosed symptom. Neurosurg Focus. 2010;28:E7.
21. Sanford RA, Muhlbauer MS. Craniopharyngioma in children. Neurol Clin. 1991;9:453–65.
22. Samii M, Bini W. Surgical treatment of craniopharyngiomas. Zentralbl Neurochir. 1991;52:17–23.
23. Smith MM, Strottmann JM. Imaging of the optic nerve and visual pathways. Semin Ultrasound CT MR. 2001;22:473–87.
24. Wisoff JH. Craniopharyngioma. J Neurosurg Pediatr. 2008;1:124–5 (discussion 5).
25. Wisoff JH. Surgical management of recurrent craniopharyngiomas. Pediatr Neurosurg 1994;21(Suppl 1):108–13.
26. Sanford RA. Craniopharyngioma: results of survey of the American Society of Pediatric Neurosurgery. Pediatr Neurosurg. 1994;21(Suppl 1):39–43.
27. Merchant TE, Kiehna EN, Sanford RA, et al. Craniopharyngioma: the St. Jude Children's Research Hospital experience 1984–2001. Int J Radiat Oncol Biol Phys. 2002;53:533–42.
28. Hoffman HJ, De Silva M, Humphreys RP, Drake JM, Smith ML, Blaser SI. Aggressive surgical management of craniopharyngiomas in children. J Neurosurg. 1992;76:47–52.
29. Elliott RE, Hsieh K, Hochm T, Belitskaya-Levy I, Wisoff J, Wisoff JH. Efficacy and safety of radical resection of primary and recurrent craniopharyngiomas in 86 children. J Neurosurg Pediatr. 2010;5:30–48.
30. Ullrich NJ, Robertson R, Kinnamon DD, et al. Moyamoya following cranial irradiation for primary brain tumors in children. Neurology. 2007;68:932–8.
31. Yang I, Sughrue ME, Rutkowski MJ, et al. Craniopharyngioma: a comparison of tumor control with various treatment strategies. Neurosurg Focus. 2010;28:E5.
32. Campbell PG, McGettigan B, Luginbuhl A, Yadla S, Rosen M, Evans JJ. Endocrinological and ophthalmological consequences of an initial endonasal endoscopic approach for resection of craniopharyngiomas. Neurosurg Focus. 2010;28:E8.
33. Curtis J, Daneman D, Hoffman HJ, Ehrlich RM. The endocrine outcome after surgical removal of craniopharyngiomas. Pediatr Neurosurg. 1994;21(Suppl 1):24–7.
34. Waber DP, Pomeroy SL, Chiverton AM, et al. Everyday cognitive function after craniopharyngioma in childhood. Pediatr Neurol. 2006;34:13–9.
35. Muller HL, Bruhnken G, Emser A, et al. Longitudinal study on quality of life in 102 survivors of childhood craniopharyngioma. Childs Nerv Syst. 2005;21:975–80.
36. Kim SK, Wang KC, Shin SH, Choe G, Chi JG, Cho BK. Radical excision of pediatric craniopharyngioma: recurrence pattern and prognostic factors. Childs Nerv Syst. 2001;17:531–6 (discussion 7).
37. Bulow B, Attewell R, Hagmar L, Malmstrom P, Nordstrom CH, Erfurth EM. Postoperative prognosis in craniopharyngioma with respect to cardiovascular mortality, survival, and tumor recurrence. J Clin Endocrinol Metab. 1998;83:3897–904.
38. Elliott RE, Moshel YA, Wisoff JH. Minimal residual calcification and recurrence after gross-total resection of craniopharyngioma in children. J Neurosurg Pediatr. 2009;3:276–83.

Dermoid: Head and Neck

14

Mark S. Volk

Introduction

Dermoid cysts may be either congenital or acquired and are most commonly diagnosed during childhood. These benign lesions can occur in multiple locations within the head and neck region. The diverse location of these cysts results in a varied presentation. Because of this, dermoid cysts often come to the attention of assorted consultants, including otolaryngologist, ophthalmologists, plastic surgeons, general surgeons, neurosurgeons, and dermatologists. This chapter will review head and neck dermoids, except those that present in the nasal region.

Occurrence

- Dermoid cysts have equal gender distribution.
- The incidence of dermoids is unknown. However, teratomas occur 1 in 4,000 births. Dermoids are a subset of teratoma and are the most common of these congenital abnormalities [1, 2].
- 7–34 % of all dermoids occur in the head and neck [3, 4].
- Most dermoids present in the first five years of life. (Fig. 14.1) [3].

Embryology

- Three proposed etiologies [1, 3]
  - *Acquired implantation.* Traumatic implantation of skin into the deeper layers resulting in formation of a dermal cyst lined with squamous epithelium and resembling epidermoid cysts.
  - *Congenital teratomas.* Technically from all three types of germinal epithelium (ectoderm, endoderm, and mesoderm), these dermoids, which are usually found in the ovaries or testes, are often included as a subset of teratoma.
  - *Congenital inclusion dermoid cysts.* Form along the lines of embryologic fusion and contain both epidermal and dermal elements. These are the lesions found in the head and neck.

Histopathology

- Dermoid cysts are benign neoplasms that are derived from epidermal and dermal elements.
- Dermoids are usually cystic lesions that contain a cheesy, keratinous substance. They can also be solid tumors, composed of a thick fibrofatty matrix.
- The walls of dermoid cysts are made up of keratinized stratified squamous epithelium along with appendages such as sweat glands sebaceous glands, hair follicles, and connective tissue elements (Fig. 14.2a, b).
- The term "dermoid cyst" can be confusing since over the years it has been used to identify several different histopathologic entities. In the head and neck, this term has been applied to (1) true dermoid cysts, (2) epidermal (epidermoid) cysts, and (3) teratoid cysts [5].
- Unlike dermoids, the wall of epidermoids contains solely squamous epithelium (Fig. 14.2c). Both of these cyst types usually contain sebaceous debris within their lumen.
- Clinically, dermoid and epidermoid cysts behave identically. Differentiation between dermoid and epidermoid cysts can be made only by pathologic examination.
- True dermoid cysts are rare. Epidermoid cysts are much more common but because of their similar appearance and location, clinicians often lump the two types of lesions together and call them dermoids.

M. S. Volk (✉)
Department of Otolaryngology and Communication Enhancement, Boston Children's Hospital, Harvard Medical School, Boston, MA, USA
e-mail: mark.volk@childrens.harvard.edu

R. Rahbar et al. (eds.), *Pediatric Head and Neck Tumors*,
DOI 10.1007/978-1-4614-8755-5_14, © Springer Science+Business Media New York 2014

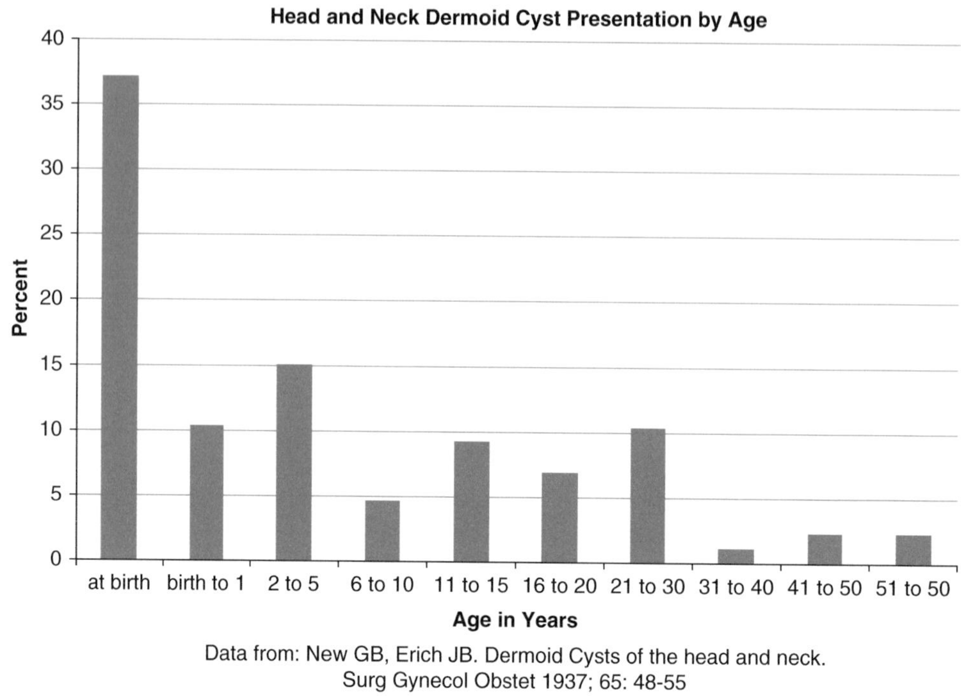

Fig. 14.1 Dermoid age presentation

- Teratoid cysts have in the past been confused with dermoids and epidermoids. However, teratoid cysts contain endodermal and/or mesodermal components in addition to their ectodermal-derived epithelium [6].

Presentation

- In the most comprehensive study on dermoids to date, New and Erich reviewed 1,495 dermoids cysts treated at the Mayo Clinic from 1910 to 1935. They noted the majority of dermoid cysts presented in the anal region (44.5 %). This was followed in frequency by the ovaries (42 %) and the head and neck (7 %) [3].
- Of the 103 head and neck dermoids reported by New and Erich, the majority were located in the orbital region (Figs. 14.3, 14.4) [3].
- Dermoid cysts of the head and neck usually present as asymptomatic masses.
- On occasion, a dermoid may present as an inflamed mass in which case it may mimic an abscess. The inflammation may occur secondary to infection. Rupture of the dermoid cyst may also cause an inflammatory reaction when the cyst contents come in contact with the surrounding soft tissue. Rupture most often occurs in dermoids located in the lateral canthal region.
- Except for the orbital region, dermoids usually present near or at the midline. Lateral cervical dermoids are rare. There have been several reports of lateral dermoids associated with midline dermoids. For this reason, many authors feel that lateral dermoid cysts are essentially a portion of a midline cyst that has migrated laterally [1, 6, 7].

Imaging

- Ultrasound has limited utility in diagnosing superficial dermoid and epidermoid cysts in the neck. This modality is able to distinguish between dermoid cysts and schwannomas, lymph nodes (benign and malignant), and Kimura's disease. However, dermoids cannot be reliably differentiated from lipomas and thyroglossal duct cysts on ultrasound [8, 9].
- Dermoid cysts imaged by magnetic resonance imaging (MRI) usually appear as a unilocular, round lesion with variable signal intensity on T1-weighted images: hyperintense or isointense in comparison to muscle. The T2-weighted images are usually hyperintense. The internal aspect of the cyst often appears heterogeneous. They generally do not enhance with gadolinium (Fig. 14.5) [10]

Differential Diagnosis

- Dermoid cysts that present in the floor of the mouth share similar characteristics with a number of other lesions. These include mucocele, ranula, foregut duplication cyst, venous/lymphatic malformation, teratoma, and thyroglossal duct cyst.

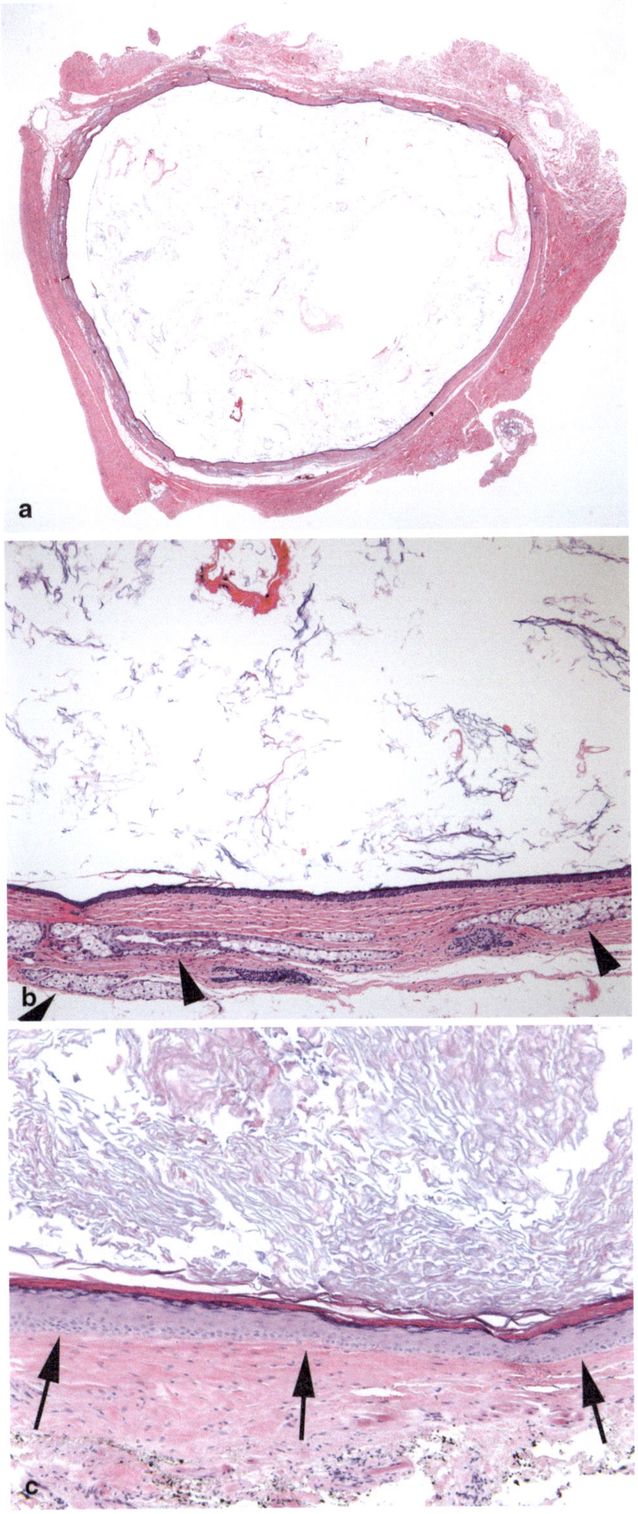

Fig. 14.2 Dermoid cyst. **a** Simple cyst lined by keratinizing squamous epithelium and containing keratin debris and fragments of hair. **b** Characteristically, the cyst wall contains dermal appendages with well-formed pilosebaceous units (*arrowheads*). **c** For comparison, an epidermal inclusion cyst is shown. The lining consists of keratinizing squamous epithelium (*arrows*) devoid of dermal appendages and the lumen (*top*) contains laminated keratin debris

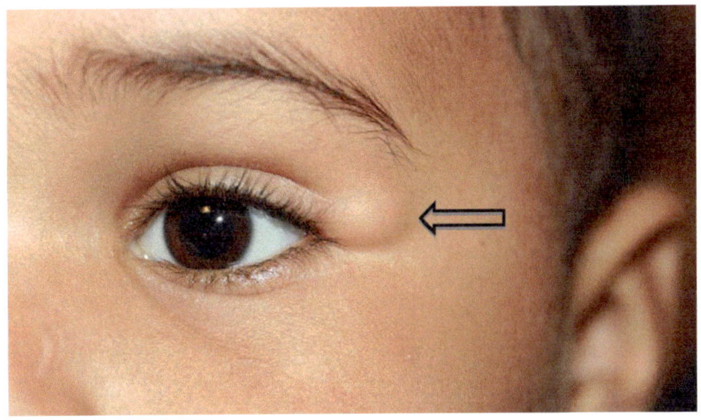

Fig. 14.3 Dermoid cyst of lateral canthus region. (Courtesy of Linda Dagi, MD)

- While not often found in the oral cavity, foregut duplication cysts are clinically almost indistinguishable from dermoids. Classified as choristomas, foregut duplication cysts consist of islands of gastrointestinal mucosa (with various proportions of stratified squamous epithelium, parietal, chief, goblet, argentaffin, and Paneth cells), with a surrounding layer of smooth muscle.
- Mucoceles or ranulas tend to be located off the midline. They often have a thin wall with a translucent appearance. These lesions are not true cysts but rather are salivary extravasations, usually emanating from minor salivary glands in the case of a mucocele or the sublingual gland in the case of a ranula.
- Venous/lymphatic malformations may present in the floor of the mouth but generally have a very different appearance from dermoids. They may mimic a mucocele by having a thin, translucent wall or they may have an irregular vascular appearance.

Treatment

- Treatment of dermoid cysts consists of surgical excision.
- Removal of the cyst allows pathologic diagnosis, corrects cosmetic deformity, prevents the possibility of future infection, and avoids possible airway obstruction or swallowing dysfunction from mass effect.
- Treating infected dermoids with antibiotics only and avoiding incision and drainage will reduce the difficulty in the cyst's subsequent removal.
- Management of ruptured dermoid cysts may benefit from a course of steroids to help reduce the inflammatory response to the cyst contents.
- The approach to excising a floor-of-mouth dermoid requires consideration of the cyst's relation to the mylohyoid muscle. Lesions rostral to the mylohyoid are amenable to intraoral excision. Those cysts located caudal to

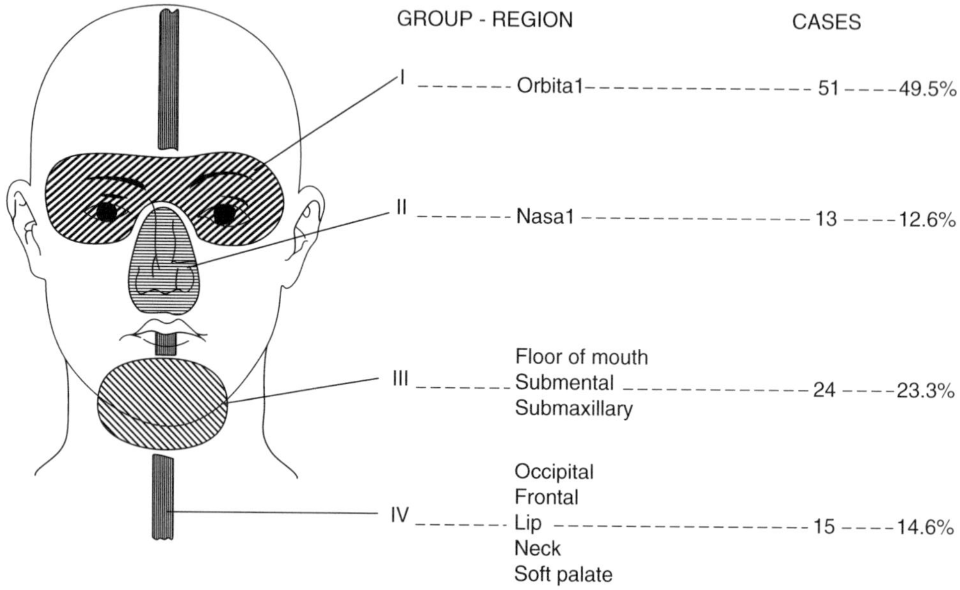

Fig. 14.4 Location of head and neck dermoid cysts [3]. (Reprinted with permission from the Journal of the American College of Surgeons, formerly Surgery, Gynecology and Obstetrics)

the mylohyoid muscle are best removed through a submandibular approach (Fig. 14.6) [11].

- For the intraoral approach, an incision is made anterior to the submandibular ducts. For additional exposure, a midline incision between the ductal orifices may be made (Fig. 14.7).

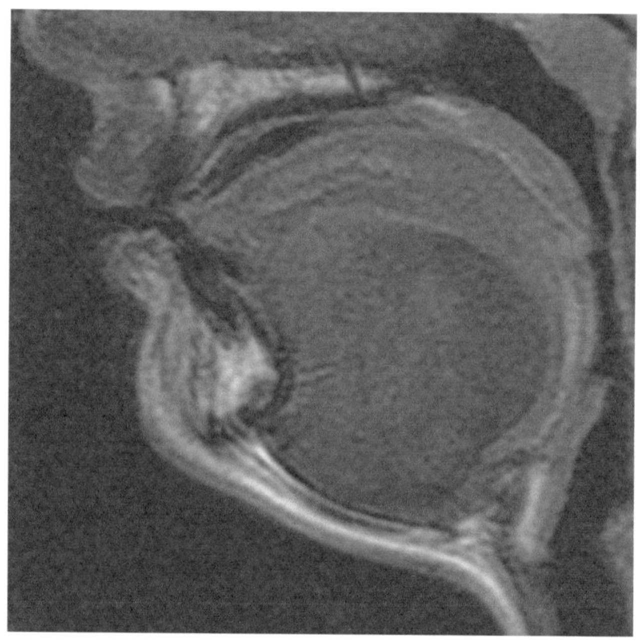

Fig. 14.5 T-1-weighted sagittal MRI of lingual dermoid cyst

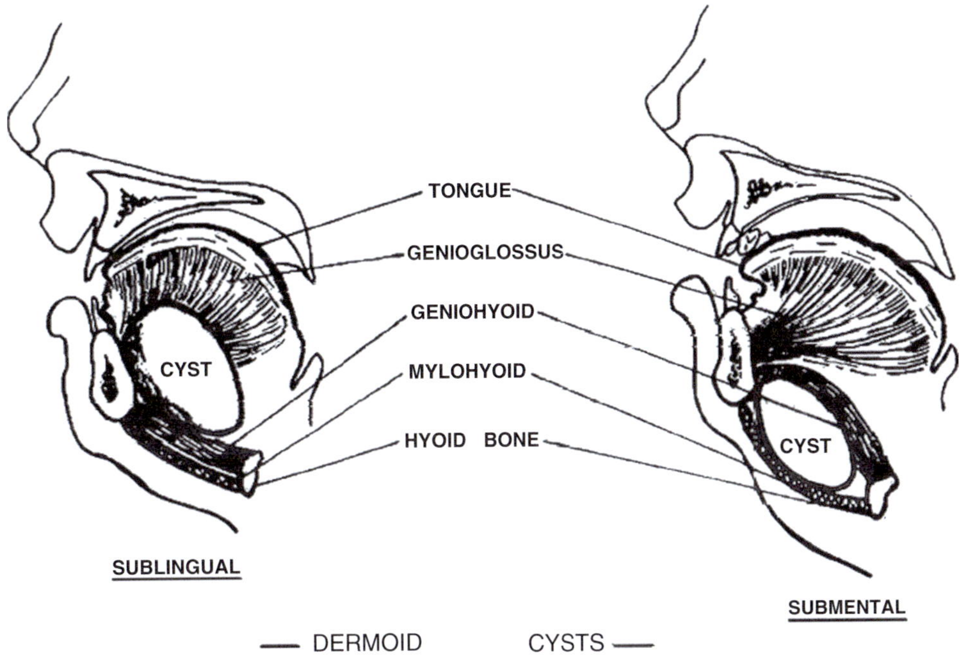

Fig. 14.6 Location of floor-of-mouth dermoid cysts above and below the mylohyoid muscle [11]. (Reprinted with permission from C.V. Mosby Co.)

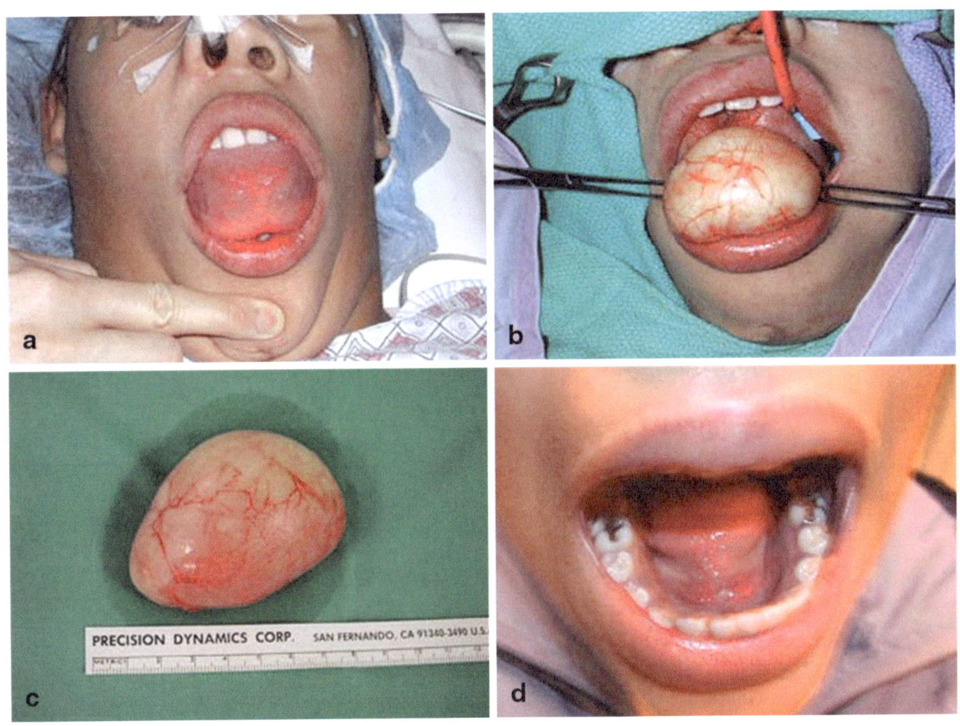

Fig. 14.7 Floor-of-mouth dermoid excision. **a** Preoperative. **b** Intraoperative. **c** Excised dermoid cyst. **d** Two weeks postoperative

References

1. Rosen D, Wirtschafter A, Rao VM, Wilcox TO. Dermoid cyst of the lateral neck: a case report and literature review. Ear Nose Throat J. 1998;77:125–32.
2. Erich JB, Johnsen DS. Congenital dermoid cyst. Am J Surg. 1953;85(1):104–7.
3. New GB, Erich JB. Dermoid cysts of the head and neck. Surg Gynecol Obstet. 1937;65:48–55.
4. Taylor BW, Erich JB, Dockerty MB. Dermoids of the head and neck. Minn Med. 1966;49:1535–40.
5. Batsakis JG. Non-odontogenic and fissural cysts. ORL. 1971;33:19.
6. Batsakis JG. Tumours of the head and neck. Clinical and pathological considerations. 2nd ed. Baltimore: Williams and Wilkins; 1979. p 226–31.
7. Leveque H, Saraceno CA, Tang CK, et al. Dermoids cysts of the floor of mouth. Laryngoscope. 1979;89:296–305.
8. Sidell DR, Shapiro NL. Diagnostic accuracy of ultrasonography for midline neck masses in children. Otolaryngol Head Neck Surg. 2011;144:431–4.
9. Yasumoto M, Shibuya H, Gomi N, et al. Ultrasonographic appearance of dermoid and epidermoid cysts in the head and neck. J Clin Ultrasound. 1991;19:455–61.
10. Koeller KK, Alamo L, Adair CF, Smirniotopoulos JG. Congenital cystic masses of the neck: radiologic-pathologic correlation. Radiographics. 1999;19(1):121–46.
11. Meyer I. Dermoid cysts (dermoids) of the floor of the mouth. Oral Surg Oral Med Oral Pathol. 1955;8(11):1149–64.

Dermoid: Nasal

15

Stephen Kieran, John G. Meara, Mark Proctor and Reza Rahbar

Introduction

First reported in 1817 by Cruvelier, congenital dermoid cysts contain ectodermal and embryonal elements, as opposed to teratomas, which contain elements from all three embryonal layers. Nasal dermoids account for 1–3 % of all dermoid cysts and approximately 10 % of all head and neck dermoid cysts [1, 2]. These benign lesions are the commonest diagnosis in a child who presents with a midline nasal defect. The differential diagnoses are nasal glioma or encephalocele.

Key Points

- Commonest congenital midline nasal defect [3].
- Potential for significant morbidity if becomes infected; brain abscess, meningitis and frontal osteomyelitis [4].
- Complete surgical excision including excision of any intracranial extension is recommended.
- The optimum surgical approach differs for each patient, depending on the site and extension of the lesion.

Biology and Epidemiology

Nasal dermoids are frontonasal inclusion cysts or tracts related to embryologic errors localized to the anterior neuropore. Grunwald described in 1910 the prenasal theory for the embryogenesis of a nasal dermoid cyst or tract. This theory was subsequently illustrated by Pratt in 1965 [5, 6].

Pathogenesis

- At 8 weeks gestation, a dural diverticulum protrudes through the nasal and frontal bones, entering the space between the nasal bones and nasal capsule.
- This diverticulum is subsequently surrounded by the frontal process of the nasal bones, hence separating the dura from the skin. Under normal circumstances, this diverticulum involutes, but incomplete closure results in a persistent attachment of the dura to the dermis.
- As the dura recedes, dermis is pulled superiorly resulting in trapped epithelium along the diverticulum path.
- These trapped elements result in a sinus tract and/ or cyst containing glands and hair follicles, located anywhere along the course of the diverticulum, from the columella to the anterior cranial fossa.
- As a consequence, the cyst may be extranasal, intranasal, or a combination of the two. Intracranial extension usually communicates through the foramen cecum or the cribriform plate with extradural adherence to the falx cerebri.

Molecular/Genetic Pathology

- Majority of dermoid cysts appear to occur spontaneously.
- Familial tendency has been suggested but no genetic cause identified [7].
- Nasal dermoids have been reported in a mother and identical twin daughters—suggesting an autosomal dominant inheritance in some rare patients [8].

R. Rahbar (✉) · S. Kieran
Department of Otolaryngology, Boston Children's Hospital, Harvard Medical School, Boston, MA, USA
e-mail: Reza.rahbar@childrens.harvard.edu

J. G. Meara
Department of Plastic and Oral Surgery, Boston Children's Hospital, Harvard Medical School, Boston, MA, USA

M. Proctor
Boston Children's Hospital, Harvard Medical School, Boston, MA, USA

R. Rahbar et al. (eds.), *Pediatric Head and Neck Tumors*,
DOI 10.1007/978-1-4614-8755-5_15, © Springer Science+Business Media New York 2014

Incidence and Prevalence

- Uncommon lesion: estimated to occur in 1 in every 20,000–40,000 live births [9].

Age Distribution

- Generally present at birth or in early childhood.
- Mean age at presentation is 14–34 months [10].
- Late presentation in adulthood does rarely occur [11].

Sex Predilection

- Slight male predominance [10].

Risk Factors—Environmental, Life Style

- None reported.

Relationships to Other Disease States, Syndromes

- Nasal dermoids are not associated with any named syndrome.
- However, other congenital anomalies have been reported in up to 41 % of cases, including cleft palate, aural atresia, hydrocephalus, craniosynostosis, hemifacial microsomia, lacrimal duct cysts, and hypertelorism [2, 12].
- In the presence of other congenital anomalies the incidence of intracranial extension of the dermoid cyst is said to increase [12].

Presentation

Nasal dermoids present in early childhood as a midline mass, anywhere from the base of the columella to the nasoglabellar region. The reported incidence of intracranial extension varies widely from 5–45 % [6].

The mass is typically noncompressible and does not enlarge with compression of the jugular vein (negative Furstenberg sign). The mass may cause broadening of the nasal dorsum. The cyst may first present when it becomes infected with pain, tenderness and erythema.

Sixty percent are located on the lower nasal dorsum, 30 % are intranasal, and 10 % are combined intra- and extranasal.

A sinus opening is best appreciated by examining the nose with magnification. The opening may express sebaceous material. The presence of a hair follicle in the sinus opening is pathognomonic for a nasal dermoid.

Rarely, a nasal dermoid may present with local extension of infection such as a recurrent septal abscess, osteomyelitis, meningitis, or brain abscess.

Table 15.1 Differential diagnosis of a congenital midline nasal mass

Nasal Dermoid
Glioma
Encephalocele
Hemangioma
Teratoma

Differential Diagnosis

The differential diagnosis of a midline nasal mass includes nasal dermoid, glioma, and encephaloceles (Table 15.1). Differentiation between these entities relies upon clinical examination and radiological findings. Clinically, encephaloceles often transilluminate whilst nasal dermoids do not. Furthermore, encephaloceles tend to enlarge with straining, crying, or jugular vein compression (Furstenburg sign), whilst lesions that do not communicate intracranially (dermoids or gliomas) do not.

Diagnosis and Evaluation

Physical Examination

- Noncompressible mass between columella and glabella.
- Does not transilluminate.
- Negative Furstenberg sign.
- Broadening of nasal dorsum.
- Widening of the anterior nasal septum.
- Sinus opening may be difficult to see unless it contains sebaceous material or a hair follicle.

Imaging Evaluation

Preoperative imaging is mandatory in order to assess for intracranial extension as well as the extent of the cyst, with computerized tomography (CT) and magnetic resonance imaging (MRI) giving complimentary information. CT provides information on boney anatomy, whilst MRI determines the soft tissue characteristics. Traditionally, many centers have performed both investigations. However, with a heightened awareness of the potential long-term complications from the radiation exposure in CT, MRI is being increasingly utilized as a solitary investigation [13].

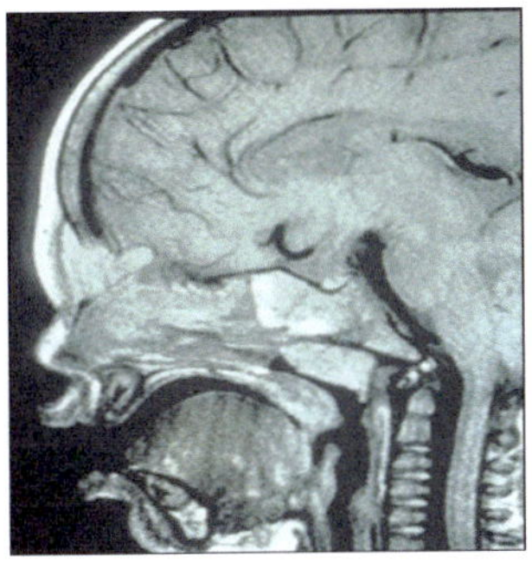

Fig. 15.1 MRI scan in sagittal section demonstrating intracranial extension of a nasal dermoid

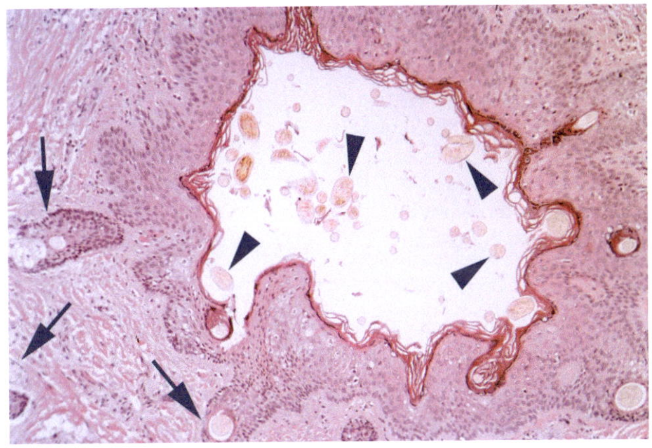

Fig. 15.2 Nasal dermoid characterized by a sinus tract lined by keratinizing squamous mucosa, dermal appendages (*arrows*), and luminal hair shafts on cross section (*arrowheads*)

Computerized Tomography

- Fine-cut CT (1–3 mm) of the anterior skull base is suggestive of intracranial extension if there is widening of the foramen cecum, a bifid crista galli, or a boney defect in the skull base. However, a fibrous attachment to the dura, without intracranial extension of the cyst may result in a widened foramen cecum and bifid crista galli, therefore mimicking intracranial extension on CT [14].
- Images should include the entire nasal, ethmoid, and orbital region from the tip of the nose through the anterior cranial fossa. Contrast should be used in cases of infection and to differentiate a boney defect from enhancing cartilage as well as to differentiate between enhancing nasal mucosa and nonenhancing dermoids.

Magnetic Resonance Imaging

- Multiplanar, high-resolution MRI using T1 images, fat-suppressed T2, fast-spin echo inversion recovery pulse sequences as gadolinium-enhanced, fat suppressed T1 images are used to deliver improved soft tissue resolution, particularly in patients who are suspected of having intracranial extension (Fig. 15.1).
- Gadolinium contrast helps differentiate dermoids from other enhancing masses such as hemangiomas or teratomas.

Pathology

Macroscopic examination reveals a well-defined cyst lined by squamous epithelium of ectodermal origin with adnexal structures (i.e., hair follicle, sebaceous glands, and sweat glands) of mesodermal origin. These adnexal structures allow differentiation of dermoid cysts from epidermoid cysts. Furthermore, unlike teratomas, nasal dermoids do not contain tissue of endodermal origin (Fig. 15.2).

Treatment

Treatment entails complete surgical excision. Conservative procedures such as incision and drainage, aspiration, curettage, and subtotal excision fail to eradicate the cyst, with consequent high rates of recurrence [15, 16].

Surgical Therapy

A wide array of surgical approaches have been described. The optimum approach for each individual patient is determined by the site of the cyst, the site of any tract opening, the presence or absence of intracranial extension, and the surgeon's experience.

Excision is performed under general anesthesia with a thorough examination of the nasal skin performed under magnification (prior to injection of local anesthesia), as a sinus tract opening may be visible that may not have been appreciated in the office.

- In the absence of intracranial extension, the external rhinoplasty approach, a vertical incision over the cyst, a horizontal incision over the cyst, facial degloving approach, endoscopic transnasal approach, and a medial canthal incision have all been described [10].
- Excision of any sinus tract opening necessitates an incision on the nasal dorsum. Excision of the underlying cyst and tract via a vertical extension of this has remained the most traditional approach. The sinus tract opening is excised using a small elliptical incision and attempts are made to confine the vertical incision to the skin overlying the cartilaginous nose, as it is the senior author's experience that skin in this area heals more satisfactorily than the skin overlying the boney nasal skeleton. Depending on the location of the cyst, this incision may be in continuity or separate from the elliptical incision around the sinus tract opening. This approach has been suggested to have superior cosmetic outcomes to lateral rhinotomy and horizontal incisions [17, 18] (Fig. 15.3).
- Cysts located near the nasal tip can be successfully approached via an external rhinoplasty incision, dissection being aided by otologic dissecting instruments and the use of a 0° sinus telescope. This approach has been suggested to have better cosmetic outcomes [19]. However, this approach is of limited utility if an external

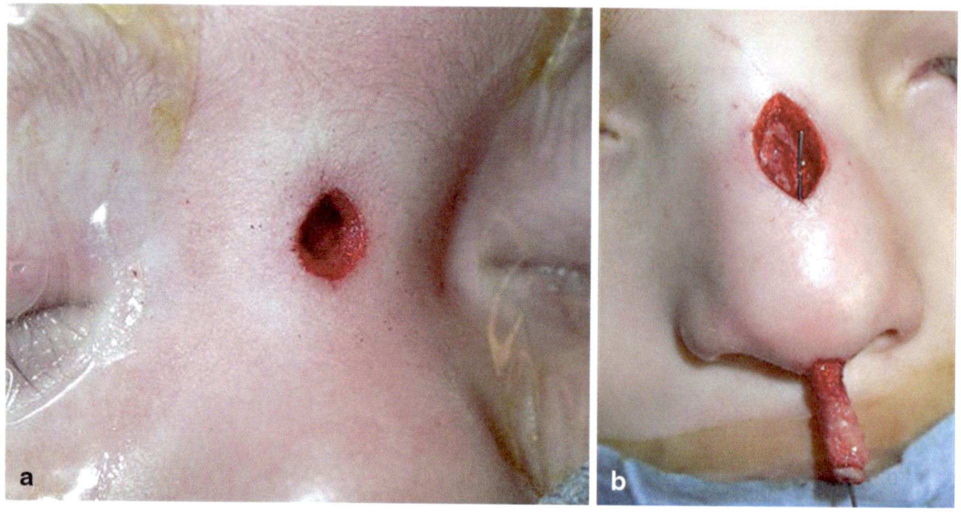

Fig. 15.3 Examples of nasal dermoids in two separate patients. **a** Small cyst that was adjacent to the sinus opening, amenable to excision via a single elliptical incision. **b** Sinus tract opening at the nasal tip, with a sinus tract extending to a more cranially located cyst. In this patient two separate incisions were necessary

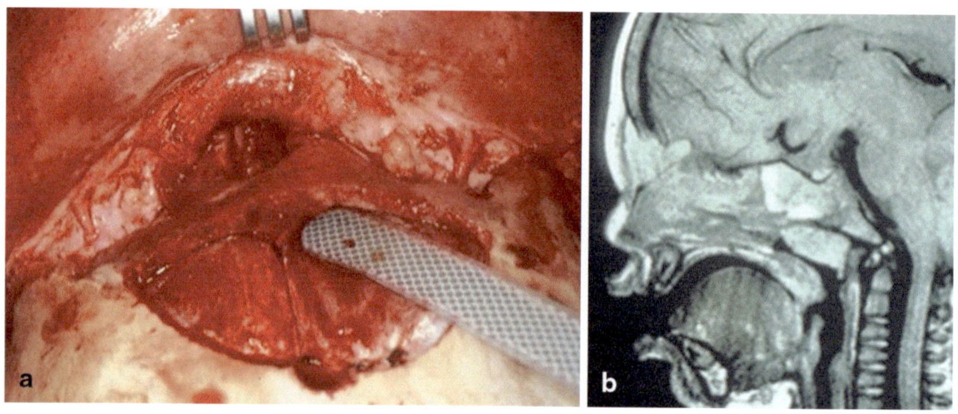

Fig. 15.4 **a** Intraoperative photograph of an intracranial dermoid cyst being excised via a bicoronal approach with bifrontal craniotomy. **b** MRI of same patient

opening exists which needs to be excised via a separate incision and only gives limited access to the superior nasal dorsum.

- If the sinus tract or cyst extends deep to the nasal bones, a nasal osteotomy is performed to improve access to the entirety of the cyst. The nasal bones are fractured and separated vertically over the dorsum of the nose at the nasofrontal suture. Meticulous care is required in following the entire tract and assessing for intracranial extension.
- In some cases the preoperative imaging will suggest a sinus tract extending to the skull base, widening of the crista galli but no intracranial cyst. This may represent a vestigial fibrous tract rather than an epithelial tract. Faced with this situation, it is recommended to confirm the absence of epithelial components with a frozen section biopsy prior to suture ligation of the fibrous tract [1].
- Definitive intracranial disease requires either a combined approach with neurosurgery utilizing a bifrontal craniotomy, or more recently a transglabellar sub cranial approach has also been described, which may obviate the need for a nasal dorsum incision [20] (Fig. 15.4).

Outcomes

Complete surgical resection is curative, however, recurrence and complicated infections can occur if epithelial tissue remains in situ following an incomplete resection. A recurrence rate of 12% has been reported, with a mean time to recurrence of 3.6 years [10].

Follow-up

Due to the potential for recurrence years after resection, prolonged annual follow-up is recommended.

References

1. Sessions RB. Nasal dermal sinuses—new concepts and explanations. Laryngoscope. 1982;92:1–28.
2. Denoyelle F, Ducroz V, Roger G, Garabedian EN. Nasal dermoid sinus cysts in children. Laryngoscope. 1997;107:795–800.
3. Bloom DC, Carvalho DS, Dory C, Brewster DF, Wickersham JK, Kearns DB. Imaging and surgical approach of nasal dermoids. Int J Pediatr Otorhinolaryngol. 2002;62:111–22.

4. Blake WE, Chow CW, Holmes AD, Meara JG. Nasal dermoid sinus cysts: a retrospective review and discussion of investigation and management. Ann Plast Surg. 2006;57:535–40.
5. Pratt LW. Midline cysts of the nasal dorsum: embryologic origin and treatment. Laryngoscope. 1965;75:968–80.
6. Zapata S, Kearns DB. Nasal dermoids. Curr Opin Otolaryngol Head Neck Surg. 2006;14:406–11.
7. Anderson PJ, Dobson C, Berry RB. Nasal dermoid cysts in siblings. Int J Pediatr Otorhinolaryngol. 1998;44:155–9.
8. Bratton C, Suskind DL, Thomas T, Kluka EA. Autosomal dominant familial frontonasal dermoid cysts: a mother and her identical twin daughters. Int J Pediatr Otorhinolaryngol. 2001;57:249–53.
9. Szeremeta W, Parikh TD, Widelitz JS. Congenital nasal malformations. Otolaryngol Clin North Am. 2007;40:97–112, vi–vii.
10. Rahbar R, Shah P, Mulliken JB, et al. The presentation and management of nasal dermoid: a 30-year experience. Arch Otolaryngol Head Neck Surg. 2003;129:464–71.
11. Hacker DC, Freeman JL. Intracranial extension of a nasal dermoid sinus cyst in a 56-year-old man. Head Neck. 1994;16:366–71.
12. Wardinsky TD, Pagon RA, Kropp RJ, Hayden PW, Clarren SK. Nasal dermoid sinus cysts: association with intracranial extension and multiple malformations. Cleft Palate Craniofac J. 1991;28:87–95.
13. Lusk RP, Lee PC. Magnetic resonance imaging of congenital midline nasal masses. Otolaryngol Head Neck Surg. 1986;95:303–6.
14. Pensler JM, Bauer BS, Naidich TP. Craniofacial dermoids. Plast Reconstr Surg. 1988;82:953–8.
15. Yavuzer R, Bier U, Jackson IT. Be careful: it might be a nasal dermoid cyst. Plast Reconstr Surg. 1999;103:2082–3.
16. Vibe P, Lontoft E. Congenital nasal dermoid cysts and fistulas. Scand J Plast Reconstr Surg. 1985;19:105–7.
17. Kelly JH, Strome M, Hall B. Surgical update on nasal dermoids. Arch Otolaryngol. 1982;108:239–42.
18. Posnick JC, Clokie CM, Goldstein JA. Maxillofacial considerations for diagnosis and treatment in Gorlin's syndrome: access osteotomies for cyst removal and orthognathic surgery. Ann Plast Surg. 1994;32:512–8.
19. Locke R, Rakhra J, Kubba H. A comparative study of two techniques for excision of midline nasal dermoids: how we do it. Clin Otolaryngol. 2011;36:252–5.
20. Goyal P, Kellman RM. Tatum SA, 3rd. Transglabellar subcranial approach for the management of nasal masses with intracranial extension in pediatric patients. Arch Facial Plast Surg. 2007;9:314–7.

Encephaloceles

16

Christian J. Vercler, Frank W. Virgin, Reza Rahbar, Edward R. Smith and John G. Meara

Introduction

Encephaloceles are the result of a congenital cranial defect that allows intracranial contents to herniate. The herniated contents may consist of the meninges (meningocele), meninges, and brain (meningoencephalocele) (see Fig. 16.1), or in severe cases meninges, brain, and part of the ventricular system (hydroencephalomeningocele). Encephaloceles are classified by their anatomic location (see Table 16.1) [1]. The vast majority (75 %) are located in the posterior cranial fossa. However, it is the anterior cranial fossa (sincipital) encephalocele that is the concern of the craniofacial team, as it is considerably more deforming.

Biology and Epidemiology

- No known genetic mutation.
- Higher incidence in Southeast Asia (1:6,000 live births) than North America (1:35,000 live births) [2].

Theories of pathogenesis

- Primary arrest of bone development allowing brain to herniate [3].
- Adhesions from brain, dura, and skin arresting bony development [4].
- Increased intracranial pressure pushes the brain through the developing cranial base, causing arrest of bone development [5].

Embryology

- Neural tube begins to close between 3rd and 4th week of fetal development.
- Neural crest cells migrate into the frontonasal and maxillary processes, differentiating into the facial bones, cartilage, and muscles.
- Abnormal development of the potential spaces between these developing structures (fonticulus frontalis, prenasal space, foramen cecum) is responsible for congenital midline masses.

Presentation

- Soft, compressible, pulsatile midline mass that transilluminates
- Occasionally may present with ulcerations and leaking CSF, which requires emergent closure

Differential Diagnosis

The three most common diagnoses of a midline mass in an infant are dermoid cyst, glioma, and encephalocele [6, 7]. History and physical exam can generally lead to the correct diagnosis; however, this is usually confirmed with imaging.

J. G. Meara (✉)
Department of Plastic and Oral Surgery, Boston Children's Hospital, Harvard Medical School, Boston, MA, USA
e-mail: john.meara@childrens.harvard.edu

C. J. Vercler
Section of Plastic Surgery, University of Michigan, Ann Arbor, MI, USA

F. W. Virgin
Department of Otolaryngology Head and Neck Surgery, Monroe Carell Jr. Children's Hospital at Vanderbilt, Nashville, TN, USA

R. Rahbar
Department of Otolaryngology, Boston Children's Hospital, Harvard Medical School, Boston, MA, USA

E. R. Smith
Department of Neurosurgery, Boston Children's Hospital, Harvard Medical School, Boston, MA, USA

R. Rahbar et al. (eds.), *Pediatric Head and Neck Tumors*,
DOI 10.1007/978-1-4614-8755-5_16,

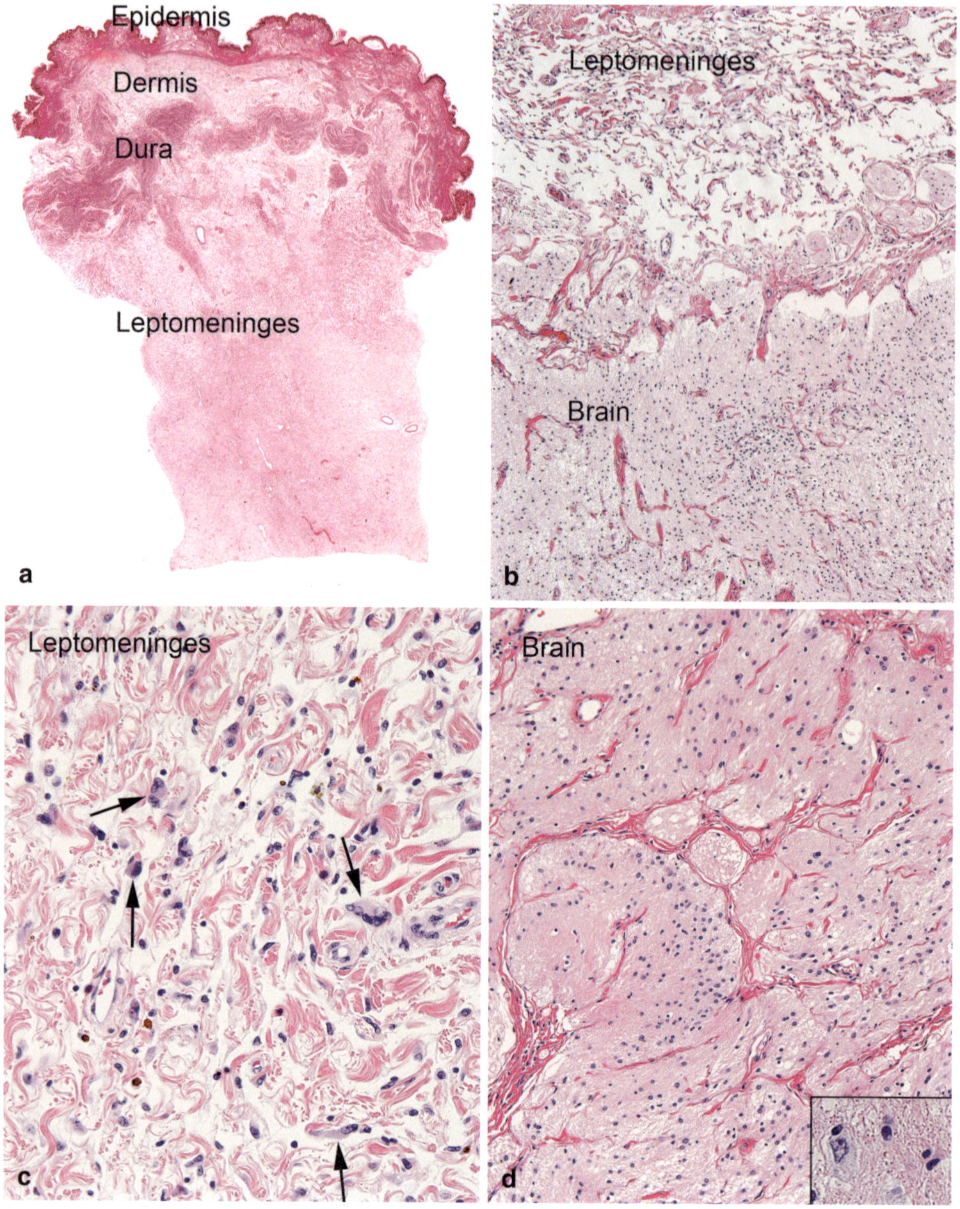

Fig. 16.1 Encephalocele. **a** Cut section of encephalocele wall showing skin surface with *dermis* and *epidermis* a dense fibrous *dura*-like band and deep-seated *leptomeninges*. **b** *Brain* tissue covered by a layer of *leptomeninges*. **c** Leptomeningeal tissue with reactive glial cells (*arrows*) and short curvilinear bands of collagen. **d** Malformed *brain* tissue. Neurons are seen in the *inset*

- Nasal dermoid cyst
  - Most common midline mass
  - Present at birth, diagnosed in early childhood
  - Composed of ectodermal and mesodermal elements
  - Hallmark is punctum with a single hair located on the nasal dorsum
  - Often become infected and can drain sebaceous material
  - Intracranial extension cannot be ruled out on exam—imaging required for accurate diagnosis
- Nasal glioma
  - Presents as firm rubbery mass with bluish or reddish appearance
  - Composed of glial cells in a connective tissue matrix
  - Often extend intranasally
  - Does not communicate with cerebral contents, so not pulsatile and does not transilluminate
- Less common entities that occur in the midline
  - Vascular malformation
  - Teratoma
  - Sebaceous cyst
  - Neurofibroma
  - Ganglioneuroma
  - Nasal fibroma
  - Adenoma
  - Chondroma
  - Carcinoma

Diagnosis and Evaluation

Patients who present with an encephalocele are most appropriately managed by a multidisciplinary craniofacial team comprised of a craniofacial surgeon, a neurosurgeon,

Table 16.1 Classification of encephaloceles [1]

Frontoethmoidal encephaloceles
Nasofrontal
Nasoethmoidal
Nasoorbital
Cranial vault encephaloceles
Interfrontal
Anterior fontanel
Interparietal
Posterior fontanel
Temporal
Cranial base encephaloceles
Transethmoidal
Sphenoethmoidal
Transsphenoidal
Frontosphenoidal
Occipital encephaloceles
Cranioschisis
Associated with cranial/upper face clefts
Associated with basal/lower face clefts
Occipitocervical clefts
Acrania and/or anencephaly

an otolaryngologist, a geneticist, and a pediatrician. Neurological and developmental assessments and evaluation by an ophthalmologist are also essential.

Physical Examination

- Soft nasal mass in midline is the most common presentation
- Bluish appearance
- Soft, compressible, and pulsatile mass that transilluminates
- Mass increases with size with crying, Valsalva, or compression of internal jugular veins (Furstenberg test)
- "Long nose hypertelorism"—patients present with long, flat, wide noses that is more pronounced after encephalocele excision [8, 9]
  –True orbital hypertelorism is rare, but telecanthus and interorbital hypertelorism are universal
- Deformational trigonocephaly

Laboratory Data

No specific laboratory test confirms the diagnosis of encephalocele. A preoperative hemoglobin is prudent.

Imaging Evaluation

- Computed tomography (CT) scan is the imaging modality of choice.
  - Analyzing both bone and brain windows in the axial, coronal, and sagittal planes, as well as three-dimensional reconstructions, are necessary for understanding the complex bony and intracranial anatomy involved.
  - Useful for assessing the potential presence of hydrocephalus.
  - Sagittal reconstructions helpful for evaluating the presence of Chiari I malformation, relevant to patients at risk for hydrocephalus (can also be seen on magnetic resonance imaging, MRI).
  - Essential for planning a successful operative intervention.
- MRI.
  - Provides the most detailed soft tissue images and is useful in distinguishing between soft tissue masses.
- Ultrasound.
  - May be useful in evaluating for hydrocephalus, but often redundant if CT or MRI performed in initial evaluation.

Pathology

Diagnosis can be made with a combination of history, physical exam, and imaging. Biopsies prior to definitive repair are unnecessary and should be discouraged. Histopathologically, meningoceles consist of leptomeningeal membranes with or without glial tissue and meningoencephaloceles of malformed brain tissue and the leptomeningeal membranes covering it (Fig. 16.1). Ependymal tissue may be be seen in hydroencephalomeningoceles.

Treatment

Medical

No medical intervention exists to treat this anatomical abnormality.

Surgical

Operative intervention provides definitive correction of this problem (see Fig. 16.2). Successful correction follows the following principles [10]:

- Accurate diagnosis, delineation of anatomy, and surgical planning

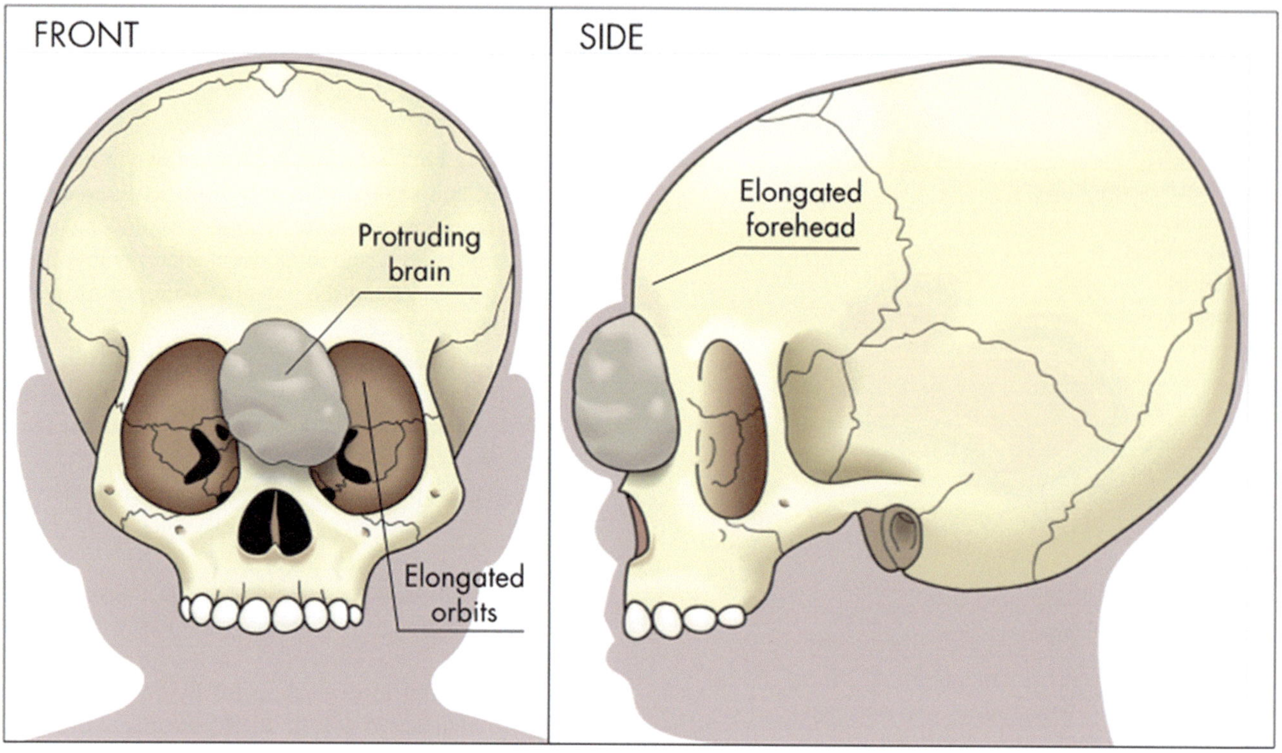

A frontoethmoidal encephalocele is a protrusion of the brain through an opening in a skull due to a birth defect. This also causes an elongation of the orbits and the forehead.

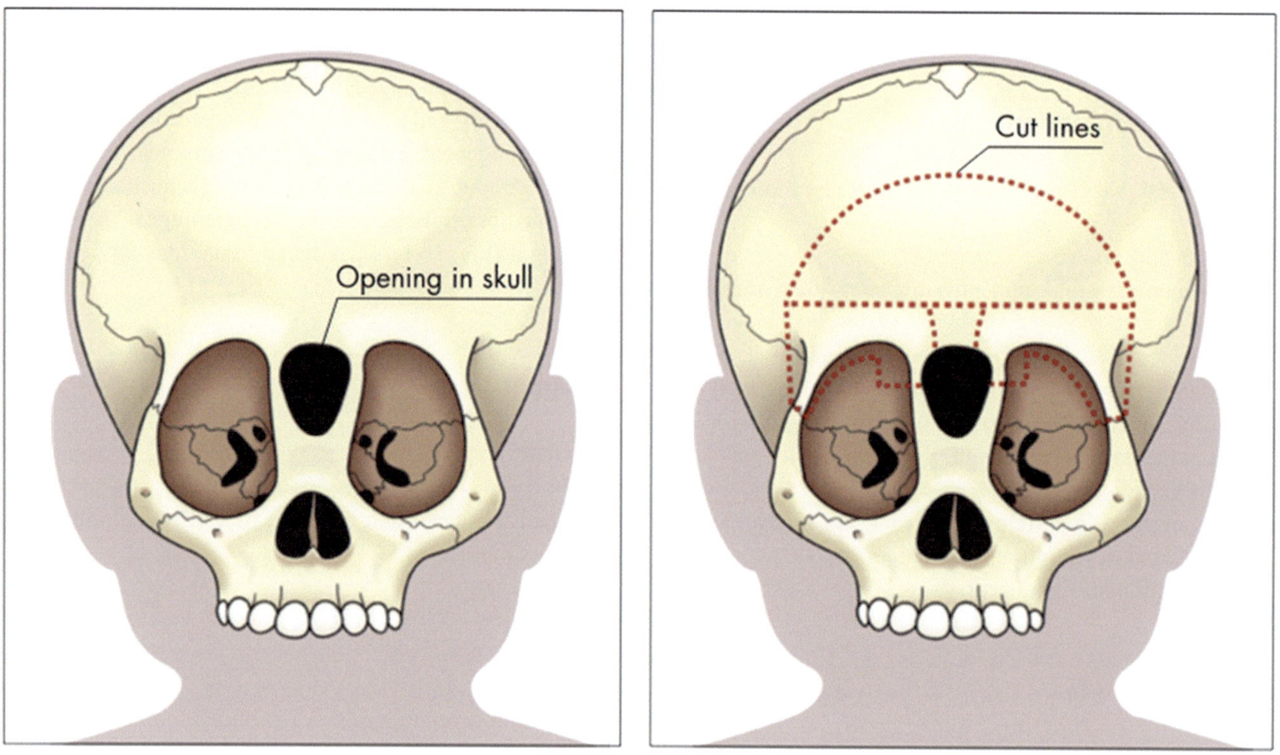

The encelphalocele is removed exposing the opening in the skull.

Lines are drawn along which the skull will be cut.

Fig. 16.2 Reconstruction of frontoethmoidal encephaloceles

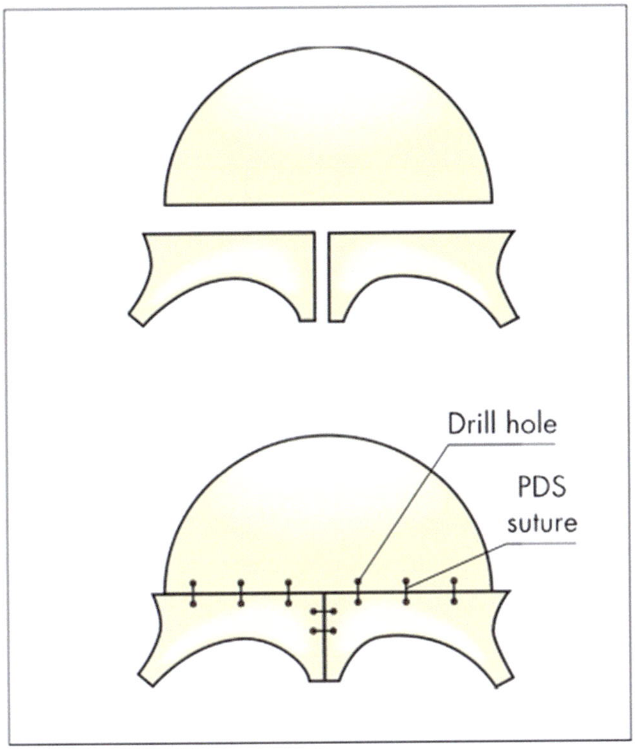

Pieces of the skull are trimmed and shaped and then held together with wire.

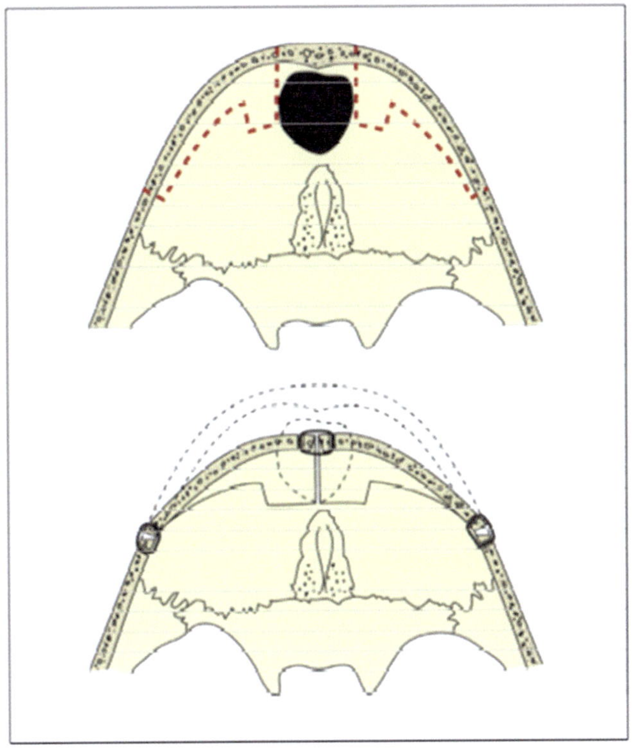

The reconstucted forehead and nose are placed back on the skull.

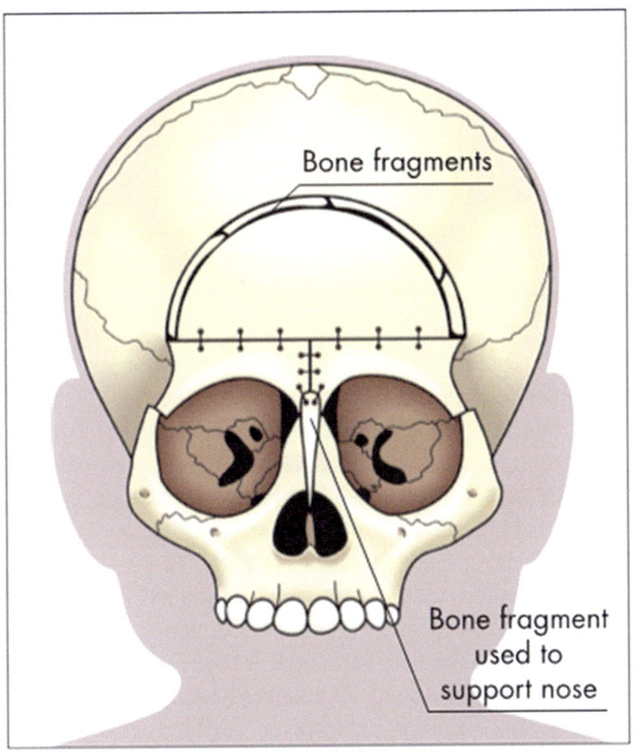

Left over bone is used to fill gaps. Another bone fragment is used to support the nose.

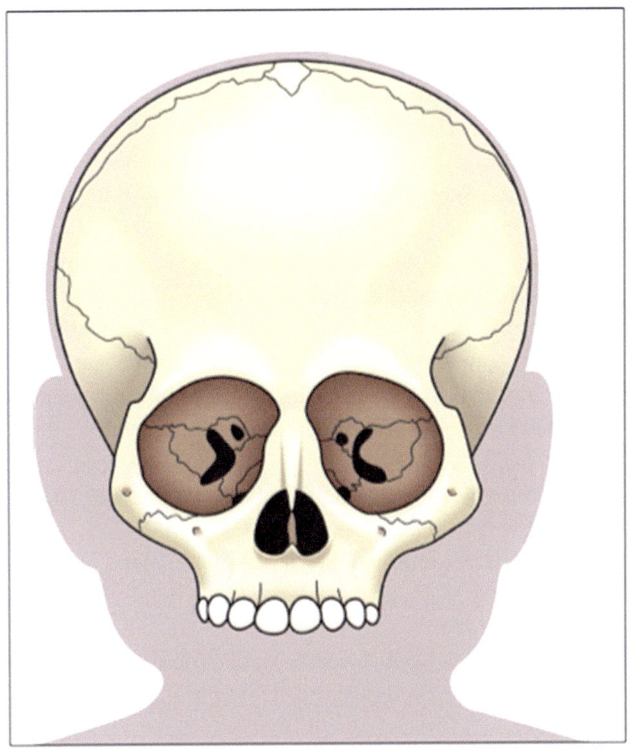

As the patient heals, the bone fragments fuse together again.

Fig. 16.2 (continued)

- Single-stage operation with both craniofacial surgeon and neurosurgeon present
- Osteotomies and bone movements that correct all deformities, including the trigonocephalic head shape and interorbital hypertelorism
- Nasal reconstruction that avoids the long-nose hypertelorism deformity
- Skin closure that removes abnormal skin and places incisions in advantageous locations

Proper anatomical relationships need to be restored. A frontonasoethmoidal encephalocele displaces the frontal bone cephalad and the nasal bones caudad; the medial orbital walls are anterolaterally displaced. Specifics of the technique used by the authors are described in the following sections [11].

Positioning

- Supine, using a Mayfield headrest to secure the cranium.
- Pins are placed posterior enough to avoid interference with the coronal flap and parietal bone graft harvest.
- Circum-mandibular 28-gauge dental wire is used to secure the endotracheal tube.
- Tarsorrhapy sutures placed for corneal protection.
- If hydrocephalus present, or if dural dissection difficult, consider placement of external ventricular drain (in mid-pupillary line, just anterior to coronal suture, preferably on right (nondominant) side, inserted perpendicular to skull to a depth of 3–5 cm then affixed in place during case).

Coronal Exposure

- Wavy-line coronal incision.
- Combination of local anesthesia with epinephrine and use of electrocautery obviate the need for hemostatic clips at the scalp edge.
- Subperiosteal dissection performed anteriorly, elevating the temporalis muscles with the flap.
- Pericranial flap based on the supraorbital vessels is preserved for potential use in closing the dural defect.
- The encephalocele sac is bluntly dissected from the pericranium of the frontal bone and the periosteum of the nasal and orbital bones.
- Periorbita elevated circumferentially taking care to preserve the lacrimal system.
- Medial canthi detached for repositioning later.

Nasal Exposure

- Circumferential skin incision made around the encephalocele, leaving enough skin to close the final defect

Frontal Craniotomy

- Marchac template used to determine the position of the craniotomy
- 1–2 cm frontoorbital bandeau preserved
- Bandeau removed before encephalocele resection
- Dura opened on superior and lateral border of sac, prepared for possible superior sagittal sinus ligation, with amputation of herniated cranial tissue (taking care to preserve arterial anatomy) and meticulous hemostasis
- Sac transected
- Dura closed primarily, reinforced with DuraGen, cadaveric dermis and pericranial flap as necessary, along with possible dural glue, such as Tisseal

Cranial Remodeling

- Trigonocephaly and interorbital hypertelorism must be corrected.
- Central segment of bandeau resected.
- Two hemibandeau segments rotated and advanced medially to close the bony defect and secured to the frontal bone.
- Calvarial defects closed with a combination of bone graft and bone mush harvested from inner table of the frontal bone.

Nasal Reconstruction

- Correction of the long-nose deformity is essential
- Dorsal onlay graft of calvarial bone or costal cartilage attached as a cantilever to bandeau/neofrontal construct with lag screws

Medial Canthal Repositioning

- 30-gauge wire used to transnasally reposition the medial canthal ligaments
- Slight overcorrection necessary as canthal height will drift caudally and laterally as swelling subsides

Skin Closure

- External ventriculostomy drain placed before skin closure.
- Coronal incision closed in two layers over a closed suction drain.
- H-shaped excision of excess skin over the encephalocele addresses both vertical and horizontal tissue excess and allows for repositioning of the medial brow.
- Gentle compression dressing placed prior to extubation.

Endoscopic Management of Encephaloceles

Basal encephaloceles are located in the anterior skull base and herniate through the cribiform plate or posterior to it. Therefore, the masses are confined to the nasal cavity and are potentially amenable to endoscopic repair. Historically these lesions have been removed and the skull base defects repaired using external approaches including lateral rhinotomy and craniotomy. However, advancements in endoscopic equipment and technique has made endoscopic repair of spontaneous cerebrospinal fluid leaks and encephaloceles involving the anterior skull base standard of care in the adult population [12, 13]. Currently there is less experience with repair of these lesions in the pediatric patient population, but there is evidence to support this treatment option in young patients.

- Successful endoscopic repair demonstrated in children as young as 1.5 months [14].
- Delay in repair can increase risk of complications such as meningitis.
- Multiple small case series have shown that endoscopic techniques are effective for repair of encephaloceles in pediatric patients [14–21].

Technique

- Localization of encephalocele by preoperative CT and MRI imaging.
- Image guidance can assist in intraoperative localization.
- 0, 30, and 70° endoscopes in 2.7 mm and 4 mm sizes depending on age of the child.
- Pediatric sinus instruments.
- Lumbar drain dependent on presence of hydrocephalus or other indicator of increased intracranial pressure [14].
- Intrathecal fluorescein can be used to identify the breach in the skull base in the setting of CSF leak; however, use in pediatric patients is limited.
- Bipolar cauterization or Coblation™ technology for reduction of the encephalocele for visualization of the skull base defect requiring repair [22].
- Repair is carried out using underlay or overlay techniques.
- Materials used include temporalis fascia, fascia lata, autologous fat, dural substitutes, bone, and cartilage.
- Pedicled septal flaps and turbinate flaps provide vascularized tissue.
- Absorbable packing such as gelfoam used to hold repair in place, followed by the placement of nonabsorbable packs which are left in place for 1–2 weeks.
- Patients left on antibiotics as long as packing in place.
- Patients should be followed up long-term with serial nasal endoscopy and repeat imaging if clinical evaluation indicates.

Postoperative Monitoring

- Intensive care unit (ICU) monitoring with frequent neurologic assessments performed for 24 h
- Closed suction drain monitored for evidence of cerebrospinal fluid (CSF) leak and removed between postoperative days 3 to 5
- External ventriculostomy usually removed by postoperative day 5 following successful clamping trial, but options of endoscopic (endoscopic third ventriculocisternostomy/choroid plexus cauterization) or CSF diversion (ventriculoperitoneal shunt) surgical treatments exist should hydrocephalus develop
- Periorbital edema universally present for first 72 h
- 3-day steroid taper used to address edema

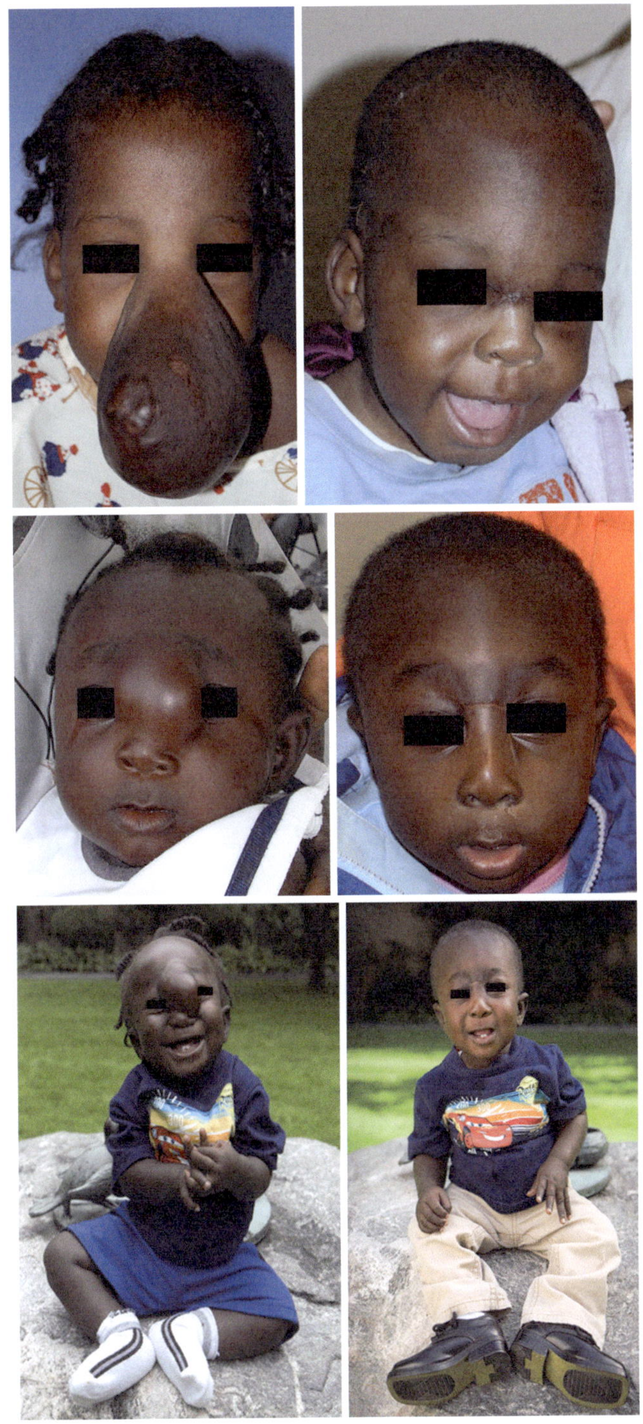

Fig. 16.3 Patients before and after operative intervention

Adjuvant Treatment

Postoperative hydrocephalus is managed by neurosurgery as necessary with conversion of external ventriculostomy to an internal shunt. Some children are at risk of seizure and a course of antiepileptic medication may be indicated.

Outcome

The prognosis of patients who have had anterior encephaloceles corrected is generally good, although mental retardation, epilepsy, and ocular problems have been reported in this population [23, 24]. Children who have the encephalocele repaired well before puberty may require further augmentation of the nasal dorsum later in life as the reconstructed nose is unlikely to grow. Current refinements in technique have shown that a one stage intracranial and extracranial approach is safe and is associated with high parental satisfaction rates of the improvement in appearance (Fig. 16.3) [11, 25, 26].

References

1. Suwanwela C, Suwanwela N. A morphological classification of sincipital encephalomeningoceles. J Neurosurg. 1972;36(2):201–11.
2. Rahman N. Nasal encephalocele: treatment by transcranial operation. J Neurosci. 1979;42:73–85.
3. Fenger C. Basal hernias of the brain. Am J M Sc. 1895;1:109.
4. Gorenstein A, Kern EB, Facer GW, Laws ER Jr. Nasal gliomas. Arch Otolaryngol. 1980;106(9):536–40.
5. Moore PM. Intranasal encephalomeningocele report of a case. Laryngoscope. 1952;62(7):659–77.
6. Birnbaum LM, Owsley JQ Jr. Frontonasal tumors of neurogenic orgin. Plast Reconstr Surg. 1968;41:462–70.
7. Griffith BH. Frontonasal tumors: their diagnosis and management. Plast Reconstr Surg. 1976;57(6):692–9.
8. Jackson IT, Tanner NS, Hide TA. Frontonasal encephalocele—"long nose hypertelorism". Ann Plast Surg. 1983;11(6):490–500.
9. Ortiz-Monasterio F, Fuente-del-Campo A. Nasal correction in hyperteleorbitism. The short and the long nose. Scand J Plast Reconstr Surg. 1981;15(3):277–86.
10. Holmes AD, Meara JG, Kolker AR, Rosenfeld JV, Klug GL. Frontoethmoidal encephaloceles: reconstruction and refinements. J Craniofac Surg. 2001;12(1):6–18.
11. Andrews BT, Meara JG. Reconstruction of frontoethmoidal encephalocele defects. Atlas Oral Maxillofac Surg Clin North Am. 2010;18(2):129–38.
12. Lund VJ. Endoscopic management of cerebrospinal fluid leaks. Am J Rhinol. 2002;16(1):17–23.
13. Senior BA, Jafri K, Benninger M. Safety and efficacy of endoscopic repair of CSF leaks and encephaloceles: a survey of the members of the American Rhinologic Society. Am J Rhinol. 2001;15(1):21–5.
14. Di Rocco F, Couloigner V, Dastoli P, Sainte-Rose C, Zerah M, Roger G. Treatment of anterior skull base defects by a transnasal endoscopic approach in children. J Neurosurg Pediatr. 2010;6(5):459–63.
15. Woodworth B, Schlosser RJ. Endoscopic repair of a congenital intranasal encephalocele in a 23 months old infant. Int J Pediatr Otorhinolaryngol. 2005;69(7):1007–9.
16. Castelnuovo P, Dallan I, Bignami M, Pistochini A, Battaglia P, Tschabitscher M. Endoscopic endonasal management of petroclival cerebrospinal fluid leaks: anatomical study and preliminary clinical experience. Minim Invasive Neurosurg. 2008;51(6):336–9.
17. Abdel-Aziz M, El-Bosraty H, Qotb M, El-Hamamsy M, El-Sonbaty M, Abdel-Badie H, Zynabdeen M. Nasal encephalocele: endoscopic excision with anesthetic consideration. Int J Pediatr Otorhinolaryngol. 2010;74(8):869–73.
18. Kanowitz SJ, Bernstein JM. Pediatric meningoencephaloceles and nasal obstruction: a case for endoscopic repair. Int J Pediatr Otorhinolaryngol. 2006;70(12):2087–92.
19. Kassam A, Thomas AJ, Snyderman C, Carrau R, Gardner P, Mintz A, Kanaan H, Horowitz M, Pollack IF. Fully endoscopic expanded endonasal approach treating skull base lesions in pediatric patients. J Neurosurg. 2007;106(2 Suppl):75–86.
20. Locatelli D, Rampa F, Acchiardi I, Bignami M, De Bernardi F, Castelnuovo P. Endoscopic endonasal approaches for repair of cerebrospinal fluid leaks: nine-year experience. Neurosurgery. 2006;58(4 Suppl 2):ONS-246–56; discussion ONS-256–7.
21. Van Den Abbeele T, Elmaleh M, Herman P, Francois M, Narcy P. Transnasal endoscopic repair of congenital defects of the skull base in children. Arch Otolaryngol Head Neck Surg. 1999;125(5):580–4.
22. Smith N, Riley KO, Woodworth BA. Endoscopic Coblator-assisted management of encephaloceles. Laryngoscope. 2010;120(12):2535–9.
23. David DJ, Sheffield L, Simpson D, White J. Fronto-ethmoidal meningoencephaloceles: morphology and treatment. Br J Plast Surg. 1984;37(3):271–84.
24. Jacob OJ, Rosenfeld JV, Watters DA. The repair of frontal encephaloceles in Papau New Guinea. Aust N Z J Surg. 1994;64:856–60.
25. Kumar A, Helling E, Guenther D, Crabtree T, Wexler AW, Bradley JP. Correction of frontonasoethmoidal encephalocele: the HULA procedure. Plast Reconstr Surg. 2009;123(2):661–9.
26. Sargent LA, Seyfer AE, Gunby EN. Nasal encephaloceles: definitive one-stage reconstruction. J Neurosurg. 1988;68(4):571–5.

Esthesioneuroblastoma

17

Karen Watters, Edward R. Smith and Reza Rahbar

Introduction

Esthesioneuroblastoma (ENB), also known as olfactory neuroblastoma, is a rare neoplasm of neuroectodermal origin. Controversy exists as to the cell of origin of ENB. The most widely accepted opinion is that it arises from olfactory epithelium, which would account for the intimate relationship of ENB with the cribriform plate, the anterior skull base, and the midline superior nasal structures, including the superior turbinate and the superior third of the nasal septum [1]. Since its first description in 1924 by Berger and Luc, approximately 1,200 cases have been reported [2, 3]. ENB has an approximate incidence of 0.4 per million population, representing 3–6 % of all sinonasal tumors.

Etiology

ENB affects men and women with equal rates. No geographic or racial predilection and no known occupational exposure have been identified to date. There also appears to be no known familial association or associated chromosomal anomaly.

Clinical Presentation

Age of presentation ranges from 2 to 94 years, with a bimodal distribution in the 2nd and 6th decade of life [1, 2]. Biologic behavior can be very variable, ranging from a slow indolent tumor growing over decades to an aggressive tumor with metastases over a few months. The average time from initial symptoms to diagnosis is typically 6 months [2]. Delay in diagnosis is often a consequence of symptoms mimicking those seen in chronic rhinosinusitis or polypoidal disease.

ENB can be locally aggressive invading the nasal cavity, paranasal sinuses, cribriform plate, intracranial cavity, brain parenchyma, and/or orbit. Metastases typically occur in the neck, thorax, and skeleton. Presenting symptoms can be categorized as nasal, neurologic, ophthalmologic, facial, and cervical (Table 17.1). Most commonly presenting symptoms include unilateral nasal obstruction (70 %) and epistaxis (50 %) [4]. Although the tumor arises from the olfactory neuroepithelium, anosmia is not a common complaint (5 %).

Evaluation

Examination

A full otolaryngologic and cranial nerve examination should be performed. This should include nasal endoscopy. ENB does not have specific distinguishing features on examination but usually appears as a unilateral polypoid, glistening, soft, red–grey mass with intact mucosa arising in the upper nasal cavity that often bleeds easily on instrumentation. Cervical lymphadenopathy may be palpable in advanced disease. Ectopic tumors within the paranasal sinuses are rare, but have been described in the sphenoid sinus, lateral nasal wall, petrous apex, maxillary sinus, and the nasopharynx [5]. Diagnosis is made via biopsy, which should not be performed until imaging studies are complete. General anesthesia is recommended for biopsy, due to the highly vascular nature of the tumor; a comprehensive endoscopic examination can also be performed at the same time.

K. Watters (✉)
Otolaryngology and Communication Enhancement, Boston Children's Hospital, Harvard Medical School, Boston, MA, USA
e-mail: Karen.Watters@childrens.harvard.edu

E. R. Smith
Department of Neurosurgery, Boston Children's Hospital, Harvard Medical School, Boston, MA, USA

R. Rahbar
Department of Otolaryngology, Boston Children's Hospital, Harvard Medical School, Boston, MA, USA

R. Rahbar et al. (eds.), *Pediatric Head and Neck Tumors*,
DOI 10.1007/978-1-4614-8755-5_17, © Springer Science+Business Media New York 2014

Table 17.1 Presenting symptoms in ENB

	Symptoms
1. Nasal	Unilateral nasal obstruction (70%)
	Epistaxis (50%)
	Unilateral nasal mass
	Rhinorrhea
	Anosmia (5%)
2. Neurologic	Headaches
	Cranial nerve paralysis
3. Ophthamologic	Proptosis
	Visual disturbance
	Excessive lacrimation
4. Facial	Facial pain/swelling
	Parathesia (rare)
5. Cervical	Neck swelling (5–7% at diagnosis)

Table 17.2 Differential diagnosis of ENB

Infectious/inflammatory	Fungal rhinosinusitis
	Inflammatory polyp
	Adenoidal hypertrophy
	Wegners' granulomatosis
Congenital masses	Dermoid cyst
	Glioma
	Encephalocoele
	Teratoma
Primary neoplasms	Rhabdomyosarcoma
	Nasopharyngeal carcinoma
	Squamous cell carcinoma
	Sinonasal undifferentiated carcinoma
	Lymphoma
	Angiofibroma
	Osteosarcoma
	Chondrosarcoma
	Ewing sarcoma / PNET
	Neuroblastoma
	Idiopathic midline granuloma
	Meningioma
	Hemangioma
	Hemangiopericytoma
	Fibrosarcoma
	Fibrous histiocytoma
	Malignant melanoma
	Neuroendocrine carcinoma
Secondary neoplasms	Metastases
	Chordoma
	Meningioma
	Lymphoma

Differential Diagnosis

All causes of pediatric sinonasal masses must be carefully excluded (Table 17.2).

Histopathology

ENB is histologically very similar to small, round, blue cell tumors. These are important to distinguish, as they respond very differently to different treatment modalities (Fig. 17.1). Tumor cells are "small, round, blue" and mitotically active. The hallmark of well-differentiated ENB is small, round neuroepithelial cells arranged in rosettes (Flexner-Wintersteiner) or pseudorosettes (Homer-Wright) patterns, separated by fibrous elements. Rosettes consist of a central space ringed by columnar cells. Immunohistochemical tests are helpful in differentiating neuroblastomas from other malignant small round cell tumors, however, to date there is no test specific to ENB. [6] (Table 17.3).

Imaging Studies

Both computed tomography (CT) and magnetic resonance imaging (MRI) are recommended for the workup of ENB. Particular attention needs to be paid to areas such as the lamina papyracea, the fovea ethmoidalis, and the cribriform plate.

CT Imaging A fine-cut CT with contrast, according to an image guidance protocol, should be performed. ENB appears as a homogeneous soft tissue mass with uniform enhancement on contrast (Fig. 17.2). Nonenhancing areas may suggest areas of necrosis. Speckled calcifications may also be present. CT is useful to evaluate for bony erosion, especially of the lamina papyracea, cribiform plate, and fovea ethmoidalis. A "dumbbell-shaped" mass extending across the cribriform plate is one of the most characteristic findings on imaging for an ENB.

MRI Imaging MRI images with and without contrast will delineate the extent of the tumor and can be extremely helpful in determining intracranial and intraorbital soft tissue extension and differentiating fluid or secretions from tumor. T1-weighted images show hypointense signal intensity. T2-weighted images show isointense or hyperintense regions (Fig. 17.3). An unusual feature of ENB may be cystic regions at the tumor–brain interface, which typically appear hyperintense.

The soft tissues of the neck should also be imaged to look for cervical nodal disease (Fig. 17.4).

Staging

Accurate staging of ENB is an important guide for treatment and prognosis. There is no universally accepted staging system for ENB that has provided consistent information

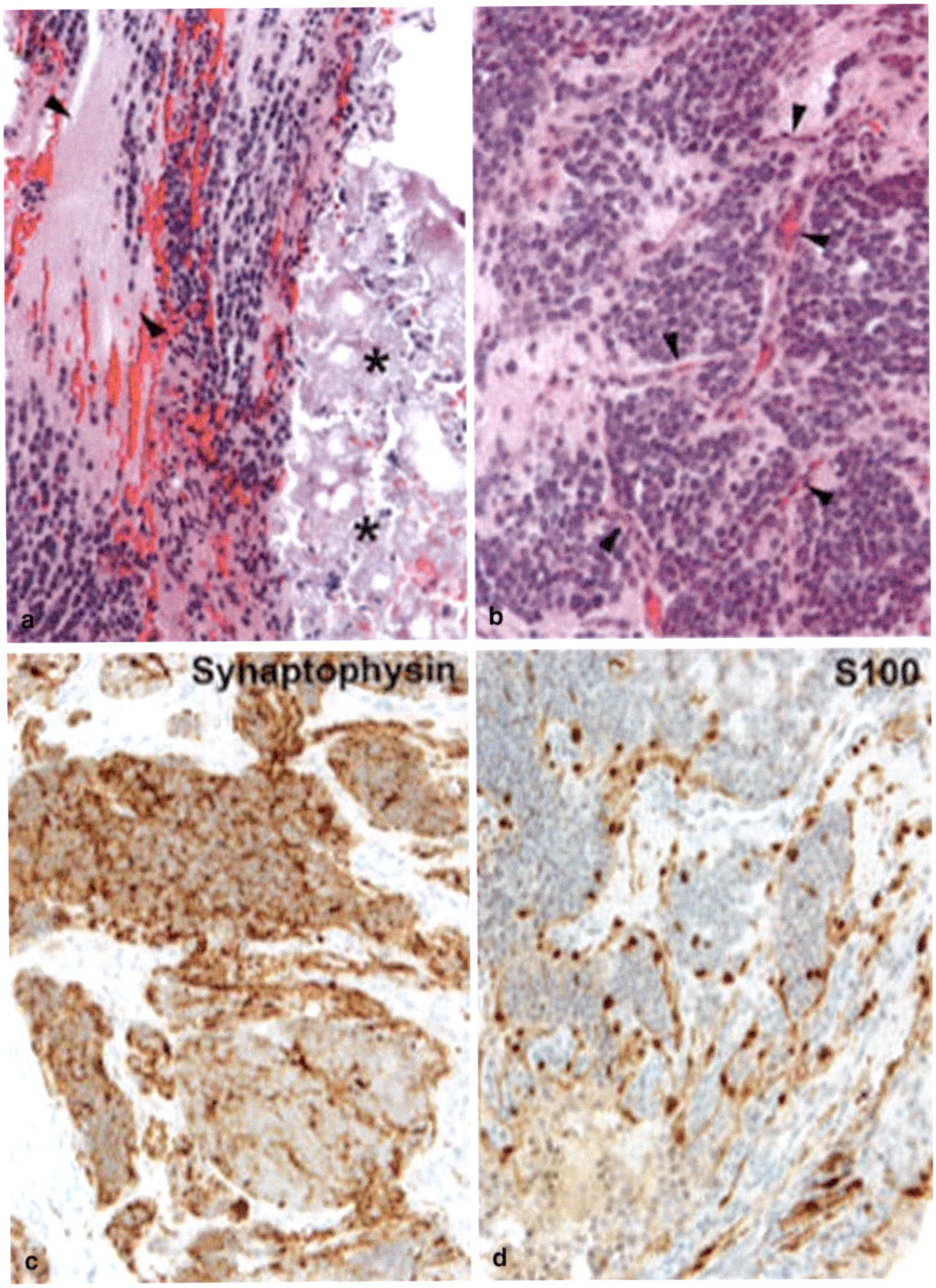

Fig. 17.1 Olphatory neuroblastoma. **a** Poorly differentiated ENB with abundant neuropil (*between arrowheads*) and a low mitotic/karyorrhectic index. Extensive dystrophic calcifications are seen on the right (*asterisks*). **b** Tumor cells are arranged in tight nests outlined by a delicate capillary network (*arrowheads*). **c** Tumor cells are strongly and diffusely immunoreactive for *synaptophysin*. **d** A network of Schwannian sustentacular cells strongly immunoreactive for *S100* protein invests nests and cords of tumor cells

on prognosis, including overall survival. All staging systems are based on radiological findings. The Kadish staging system proposed in 1976 is still the most frequently used (Table 17.4) [7]. The main limitation of this staging system is that it fails to account for metastases. This was addressed by Morita et al., who amended the Kadish staging system by establishing a Stage D for tumors with regional and distant metastasis [4]. A TNM-type classification was more recently proposed by Dulguerov and Calcaterra [8, 9].

A histologic grading system (I–IV) was described by Hyams [10]. This system is based upon six features including architectural findings, the mitotic index, the degree of nuclear polymorphism, the presence of rosettes, and the degree of necrosis. This staging system appears to offer more useful prognostic data but has been less well accepted in clinical practice.

Treatment

Open surgery was previously regarded as the gold standard for treatment of ENB, however, since the advent of endoscopic techniques for anterior skull base surgery in the early 1990s, there has been considerable refinement in techniques

Table 17.3 Immunohistochemical features of ENB and other sinonasal tumors

	Immunohistochemistry	Other tests
ENB	Positive for S-100, neuron-specific enolase (NSE), synaptophysin, NFP, CD56, chromogranin	Ki-67 positive—high proliferation index
	Negative for cytokeratin, vimetin, desmin, myogenin, common leukocytic antigen (CD 45RB), CD99 (MIC2 antigent)	
Neuroblastoma	Positive synaptophysin, Leu7, neurofilament protein, NSE	Elevated catecholamines
Rhabdomyosarcoma	Positive for desmin, muscle-specific actin, myoglobin	Loss of chromosome 11
Lymphoma	Positive for C45	
Ewing sarcoma	Positive for MI22/CD99	11:22 translocation
Malignant melanoma	Positive for S-100, MART-1/Melan-A, HMB-45	

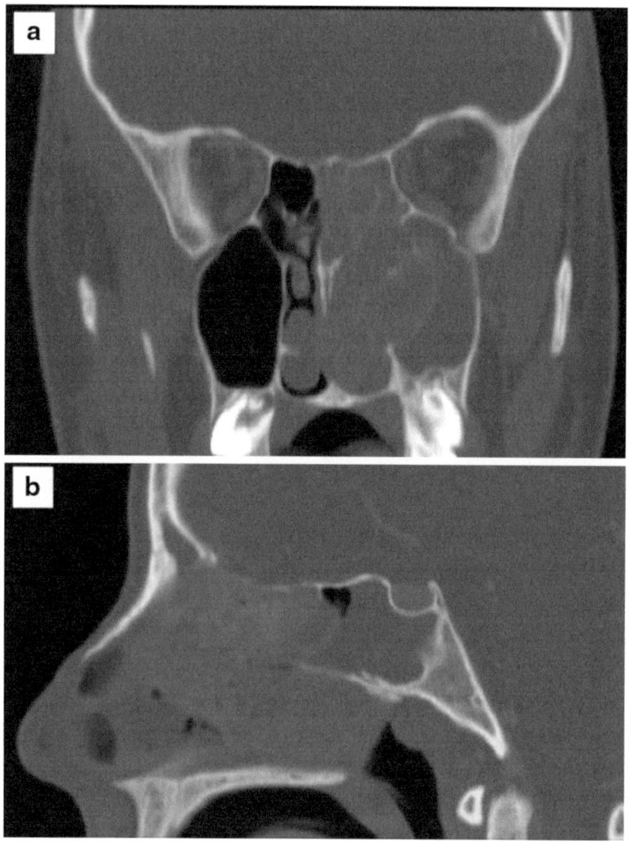

Fig. 17.2 A coronal (**a**) and axial (**b**) postcontrast CT image of the paranasal sinuses in a 16-year-old girl who presented with a 6-week history of nasal obstruction. A large heterogeneously enhancing soft tissue mass completely fills and opacifies the left maxillary antrum. There is thinning of the bony margins of the sinonasal cavity and left maxillary sinus consistent with areas of bone resorption. The left lamina papyracea is thinned but intact. The tumor abuts the skull base but there is no evidence of soft tissue extension into the anterior cranial fossa. Biospy of this tumor was consistent with an ENB

and adjuvant therapies. Considerable heterogeneity continues to exist regarding the optimal treatment modality. The data-guiding treatment type is based upon small, single-institution retrospective series and meta-analyses of combinations of treatment data. The most effective strategy for prolonged disease-free survival appears to be the combined approach of complete surgical resection followed by radiation therapy [11]. Chemotherapy does not appear to offer any advantage over dual-modality treatment and it is associated with more side effects.

Surgery

The aim of surgery is to achieve complete surgical resection with tumor-free margins. The advent of craniofacial resection (CFR) in the 1970s has led to a significant improvement in surgical outcome. CFR via open and endoscopic approaches can achieve complete resection. The surgical approach is dependent on the stage of the tumor, primarily the extent of involvement of the cribiform plate.

- **Open craniofacial resection:** As ENB usually arises from the cribriform plate, it is important that the dura overlying the tumor is removed to ensure complete resection. This is usually performed via a bilobed coronal flap and midfacial approach in combination with the neurosurgical team (Fig. 17.5a, b). Advantages of open resection include en bloc resection, margins for histology, and analysis of intracranial extension with preservation of cranial nerves. Disadvantages include incision and functional status changes related to frontal lobe retraction.
- **Endoscopic craniofacial resection (ECFR):** This involves a Draf type III, Lothrop type, frontal sinusotomy communicating both frontal sinuses across the midline to expose a common frontal sinus cavity. One of the main disadvantages of the endoscopic approach is the inability to achieve an en bloc resection. Numerous studies report comparable success using a purely endoscopic approach for the treatment of ENB with using an open surgical approach. A recent meta-analysis by Devaiah et al. in 2009 suggests that the endoscopic approach is a valid treatment of ENB, producing better survival rates than open approach [12]. However, most of the tumors removed via an open surgical approach in these studies belonged to the Kadish C and D stages, whereas endoscopic techniques were more commonly used for Kadish A and B stage tumors, contributing, at least partially, to the better survival found for the endoscopic approach. Additional

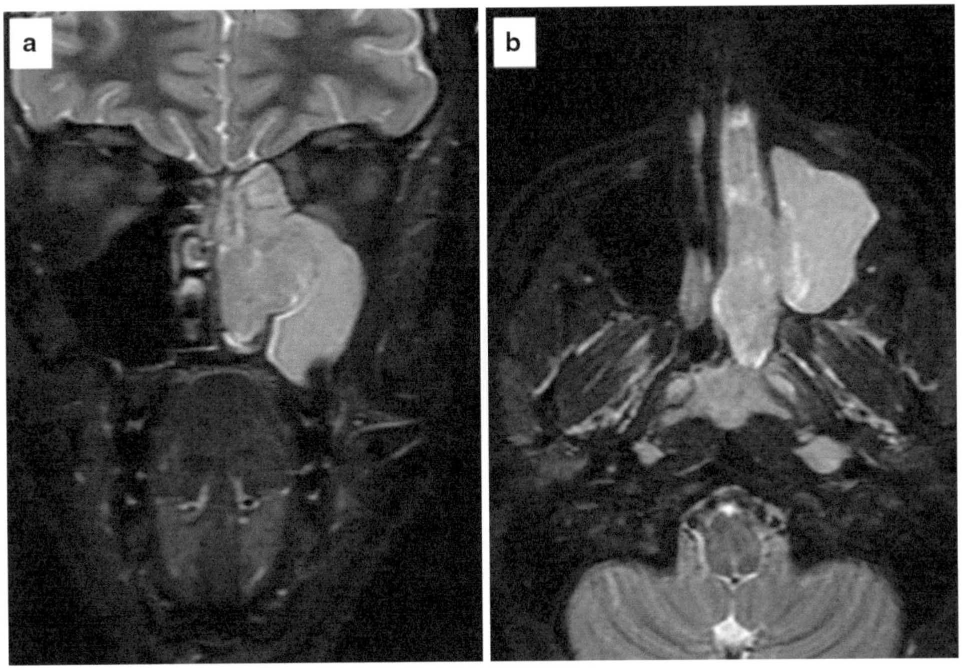

Fig. 17.3 A coronal (**a**) and axial (**b**) T1-weighted post gadolinium MR image of the same patient in Fig. 17.1, showing a multilobulated solid mass centered in the left nasal cavity that extends laterally into the left maxillary sinus, cephalad into the ipsilateral ethmoid sinus, and posteriorly into the nasopharynx. Retained left maxillary secretions are seen in the coronal image. There is no evidence of intraorbital or intracranial extension

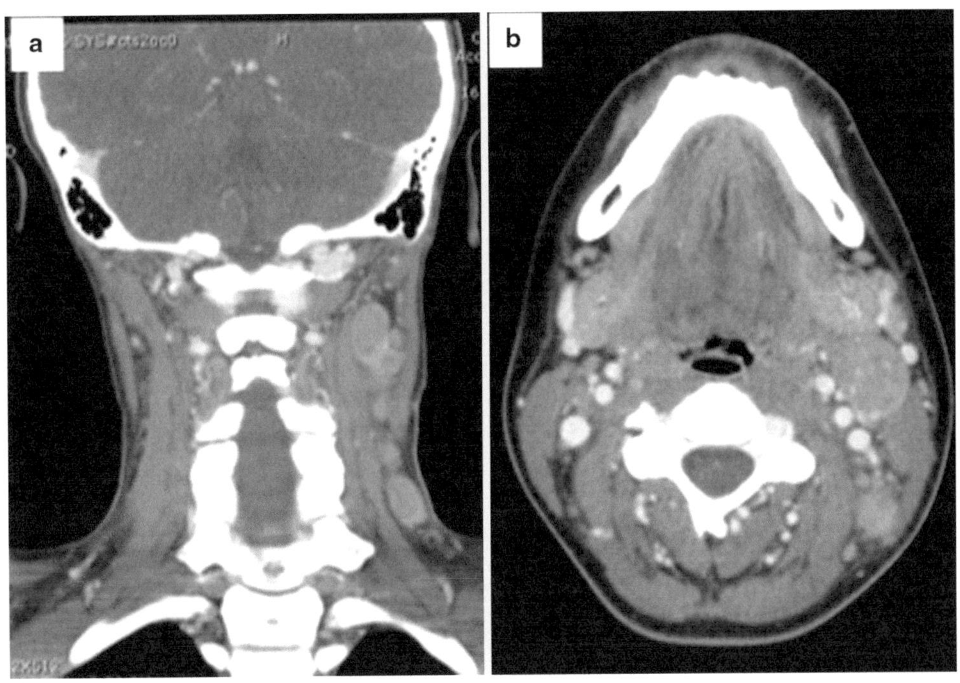

Fig. 17.4 Postcontrast coronal (**a**) and axial (**b**) CT images of neck soft tissues of the patient described in Fig. 17.1. There is significant heterogeneous lymphadenopathy in the left cervical chain, left retropharyngeal space, and posterior triangle. The largest node measures 3 × 2.2 cm

studies are required to definitively address the utility of endoscopic surgery for patients with ENB.

- **Neck dissection:**

  N+ Neck: Given the significant decrease in survival for node-positive disease in ENB, aggressive treatment by neck dissection at the time of treatment of the primary surgery followed by adjuvant radiotherapy is recommended for clinically or radiologically evident nodal disease [13]. There are no data to support the extent of neck dissection; typically, a selective neck dissection is performed. Patients presenting with late neck disease following primary treatment have been shown to have a clear survival advantage (59 vs. 14 %) when treated with a combination of surgery and radiotherapy relative to single-modality methods alone [14].

  N0 Neck: Even though 20–25 % of patients with ENB will eventually develop neck metastasis, elective neck dissection in the absence of neck disease is not recommended [13].

Table 17.4 Kadish tumor staging

Stage	Definition	5-year survival (%)
A	Tumor limited to nasal cavity	75–91
B	Tumor confined to nasal cavity and paranasal sinuses	68–71
C	Tumor extending to cribriform plate, base of skull, orbit, or intracranial	41–47
D	Tumor with cervical node or distant metastasis	–

Postoperative Care

Regardless of the surgical approach, the patient typically receives intensive care unit (ICU) neurosurgical monitoring for at least 24 h. Antibiotics (typically ceftriaxone) are administered intravenously. A lumbar drain is placed for removal of Cerebrospinal fluid (CSF) during reconstruction of the skull base and is often left in situ for 24 h postoperatively.

Radiation

Surgical margins are often difficult to analyze and clear margins cannot be guaranteed. Postoperative radiation is optimal to prevent recurrence and has also been shown to increase survival. Patients typically receive between 55–65 Gy, making them susceptible to radiation-induced toxicity, especially cataract formation and glaucoma. Intensity-modulated radiotherapy (IMRT) techniques have shown good tumor control with low rates of radiation-induced toxicity [15]. Neoadjuvant radiotherapy has not demonstrated any advantage over postoperative radiation.

Chemotherapy

The role of chemotherapy continues to evolve. As a primary treatment modality, it is reserved for unresectable, recurrent, or metastatic disease. Although there is no standard chemotherapy regimen used for ENB, the agents used are chiefly cisplatin and etoposide, or doxorubicin and vincristine with an alkylating agent [16]. Studies investigating benefit of neoadjuvant chemotherapy remain unclear, as patients in these studies also received concurrent radiation therapy [17].

Multidisciplinary Management

Treatment should be multidisciplinary in all cases, with involvement of head and neck surgery, neurosurgery, radiation and medical oncology, speech and language therapy, and nutrition. A prosthetic consultant may also have a role if maxillectomy is anticipated. A preoperative ophthalmology assessment is essential in all patients undergoing surgical intervention due to the close proximity of the optic nerves to the tumor. Partial intraorbital resection may be necessary in rare cases.

Complications

- **From tumor growth:** Direct extension into anterior cranial fossa can result blindness and functional status changes.
- **From surgery:** Reported as occurring in 10–15% of cases regardless of surgical approach, with higher rates in cases of revision or salvage surgery [18]. Early complications include meningitis, abscess around the bone flap, pneumocephalus, CSF leak (<10%), and epidural or subdural abscess. Later complications include anosmia, nasal crusting, frontal sinus mucocoele, and epiphora. Rare but potential events include that of blindness from optic

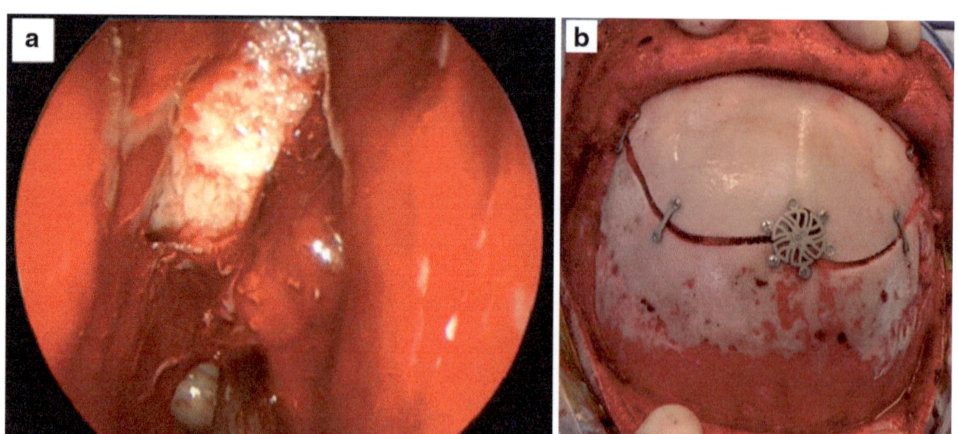

Fig. 17.5 CFR of the ENB in Figs. 17.1, 17.2, and 17.3 was performed using a bifrontal craniotomy and transnasal approach. The dura and bone overlying the tumor was completely removed. The skull base defect is seen endoscopically. **a** The closed cranial incision is shown. **b** A left modified radical neck dissection was also performed on this patient

nerve injury and death from intracerebral hemorrhage. Functional status changes and epilepsy can result from excessive pressure on the frontal lobe during open resection.

- **From radiation**: Cataract formation, glaucoma, epiphora, and radiation retinopathy may occur following radiation therapy. Late toxicity includes osteoradionecrosis of the frontal bone flap.

Prognosis

The most important factor influencing survival is **the extent of disease at initial diagnosis**. The average 5-year survival for combination treatment (surgery and radiotherapy) is 65 %. The prognostic value of the Kadish staging system is unclear, but 5-year survival rates for the respective stages A, B, and C are 72, 59, and 47 %, respectively (Table 17.4). Recurrence is local in the majority of cases with reported rates of 20–40 %, and can occur up to 10 years after treatment [19, 20]. Patients should therefore remain under close long-term follow-up [21].

Given the high rate of late neck metastases (20–25 %), it is reasonable to screen patients who do not have neck disease at the time of initial diagnosis, for recurrence or nodal disease 6 months and 1 year after diagnosis with neck CT or MRI: The necessity of regular imaging studies following that period to assess for recurrence has not been clearly defined. Salvage surgery after local recurrence is possible in up to 50 % of cases [14].

References

1. Unger F, Haselsberger K, Walch C, Stammberger H, Papaefthymiou G. Combined endoscopic surgery and radiosurgery as treatment modality for olfactory neuroblastoma (esthesioneuroblastoma). Acta Neurochir (Wien). 2005;147:595–601; discussion 601–2.
2. Broich G, Pagliari A, Ottaviani F. Esthesioneuroblastoma: a general review of the cases published since the discovery of the tumor in 1924. Anticancer Res. 1997;17:2683–706.
3. Berger L, Luc G, Richard D. The olfactory esthesioneuroepithelioma. Bull Assoc Fr Etud Cancer. 1924;13:410–21.
4. Morita A, Ebersold MJ, Olsen KD, Foote RL, Lewis JE, Quast LM. Esthesioneuroblastoma: prognosis and management. Neurosurgery. 1993;32:706–14; discussion 714–5.
5. Wormald R, Lennon P, O'Dwyer TP. Ectopic olfactory neuroblastoma: report of four cases and a review of the literature. Eur Arch Otorhinolaryngol. 2011;268(4):555–60.
6. Thompson LD. Olfactory neuroblastoma. Head Neck Pathol. 2009;3(3):252–9.
7. Kadish S, Goodman M, Wang CC. Olfactory neuroblastoma. A clinical analysis of 17 cases. Cancer. 1976;37(3):1571–6.
8. Dulguerov P, Calcaterra T. Esthesioneuroblastoma: the UCLA experience 1970–1990. Laryngoscope. 1992;102(8):843–9.
9. Dulguerov P, Allal AS, Calcaterra TC. Esthesioneuroblastoma: a meta-analysis and review. Lancet Oncol. 2001;2:683–90.
10. Hyams VJ. Olfactory neuroblastoma. In: Hyams VJ, Baksakis JG, Michaels L, editors. Tumors of the upper respiratory tract and ear. Washington: Armed Forces Institute of Pathology; 1988. pp 240–8.
11. Ward PD, Heth JA, Thompson BG, Marentette LJ. Esthesioneuroblastoma: results and outcomes of a single institution's experience. Skull Base. 2009;19(2):133–40.
12. Devaiah AK, Andreoli MT. Treatment of esthesioneuroblastoma: a 16-year meta-analysis of 361 patients. Laryngoscope. 2009;119(7):1412–6.
13. Zanation AM, Ferlito A, Rinaldo A, Gore MR, Lund VJ, McKinney KA, Suárez C, Takes RP, Devaiah AK. When, how and why to treat the neck in patients with esthesioneuroblastoma: a review. Eur Arch Otorhinolaryngol. 2010;267(11):1667–71.
14. Gore MR, Zanation AM. Salvage treatment of late neck metastasis in esthesioneuroblastoma: a meta-analysis. Arch Otolaryngol Head Neck Surg. 2009;135:1030–4.
15. Bachar G, Goldstein D, Shah M, Tandon A, Ringash J, Pond G, Gullane P, Perez-Ordonez B, Gilbert R, Brown D, Irish J. Esthesioneuroblastoma: the Princess Margaret Hospital experience. Head Neck. 2008;30:1607–14.
16. Sohrabi S, Drabick JJ, Crist H, Goldenberg D, Sheehan JM, Mackley HB. Neoadjuvant concurrent chemoradiation for advanced esthesioneuroblastoma: a case series and review of the literature. J Clin Oncol. 2011;29(13):e358–61.
17. Polin RS, Sheehan JP, Chenelle AG, et al. The role of preoperative adjuvant treatment in the management of esthesioneuroblastoma: the University of Virginia experience. Neurosurgery. 1998;42:1029–37.
18. Greenfield JP, Anand VK, Kacker A, Seibert MJ, Singh A, Brown SM, Schwartz TH. Endoscopic endonasal transethmoidal transcribriform transfovea ethmoidalis approach to the anterior cranial fossa and skull base. Neurosurgery. 2011;66:883–92; discussion 892.
19. Gabory L de, Abdulkhaleq HM, Darrouzet V, Bébéar JP, Stoll D. Long-term results of 28 esthesioneuroblastomas managed over 35 years. Head Neck. 2011;33(1):82–6.
20. Bäck L, Oinas M, Pietarinen-Runtti P, Saarilahti K, Vuola J, Saat R, Ohman J, Haglund C, Niemelä M, Leivo I, Hagström J, Mäkitie AA. The developing management of esthesioneuroblastoma: a single institution experience. Eur Arch Otorhinolaryngol. 2012;269:213–21.
21. Gallia GL, Reh DD, Salmasi V, Blitz AM, Koch W, Ishii M. Endonasal endoscopic resection of esthesioneuroblastoma: the Johns Hopkins Hospital experience and review of the literature. Neurosurg Rev. 2011;34(4):465–75.

18 Fibrous Dysplasia

Melissa S. Putman, Karen Watters, Reza Rahbar and Catherine M. Gordon

Introduction

Fibrous dysplasia (FD) is a noninheritable genetic disease characterized by overgrowth of fibrous tissue within bone. FD can occur in monostotic forms, affecting a single bone, or can be polyostotic in which more than one skeletal site is affected. The combination of FD with café au lait skin lesions and endocrinopathies is referred to as the McCune–Albright syndrome. Clinical manifestations of FD range from asymptomatic bone lesions that are incidentally discovered to significant bone pain, pathologic fracture, and bony deformities. When craniofacial bones are involved, cranial nerve impingement from compression by affected bony lesions can lead to blindness or nerve palsies. The diagnosis of FD can usually be made by classic findings on radiologic imaging, and biopsies are reserved for unusual or complicated cases. Treatment options include medical management with antiresorptive therapies such as bisphosphonates, and surgical intervention is indicated for repair of fracture or bony deformities. Prognosis varies depending primarily on the number and location of affected sites, as well as association with underlying endocrinopathies.

R. Rahbar (✉) · K. Watters
Department of Otolaryngology and Communication Enhancement, Boston Children's Hospital, Harvard Medical School, 300 Longwood Avenue, LO-367, Boston, MA 02115, USA
e-mail: reza.rahbar@childrens.harvard.edu

M. S. Putman
Department of Endocrinology, Boston Children's Hospital, Harvard Medical School, 333 Longwood Avenue, 6th Floor, Boston, MA 02115, USA

C. M. Gordon
Department of Adolescent Medicine, Hasbro Children's Hospital, 593 Eddy St., Providence, RI 02903, USA

Pathophysiology and Genetics

FD is caused by post-zygotic missense mutations occurring in a specific gene on chromosome 20q13 that encodes for the alpha subunit of the stimulatory G-protein (Gs) within the GNAS complex, resulting in constitutive activation of this receptor complex [1–3]. Specifically, decreased GTPase activity leads to the overproduction of cAMP from constitutive activation of adenylyl cyclase. Intracellular signaling pathways are activated leading to multiple downstream effects (Fig. 18.1). Clinical effects of this constitutive receptor activation depend on the tissues in which the affected receptors are located. The distribution and degree to which various tissues are affected then depend on the pattern of somatic mosaicism and possibly the stage of embryonic development when the mutation occurred [4, 5].

In bone, constitutive receptor activation results in increased expression of *c-fos* proto-oncogene and increased interleukin-6 production, leading to abnormal proliferation and differentiation of osteoblast precursors [6, 7]. These poorly differentiated osteoblasts generate abnormal fibrous tissue in the bone marrow space. There is also activation of nearby osteoclasts, increasing bone resorption that further alters bone architecture at the site of the lesion [7]. The net result of these alterations of bone formation and resorption is the proliferation and accumulation of fibrous tissue replacing normal bone in cyst-like spaces. Lesions can occur in a single discrete site (monostotic FD), or involve multiple bones (polyostotic FD). In some patients, FD lesions also produce fibroblast growth factor 23 (FGF-23), leading to excessive loss of urinary phosphate that can complicate this disorder [8]. Renal phosphate wasting can result in concomitant osteomalacia, further weakening bones and contributing to fracture risk [9].

This constitutive receptor activation can also affect tissues other than bone. Within skin, the constitutive activation of melanocytes leads to hyperpigmented macules, termed café au lait macules (Fig. 18.2). Unlike the smooth borders of café au lait macules seen in neurofibromatosis, the characteristic

R. Rahbar et al. (eds.), *Pediatric Head and Neck Tumors*,
DOI 10.1007/978-1-4614-8755-5_18, © Springer Science+Business Media New York 2014

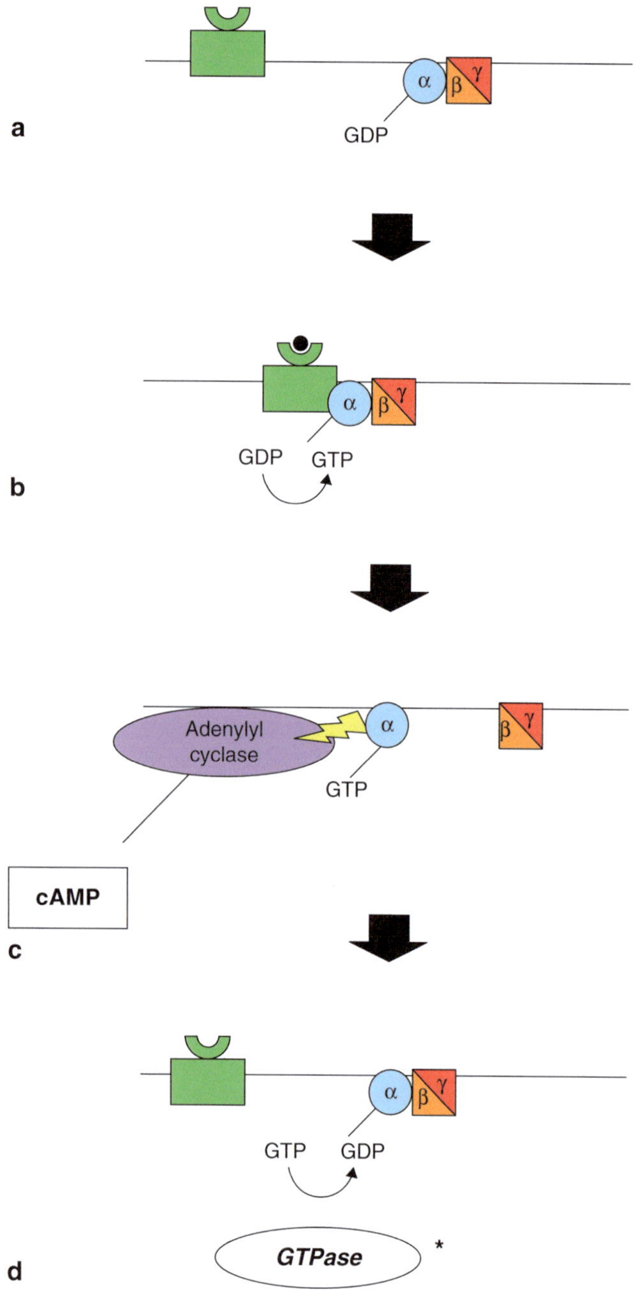

Fig. 18.1 G Protein-coupled receptor activation and inactivation pathway. **a** In its inactive state, the Gsα is bound to guanosine diphosphate (GDP) and βγ subunits. **b** Agonist binding to the receptor results in conversion of GDP to hydrolyze guanosine triphosphate (GTP). **c** Gsα bound to GTP is in its active form and activates adenylyl cyclase, which generates cAMP. **d** GTPase inactivates Gsα by converting GTP to GDP. Gsα then reassociates with βγ subunits. * In FD and macrophage activation syndrome (MAS), GTPase is mutated, leading to constitutive activation of Gsα

macules are distinguished by their more irregular borders, sometimes referred to as "Coast of Maine" lesions, with the borders resembling the ragged Maine coastline.

Endocrine organs may also be involved in cases of FD, with the combination of FD with café au lait macules and

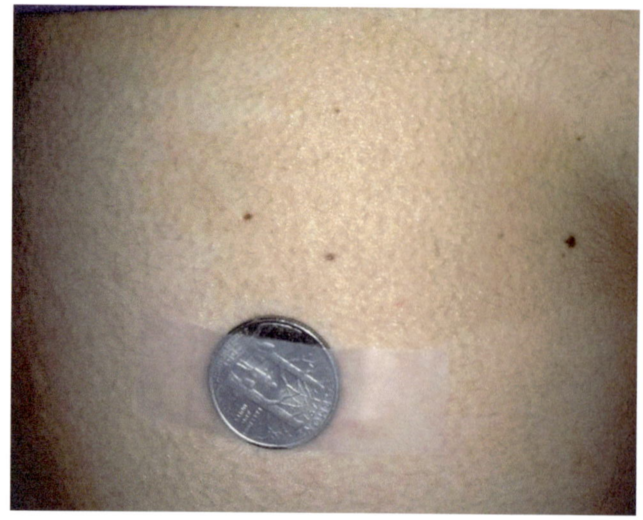

Fig. 18.2 Café au lait macule. Classic "coast of Maine" appearance marked by irregular borders

endocrinopathies referred to as the McCune–Albright syndrome [10]. The most well known endocrinopathy associated with McCune–Albright syndrome is gonadotropin-independent, precocious puberty caused by primary ovarian or testicular hyperfunction. Pituitary gland involvement can lead to acromegaly, Cushing's disease, and nonfunctioning pituitary adenomas. Constitutive activation of the thyrotropin (TSH) receptor can lead to hyperthyroidism and/or thyroid nodules. Primary adrenal involvement manifests as adrenal nodules and/or hypercortisolemia (Table 18.1).

FD can rarely occur in combination with benign intramuscular myxomas without associated endocrinopathies, referred to as Mazabraud's syndrome.

Epidemiology

The prevalence is difficult to estimate, but FD has been reported to comprise up to 7 % of all benign bone tumors [11]. Because this mutation occurs post-zygotically, FD and the McCune–Albright syndrome are noninheritable. Males and females tend to be similarly affected. Approximately 60 % of affected patients have the monostotic form of FD, which typically presents during young adulthood. The less common polyostotic form tends to be more severe and presents at a younger age, often in children under 10 years of age. Craniofacial bones are affected in approximately 10 % of cases of monostotic FD and more than 50 % of cases of polyostotic FD. McCune–Albright syndrome occurs in a small subset of patients with polyostotic FD, comprising less than 5 % of all affected patients [12–15].

Table 18.1 Endocrine tissues expressing GNAS receptors and the resulting clinical manifestations of constitutive activation

Bone	*Adrenal glands*
Fibrous dysplasia	Adrenal nodules
FGF-23 overproduction leading to renal phosphate wasting	Cushing's syndrome
Ovarian/testicular tissue	*Pituitary gland*
Precocious puberty	Acromegaly
Testicular mass (Leydig and/or Sertoli cell hyperplasia)	Hyperprolactinemia
	Cushing's disease
	Pituitary adenoma
Thyroid	*Parathyroid glands*[a]
Thyroid nodules	Primary hyperparathyroidism
Hyperthyroidism	

[a] Reported association, but not confirmed

Clinical Presentation

The clinical presentation of FD includes a spectrum, ranging from asymptomatic to severe depending on the number and anatomical location of affected sites. Any bone can be involved, although the femur and skull base are the most commonly affected. FD may be incidentally discovered as a bony lesion found on unrelated radiology images. Patients may also present with bone pain or tenderness corresponding to the affected region. If the long bones are affected, patients may also develop an abnormal skeletal angulation that is often referred to as a "shepherd's crook" deformity. In addition, patients can present with a pathologic fracture at the site of the FD lesion due to weakening of the bone from an abnormal architecture. In one study, peak fracture rate occurred between the ages of 6 and 10 years, with a decline in rate of fracture thereafter [9]. Craniofacial involvement can lead to asymmetry and disfigurement of affected areas, as well as abnormal tooth development and jaw issues. Compression of important intracranial structures can cause visual impairment or cranial nerve palsies. Scoliosis can be a presenting sign of spine involvement [16]. The McCune–Albright syndrome can present either with the above bone manifestations or from effects of associated endocrinopathies, most commonly precocious puberty.

Differential Diagnosis

FD lesions display characteristic findings on imaging as described in more detail below, and few other disease processes produce a similar clinical picture. Paget's disease of bone, a disease characterized by expansive bony lesions, can occur in one or more discrete bony regions and result in expansion of the cortical envelope similar to FD. These lesions are distinct from FD lesions in that they typically occur later in life and can typically be distinguished on imaging. Solitary lesions seen in monostotic FD can resemble other bony tumors or processes. For example, simple bone cysts, nonossifying fibromas, osteofibrous dysplasia, bone angiomas, and low-grade, intramedullary osteosarcoma or other sarcomas can resemble an isolated FD lesion. In addition, craniofacial FD lesions may appear similar to a calcified meningioma. In cases where imaging does not confirm the diagnosis, biopsy of the lesion can be performed [17, 18].

Diagnosis and Evaluation

Physical Examination

Distinct findings on physical examination may be subtle or absent. Bone deformities, such as abnormal long bone angulation or asymmetric craniofacial swelling, may be identified on close inspection. Tenderness to palpation of affected bones may be present. In craniofacial FD, impingement of cranial nerves can result in visual abnormalities or cranial nerve palsies. Consultation with an ophthalmologist for regular complete ophthalmologic examinations is indicated in craniofacial cases. Careful skin examination may reveal café au lait macules. In the McCune–Albright syndrome, evidence of hormonal excess may also be apparent on exam. Palpable masses within the thyroid or testis may be noted, or the clinical stigmata of Cushing's syndrome, acromegaly, or hyperthyroidism. Lastly, premature pubertal development in children may be noted if precocious puberty is present.

Laboratory Evaluation

In monostotic and polyostotic FD, laboratory evaluation may reveal abnormalities in bone turnover, with increased markers of bone resorption and formation. Serum alkaline phosphatase may also be elevated due to an increase in bone-specific alkaline phosphatase. Electrolytes, calcium, and renal function are typically normal. If excess FDF-23 is produced by FD lesions, phosphate levels may be low, associated with high urinary phosphate levels and low tubular

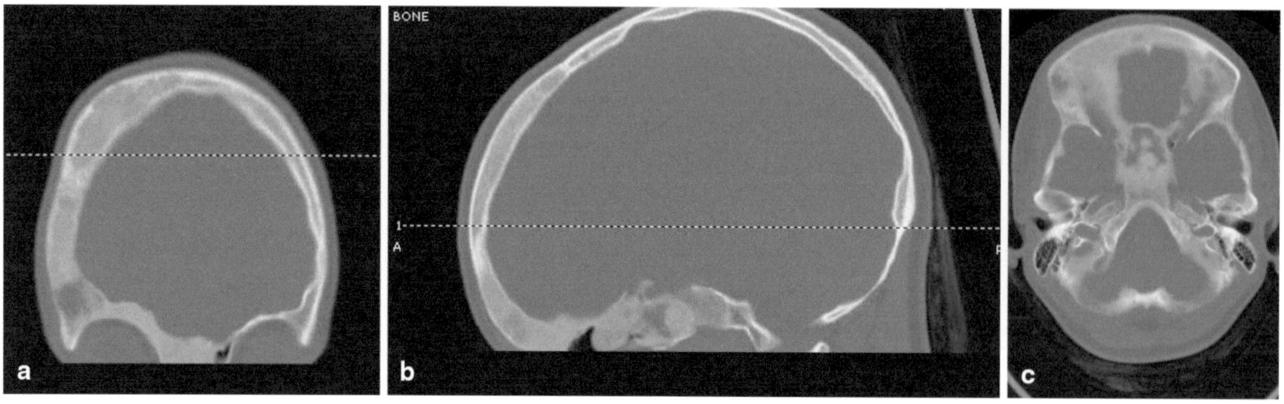

Fig. 18.3 Head CT images in a patient with craniofacial FD. Images reveal heterogeneous appearance of the skull with both sclerotic, as well as lytic changes and the characteristic a ground glass appearance. Multiple bones are involved, including right frontal bone, the body of sphenoid, the right pterygoid bone, the medial right orbital wall, the ethmoidal bone, the ethmoid air cells, the right orbital roof, and the medial aspect left frontal bone

resorption of phosphate (TRP) due to renal phosphate wasting. Serum 25-hydroxyvitamin D levels should be measured, since previous studies have shown that vitamin D deficiency is not uncommon in this patient population [19].

All patients with polyostotic FD should also undergo evaluation for underlying endocrinopathies to evaluate for McCune–Albright syndrome, including evaluation for hyperthyroidism, cortisol excess, and acromegaly. In prepubertal children, this evaluation should also include an assessment for physical or biochemical evidence of precocious puberty as suggested by the history, physical examination or results of laboratory tests [20].

Imaging

Findings on imaging studies can be diagnostic of FD. Appearance on plain radiographs can vary, but typically reveal expansion of bone from the medullary space outward to the cortex in discrete well-defined regions. Cortices are often thinned and can appear sclerotic. The center of the lesion may have a radiolucent or ground glass appearance. The lesions can develop an increasingly sclerotic appearance with advancing age. Associated deformities can be seen in long bones, including abnormal angulation or bowing [21]. In polyostotic forms, a hemimelic distribution of lesions may often, although not always, be seen. Monostotic lesions may be more difficult to distinguish from other potential disorders, and additional imaging with computed tomography (CT) or magnetic resonance imaging (MRI) can be helpful, particularly in craniofacial cases. CT can provide additional detail illustrating the characteristic sclerotic and lytic changes and ground glass appearance seen within FD lesions (Fig. 18.3). MRI can add complementary information regarding content, size, and shape of lesions and can also be used to visualize important nearby neurovascular structures in craniofacial cases [22]. In addition, given the underlying pathophysiology of increased osteoblast activity, FD lesions are easily visualized on nuclear medicine bone scans, with areas of increased uptake corresponding to each bony lesion (Fig. 18.4). This type of imaging can be helpful to localize all potential affected areas and distinguish monostotic and polyostotic forms [23].

Pathology

In most cases, a biopsy of the bony lesion is not required to make the diagnosis of FD, since characteristic findings on imaging can be diagnostic. Biopsy can potentially contribute to pathologic fracture and, therefore, should be performed with caution and only in situations where the diagnosis remains unclear, after appropriate imaging and consultation with expert radiologists have been pursued.

Pathologic findings pathognomonic for FD include the accumulation of fibrous tissue within the bone marrow, associated with abnormal osteoblasts shaped like immature spindle fibroblast-like cells arranged in parallel arrays or whirls (Fig. 18.5 and 18.6). Lesions typically expand from the medullary cavity outward to the cortical bone. Sequence analysis of the *GNAS* gene from a sample of the affected bone can confirm the disease-causing mutation [24].

Treatment

Medical Treatment

Medical therapy for all patients with FD includes optimizing factors known to affect their bone health. Most experts

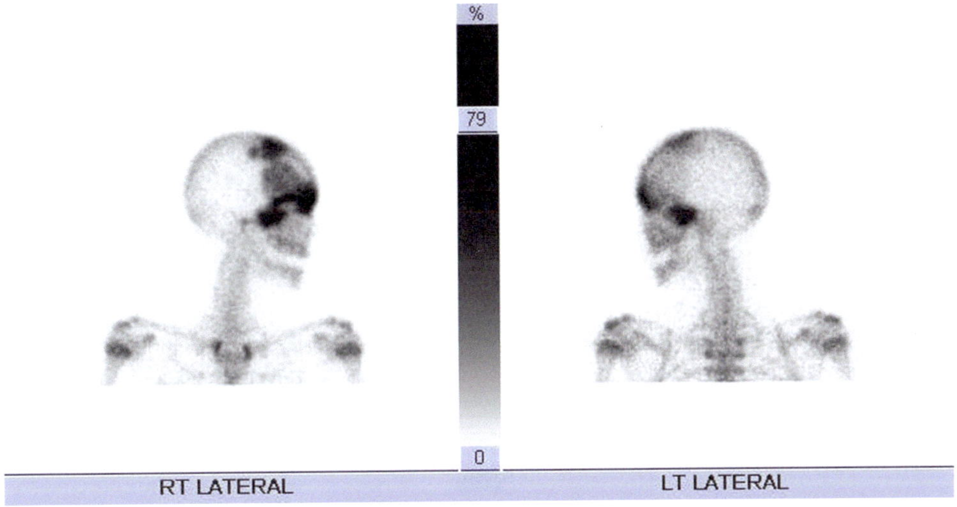

Fig. 18.4 Radionuclide bone scan in a patient with craniofacial FD. Images reveal increased uptake in multiple sites corresponding to FD lesions

recommend that patients receive adequate amounts of daily vitamin D and calcium in order to prevent secondary hyperparathyroidism that can ultimately lead to concomitant rickets or osteomalacia and further weaken bones. In addition, subjects with renal phosphate wasting and hypophosphatemia may benefit from phosphate supplementation and calcitriol, although the efficacy of this approach has not been confirmed in clinical trials.

Nonpainful FD lesions that do not impinge on associated structures and are not associated with fracture or deformity can usually be followed expectantly. However, patients with FD can suffer significant pain related to the lesion itself or underlying pathologic fracture. Significant bone deformities caused by FD can also lead to disability and disfigurement. In addition, craniofacial lesions may expand to compromise the nearby important neurovascular structures. In these cases, additional medical therapy or surgical intervention may be indicated.

Bisphosphonates are antiresorptive agents that are classically used for the treatment of osteoporosis in adults. When used in patients with FD, bisphosphonates function to inhibit the osteoclastic bone resorption that takes place around abnormal fibrous tissue. Pamidronate administered by intravenous infusion has been studied to the greatest extent in this patient population. The initial report of clinical improvement after treatment with pamidronate came in 1994 in an open-label study involving nine patients [26]. Since that time, additional studies have shown improved bone pain, decreased markers of bone turnover, and increased bone density with pamidronate treatment [19, 27, 28]. Although some studies report improvement in the radiologic appearance of FD lesions, the effect of bisphosphonates on disease progression, inhibition of new lesion development, or prevention of pathologic fracture has not been established. In addition, data in children are more limited, suggesting improvement in pain with treatment, but without consistent effect on radiographic or fracture outcomes [29–32].

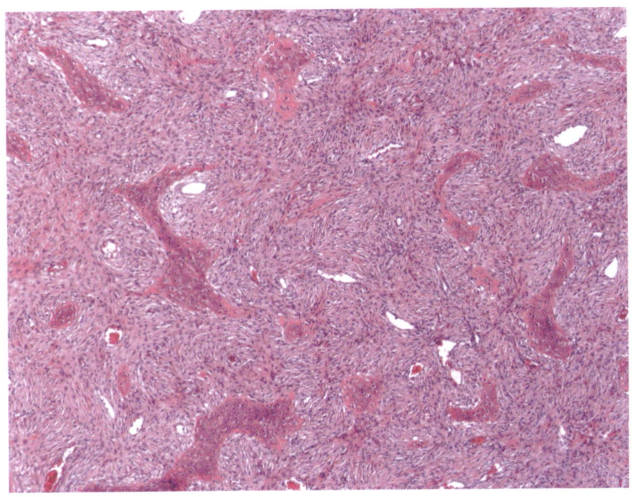

Fig. 18.5 Representative histological image. The tumor is composed of well-differentiated cords and sheets of spindle shaped fibroblast-like cells, which have been shown to have osteoblast proteins by immunocytochemistry. Embedded within this tissue are irregular, mineralized, woven bone trabeculae. There are no cuboidal osteoblasts rimming the bone trabeculae. There are a few large vascular channels. The tumor cells immunohistochemically express perostin [25]. (Picture and description provided by Sanford I. Roth MD)

In addition to pamidronate, other bisphosphonates have been used in the treatment of FD. Several case reports and case series suggest that oral alendronate may be effective in improving bone pain associated with FD lesions in adults, either alone or following treatment with intravenous pamidronate [33–35]. In one case series, high-dose, oral alendronate was effective in the treatment of intractable headache from skull involvement in three patients [36]. Zoledronic acid has also been prescribed with variable results in several reports, and is typically reserved for patients unresponsive to pamidronate [37–39].

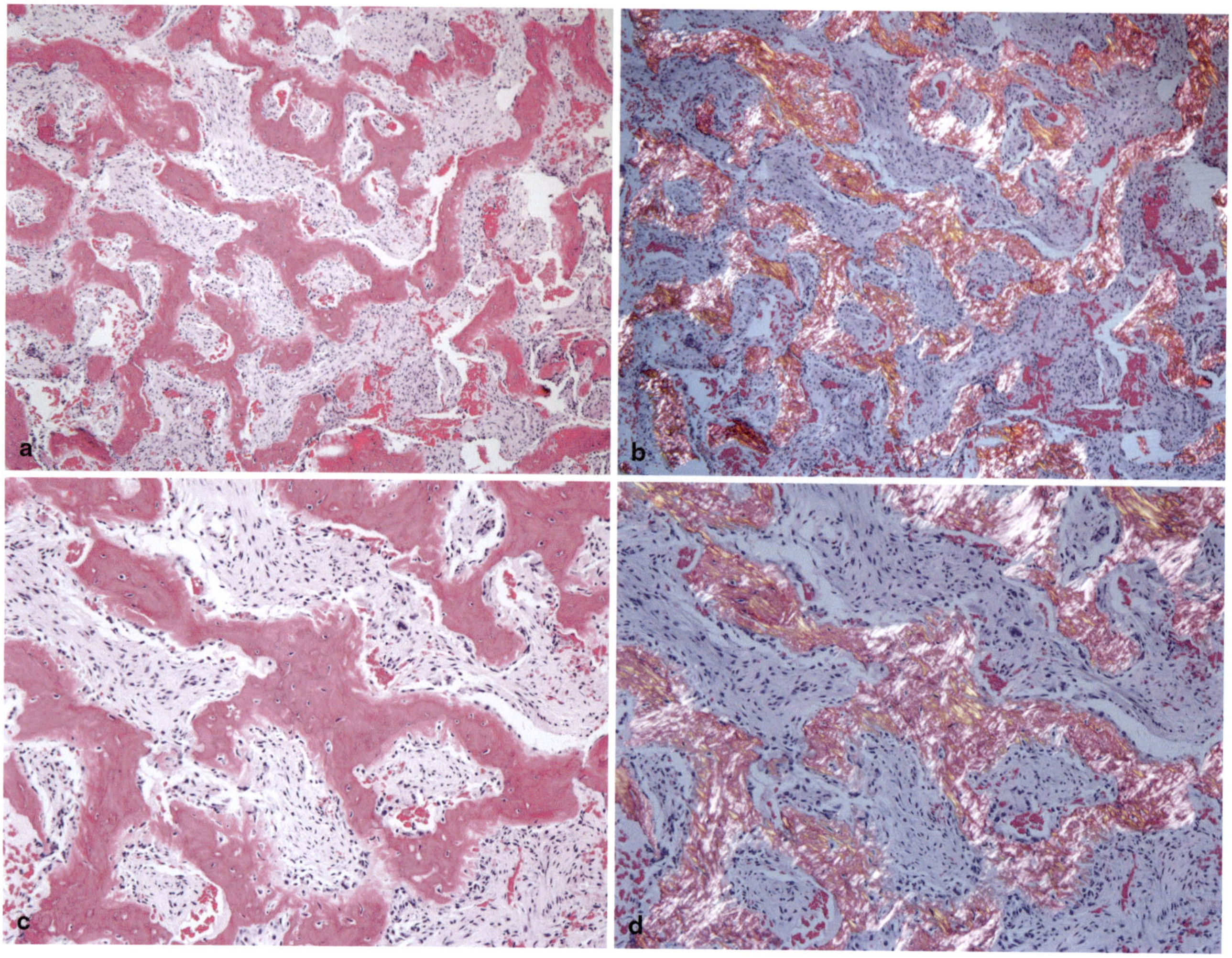

Fig. 18.6 Additional histological images. **a** Complex trabeculae of woven bone separated by a moderately cellular fibrous stroma. Anastomosing branching trabeculae of bone mimic Chinese characters. **b** Same image as **a** under polarizing lenses showing woven bone with absent lamellae. **c** At higher magnification, trabeculae of woven bone lack osteoblastic rimming. The fibrous stroma cells are bland, lacking nuclear hyperchromatism or pleomorphism. **d** Same image as **c** under polarizing lenses showing the characteristic woven bone with absence of osteoblastic rimming

Potential side effects of intravenous bisphosphonates include myalgias, fever, and flu-like symptoms after infusion. Of note, these side effects are primarily seen after the initial infusion and typically do not recur with subsequent infusions. Hypocalcemia after the infusion is seen, but can usually be prevented by treating any preexisting vitamin D deficiency and ensuring adequate provision of dietary calcium prior to the infusion. Osteonecrosis of the jaw has been seen with bisphosphonate use as well, particularly when given in high doses in patients treated for bony metastases. There is one published report in the literature of a case of osteonecrosis of the jaw in an adult with FD treated with zoledronic acid [40]. In addition, long-term consequences of treatment in children with growing bones are largely unknown. Lastly, caution should be taken in treating girls and women of childbearing age, since bisphosphonates deposit in bone for many years and the effects on fetal skeleton in future pregnancies are not clear.

In addition to bisphosphonates, denosumab is a new antiresorptive medication that may potentially have a future role in the medical management of FD. Denosumab is a monoclonal antibody against receptor activated nuclear kappa (RANK) ligand that results in inhibition of osteoclast differentiation and activation. One case report suggested that denosumab resulted in clinical improvement in pain and decreased lesion expansion in a child previously unresponsive to bisphosphonates [41]. Whether this will become an established treatment option for FD requires additional study.

In summary, medical management of FD includes optimizing calcium and vitamin D intake, treating concurrent osteomalacia, and considering antiresorptive therapy in cases complicated by significant pain. Phosphate supplementation should also be considered for those patients with FD who exhibit hypophosphatemia. Many questions remain regarding the use of antiresorptive therapy in the treatment of FD. Most importantly, whether bisphosphonates prevent pathologic fracture, deformities, and disease progression over time in FD patients has yet to be established. Multiple different regimens and drug choices are available, and it is unclear which represents the optimal treatment choice. In addition, duration of treatment remains controversial. Additional trials will be required to clarify these issues.

Surgical Treatment

Surgical Indications

Difficulties in establishing surgical indications for FD result from the benign nature of the disease and the unpredictable natural history. In general, FD lesions in the head and neck are not treated surgically. The primary aim of surgery is symptomatic relief, functional restoration and aesthetic improvement. Surgical therapy may be indicated in the following situations:

1. In cases of significant functional compromise secondary to compression of adjacent structures or cosmetic concern.
2. If complete resection is surgically possible, without significant morbidity—this is the ideal situation.
3. However, where surgery is indicated but complete resection will not be possible, partial excision or surgical recontouring may be performed, noting that there may be a high incidence of recurrence and the need for further surgical procedures.

Timing of Surgery

It was previously recommended that surgery for FD be delayed until after completion of skeletal growth after puberty and a possible arrest of further disease progression, allowing for a more definitive procedure at that point. However, the growth rate of normal residual tissue and even dysplastic tissue has been found to be unaffected by early surgical intervention. Therefore, the decision to proceed with surgical treatment should be based on careful assessment of the impact of the disease on each individual patient [42]. For example, the development of cystic degeneration may be associated with significant expansion, pain, and associated functional and aesthetic problems that may compel surgery at a younger age. The possibility of reactivation of disease later in life, especially during pregnancy, should be clearly explained.

Technique

Surgical technique and the extent of the resection depend primarily on the location and size of the lesion, its proximity to critical anatomic structures (carotid artery, optic nerve, middle and anterior cranial fossae), the severity of symptoms, patient age, and the possibility of sarcomatous degeneration. Over recent decades, traditional and more invasive external approaches such as craniofacial resection, Caldwell–Luc, and lateral rhinotomy with external ethmoidectomy for sinus lesions, have now largely been replaced by minimally invasive transnasal endoscopic approaches, used in conjunction with image-guided navigational tools [43]. Particularly in young patients, endoscopic techniques interfere less with the growth of maxillary skeleton compared to open techniques.

For lesions of the facial and skull bones, surgical recontouring of expanded bone back to near normal dimensions, especially in the nasoethmoidal and orbitozygomatic units, allows preservation of function and facial appearance. Although the recurrence rate has been reported as high as 50 %, periodic bony recontouring is sometimes necessary until the disease becomes stable. Partial excision of large bony lesions of the mandible and zygoma and around the orbit should be considered only at the time of functional or cosmetic concern. Autologous bone grafting with blocks of resected, contoured, dysplastic bone are occasionally used in reconstruction, reportedly without any increased risk of regrowth of diseased bone [44].

Prophylactic optic nerve decompression of FD lesions encasing the optic nerves in patients who do not have vision loss is not recommended. A recent meta-analysis investigating the outcome of 368 optic nerves showed that while patients with radiographic optic nerve compression secondary to FD are at potential risk for visual deterioration, most of them are asymptomatic and will remain that way [45]. Surgical decompression should be reserved for symptomatic patients only, the majority of whom will show an improvement in vision and good, long-term results after optic nerve decompression. Expectant management is recommended in asymptomatic patients with optic nerve encasement, provided growth hormone excess is not present [46].

It is recommended that patients surgically treated for FD should be closely followed with serial MRI every 6 months during the first year after surgery and at yearly intervals thereafter in order to detect possible residual lesions.

Prognosis

Overall, the prognosis of FD depends on the site and degree of bony involvement. FD lesions do not spontaneously regress, and the natural history of these lesions is variable, ranging from asymptomatic stability to unremitting progression over time. The primary complications of this disease consist of pathologic fracture, bone deformities, and nerve compression from craniofacial involvement. Disease progression may occur more rapidly in children, and pregnancy has been reported as a risk factor for worsening disease burden, possibly related to estrogen receptors located within FD lesions [47]. In craniofacial FD, those patients with concurrent growth hormone excess may have the highest risk for disease progression leading to vision or hearing loss [46].

Rarely, FD lesions can undergo malignant transformation, with reported incidence 0.5–4 %, primarily occurring in patients over the age of 30 years. Malignancies include osteosarcoma (most commonly), fibrosarcoma, chondrosarcoma, or malignant fibrohistiocytoma. Radiation therapy increases the risk of malignancy, which is why this treatment is currently contraindicated in patients with FD. The overall prognosis of malignancy arising from FD is poor [48, 49].

Summary

FD is a genetic skeletal disorder caused by a post-zygotic activating mutation in the *GNAS* gene resulting in a wide array of clinical phenotypes. Characterized by expanding bony lesions composed of abnormal fibrous tissue, FD can occur as a single lesion in the monostotic form or in multiple bones in the polyostotic form. The combination of FD, café au late macules, and endocrinopathies comprises the McCune–Albright syndrome. Treatment options are limited and require further study, but antiresorptive therapies show promise in treating the pain associated with this disorder. Prognosis depends on the number, anatomic location, and degree of involvement of bony lesions as well as the association with coexisting endocrinopathies and renal phosphate wasting.

References

1. Weinstein LS, Shenker A, Gejman PV, Merino MJ, Freidman E, SPeigel MA. Activation mutations of the stimulatory G protein in the McCune–Albright syndrome. N Engl J Med. 1991;325:1688–95.
2. Shenker A, Weinstein LS, Sweet DE, Spiegel AM. An activating Gs alpha mutation is present in fibrous dysplasia of bone in the McCune–Albright syndrome. J Clin Endocrinol Metab. 1994;79:750–5.
3. Shenker A, Chanson P, Weinstein LS, Chi P, Spiegel AM, Lomri A, Marie PJ. Osteoblastic cells derived from isolated lesions of fibrous dysplasia contain activating somatic mutations of the Gs alpha gene. Hum Mol Gent. 1995;4:1675–6.
4. Bianco P, Riminucci M, Majolagbe A, Kuznetsov SA, Collins MT, Mankani MH, Corsi A, Bone HG, Wientroub S, Speigel AM, Fisher LW, Robey PG. Mutations of the GNAS1 gene, stromal cell dysfunction and osteomalacic changes in the non-McCune–Albright fibrous dysplasia of bone. J Bone Min Res. 2000;15:120–8.
5. Happle R. The McCune–Albright syndrome: a lethal gene surviving by mosaicism. Clin Genet. 1986;29:321–4.
6. Candeliere GA, Glorieux FH, Prudhomme J, St Arnaud R. Increased expression of the c-fos proto-oncogene in bone from patients with fibrous dysplasia. N Engl J Med. 1995;332:1546–51.
7. Yamamoto T, Ozono K, Kasayama S, Yoh K, Hiroshima K, Takagi M, Matsumoto S, Michigami T, Tamaoka K, Kishimoto T. Okada S. Increased IL-6-production by cells isolated from the fibrous bone dysplasia tissues in patients with McCune–Albright syndrome. J Clin Invest. 1996;98:30–5.
8. Collins MT, Chebli C, Jones J, Kushner H, Consugar M, Rinaldo P, Wientroub S, Bianco P, Robey PG. Renal phosphate wasting in fibrous dysplasia of bone is part of a generalized renal tubular dysfunction similar to that seen in tumor-induced osteomalacia. J Bone Miner Res. 2001;16(5):806–13.
9. Leet AI, Chebli C, Kushner H, Chen CC, Kelly MH, Brillante BA, Robey PG, Bianco P, Wientroub S, Collins MT. Fracture incidence in polyostotic fibrous dysplasia and the McCune–Albright syndrome. J Bone Miner Res. 2003;88:4569–75.
10. Albright F, Butler AM, Hamstra AJ, Smith R. Syndrome characterized by osteitis fibrosis disseminate, areas of pigmentation and endocrine dysfunction, with precocious puberty in females. New Engl J Med. 1937;216:727–46.
11. Dorfman HD, Czerniak B. Fibroosseious lesions. In: Dorkman HD, Czerniak B, editors. Bone tumors. St Louis: Mosby; 1998. pp 441–91.
12. Firat D, Stutzman L. Fibrous dysplasia of the bone, review of 24 cases. Am J Med. 1968;44:421–9.
13. Lustig LR, Holliday MJ, McCarthy EF, Nager GT. Fibrous dysplasia involving the skull base and temporal bone. Arch Otolaryngol Head Neck Surg. 2001;127:1239–47.
14. Panda NK, Parida PK, Sharma R, Jain A, Bapuraj JR. A clinicoradiologic analysis of symptomatic craniofacial fibro-osseous lesions. Otolaryngol Head Neck Surg. 2007;136:928–33.
15. Yetiser S, Gonul E, Tosun F, Tasar M, Hidir Y. Monostotic craniofacial fibrous dysplasia: the Turkish experience. J Craniofac. 2006;171:62–7.
16. Leet AI, Magur E, Lee JS, Wientroub S, Robey PG, Collins MT. Fibrous dysplasia in the spine: prevalence of lesions and association with scoliosis. J Bone Joint Surg Am. 86:531–7.
17. Ippolito E, Bray EW, Corsi A, De Maio F, Exner UG, Robey PG, Grill F, Lala R, Massobrio M, Pinggera O, Riminucci M, Snela S, Zamakidis C, Bianco P. Natural history and treatment of fibrous dysplasia of bone: a multicenter clinicopathologic study promoted by the European Pediatric Orthopaedic Society. J Pediatr Ortho B. 2003;12:155–77.
18. DiCaprio MR, Enneking WF. Current concepts review: fibrous dysplasia. J Bone Joint Surg. 2005;87:1848–64.
19. Chapurlat RD, Hugueny P, Delmas PD, Meunier PJ. Treatment of fibrous dysplasia of bone with intravenous pamidronate: long term effectiveness and evaluation of predictors of response to treatment. Bone. 2004;35:235–42.
20. Hannon TS, Noonan K, Steinmetz R, Eugster EA, Levine MA, Pescovitz OH. Is McCune–Albright syndrome overlooked in subjects with fibrous dysplasia of bone? J Pediatr. 2003;142:532–8.
21. Fitzpatrick KA, Taljanovic MS, Speer DP, Graham AR, Jacobson JA, Barnes GR, Hunter TB. Imaging findings of fibrous dysplasia with histopathologic and intraoperative correlation. Am J Roentgenol. 2004;182:1389–98.
22. Jee WH, Choi KH, Choe BY, Park JM, Shinn KS. Fibrous dysplasia: MR imaging characteristics with radiopathologic correlation. AM J Roentgenol. 1996;73:1523–7.
23. Zhibin Y, Quanyong L, Libo C, Jun Z, Hankul L, Jifang Z, Ruisen Z. The role of radionuclide bone scintigraphy in fibrous dysplasia of bone. Clin Nucl Med. 2004;29:177–80.
24. Candeliere GA, Roughly PG, Glorieux FH. Polymerase chain reaction-based technique for the selective enrichment and analysis of mosaic arg201 mutation in the G alpha s from patients with fibrous dysplasia of bone. Bone. 1997;21:201–6.
25. Kashima TG, Nishiyama T, Shimazu k, et al. Periostin, a novel marker of intramembranous ossification is expressed in fibrous dysplasia and in c-Fos overexpressing bone lesions. Hum Pathol. 2009;40:226–37.
26. Liens D, Delmas PD, Meunier PJ. Long term effects of intravenous pamidronate in fibrous dysplasia of bone. Lancet. 1994;232(8903):953–4.
27. Chapurlat RD, Delmas PD, Liens D, Meunier PJ. Long term effects of intravenous pamidronate in fibrous dysplasia of bone. J Bone Miner Res. 1997;12:1746–52.
28. Parisi MS, Olivieri B, Mautalen CA. Effect of intravenous pamidronate on bone makers and local bone mineral density in fibrous dysplasia of bone. Bone. 2003;33:582–8.

29. Pfeilschifter J, Ziegler R. Effect of pamidronate on clinical symptoms and bone metabolism in fibrous dysplasia and McCune–Albright syndrome. Med Klin. 1998;93:352–9.
30. Lala R, Matarazzo P, Bertelloni S, Buzi F, Rigon F, de Sanctis C. Pamidronate treatment of bone fibrous dysplasia in nine children with McCune–Albright syndrome. Acta Paediatr. 2000;89:188–93.
31. Zacharin M, O'Sullivan M. Intravenous pamidronate treatment of polyostotic fibrous dysplasia associated with the McCune–Albright syndrome. J Pediatr. 2000;137:403–9.
32. Plotkin H, Rauch F, Zeitlin L, Munns C, Travers R, Glorieux FH. Effect of pamidronate treatment in children with polyostotic fibrous dysplasia of bone. J Clin Endocrinol Metab. 2003;88:4569–75.
33. Weinstein RS. Long-term aminobisphosphonate treatment of fibrous dysplasia: spectacular increase in bone density. J Bone Miner Res. 1997;12:1314–5.
34. Kitagawa Y, Tamai K, Ito H. Oral alendronate treatment for polyostotic fibrous dysplasia of bone: a case report. J Ortho Sci. 2004;9:521–5.
35. Lane JM, Khan SF, O'Connor WJ, Nydick M, Hommen JP, Schneider R, Tomin E, Brand J, Curtin J. Bisphosphonate therapy in fibrous dysplasia. Clin Orthop Rel Res. 2001;382:6–12.
36. Chao K, Katznelson L. Use of high-dose oral bisphosphonate therapy for symptomatic fibrous dysplasia of the skull. J Neurosurg. 2008;109:889–92.
37. Chapurlat RD. Medical therapy in adults with fibrous dysplasia of bone. J Bone Miner Res. 2006;21(Suppl 2):P114–8.
38. Mansoori LS, Catel CP, Rothman MS. Bisphosphonate treatment in polyostotic fibrous dysplasia of the cranium: case report and literature review. Endocr Pract. 2010;16:851–4.
39. Mrabet D, Rekik S, Sahli H, Ben Amor M, Meddeb N, Sellami S. An extensive hemimelic polyostotic fibrous dysplasia: a case report. Rheumatol Int. 2012;32:1075–8.
40. Dimitrakopoulos A, Magopoulos C, Karakasis D. Bisphosphonate-induced avascular osteonecrosis of the jaws: a clinical report of 11 cases. Int J Oral Maxillofac Surg. 2006;35:588–93.
41. Boyce AM, Yo J, Kelly MH, Chamberlain C, Chong W, Gafni R, Molinolo A, Cherman N, Bhattacharyya N, Ellsworth M, Kasa-Vubu J, Collins M. Denosumab treatment of fibrous dysplasia of bone. Abstract, 2011 American Society of Bone and Mineral Research annual meeting proceedings; 2011.
42. Schreiber A, Villaret AB, Maroldi R, Nicolai P. Fibrous dysplasia of the sinonasal tract and adjacent skull base. Curr Opin Otolaryngol Head Neck Surg. 2011;20(1):45–52.
43. Berlucchia M, Salsib D, Farinac D, Nicolaib P. Endoscopic surgery for fibrous dysplasia of the sinonasal tract in pediatric patients. Int J Pediatr Otorhino. 2005;69:43–8.
44. Kim DD, Ghali GE, Wright JM, Edwards SP. Surgical treatment of giant fibrous dysplasia of the mandible with concomitant craniofacial involvement. J Oral Maxillofac Surg. 2012 Jan;70(1):102–18.
45. Amit M, Collins MT, FitzGibbon EJ, Butman JA, Fliss DM, Gil Z. Surgery versus watchful waiting in patients with craniofacial fibrous dysplasia—a meta-analysis. PLoS One. 2011;6(9):e25179.
46. Cutler CM, Lee JS, Butman JA, FitzGibbon EJ, Kelly MH, Brillante BA, Feuillan P, Robey PG, DuFresne CR, Collins MT. Long-term outcome of optic nerve encasement and optic nerve decompression in patients with fibrous dysplasia: risk factors for blindness and safety of observation. Neurosurgery. 2006;59:1011–7.
47. Kaplan FS, Fallon MD, Boden SD, Schmidt R, Senior M, Haddad JG. Estrogen receptors in bone in a patient with polyostotic fibrous dysplasia (McCune–Albright syndrome). New Engl J Med. 1988;319:421–5.
48. Ruggieri P, Sim FH, Bond JR, Unni KK. Malignancies in fibrous dysplasia. Cancer. 1994;73:1411–24.
49. Yabut SM, Kenan S, Sissons HA, Lewis MM. Malignant transformation of fibrous dysplasia: a case report and review of the literature. Clin Ortho Rel Res. 1988;228:281–9.

19 Foregut Duplication Cysts

Stephen Kieran, Antonio R. Perez-Atayde and Reza Rahbar

Introduction

Foregut duplication cysts most commonly occur in the thorax. Whilst rarely encountered in the head and neck, their wide spectrum of presentation renders these cysts clinically important, as they can masquerade as other congenital head and neck lesions.

Embryology and Epidemiology

- In the developing embryo, the foregut gives rise to the pharynx, lower respiratory tract and upper gastrointestinal tract (esophagus, stomach, duodenum and hepatobiliary system). During the first trimester, heterotopic rests of foregut-derived epithelium may persist resulting in what are termed foregut duplication cysts. Such cysts can occur anywhere along the alimentary tract from the mouth to the anus.
- Based on their epithelial type and other features, foregut duplication cyst may appear to closely recapitulate airway, esophagus or small intestine. Therefore, the term "foregut duplication cyst" encompasses "bronchogenic cyst", "esophageal duplication cyst" and "enteric duplication cyst". Bronchogenic cysts represent 50–60 % of all mediastinal cysts. They have a ciliated columnar, cuboidal or pseudostratified epithelial cell layer, with cartilage and respiratory glands, and a fibromuscular connective tissue, which identifies this cyst as bronchial in origin. An esophageal duplication cyst has a mucosa with either ciliated columnar epithelium or stratified squamous epithelium, and a layer or two of muscularis propria. Enteric duplication cyst may be lined by gastric and/or respiratory mucosa and are located in the posterior mediastinum, distinct from the esophagus [1].
Three embryological theories exist as to the etiology of foregut duplication cysts:

1. Duplication abnormalities may occur because of disturbed recanalization with abnormal foregut rests forming cysts [2].
2. Cystic duplications arise from a supernumerary lung bud found in the foregut during the 5th and 7th week of embryogenesis [3].
3. Part of the developing stomach may become trapped between the lateral lingual swellings as they close over the tuberculum impar [4].

The third theory is supported by the finding that columnar and goblet cells in foregut duplication cysts tend to be well differentiated with local inductive factors possibly acting upon primitive endothelial cell rests [5].

Presentation

- Head and neck: foregut duplication cysts are most commonly located in the floor of mouth or tongue; however, other anatomical sub-sites have been described (Table 19.1).
- Approximately 50 % of patients with foregut duplication cysts have no symptoms at presentation. Of those who present with symptoms, the most common presenting clinical features are feeding difficulties, odynophagia, stridor, tongue edema and speech difficulties. The neonate, however, may present with frank respiratory distress secondary to airway obstruction from the mass [6].

R. Rahbar (✉)
Department of Otolaryngology, Boston Children's Hospital, Harvard Medical School, Boston, MA, USA
e-mail: reza.rahbar@childrens.harvard.edu

S. Kieran
Department of Otolaryngology and Communication Enhancement, Boston Children's Hospital, Harvard Medical School, Boston, MA, USA

A. R. Perez-Atayde
Department of Pathology, Boston Children's Hospital, Harvard Medical School, Boston, MA, USA

R. Rahbar et al. (eds.), *Pediatric Head and Neck Tumors*,
DOI 10.1007/978-1-4614-8755-5_19, © Springer Science+Business Media New York 2014

Table 19.1 Anatomical sites of foregut duplication cysts in the head and neck [6]

Anatomical site	Percentage (%)
Floor of mouth	30
Tongue	26
Oropharynx	17
Anterior neck	13
Epiglottis/Vallecula	9
Retropharynx	4

Differential Diagnosis

The differential diagnosis of these lesions is that of any congenital cystic mass in the head and neck, the anatomical subsite indicating a more specific differential. Therefore, the following differential should be considered:

- Mucocoele
- Rannula
- Dermoid
- Lymphatic malformation
- Venous malformation
- Teratoma
- Thyroglossal duct cyst
- Epidermoid cyst
- Lymphoepithelial cyst

Diagnosis and Evaluation

Physical Examination

- The commonest site for a foregut duplication cyst to arise is from the floor of mouth or anterior tongue [6]. Such a lesion should be obvious on routine oral cavity examination in the neonatal period (Fig. 19.1).
- Those rarer lesions in the oropharynx, hypopharynx and supraglottis are either visible on oral cavity examination, fiberoptic laryngoscopy or at the time of a direct laryngoscopy (being performed for feeding or airway symptoms).

Imaging Evaluation

In evaluating these lesions, imaging (computed tomography, CT, or magnetic resonance imaging, MRI) is invaluable. Although a foregut duplication cyst is indistinguishable from thyroglossal duct cyst and dermoid cyst in terms of appearance on CT and routine MRI pulse sequences, the presence of a cystic mass in the anterior floor of mouth or anterior third of the tongue is suggestive of the diagnosis (Fig. 19.2). Anatomically, thyroglossal duct cysts are usually located between the foramen cecum and hyoid bone or within the infrahyoid neck, whereas vallecular cysts are located between the epiglottis and tongue base in the supraglottic larynx. Mucous retention cyst may, however, appear indistinguishable from foregut duplication cyst in terms of both imaging characteristics and location, especially in the floor of mouth.

- Studies have noted the association of vertebral anomalies with foregut duplication cysts, termed neurenteric cysts, since the cyst interferes with anterior fusion of the vertebral mesoderm. However, in the largest reported series of head and neck foregut duplication cysts, no patient had any vertebral or spinal anomalies noted on CT or MRI.
- With the increased use of maternal ultrasound, cystic lesions are being diagnosed antenatally. Foregut duplication cysts have been identified in this manner and may potentially warrant emergent airway management at birth including consideration of a potential EXIT procedure [7].

Pathology

Traditionally, there are three pathological criteria (Fig. 19.3) that must be met in order to make a diagnosis of foregut duplication cyst [8]:

1. Covered by a smooth muscle layer
2. Contain epithelium derived from the foregut
3. Attached to a portion of the foregut

- Duplication cysts are lined by one or more types of epithelium; gastric mucosa, ciliated respiratory-type epithelium, stratified squamous epithelium and/or simple cuboidal epithelium can be present. All types of cysts may show squamous metaplasia, mucosal ulceration, inflammation and necrosis, making distinction between bronchogenic or esophageal cysts sometimes impossible. In head and neck foregut duplication cysts, respiratory type mucosa predominates over gastric mucosa [6].
- In the head and neck, foregut duplication cysts may contain only a mucosal lining or a mucosa, submucosa and muscularis propria. The mucosal lining may be squamous, respiratory, intestinal or mixed with secretory epithelium causing gradual enlargement [9].

Treatment

- The treatment options traditionally proposed for foregut duplication cysts include observation, resection and aspiration. However, if left untreated there is potential for complications to develop. In particular, malignancy has been reported to occur in a longstanding foregut duplication cyst, with one case report of an adenocarcinoma and one case of metaplasia arising within longstanding foregut duplication cysts of the head and neck [10, 11].

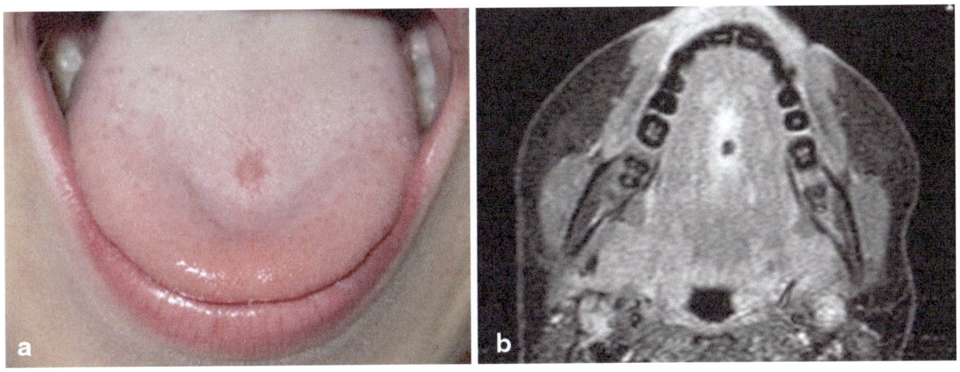

Fig. 19.1 Clinical photograph (**a**) and MRI (**b**) from the same patient of a foregut duplication cyst located in the anterior tongue

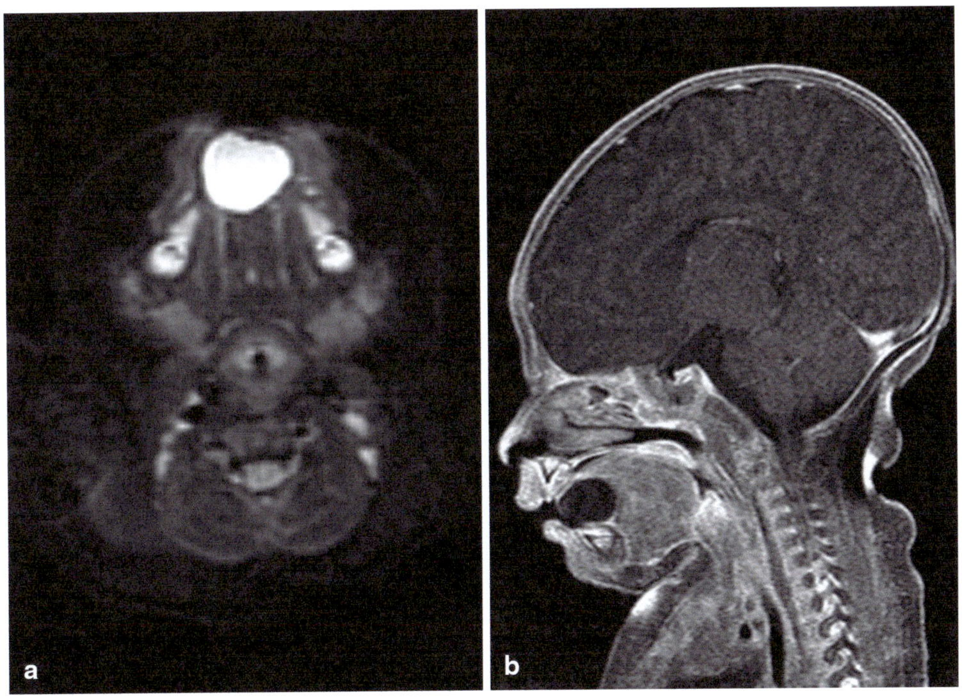

Fig. 19.2 A 7-week-old girl with a tongue foregut duplication cyst. **a** An axial fast spin-echo inversion recovery MRI reveals a unilocular, sharply circumscribed midline lesion that is isointense with cerebrospinal fluid located within the anterior aspect of the floor of the mouth. **b** A gadolinium-enhanced, fat-suppressed sagittal T1-weighted image reveals a cystic mass that does not enhance

- In the chest where foregut duplication cysts are more frequently encountered, early excision has traditionally been recommended in order to avoid serious complications [12]. Gastric epithelium may be a component; hence, peptic ulceration can occur resulting in bleeding or tissue perforation [13]. Left untreated, sinus formation with chronic mucus secretion may also occur [14].
- In certain circumstances, temporary aspiration of the cyst may be performed as it may confirm a benign diagnosis and temporarily alleviate symptoms such as respiratory distress and feeding difficulties. Asymptomatic simple cysts, if observed, have the potential to grow and potentially result in higher rates of peri-operative complications upon becoming symptomatic. Therefore, in view of the need for definitive histological diagnosis, the risk of malignant potential if left untreated and in order to relieve associated symptoms, surgical resection is the definitive treatment of choice.

Outcome

In one series of 22 patients undergoing simple surgical excision of head and neck foregut duplication cysts, none had evidence of recurrence at follow-up. One patient was reported to suffer from a post-operative complication (tongue wound dehiscence) [6].

Conclusion

Foregut duplication cysts of the head and neck may present a diagnostic dilemma and should be included in the differential diagnosis of a congenital lesion of the head and neck, particularly for lesions involving the floor of mouth or anterior tongue. Surgical intervention in the form of simple excision is recommended, as it is both diagnostic and therapeutic. Pre-operative imaging is used to provide a narrow

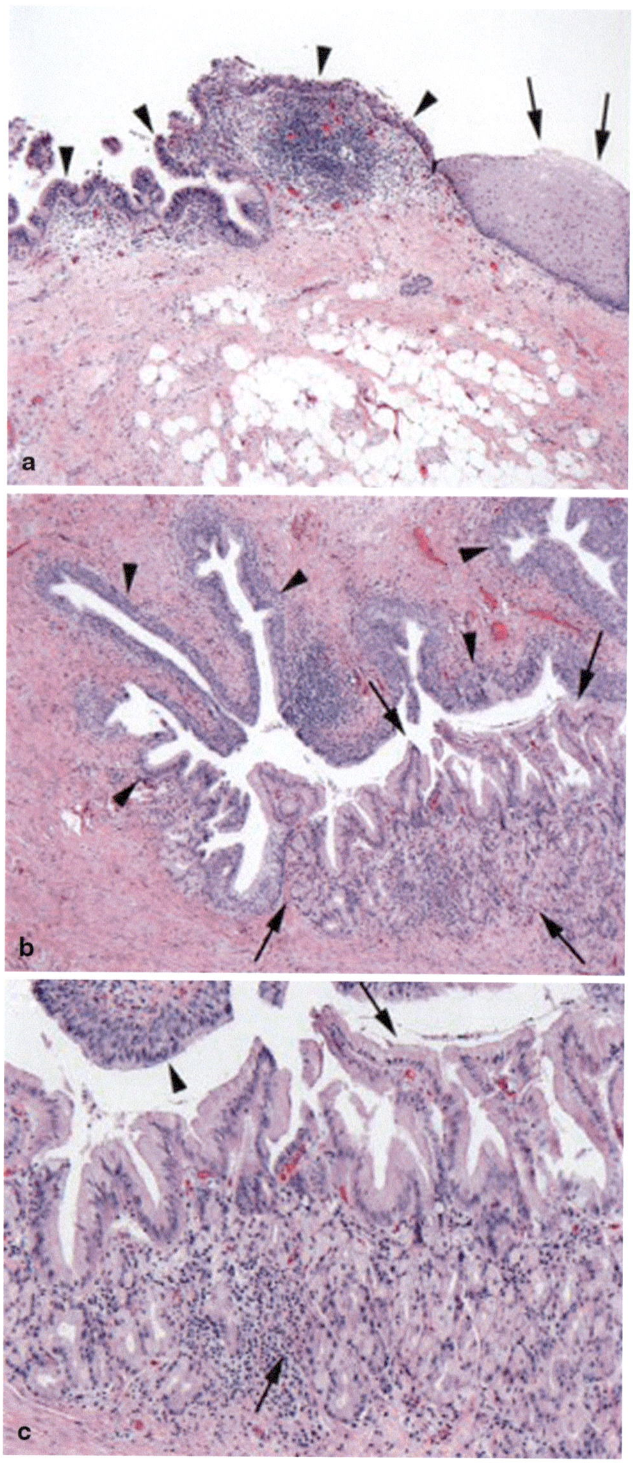

Fig. 19.3 Foregut duplication cyst of the floor of the mouth. **a** The cyst wall is composed of mature fibroadipose tissue and is lined by respiratory type ciliated mucosa (*arrowheads*) and non-keratinizing squamous mucosa (*arrows*). Chronic inflammation is focally present. **b** In some areas, the mucosa of the cyst consists of respiratory epithelium (*arrowheads*) adjacent to well-differentiated gastric antral mucosa (*between arrows*). Chronic inflammation is focally present. **c** Gastric antral mucosal lining shown in **b** is at higher magnification (*between arrows*). A portion of respiratory mucosa is seen in the *upper left corner* (*arrowhead*)

differential diagnosis and assists with surgical planning. Surgical excision has been shown to be both diagnostic and curative.

References

1. Strollo DC, Rosado-de-Christenson ML, Jett JR. Primary mediastinal tumors: part II. Tumors of the middle and posterior mediastinum. Chest. 1997 Nov 5;112(5):1344–57.
2. Bremner JL. Diverticula and duplications of the intestinal tract. Arch Pathol Lab Med. 1944;1944(38):132.
3. Teele RL, Henschke CI, Tapper D. The radiographic and ultrasonographic evaluation of enteric duplication cysts. Pediatr Radiol. 1980 Sep;10(1):9–14.
4. Gorlin RJ, Kalnins V, Izant RJ Jr. Occurrence of heterotopic gastric mucosa in the tongue. J Pediatr. 1964 Apr;64:604–6.
5. Woolgar JA, Smith AJ. Heterotopic gastrointestinal cyst of oral cavity: a developmental lesion? Oral Surg Oral Med Oral Pathol. 1988 Aug;66(2):223–5.
6. Kieran SM, Robson CD, Nose V, Rahbar R. Foregut duplication cysts in the head and neck: presentation, diagnosis, and management. Arch Otolaryngol Head Neck Surg. 2010 Aug;136(8):778–82.
7. Chen MK, Gross E, Lobe TE. Perinatal management of enteric duplication cysts of the tongue. Am J Perinatol. 1997 Mar;14(3):161–3.
8. Qi BQ, Beasley SW, Williams AK. Evidence of a common pathogenesis for foregut duplications and esophageal atresia with tracheo-esophageal fistula. Anat Rec. 2001 Sept 1;264(1):93–100.
9. Tucker R, Maddalozzo J, Chou P. Sublingual enteric duplication cyst. Arch Pathol Lab Med. 2000 Apr;124(4):614–5.
10. Volchok J, Jaffer A, Cooper T, Al-Sabbagh A, Cavalli G. Adenocarcinoma arising in a lingual foregut duplication cyst. Arch Otolaryngol Head Neck Surg. 2007 Jul;133(7):717–9.
11. Kim YS, Ahn SK, Lee SH. Sublingual foregut cyst. J Dermatol. 1998 Jul;25(7):476–8.
12. Parikh D, Samuel M. Congenital cystic lung lesions: is surgical resection essential? Pediatr Pulmonol. 2005 Dec;40(6):533–7.
13. Burgner DP, Carachi R, Beattie TJ. Foregut duplication cyst presenting as neonatal respiratory distress and haemoptysis. Thorax. 1994 Mar;49(3):287–8.
14. Eaton D, Billings K, Timmons C, Booth T, Biavati JM. Congenital foregut duplication cysts of the anterior tongue. Arch Otolaryngol Head Neck Surg. 2001 Dec;127(12):1484–7.

Germ Cell Tumors/Teratoma

20

Jacob R. Brodsky, Vikramjit S. Kanwar, Lisa M. Stafford,
Reza Rahbar and A. Lindsay Frazier

Introduction

Pediatric germ cell tumors (GCT) of the head and neck are rare. Malignant pediatric GCT overall account for 3% of childhood cancers and are categorized as either benign or with malignant elements and as either extragonadal or gonadal [1]. Extragonadal sites are predominant in childhood, although extracranial head and neck GCT are the least common extragonadal sites, representing approximately 10% of benign teratomas and only 2.5% of malignant pediatric GCT [2, 3]. Most head and neck GCT diagnosed at birth or during the first 3 months of life are benign teratomas; however, after the age of 12 months, malignant GCT is the almost exclusive diagnosis [2].

The name teratoma originates from the Latin for "monster-like tumor," probably in reference to its potential to contain an assortment of unusual structural elements often in advanced stages of maturation. Teratomas most commonly present in the sacrococcygeal region [3]. Although it is typically a benign congenital neoplasm, teratomas presenting in the neonatal period can be associated with a considerable risk of mortality due to its potential for causing fetal hydrops and premature delivery resulting from the sheer volume of the tumor. The risk of partial or complete airway obstruction at birth provides an additional source of potential mortality when teratomas present in the head and neck. Recent advances in prenatal imaging techniques now provide a degree of detail adequate to both diagnose potentially obstructing teratomas and to plan airway and tumor management strategies before the child is born. Furthermore, the advent of the *ex utero* intrapartum treatment (EXIT) procedure has allowed for the successful management of neonates with obstructive teratomas that would have been unlikely to survive without such technology.

One-fifth of pediatric head and neck GCT are malignant. Pathologically these are usually yolk sac tumors, also known as endodermal sinus tumors (EST), and respond well to therapy with surgery and cis-platinum-based chemotherapy [3]. Head and neck GCT in childhood occurs most commonly before 3 years of age, and with an overall female predominance [4]. With such an assortment of diagnostic and treatment modalities available, GCT of the head and neck are best managed by a multidisciplinary team, which may include some or all of the following members, depending on whether the tumor is detected pre- or postnatally: pediatric otolaryngologist, pediatric general surgeon, pediatric oncologist, neonatologist, obstetrician, radiologist, and anesthesiologist. A good understanding of the development, diagnosis, and management of these lesions is paramount to ensuring that such patients are given the best possible chance at survival with a minimum of long-term morbidity.

Epidemiology

Teratoma is the most common neonatal tumor (including all benign and malignant tumors), accounting for approximately 25% of tumors presenting in infancy [5], and it is the most common extragonadal GCT in children. The most frequent anatomic site is the sacrococcygeal region with an incidence of approximately 1 in 40,000 live births [6]. Head and neck teratomas are predominantly cervical in location and account for 2–9% of all congenital teratomas. The incidence is greater in females with a female to male ratio of approximately 3:1 [5, 7].

R. Rahbar (✉) · J. R. Brodsky
Department of Otolaryngology and Communication Enhancement, Boston Children's Hospital, Harvard Medical School, Boston, MA, USA
e-mail: reza.rahbar@childrens.harvard.edu

V. S. Kanwar
Pediatric Hematology-Oncology, Albany Medical Center, Albany, NY, USA

L. M. Stafford
College of Nanoscale Engineering, Albany, NY, USA

A. L. Frazier
Department of Pediatric Oncology, Dana-Farber Cancer Institute, Boston, MA, USA

R. Rahbar et al. (eds.), *Pediatric Head and Neck Tumors*,
DOI 10.1007/978-1-4614-8755-5_20, © Springer Science+Business Media New York 2014

In general, GCT of the head and neck are extremely rare in infancy and childhood, and Bernbeck et al. [2] reported 32 GCT of the head and neck region out of all pediatric GCT registered on the German MAKEI protocols: 26 of 611 (4 %) teratomas and 6 of 655 (1 %) malignant GCT. Based on these data, head and neck malignant GCT occurs with an estimated annual incidence of 0.08 per million children under 15 years of age, which explains its rarity in the published medical literature.

Biology

The pathogenesis of teratoma is unclear and multiple theories have been proposed. Batsakis et al. in 1964 proposed that the lesions derive from a sequestration of pluripotent stem cells isolated during embryologic development [8]. Kountakis et al. in 1994 suggested that teratomas originate from foci of embryonic tissue that fail to migrate appropriately during development and escape the influence of their regional primary organizer [9]. They note that the most common presenting sites of teratomas within the head and neck can be predicted by the areas where all three germ cell layers closely approximate during embryological migration. Thus, the abnormal descent of Rathke's pouch endoderm and neuroectoderm with trapped elements of adjacent endoderm and mesoderm may result in the formation of a nasopharyngeal teratoma, while the abnormal descent of primitive thyroid tissue from the foramen cecum in conjunction with trapped elements of adjacent ectoderm and mesoderm may result in the formation of a cervical teratoma.

Primordial germ cells appear in the wall of the yolk sac of the 4–5-week-old embryo and migrate along the dorsal mesentery to the genital ridge; aberrant retention of germ cells near the midline is thought to account for many extragonadal GCT, which often have a midline location. However, many head and neck GCT are not in the midline, therefore another hypothesis is that these GCT arise from totipotential cells scattered throughout various parts of the body during embryonic development that are capable of differentiation in a germ-cell lineage [1].

The tendency of cervical teratomas to contain thyroid tissue or to even replace part of the thyroid gland has led to much speculation about whether such tissue simply represents a well-differentiated component of the tumor or demonstrates that these lesions actually arise from the thyroid gland itself [10–12]. Riedlinger et al. proposed in 2005 that both situations exist, but that teratomas truly originating from the thyroid anlage may be overreported in the literature, since many cases actually demonstrate a clear separation from the gland by a capsule or pseudocapsule on close histological examination [10].

Teratomas have been reported in conjunction with an assortment of other chromosomal anomalies, such as trisomy 13 [13], ring-X chromosome mosaicism with inactive ring-X chromosome [14], and gonosomal pentasomy 49,XXXXY karyotype [15], as well as with genetic syndromes, such as Aicardi syndrome [16]. Kosmadidou-Aravidou et al. in 2006 performed cytogenetic analysis of a cervical teratoma from a fetus that was terminated *in utero* and found two clones of cells with one demonstrating a normal 46,XY karyotype and the other demonstrating an additional marker chromosome, the origin of which could not be identified [17]. A consistent genetic abnormality associated with teratoma has not been demonstrated in the literature, and the etiology of these lesions is likely multifactorial [7].

Presentation

The presentation of teratoma of the head and neck varies by anatomic site and by whether the lesion is diagnosed in the pre- or postnatal period. The exact distribution of anatomic sites among teratomas of the head and neck is not well established due to the fact that the majority of the literature on these lesions consists of case reports and a few small case series. In general, approximately half of teratomas presenting in the head and neck are cervical in origin [5]. The remainder primarily present in the oral cavity, oropharynx, and nasopharynx, where they are often referred to by the term "epignathus" (Latin for "on the jaw"). An assortment of other reported locations include the ear [18], skull base [19], nasal septum [20], and parotid gland [21].

With the development of increasingly advanced prenatal imaging techniques, a patient with a suspected teratoma of the head and neck may need to be evaluated prenatally. This creates the unique situation of having to predict the patient's presentation prior to delivery based exclusively on prenatal imaging studies (see "Diagnosis"). The risk of airway compromise with large cervical, oral, and pharyngeal teratomas is significant, and may result in rapid respiratory decompensation and death if not predicted prenatally and addressed with a well-planned airway management strategy. The degree of airway obstruction can vary greatly depending on the size and location of the lesion. Rarely, oral and pharyngeal teratomas may grow large enough *in utero* to extend up into the intracranial space resulting in obstructive hydrocephalus and even impeding development of the fetal brain [22]. Indirect intrauterine findings associated with fetal teratoma of the head and neck can include polyhydramnios, likely due to obstruction of fetal swallowing, fetal hydrops, and preterm labor.

Teratomas of the head and neck that are not diagnosed prenatally are typically identified early in the postnatal period, though some smaller lesions do not present until later in childhood. Oral teratomas, particularly those of the tongue and palate, often prevent fusion of the palatal shelves resulting in a cleft palate [23]. Cervical teratomas identified postnatally typically present as an isolated neck mass [24].

Teratomas presenting in infancy are considered to be almost universally benign, but the risk of malignancy increases with age. A systematic review of 217 cervical teratomas by Jordan and Gauderer in 1988 demonstrated a total of 4 patients with malignant lesions out of 126 presenting in the prenatal period (3 %), while 16 out of 23 adults (70 %) had malignant lesions [25].

In infants and young children, head and neck GCT commonly present as soft to firm masses that may exhibit relatively rapid growth. They are found in various locations including the oropharynx [26–28], hypopharynx [2], face [29–31], mandible [32], parotid gland [33], ear or Eustachian tube [34–36], floor of mouth [37–39], and orbit [40–46]. There may be symptoms secondary to mass effect (e.g., proptosis with orbital GCT) [40], or bony destruction (e.g., temporal bone involvement) [34].

Differential Diagnosis

Teratoma of the head and neck is a rare entity. A more common congenital mass of the head and neck that may be detected on prenatal ultrasound is a lymphatic malformation (LM). Differentiating between a teratoma and LM is important, since LM can often be treated with sclerotherapy, while teratoma requires surgical resection. Teratoma characteristically demonstrates calcifications on ultrasound [47], which are not typically seen in an LM. Additionally, LM tends to demonstrate a multicystic appearance with fluid levels on MRI, which is uncharacteristic of a teratoma [48].

The differential diagnosis of neck masses presenting in a child postnatally is extensive, but more common lesions include a thyroglossal duct cyst and branchial cleft cyst, neither of which are typically enlarged at birth, but may show gradual enlargement over time or intermittent waxing and waning in size as they become inflamed or infected. Thyroglossal duct cysts and branchial cleft cysts typically demonstrate a characteristic monocystic appearance on imaging studies, in contrast to the multilobulated, heterogeneous appearance of a teratoma [48].

Extracranial masses of the head and neck presenting in childhood need to be differentiated from congenital malformations and from other malignancies. These include hemangiomas, LM, dermoid cysts, rhabdomyosarcoma, metastatic neuroblastoma, and parotid gland tumors. CT or MRI imaging is sometimes helpful in differentiating these lesions from GCT, but surgical biopsy may be needed, and the presence of elevated serum alpha-fetoprotein (AFP) is an extremely useful marker for GCT when malignant elements are present [1].

Diagnosis and Evaluation

Physical Examination

The role of the physical examination is often limited in the evaluation of teratomas of the head and neck, since so many cases are now diagnosed radiologically *in utero*. Signs of upper airway obstruction depend on the size and location of the lesion and can range from mild stertor or stridor to complete apnea. Lesions not diagnosed prenatally and not causing immediate postnatal airway obstruction may demonstrate evidence of a laterally based neck mass often extending to cross the midline. Oral lesions may be associated with cleft palate. On gross examination, the lesions are usually mobile and multilobulated. They are frequently described as having a rubbery consistency on palpation, often with cystic components [25].

Malignant GCT of the extracranial head and neck commonly present as soft to firm masses in various locations such as the pharynx, face, orbit, mandible, parotid gland, or Eustachian tube. Regional lymph node enlargement is not commonly seen, but there may be findings secondary to mass effect such as proptosis.

Laboratory Data

Elevated AFP levels are sometimes seen on amniocentesis in the setting of a fetus with a teratoma, though this finding is inconsistent and rarely of significant clinical utility. Elevated human chorionic gonadotropin (hCG) and AFP levels may signal the presence of regional recurrence or metastatic disease in the setting of malignant teratoma and these levels can be followed postoperatively for malignant GCT [49]. Thyroid function tests and calcium levels are important in the postnatal management of cervical teratomas, which frequently involve the thyroid gland, occasionally resulting in significant postoperative hypothyroidism and hypoparathyroidism with associated hypocalcemia [10].

Imaging

High quality prenatal imaging is paramount to a successful outcome in the evaluation and management of large teratomas of the head and neck. These studies play a key role in identifying such lesions, in determining an appropriate airway management strategy, and in planning for surgical resection.

The high resolution of modern ultrasound techniques allows for the direct visualization of large teratomas of the head and neck on routine prenatal ultrasound studies in some cases (Fig. 20.1), though often only secondary findings, such as polyhydramnios, are seen. The identification

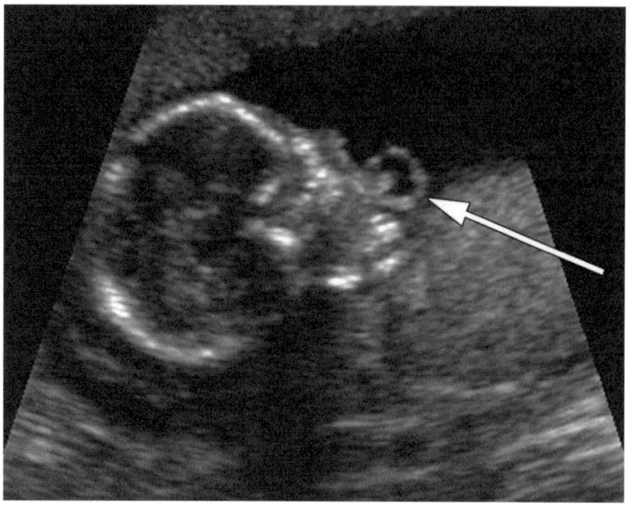

Fig. 20.1 Oblique sonogram of a 16-week gestational age fetus demonstrates a 1 cm teratoma emanating from the right cheek into the amniotic fluid of an otherwise healthy 30-year-old gravida 4, para 1 woman

of calcifications within the lesion suggests the diagnosis of teratoma over other neonatal masses of the head and neck, such as a LM, and may be easier to identify on ultrasound than on MRI. Doppler ultrasound may demonstrate vascular flow within the lesion. Although ultrasound plays a primarily diagnostic role in the evaluation of teratomas of the head and neck, high-resolution three-dimensional ultrasound provides a degree of detail that may contribute to prenatal treatment planning [47].

The development of fetal MRI has allowed for the imaging of fetal masses with an exceptional degree of detail (Fig. 20.2). This degree of detail is essential for determining the appropriate management of large teratomas of the head and neck, particularly in regard to whether an EXIT procedure is indicated and to establish what should be done to secure the airway and manage the tumor during and after the EXIT is performed. T2-weighted MRI images in a normal fetus should demonstrate a hyperintense signal throughout the tracheal column, indicating a patent, fluid-filled airway. The absence of such a signal suggests complete high airway obstruction syndrome (CHAOS) as a result of the lesion, indicating that tracheostomy in conjunction with an EXIT may be required. If a tracheostomy is determined to be necessary, then the path of a severely deviated trachea may be predicted from the fetal MRI images [48].

Though there is no evidence of risks to the fetus from MRI, the safety of MRI in pregnancy has not yet been clearly defined. Thus, the Safety Committee of the Society of MRI has deemed fetal MRI to be appropriate only in cases where other imaging methods, such as ultrasound, are determined to be inadequate or when the MRI will provide important additional information [50, 51].

MRI is helpful in delineating the tumor prior to surgery. In malignant GCT of the head and neck in infants and older children, MRI has a characteristic appearance with uniform signal intensity within a well-defined mass, hypointense on T1-weighted imaging and hyperintense on T2-weighted imaging [43]. This differentiates these tumors from vascular lesions such as LM which have a multilocular appearance and poorly defined margins, and from rhabdomyosarcomas which infiltrate surrounding structures.

The role of CT in prenatal imaging is greatly limited, due to the risk of radiation exposure to the fetus and limited soft-tissue detail in comparison to MRI. Its prenatal use has been reported where a high suspicion for progressive bony destruction of the face exists, allowing for determination of the need for early delivery and resection to prevent further facial destruction [52]. CT does play a role in identifying invasion of bone when planning for the resection of lesions diagnosed in the postnatal period that are adjacent to the skull base, palate, or facial bones.

PET scanning is not routinely used in the evaluation of pediatric GCT, but malignant GCT of head and neck are PET-avid and extrapolating from experience with adult non-germinomatous GCT; this modality may have an increasing role to play in monitoring response to therapy [53].

Pathology

Grossly, teratomas typically have a multinodular outer appearance with a fleshy whitish yellow interior with dark brown areas and foci of hemorrhage (Fig. 20.3). Microscopically, a teratoma is a true congenital neoplasm, and, by definition, contains tissues originating from each of the three major germ cell layers, namely ectoderm, mesoderm, and endoderm (Fig. 20.4). Approximately 68 % of cervical teratomas also contain neuroectodermal elements, such as neural tissue [25]. These tissues present in a variety of degrees of differentiation, ranging from immature cells to highly developed tissue structures, such as pancreas and intestine. In children and adults, tumors with an increased proportion of immature elements often have elevated levels of AFP and are more prone to recurrence. Teratoid cysts are poorly differentiated tumors developed from all three germ layers, and an epignathus is an intraoral teratoma originating from the base of the skull that may have completely developed fetal organs or limbs [54]. Cervical teratomas also frequently contain thyroid tissue, though their relationship to the thyroid gland itself varies.

Histopathologically, malignant GCT of the head and neck with a component of endodermal sinus tumor were first described by Teilum in 1959, and are typically characterized by Schiller-Duval bodies that consist of a single row of tumor cells surrounding a blood vessel that is in turn surrounded

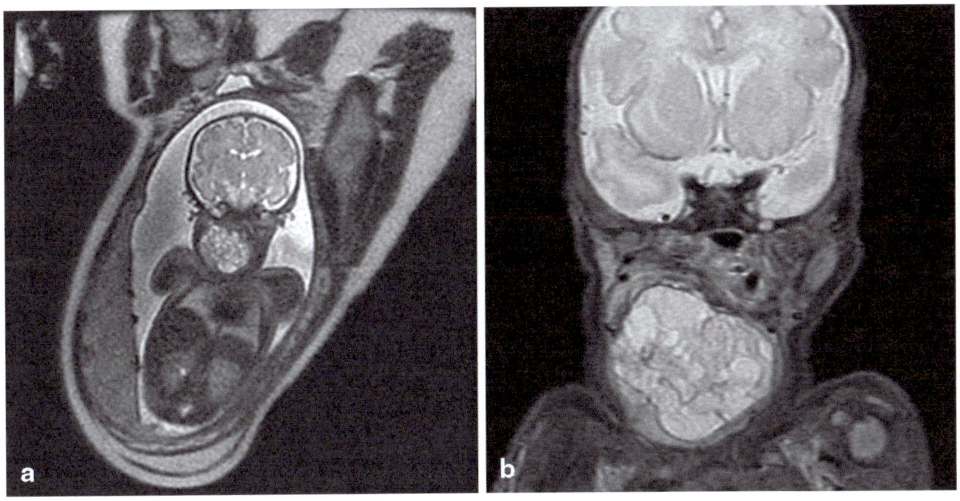

Fig. 20.2 **a** Prenatal MRI of a patient obtained at 34 weeks gestational age showing a large heterogeneous mass emanating from the right neck. A bronchoscopy and intubation were performed in conjunction with an EXIT procedure. **b** A postnatal MRI of the same patient obtained on the first day of life showing similar findings. The mass was resected 2 weeks later

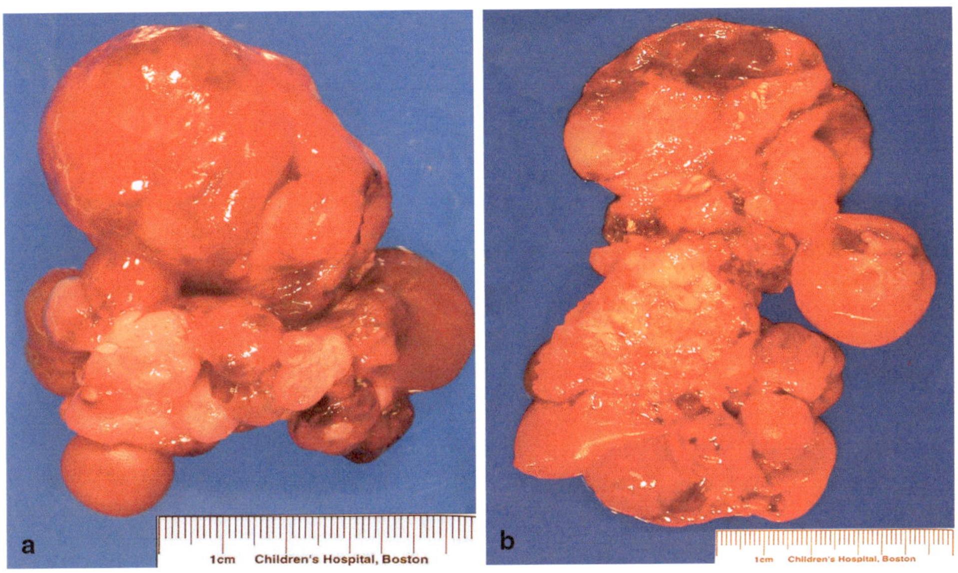

Fig. 20.3 Macroscopy of palatal solid immature teratoma. **a** Large soft-tissue mass with red brown smooth surface and a multinodular appearance. **b** On cut surface, the mass is fleshy with whitish yellow and dark brown areas as well as foci of hemorrhage

by a cystic space (Fig. 20.5) [1]. Immunohistochemical tests find that the cytoplasm of the tumor cells usually stains strongly positive for AFP and Lin28. Cytogenetic changes in chromosome 1, 3, and 6 may be found, but, unlike adult yolk sac tumors, isochromosome 12p is rarely seen [55].

Treatment

Medical

Despite their benign histology, teratomas of the head and neck region constitute a life-threatening and potentially fatal disease. The main intervention is surgical, and modern surgical techniques, accompanied by innovative supportive care, have resulted in survival rates in excess of 80 %.

During infancy, the risk of a GCT being malignant increases with age, and GCT of the head and neck in children in the first decade of life that are older than 1 year of age are primarily likely to be malignant. Due to concern about a biological switch from histologically benign teratomas in the perinatal period to mixed malignant GCT in older children, complete resection of these tumors is considered crucial [56].

A MEDLINE review revealed 45 cases of malignant GCT of the head and neck in children, published in a variety of case reports and case series (Table 20.1). Complete surgical resection is considered a keystone to cure [57]. Earlier chemotherapy regimens that included vincristine, actinomycin D, and cyclophosphamide improved survival; however, it was the introduction of Einhorn's cis-platinum-based therapy, which included etoposide and bleomycin, that produced significant improvement in disease-free survival rates in children with malignant GCT [2, 3, 58]. Given the rarity of pediatric GCT, recent progress in treating patients has occurred largely as a result of several multi-institutional trials around the world.

Fig. 20.4 Light microscopy of palatal solid immature teratoma. **a** Ectodermal and mesodermal components with developing skin (*on top*) and immature subcutaneous tissue with islands of developing adipose tissue (*arrows and inset*). **b** Endodermal and mesodermal components with well-formed intestinal structure including intestinal mucosa, muscularis mucosae, submucosa, and muscularis propria. **c** Neurectodermal component with disorganized developing brain tissue. **d** Poorly differentiated neuroblastic elements with abundant neuropil (*center*). Neuroblasts at higher magnification are seen in the inset; occasional cells are undergoing mitoses

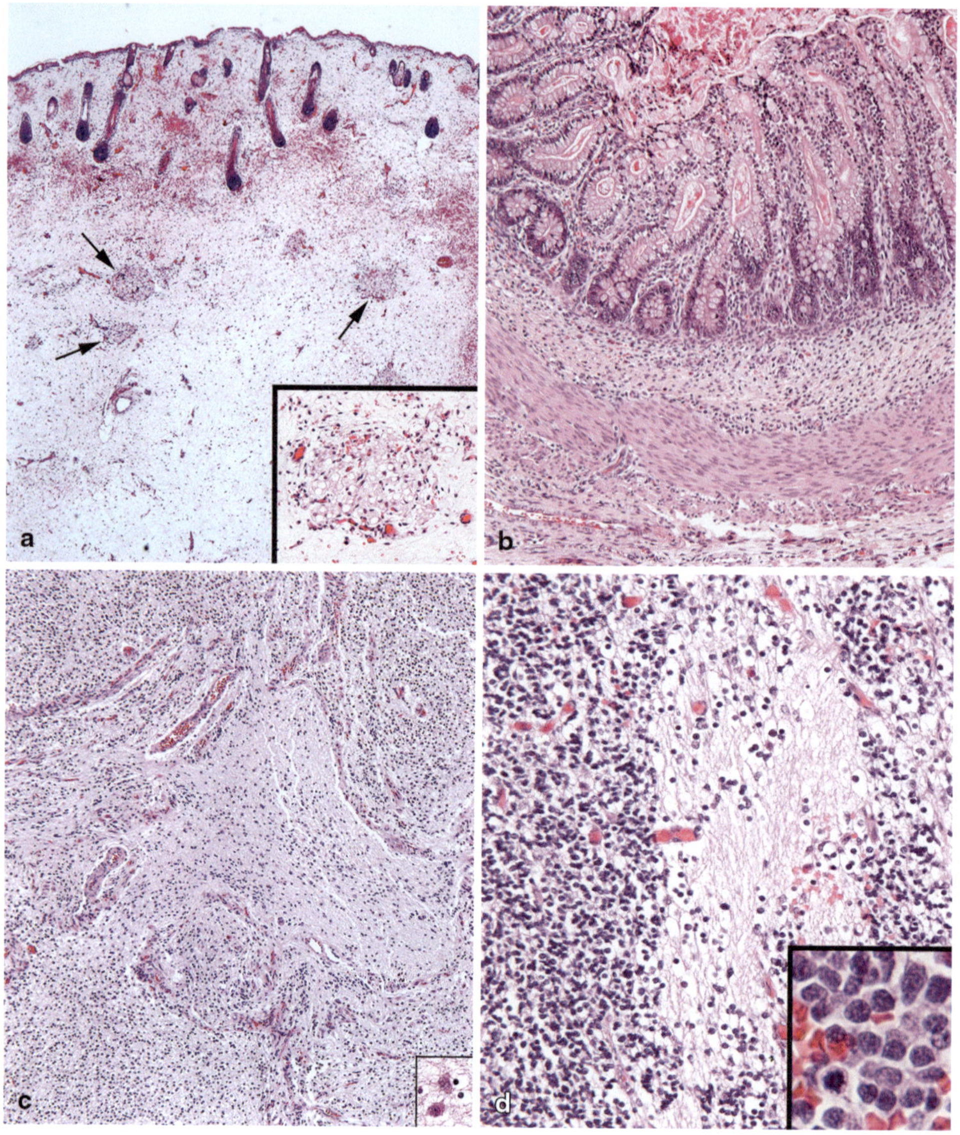

In North America, this includes the collaborative efforts of the Children's Oncology Group (COG), the merged entity of the former Children's Cancer Group (CCG) and the Pediatric Oncology Group (POG) [59]. For patients with head and neck malignant GCT who recur prior to or after surgery, the choice of salvage therapy includes TIP (i.e., paclitaxel (Taxol®) 250 mg/m^2 + ifosfamide 1.2 g/m^2 × 5 + cisplatin 20 mg/m^2 × 5), high-dose chemotherapy (HD-CT) and autologous stem cell transplant (ASCT), and TIC (i.e., paclitaxel (Taxol®) (135 mg/m^2 × 1), ifosfamide (3 g/m^2 × 5) and carboplatin (560 mg/m^2 × 1)) [60].

Surgical

Prenatally diagnosed teratomas of the head and neck are best managed by a multidisciplinary fetal treatment team, which includes not only a pediatric otolaryngologist, but also an anesthesiologist, obstetrician, neonatologist, radiologist, geneticist, and pediatric surgeon. If fetal imaging determines that there is a high likelihood of severe or complete upper airway obstruction, then an EXIT (ex utero intrapartum treatment) procedure should be considered. The EXIT procedure allows for partial fetal delivery with continued maintenance of uteroplacental perfusion and gas exchange while measures are taken to secure the fetal airway prior to completion of the delivery. This requires a delicate anesthetic balance to obtain a degree of uterine relaxation adequate for maintenance of fetal perfusion while avoiding complete, prolonged uterine atony resulting in hemorrhage that could be life-threatening for both the mother and the fetus.

During an EXIT procedure, the mother is maintained under general anesthesia while a hysterotomy is performed, and only the head and shoulders of the fetus are exposed. Direct laryngoscopy and rigid bronchoscopy are first performed with an attempt at orotracheal intubation. If the

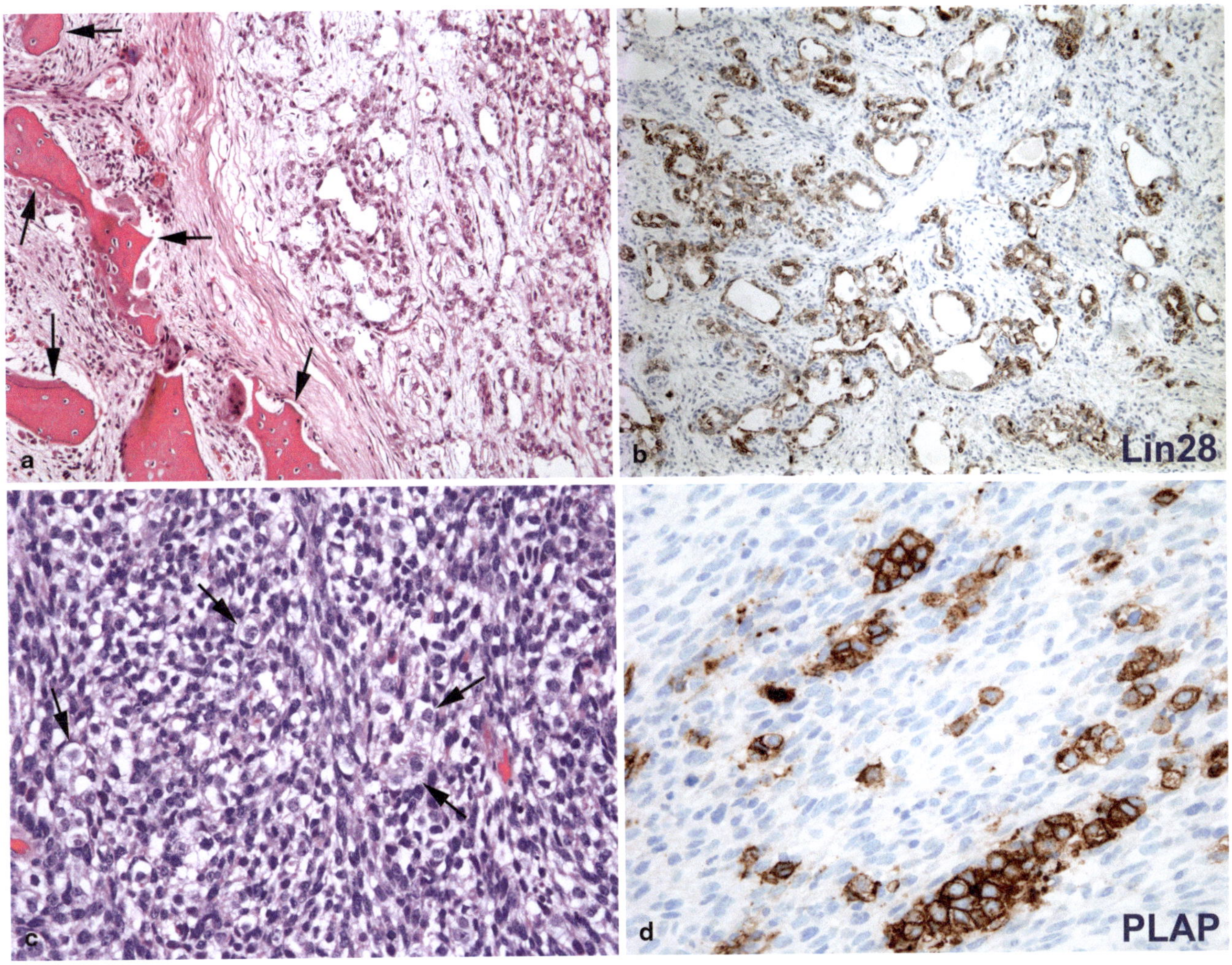

Fig. 20.5 **a** Endodermal sinus tumor (yolk sac tumor) arising within the maxillary bone (*arrows*). The tumor (*right*) is composed of irregular anastomosing glands in a loose myxoid stroma. **b** Tumor cells show diffuse and strong immunoreactivity for Lin28, a highly sensitive and useful marker for the diagnosis of these tumors. **c** Sarcomatous component of a germ cell tumor primary of the central nervous system. The tumor is predominantly composed of poorly differentiated spindled cells. Scattered large round dysgerminoma cells with clear cytoplasm are indicated by *arrows*. **d** The cytoplasm of dysgerminoma cells is strongly immunoreactive for placental alkaline phosphatase

degree of obstruction prohibits orotracheal intubation then tracheostomy is performed (Fig. 20.6). Rarely, the mass will be large and compressive enough to prevent adequate access even for tracheostomy. In this setting, an attempt at a partial resection of the mass adequate to allow for tracheostomy is appropriate [70]. Uteroplacental gas exchange can be maintained for approximately 60 min during an EXIT procedure, so complete resection of the tumor should not be attempted until the postpartum period, and access for airway stabilization should remain the focus during an EXIT procedure [71]. The trachea can be difficult to localize in these patients, due to their small size, distortion of landmarks by the mass, and the limited time frame allowed by the EXIT procedure. The use of intraoperative ultrasound has been described as a useful adjunct for identification of the trachea during an EXIT procedure for a large cervical teratoma and may be considered in such circumstances.

A successful EXIT procedure requires careful coordination and timing, and is often not feasible in the setting of an emergent premature delivery. In such a setting, the pediatric otolaryngologist must be prepared to do an immediate direct laryngoscopy and bronchoscopy with intubation at the time of delivery. Emergent tracheostomy is rarely successful in this situation, and a newborn infant with a teratoma completely obstructing the upper airway is unlikely to survive when orotracheal intubation is not possible. Realistic expectations reflecting this possibility must be clearly outlined to the parents prior to delivery.

Teratomas are frequently highly vascularized tumors and can often result in hemodynamic instability [70, 72]. They can also often rapidly enlarge due to cystic components resulting in airway obstruction, even when none was present initially [25]. For these reasons, early resection is recommended, even in the absence of upper airway obstruction

Table 20.1 Outcome for pediatric patients with extracranial malignant GCT of the head and neck

Age	Sex	Location	Surgery	RT	Chemotherapy	Outcome	Ref.
NB	F	OP	PR	Yes	Actinomycin D, 5FU, thio-TEPA	DOD 15 m	[28]
NB	ND	Hypopharynx, neck	Resection	No	VAC × 3 cycles	NED 5 y	[2]
NB	ND	Hypopharynx, neck	Resection	No	VAC × 3 cycles	NED 5 y	[2]
NB	M	Anterior neck	Resection	No	None	NED 13 y	[26]
6 w	F	Forehead	PR	52 Gy	Actinomycin D, PVB, CTX	DOD 4.5 m	[26]
3 m	ND	Orbit	Biopsy	No	Chemo NOS	ND	[42]
4 m	F	Mandible	Resection	No	PEB × 4 cycles, TIP × 4 cycles	NED 5 y	[32]
4.5 m	F	Face	Resection	No	None	NED 10.5 m	[26]
6 m	F	Floor of mouth	PR	Yes	None	DOD, 7 m	[28]
6 m	F	Orbit, maxilla, PS	PR	No	None	DOD 5 m	[39]
6 m	M	Orbit, nasal cavity, PS	Biopsy	No	PEB × 4 cycles	NED 6 m	[44]
7 m	F	OP	PR	No	None	DOD 17 d	[27]
8 m	F	Ear	Resection	No	PEB	NED 13 m	[61]
9 m	F	Masticator space	None	No	PEB × 4 cycles	ND	[30]
10 m	F	PS	Biopsy	No	None	DOD 1 m	[31]
10 m	F	Nasopharynx	Biopsy	Yes	Chemo NOS	DOD 9 m	[28]
12 m	F	Neck	Biopsy	No	PVB	DOI	[39]
12 m	M	Orbit	PR	No	PEB × 3 cycles	NED 4 m	[45]
13 m	F	Orbit	Exenteration	No	VAC	DOD 10 m	[42]
13 m	F	Orbit	None	Yes	None	NED 8 m	[42]
13 m	ND	Hypopharynx, neck	Resection	No	PVB/EI	NED 5 y	[2]
15 m	M	Orbit, nasopharynx	None	60 Gy	C5V × 12 cycles, VCR, CTX, 5FU	NED 8.5 y	[41]
18 m	ND	Hypopharynx, neck	Resection	No	PVB/EI	NED 5 y	[2]
18 m	F	Ear	Biopsy	No	VAC/PVB	NED 15 m	[36]
18 m	F	External auditory canal	Biopsy	No	PEB × 10 cycles	NED 36 m	[62]
18 m	M	Palate, alveolus, OP	Biopsy	No	VAC	ND	[39]
18 m	M	Orbit	Exenteration	No	C5V	NED 8 y	[42]
19 m	F	Submandibular region	Biopsy	Yes	Chemo NOS	DOD 5 m	[38]
20 m	F	Temporal area	PR	No	PEB × 6 cycles	NED 5 m	[63]
23 m	F	Temporomandibular	PR	No	Chemo NOS	NED 40 m	[64]
24 m	F	Parotid space	Resection	Yes	Chemo NOS	DOD 18 m	[33]
24 m	M	Nasal cavity	Resection	Yes	Chemo NOS	NED 4y	[65]
26 m	F	Ear	Resection	No	None	DOD 3 m	[66]
30 m	F	Postauricular region	None	Yes	Chemo NOS	NED 3 y	[26]
30 m	F	Orbit	PR	No	PEB × 6 cycles	NED 9 y	[67]
33 m	ND	Hypopharynx, neck	Resection	No	PVB/EI	DOD 9 y	[2]
3 y	F	Nasopharynx, PS	None	Yes	Chemo NOS	DOD 18 m	[68]
3 y	F	Nasal cavity	PR	50.5 Gy	VAC × 2 years	NED 14 y	[69]
3 y	F	Orbit, PS	PR	30 Gy brachy	PEI × 3 cycles, VCR, dactinomycin	DOD 3 m	[40]
4 y	F	Orbit	PR	No	VCR, Doxorubicin, PEB, VAC	NED 10 y	[42]
4 y	M	Cheek region	PR	Yes	Chemo NOS	NED 5.5 y	[29]
6 y	F	Perimandibular region	PR	Yes	Chemo NOS	DOD 18 m	[29]
6 y	F	Floor of mouth	PR	No	None	DOD 2 m	[37]
9 y	M	Nasopharynx	Resection	No	PEB	NED 6 m	[57]
12 y	ND	Hypopharynx, neck	Biopsy	No	PVB, EI	NED 5 y	[2]

5FU 5-fluoro-uracil, *C5V* cis-platinum/5-FU/vincristine, *chemo NOS* chemotherapy not otherwise specified, *CTX* cyclophosphamide, *d* days, *DOD* dead of disease, *DOI* dead of infection, *EI* etoposide/ifosfamide, *F* female, *Gy* gray, *m* months, *M* male, *NB* newborn, *ND* not determined, *NED* no evidence of disease, *OP* oropharynx, *PEB* cisplatin/etoposide/bleomycin, *PEI* cisplatin/etoposide/ifosfamide, *PR* partial resection, *PS* paranasal sinuses, *PVB* cisplatin/vinblastine/bleomycin, *RT* radiation therapy, *TIP* paclitaxel/ifosfamide/cis-platinum, *VAC* vincristine/actinomycin/cyclophosphamide, *VACA* vincristine/actinomycin/cyclophosphamide/adriamycin, *VCR* vincristine, *y* years

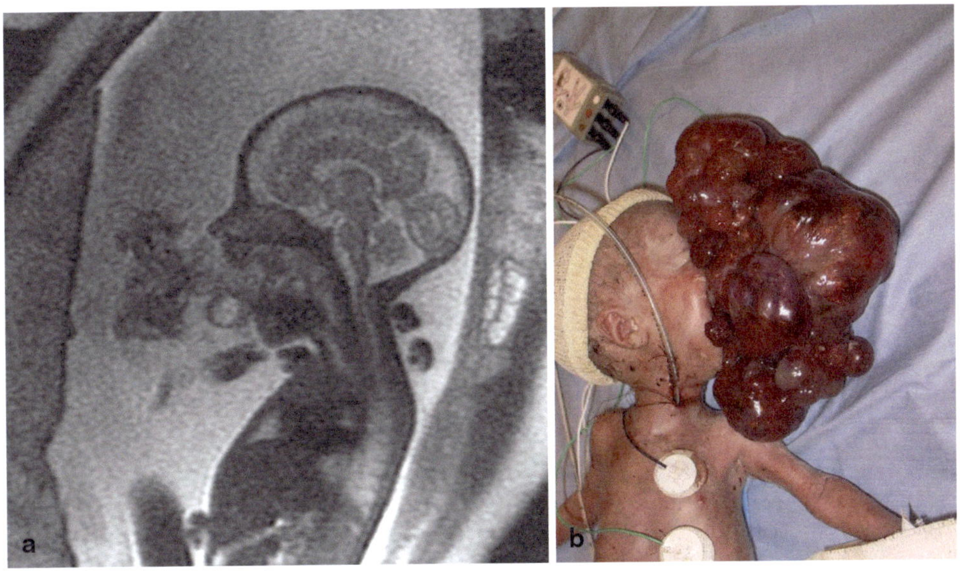

Fig. 20.6 **a** MRI of patient from Fig. 20.1 demonstrating a large, heterogeneous mass filling the oropharynx and oral cavity and emanating out from the oral cavity into the amniotic fluid. **b** The same patient now pictured immediately following successful EXIT procedure with tracheostomy tube in place and large oral teratoma. The patient underwent a series of three staged resections to remove the tumor

at the time of presentation. The surgical approach varies depending on the location of the tumor. Cervical teratomas involving the anterior neck frequently require an ipsilateral thyroid lobectomy due to their intimate relationship with or even partial replacement of the thyroid gland [10, 12, 72].

Adjuvant Treatment

Success with external beam radiotherapy has not been established in children with malignant teratoma of the head and neck, and results in the adult population have been inconsistent [73].

Outcome

The postoperative morbidity associated with teratoma of the head and neck varies by the site of tumor origin. There is a significant potential for morbidity and mortality associated with long-term tracheostomy in the pediatric population due to complications, such as mucus-plugging, granulation tissue formation, fistulization with the esophagus or innominate artery, and accidental decannulation, among others [74, 75]; thus, planned decannulation should be pursued as early as possible following complete tumor excision. Resection of cervical teratoma frequently requires thyroid lobectomy, often resulting in postoperative hypothyroidism and hypoparathyroidism, thus requiring careful monitoring and supplementation of thyroid hormone and calcium levels where appropriate. Large oral teratomas frequently prevent fusion of the palatal shelves *in utero* resulting in cleft palate and its associated morbidities, including Eustachian tube dysfunction, feeding difficulties, and speech impairment. Palatoplasty, either at the time of tumor resection or in a delayed fashion, is required in these cases.

Reported recurrences of benign teratoma of the head and neck following complete surgical resection are rare, and the long-term prognosis is excellent. Recurrence in the neonatal period associated with malignant transformation has been reported, however, and postoperative surveillance is recommended [49].

Teratomas of the head and neck presenting in the perinatal period are associated with a high mortality risk due to airway obstruction and hemodynamic compromise, particularly when not diagnosed prenatally or when an EXIT procedure is not feasible. Historically, a perinatal mortality rate of approximately 50 % has been reported [25, 76]. An updated mortality rate with the increasing use of prenatal imaging techniques and the EXIT procedure has not yet been established, though it is likely much lower.

Bernbeck et al., in their recently reported series of pediatric head and neck GCT, had an overall survival of 95 ± 5 % with an event-free survival of 81 ± 7 % [2]. The survival rate for head and neck malignant GCT based on recent case reports and small series, with surgical resection and cis-platinum-based chemotherapy, is approximately 75–80 %.

Key Points

- GCT of the head and neck presenting in the neonatal period are typically benign teratomas.
- Malignant GCT are rare in infancy, but the risk of a GCT being malignant increases with age, and most pediatric GCT of the head and neck presenting after 1 year of age will be malignant.
- The presentation of pediatric GCT varies depending on the location and the age at presentation, though many teratomas of the head and neck are now diagnosed prenatally.

- Most fetal head and neck masses can be detected on routine prenatal ultrasound, but fetal MRI is essential for determining the nature of the lesion and the need for an EXIT procedure.
- The primary treatment for pediatric GCT of the head and neck is surgical resection, though the addition of chemotherapy is recommended in cases of malignancy.
- An EXIT procedure is often necessary to allow for adequate stabilization of the airway at birth when a teratoma of the head and neck is large enough to result in airway obstruction.
- A multidisciplinary team approach is paramount to the successful management of pediatric GCT.

References

1. Rescorla FJ, Breitfeld PP. Pediatric germ cell tumors. Curr Probl Cancer. 1999;23:257–303.
2. Bernbeck B, Schneider DT, Koch S, et al. Germ cell tumors of the head and neck: report from the MAKEI Study Group. Pediatr Blood Cancer. 2009;52:223–6.
3. Pinkerton CR, Pritchard J, Spitz L. High complete response rate in children with advanced germ cell tumors using cisplatin-containing combination chemotherapy. J Clin Oncol. 1986;4:194–9.
4. Marina N, London WB, Frazier AL, et al. Prognostic factors in children with extragonadal malignant germ cell tumors: a pediatric intergroup study. J Clin Oncol. 2006;24:2544–8.
5. Forrester MB, Merz RD. Descriptive epidemiology of teratoma in infants, Hawaii, 1986–2001. Paediatr Perinat Epidemiol. 2006;20:54–8.
6. Heerema-McKenney A, Harrison MR, Bratton B, Farrell J, Zaloudek C. Congenital teratoma: a clinicopathologic study of 22 fetal and neonatal tumors. Am J Surg Pathol. 2005;29:29–38.
7. Tonni G, De Felice C, Centini G, Ginanneschi C. Cervical and oral teratoma in the fetus: a systematic review of etiology, pathology, diagnosis, treatment and prognosis. Arch Gynecol Obstet. 2010;282:355–61.
8. Batsakis JG, Littler ER, Oberman HA. Teratomas of the neck. A clinicopathologic appraisal. Arch Otolaryngol. 1964;79:619–24.
9. Kountakis SE, Minotti AM, Maillard A, Stiernberg CM. Teratomas of the head and neck. Am J Otolaryngol. 1994;15:292–6.
10. Riedlinger WF, Lack EE, Robson CD, Rahbar R, Nose V. Primary thyroid teratomas in children: a report of 11 cases with a proposal of criteria for their diagnosis. Am J Surg Pathol. 2005;29:700–6.
11. Bale GF. Teratoma of the neck in the region of the thyroid gland; a review of the literature and report of 4 cases. Am J Pathol. 1950;26:565–79.
12. Thompson LD, Rosai J, Heffess CS. Primary thyroid teratomas: a clinicopathologic study of 30 cases. Cancer. 2000;88:1149–58.
13. Yapar EG, Ekici E, Gokmen O. Sonographic diagnosis of epignathus (oral teratoma), prosencephaly, meromelia and oligohydramnios in a fetus with trisomy 13. Clin Dysmorphol. 1995;4:266–71.
14. Witters I, Moerman P, Louwagie D, Van Assche FA, Migeon BR, Fryns JP. Second trimester prenatal diagnosis of epignathus teratoma in ring X chromosome mosaicism with inactive ring X chromosome. Ann Genet. 2001;44:179–82.
15. Staboulidou I, Miller K, Gohring G, Hillemanns P, Wustemann M. Prenatal diagnosis of an epignathus associated with a 49,XXXXY karyotype—a case report. Fetal Diagn Ther. 2008;24:313–7.
16. Goldstein I, Drugan A. Congenital cervical teratoma, associated with agenesis of corpus callosum and a subarachnoid cyst. Prenat Diagn. 2005;25:439–41.
17. Kosmaidou-Aravidou Z, Siabalioti G, Karpathios S, Grigori P, Panani A. Prenatal diagnosis of a cervical teratoma with a cytogenetic study. J Matern Fetal Neonatal Med. 2006;19:377–9.
18. Roncaroli F, Scheithauer BW, Pires MM, Rodrigues AS, Pereira JR. Mature teratoma of the middle ear. Otol Neurotol. 2001;22:76–8.
19. Loveren H van, Youseff S, Morcos JJ. Malignant skull base teratoma. Skull Base. 2002;12:221–5.
20. Huth ME, Heimgartner S, Schnyder I, Caversaccio MD. Teratoma of the nasal septum in a neonate: an endoscopic approach. J Pediatr Surg. 2008;43:2102–5.
21. Ohta M, Imamura Y, Mori M, Maegawa H, Kojima A, Fujieda S. Benign cystic teratoma of the parotid gland: a case report. Acta Cytol. 2009;53:427–30.
22. Clement K, Chamberlain P, Boyd P, Molyneux A. Prenatal diagnosis of an epignathus: a case report and review of the literature. Ultrasound Obstet Gynecol. 2001;18:178–81.
23. Becker S, Schon R, Gutwald R, et al. A congenital teratoma with a cleft palate: report of a case. Br J Oral Maxillofac Surg. 2007;45:326–7.
24. Elmasalme F, Giacomantonio M, Clarke KD, Othman E, Matbouli S. Congenital cervical 2 in neonates. Case report and review. Eur J Pediatr Surg. 2000;10:252–7.
25. Jordan RB, Gauderer MW. Cervical teratomas: an analysis. Literature review and proposed classification. J Pediatr Surg. 1988;23:583–91.
26. Dehner LP, Mills A, Talerman A, Billman GF, Krous HF, Platz CE. Germ cell neoplasms of head and neck soft tissues: a pathologic spectrum of teratomatous and endodermal sinus tumors. Hum Pathol. 1990;21:309–18.
27. Kutluhan A, Ugras S, Akman E. Endodermal sinus (yolk sac) tumor of oral cavity originating from gingiva. Auris Nasus Larynx. 1998;25:459–62.
28. Lack EE. Extragonadal germ cell tumors of the head and neck region: review of 16 cases. Hum Pathol. 1985;16:56–64.
29. Shebib S, Sabbah RS, Sackey K, Akhtar M, Aur RJ. Endodermal sinus (yolk sac) tumor in 2 and children. A clinical and pathologic study: an 11 year review. Am J Pediatr Hematol Oncol. 1989;11:36–9.
30. Pasricha S, Gupta A, Shah M, Vadodaria H. Extragonadal yolk sac tumor of face in a female infant: a case report. Indian J Pathol Microbiol. 2010;53:592–3.
31. Weedon D, Musgrave J. Endodermal sinus tumour of the face. Pathology. 1974;6:365–9.
32. Steinbacher DM, Upton J, Rahbar R, Ferraro NF. Yolk sac tumor of the mandible. J Oral Maxillofac Surg. 2008;66:151–3.
33. Viva E, Zorzi F, Annibale G, Stefini S, Baronchelli C, Bonetti MF. Endodermal sinus (yolk sac) tumor of the parotid gland: a case report. Int J Pediatr Otorhinolaryngol. 1992;24:269–74.
34. Devaney KO, Ferlito A. Yolk sac tumors (endodermal sinus tumors) of the extracranial head and neck regions. Ann Otol Rhinol Laryngol. 1997;106:254–60.
35. Devaney KO, Ferlito A, Rinaldo A. Endodermal sinus tumor (yolk sac tumor) of the temporal bone: an exotic disease for otorhinolaryngologists and head and neck surgeons. Acta Otolaryngol. 2003;123:747–8.
36. Stanley RJ, Scheithauer BW, Thompson EI, Kispert DB, Weiland LH, Pearson BW. Endodermal sinus tumor (yolk sac tumor) of the ear. Arch Otolaryngol Head Neck Surg. 1987;113:200–3.
37. Jin X, Han C, Sun H. Primary yolk sac tumor in floor of mouth in a child. J Oral Maxillofac Surg. 2011;69:1973–7.
38. Fonseca I, Martins AG, Soares J. Submandibular endodermal sinus (yolk sac) tumor in a female infant. A case report. Int J Oral Maxillofac Surg. 1991;20:46–7.

39. Kusumakumari P, Geetha N, Chellam VG, Nair MK. Endodermal sinus tumors in the head and neck region. Med Pediatr Oncol. 1997;29:303–7.
40. Bresters D, Zwaan CM, Veerman AJ, Leemans CR, Westerveld GJ, Linden JC van der. A three-year-old girl with a yolk sac tumor in the orbit/maxillary sinus. Med Pediatr Oncol. 2003;40:70–1.
41. Katz NN, Ruymann FB, Margo CE, Popejoy LA, LaPiana FG. Endodermal sinus tumor (yolk-sac carcinoma) of the orbit. J Pediatr Ophthalmol Strabismus. 1982;19:270–4.
42. Margo CE, Folberg R, Zimmerman LE, Sesterhenn IA. Endodermal sinus tumor (yolk sac tumor) of the orbit. Ophthalmology. 1983;90:1426–32.
43. Appignani BA, Jones KM, Barnes PD. Primary endodermal sinus tumor of the orbit: MR findings. AJR Am J Roentgenol. 1992;159:399–401.
44. Yih JP, Sullivan P, Taylor D. Alpha fetoprotein as marker for a case of orbital yolk sac tumour. Br J Ophthalmol. 1995;79:787–8.
45. Mogaddam AS, Memar B, Aledavood A, Eslampoor A. Isolated orbital endodermal sinus tumor. Ophthal Plast Reconstr Surg. 2007;23:477–9.
46. Dragan LR, Aghaian E, Vora R, Kim GE, Seiff SR. Orbital, middle cranial fossa, and pterygopalatine fossa yolk sac tumor in an infant. Ophthal Plast Reconstr Surg. 2004;20:469–71.
47. Araujo Junior E, Guimaraes Filho HA, Saito M, et al. Prenatal diagnosis of a large fetal cervical teratoma by three-dimensional ultrasonography: a case report. Arch Gynecol Obstet. 2007;275:141–4.
48. Rahbar R, Vogel A, Myers LB, et al. Fetal surgery in otolaryngology: a new era in the diagnosis and management of fetal airway obstruction because of advances in prenatal imaging. Arch Otolaryngol Head Neck Surg. 2005;131:393–8.
49. Muscatello L, Giudice M, Feltri M. Malignant cervical teratoma: report of a case in a newborn. Eur Arch Otorhinolaryngol. 2005;262:899–904.
50. Kathary N, Bulas DI, Newman KD, Schonberg RL. MRI imaging of fetal neck masses with airway compromise: utility in delivery planning. Pediatr Radiol. 2001;31:727–31.
51. Shellock F. Policies, guidelines, and recommendations for MR imaging safety and patient management. J Magn Reson Imaging. 1991;1:97–101.
52. Morof D, Levine D, Grable I, et al. Oropharyngeal teratoma: prenatal diagnosis and assessment using sonography, MRI, and CT with management by ex utero intrapartum treatment procedure. AJR Am J Roentgenol. 2004;183:493–6.
53. Franzius C. FDG-PET/CT in pediatric solid tumors. Q J Nucl Med Mol Imaging. 2010;54:401–10.
54. Kerner B, Flaum E, Mathews H, et al. Cervical teratoma: prenatal diagnosis and long-term follow-up. Prenat Diagn. 1998;18:51–9.
55. Echten J van, Timmer A, Veen AY van der, Molenaar WM, Jong B de. Infantile and adult testicular germ cell tumors. a different pathogenesis? Cancer Genet Cytogenet. 2002;135:57–62.
56. Ueno S, Hirakawa H, Matsuda H, et al. A case of neonatal mature teratoma transformed to malignancy in the neck extending to the mouth floor. Tokai J Exp Clin Med. 2009;34:130–4.
57. Davidoff AM, Hebra A, Bunin N, Shochat SJ, Schnaufer L. Endodermal sinus tumor in children. J Pediatr Surg. 1996;31:1075–8 (discussion 1078–9).
58. Marina N, Fontanesi J, Kun L, et al. Treatment of childhood germ cell tumors. Review of the St. Jude experience from 1979 to 1988. Cancer. 1992;70:2568–75.
59. Cushing B, Giller R, Cullen JW, et al. Randomized comparison of combination chemotherapy with etoposide, bleomycin, and either high-dose or standard-dose cisplatin in children and adolescents with high-risk malignant germ cell tumors: a pediatric intergroup study—Pediatric Oncology Group 9049 and Children's Cancer Group 8882. J Clin Oncol. 2004;22:2691–700.
60. Kondagunta GV, Bacik J, Donadio A, et al. Combination of paclitaxel, ifosfamide, and cisplatin is an effective second-line therapy for patients with relapsed testicular germ cell tumors. J Clin Oncol. 2005;23:6549–55.
61. Fukunaga M, Miyazawa Y, Harada T, Ushigome S, Ishikawa E. Yolk sac tumor of the ear. Histopathology. 1995;27(6):563–7.
62. Frank TC, Anand VK, Subramony C. Yolk sac tumor of the temporal bone: report of a case. Ear Nose Throat J. 2000;79:183, 187–8, 191–2 passim.
63. Kebudi R, Ayan I, Darendeliler E, et al. Non-midline endodermal sinus tumor in the head and neck region: a case report. Med Pediatr Oncol. 1993;21:685–9.
64. Stephenson JA, Mayland DM, Kun LE, Etcubanas E, Thompson EI, Gross CW. Malignant germ cell tumors of the head and neck in childhood. Laryngoscope. 1989;99:732–5.
65. Sungur A, Ozbay G, Dogan A, Ozyilmaz F, Ataman M. An endodermal sinus tumor of the head and neck region. Int J Pediatr Otorhinolaryngol. 1993;26:177–80.
66. Choufani G, Saussez S, Detemmerman D, et al. Yolk sac tumor of the ear in a child. Am J Otol. 1998;19:298–300.
67. Kiratli H, Erkan Balci K, Guler G. Primary orbital endodermal sinus tumor (yolk sac tumor). J AAPOS. 2008;12:623–5.
68. Byard RW, Smith CR, Chan HS. Endodermal sinus tumor of the nasopharynx and previous mature congenital teratoma. Pediatr Pathol. 1991;11:297–302.
69. Gabris K, Orosz M, Suba Z. The effects on teeth of radiotherapy for nasal endodermal sinus tumor (yolk sac tumor) in childhood. Int J Oral Maxillofac Surg. 2001;30:356–8.
70. Hirose S, Sydorak RM, Tsao K, et al. Spectrum of intrapartum management strategies for giant fetal cervical teratoma. J Pediatr Surg. 2003;38:446–50 (discussion 446–50).
71. Myers LB, Bulich LA, Mizrahi A, et al. Ultrasonographic guidance for location of the trachea during the EXIT procedure for cervical teratoma. J Pediatr Surg. 2003;38:E12.
72. De Backer A, Madern GC, Ven CP van de, Tibboel D, Hazebroek FW. Strategy for management of newborns with cervical teratoma. J Perinat Med. 2004;32:500–8.
73. Djalilian HR, Linzie B, Maisel RH. Malignant teratoma of the thyroid: review of literature and report of a case. Am J Otolaryngol. 2000;21:112–5.
74. Das P, Zhu H, Shah RK, Roberson DW, Berry J, Skinner ML. Tracheotomy-related catastrophic events: results of a national survey. Laryngoscope. 2012;122:30–7.
75. Shah RK, Lander L, Berry JG, Nussenbaum B, Merati A, Roberson DW. Tracheotomy outcomes and complications: a national perspective. Laryngoscope. 2012;122:25–9.
76. Trecet JC, Claramunt V, Larraz J, Ruiz E, Zuzuarregui M, Ugalde FJ. Prenatal ultrasound diagnosis of fetal teratoma of the neck. J Clin Ultrasound. 1984;12:509–11.

Giant Cell Tumor

21

Bonnie L. Padwa

Introduction

Giant cell lesions (GCLs) are benign primary bone tumors of mesenchymal origin. They consist of a stroma with fibroblast-like spindle cells, multinucleated giant cells, and a dense vascular network composed of endothelial cell-lined capillaries. Although the neoplastic cell of origin has not been identified, it is probably not the giant cell, because these cells are present in a variety of bone tumors, particularly in children [1]. GCLs are classified as nonaggressive or aggressive based on clinical and radiographic criteria [1–6]. Nonaggressive lesions can be treated successfully by simple curettage, with a low-recurrence rate, while aggressive lesions have recurrence rates as high as 70 % after enucleation or curettage [1, 3–11]. Regardless of clinical behavior, both aggressive and nonaggressive GCLs have a similar histological appearance [1, 3–8, 12]. Furthermore, there are no currently available biological markers to predict clinical behavior, and standard histological techniques do not help the clinician determine prognosis [1, 3–6, 8, 12].

Biology and Epidemiology

Age Distribution

- The peak incidence of GCL is between 10 and 20 years of age.

Sex Predilection

- The female to male ratio is 2:1.

B. L. Padwa (✉)
Department of Plastic and Oral Surgery, Boston Children's Hospital, Harvard Medical School, 300 Longwood Avenue, Boston, MA 02115, USA
e-mail: bonnie.padwa@childrens.harvard.edu

Site Distribution

- The lesions occur more often in the mandible than in the maxilla.
- More often in the anterior mandible, with the canine-premolar area being the most common site.

Risk Factors—Environmental, Life Style

- None

Relationships to Other Disease States, Syndromes

- GCLs are usually unifocal. Multifocal lesions should alert the clinician to the possibility of hyperparathyroidism or, if bilateral, cherubism or Noonan syndrome [2, 3]. GCLs are osteoclast-rich tumors that are histopathologically indistinguishable from those seen in cherubism and Noonan syndrome. Nevertheless, patients with isolated GCLs do not have the cherubism-related germline SH3BP2 mutation, and the lesions do not contain somatic SH3BP2 mutations [4]. This suggests that even though all GCLs may appear the same histologically they likely have a different etiopathogenesis.
- Brown tumor of hyperparathyroidism occurs in children in association with chronic renal failure and secondary hyperparathyroidism. Primary hyperthyroidism is rare in children.

Presentation

There is variability in the clinical behavior of GCLs. Rapidly growing expansile lesions with an aggressive appearance (e.g., pain, paresthesia, root resorption) are at one end of the spectrum and small asymptomatic slow growing

R. Rahbar et al. (eds.), *Pediatric Head and Neck Tumors*,
DOI 10.1007/978-1-4614-8755-5_21, © Springer Science+Business Media New York 2014

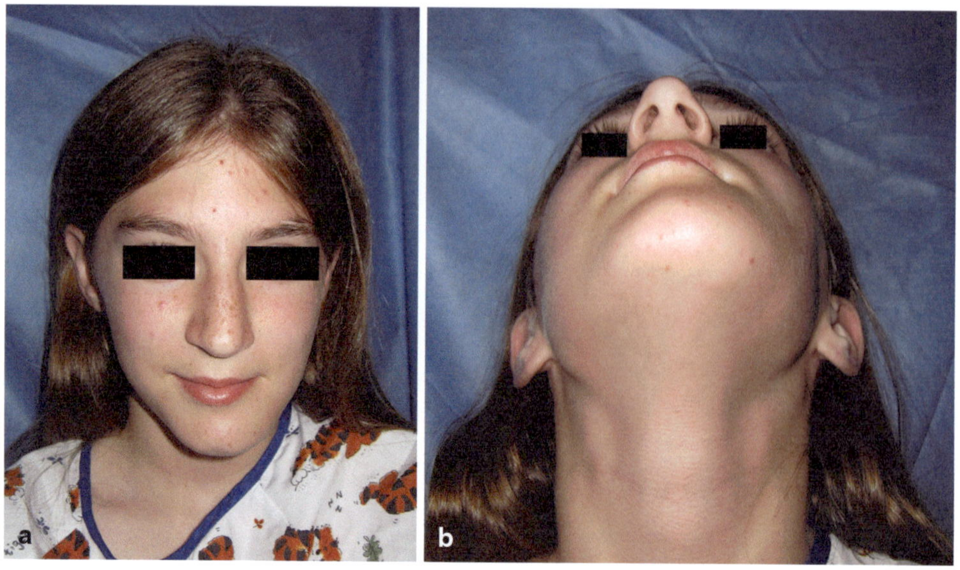

Fig. 21.1 Frontal (**a**) and submental (**b**) photograph of 12-year-old girl with left mandibular swelling

lesions at the other end. Chuong et al. categorized the clinical and radiographic features of aggressive GCLs: (1) size greater than 5 cm, (2) rapid growth, (3) recurrence after curettage, (4) cortical bone thinning and/or perforation, and (5) tooth displacement and/or resorption [13]. Tumors greater than or equal to 5 cm in size and/or recurring after curettage or resection were considered aggressive tumors based on these characteristics. Tumors with at least 3 of the other criteria were also classified as aggressive [1]. A GCL is designated as nonaggressive if it is asymptomatic and incidentally discovered and/or if it does not meet aggressive criteria [1].

- Patients with nonaggressive lesions are usually asymptomatic and the lesions are discovered as an incidental finding on routine diagnostic radiographs. Patients can have local swelling usually without pain or paresthesia.
- Aggressive lesions usually occur in younger patients, cause pain and grow rapidly.

Differential Diagnosis

The differential diagnosis should include radiolucent lesions of the jaw.

- Brown tumor of hyperparathyroidism
- Keratinizing odontogenic tumor
- Ameloblastoma
- Myxoma
- Fibro-osseous lesions
- Aneurysmal bone cyst
- Simple bone cyst

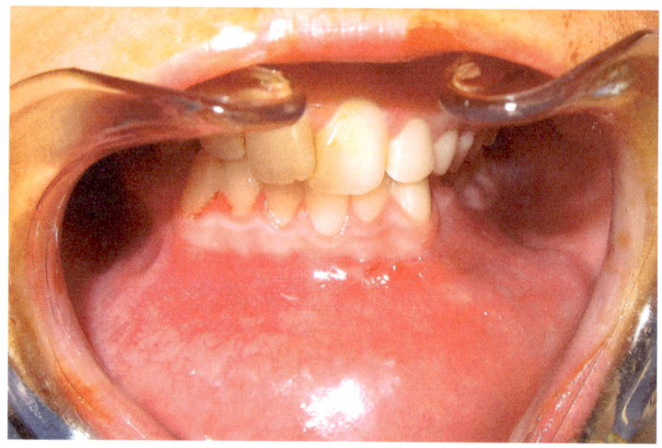

Fig. 21.2 Intraoral photograph demonstrates fullness in left buccal vestibule

Diagnosis and Evaluation

Physical Examination

- Facial swelling with asymmetry (Fig. 21.1a, b)
- Fullness in vestibule (Fig. 21.2)
- Loose teeth

Laboratory Data

- Blood studies to rule our hyperparathyroidism include parathyroid hormone, serum calcium, and phosphorous

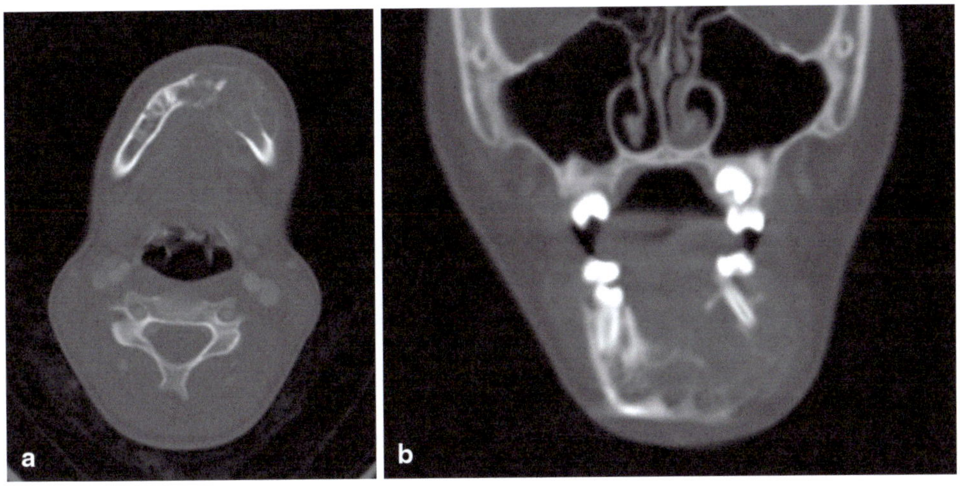

Fig. 21.3 Axial (**a**), coronal (**b**), sagittal (**c**) computed tomography (CT) images show cortical thinning and/or perforation, periosteal reaction, and root displacement consistent with aggressive GCL

Imaging Evaluation

- Panoramic radiograph: radiolucent lesion with cortical bone thinning, periosteal reaction, tooth displacement, and root resorption
- CT scan: cortical thinning and/or perforation, periosteal reaction, tooth displacement, and root resorption (Fig. 21.3a, b, c)

Pathology

The histopathologic features of GCLs are a large number of multinucleated giant cells and mononuclear cells within a fibrous stroma. (Fig. 21.4a, b) The giant cells in GCLs may be reactive or secondary, not the cell of origin. Macrophages, mesenchymal cells, and fibroblasts have also been proposed as being responsible for the lesion [14]. The lesions of brown tumor, nonaggressive and aggressive GCLs appear indistinguishable by standard histologic techniques.

Because the cell of origin is unknown and histologically aggressive and nonaggressive GCLs appear the same through the microscope (Fig. 21.5a, b), many groups have looked at biomarkers as a means of identifying aggressive/nonaggressive lesions and correlating these with clinical behavior and treatment outcome. A wide variety of parameters, including the number and size of giant cells, mean number of nuclei per giant cell, fractional surface area occupied by giant cells, DNA content, mitotic activity, and immunohistological features, have been studied in an attempt to distinguish aggressive and nonaggressive subtypes and to predict prognosis and response to treatment [13, 15–18]. Aggressive/recurring lesions have been found to have a higher number and relative size index of giant cells and a greater fractional surface area occupied by giant cells [13, 16]. Additionally, aggressive subtypes have been shown to express a greater count of nucleolar organization regions [18].

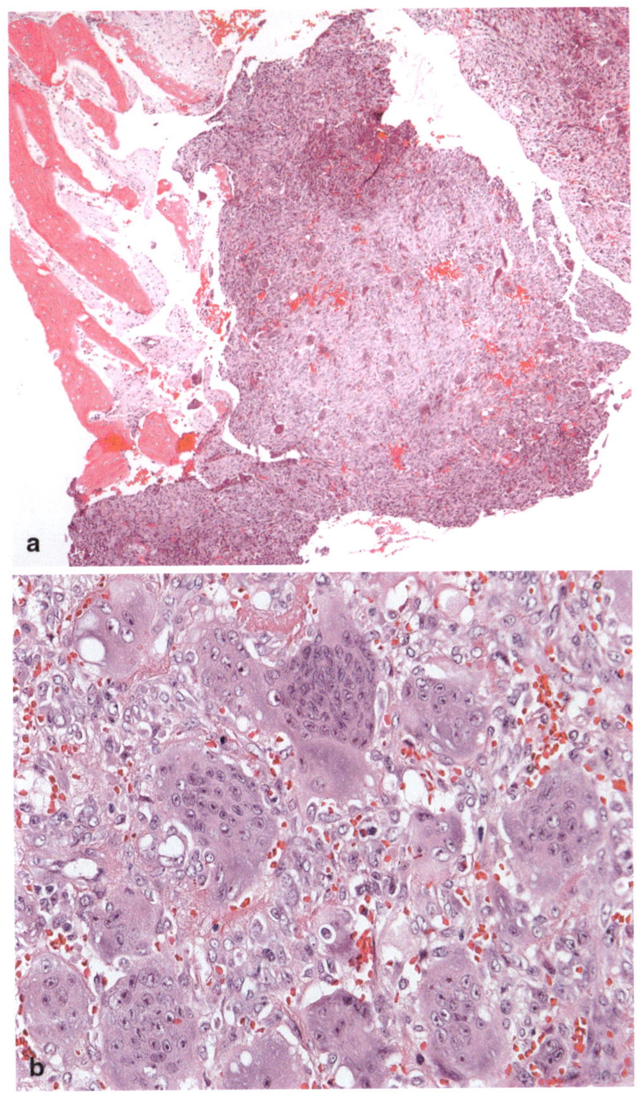

Fig. 21.4 Central giant cell reparative granuloma. **a** Intraosseous lesion composed of unevenly distributed osteoclast-like multinucleated giant cells in vascular stroma; bone trabecules are shown on the *upper* and *mid left* of the photograph. **b** Between giant cells there are plump mononuclear cells, extravasated erythrocytes, and occasional lymphocytes

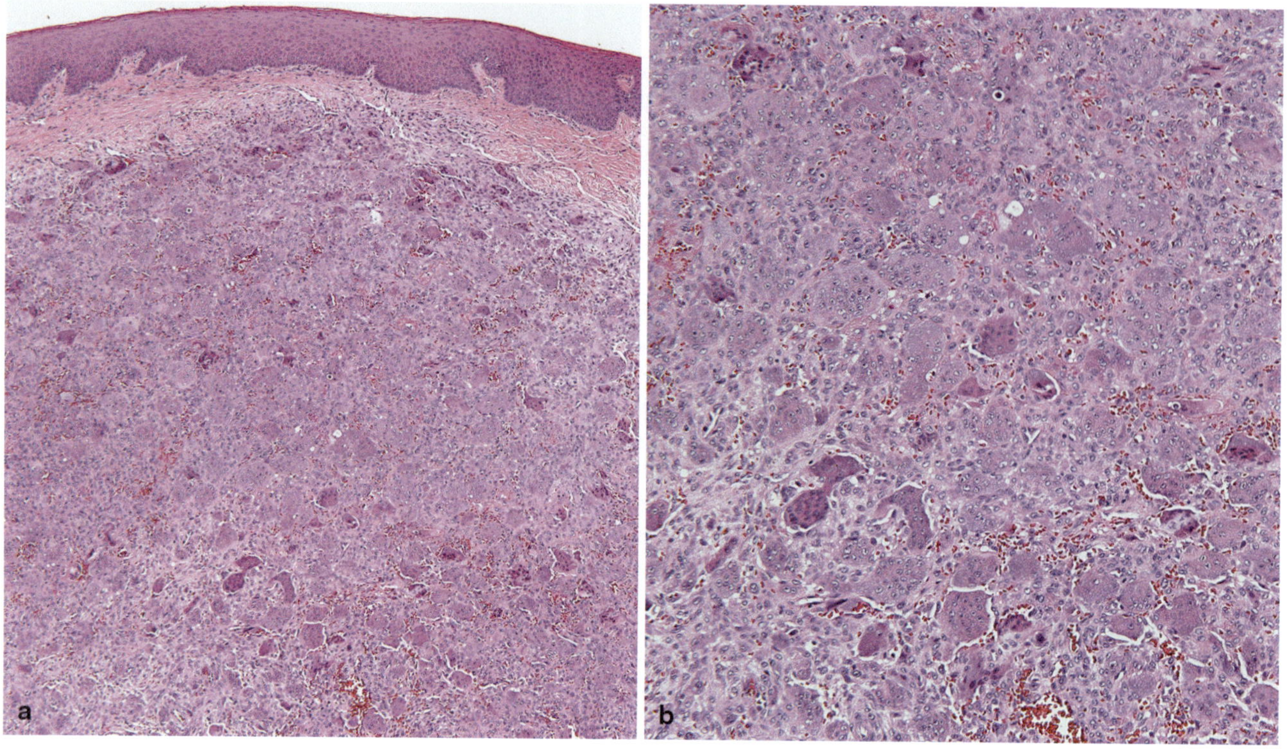

Fig. 21.5 Peripheral giant cell reparative granuloma (giant cell epulis). **a** Nonencapsulated mass primarily composed of numerous osteoclast-like multinucleated giant cells; overlying the lesion there is nonkeratinizing squamous mucosa and a spared zone of submucosa. **b** Multinucleated giant cells in a vascular stroma with plump mononuclear cells and interspersed lymphocytes

Recent advances in diagnostic techniques for GCLs may further help identify the aggressive nature of a particular lesion. Susarla and colleagues described a cell–cell adhesion factor CD34 which can be used to identify aggressive lesions; a CD34 staining density equal to or greater than 2.5 % is 100 times more likely to be associated with an aggressive GCL than a nonaggressive lesion [5].

Treatment

Medical

- Medical therapy is not indicated for treatment of GCLs.

Surgical

- Nonaggressive GCLs of the jaws predictably respond to enucleation/curettage with a low-recurrence rate [1, 10]. The use of adjuvant or alternative therapies such as intralesional steroids [19, 20], systemic [21, 22], or nasal [22, 23] calcitonin is unnecessary as patients with nonaggressive lesions can be predictably cured with curettage/enucleation. However, aggressive lesions treated in this manner have a recurrence rate of 70 % [1].
- The gold standard for treatment of aggressive GCLs is en bloc resection [7]. Given that these lesions frequently occur in children and resection of vital structures for treatment of a benign lesion can result in functional, esthetic, and psychological problems, alternatives to resection have been tried [8]. These include intralesional steroids, systemic calcitonin, and systemic interferon alpha-2a in combination with curettage [9–11]. The giant cells of GCL stained for both glucocorticoid and calcitonin receptors [8]. Intralesional corticosteroids have been tried because these multinucleated giant cells are osteoclasts and dexamethasone has been shown to inhibit osteoclast-like cells in marrow cultures. Giant cells in GCL have also been shown to have calcitonin receptors [24]. Calcitonin inhibits osteoclast/giant cell function and has also been suggested as a treatment modality. Kaban and colleagues proposed that GCL are proliferative vascular lesions that are in part angiogenesis dependent, and they theorized that aggressive GCL would respond to antiangiongenic therapy [1]. Interferon inhibits osteoclastic bone resorption and stimulates osteoblasts and preosteoblasts in cell culture [1, 25, 26].

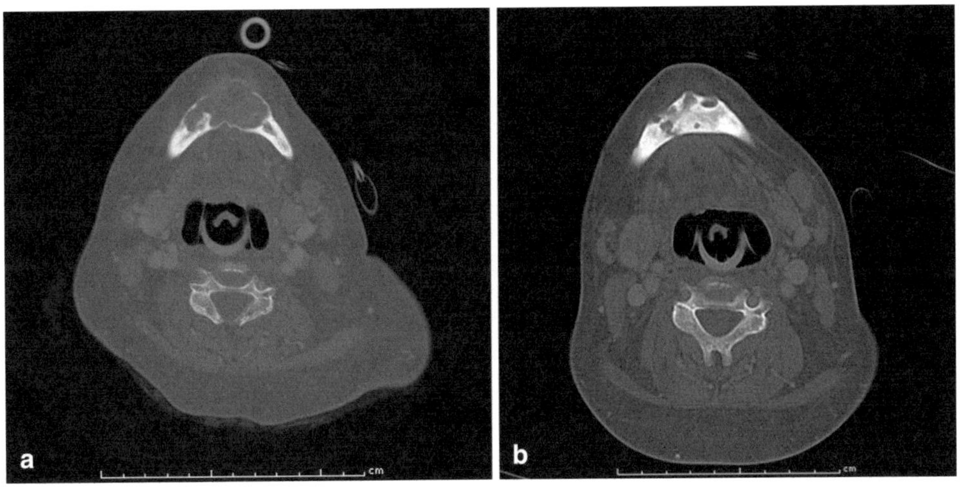

Fig. 21.6 Axial CT of aggressive GCL at time of diagnosis (**a**) and 1 year after enucleation, maintaining vital structures (teeth and nerve) and adjuvant therapy with interferon alpha-2a; there is bone fill and resolution of the lesion (**b**)

Adjuvant Treatment

- Intralesional steroids
- Systemic calcitonin
- Systemic interferon alpha-2a in combination with curettage

Outcome

The first description of GCL was by Jaffe in 1953 [27]. Yet confusion persists regarding the nature of the lesion (reactive/inflammatory, neoplastic), the cell of origin, and the variability in clinical behavior. Thus, an assortment of treatment modalities, with different mechanisms of action, have been tried in patients with a variety of lesions with inconsistent outcomes; all of which has made deciphering the best treatment option difficult for the practitioner.

Currently, the most promising treatment for aggressive GCL combines enucleation, maintaining vital structures (teeth and nerve), and adjuvant therapy with interferon alpha-2a (Fig. 21.6a, b) [10]. The combined treatment allows for successful control of tumor with decreased operative morbidity compared with en bloc resection. Kaban and colleagues reported that sixteen of 26 patients were cured of disease, 6 were in remission, and 4 were in active treatment [10].

References

1. Kaban LB, Troulis MJ, Wilkinson MS, Ebb D, Dodson TB. Adjuvant antiangiogenic therapy for giant cell tumors of the jaws. J Oral Maxillofac Surg. 2007 Oct;65(10):2018–24; discussion 2024.
2. Eisenbud L, Stern M, Rothberg M, Sachs SA. Central giant cell granuloma of the jaws: experiences in the management of thirty-seven cases. J Oral Maxillofac Surg. 1988 May;46(5):376–84.
3. Cohen MM Jr, Gorlin RJ. Noonan-like/multiple giant cell lesion syndrome. Am J Med Genet. 1991 Aug 1;40(2):159–66.
4. Idowu BD, Thomas G, Frow R, Diss TC, Flanagan AM. Mutations in SH3BP2, 2 cherubism gene, were not detected in central or peripheral giant cell tumours of the jaw. Br J Oral Maxillofac Surg. 2008 April;46(3):229–30.
5. Susarla SM, August M, Dewsnup N, Faquin WC, Kaban LB, Dodson TB. CD34 staining density predicts giant cell tumor clinical behavior. J Oral Maxillofac Surg. 2009 May;67(5):951–6.
6. Webb DJ, Brockbank J. Combined curettage and cryosurgical treatment for the aggressive "giant cell lesion" of the mandible. Int J Oral Maxillofac Surg. 1986 Dec;15(6):780–5.
7. Tosco P, Tanteri G, Iaquinta C, et al. Surgical treatment and reconstruction for central giant cell granuloma of the jaws: a review of 18 cases. J Craniomaxillofac Surg. 2009 Oct;37(7):380–7.
8. Vered M, Buchner A, Dayan D. Immunohistochemical expression of glucocorticoid and calcitonin receptors as a tool for selecting therapeutic approach in central giant cell granuloma of the jawbones. Int J Oral Maxillofac Surg. 2006 Aug;35(8):756–60.
9. de Lange J, Rosenberg AJ, van den Akker HP, Koole R, Wirds JJ, van den Berg H. Treatment of central giant cell granuloma of the jaw with calcitonin. Int J Oral Maxillofac Surg. 1999 Oct;28(5):372–6.
10. Kaban LB, Troulis MJ, Ebb D, August M, Hornicek FJ, Dodson TB. Antiangiogenic therapy with interferon alpha for giant cell lesions of the jaws. J Oral Maxillofac Surg. 2002 Oct;60(10):1103–11; discussion 1111–3.
11. Kermer C, Millesi W, Watzke IM. Local injection of corticosteroids for central giant cell granuloma. A case report. Int J Oral Maxillofac Surg. 1994 Dec;23(6 Pt 1):366–8.
12. Flanagan AM, Nui B, Tinkler SM, Horton MA, Williams DM, Chambers TJ. The multinucleate cells in giant cell granulomas of the jaw are osteoclasts. Cancer. 1988 Sep 15;62(6):1139–45.
13. Chuong R, Kaban LB, Kozakewich H, Perez-Atayde A. Central giant cell lesions of the jaws: a clinicopathologic study. J Oral Maxillofac Surg. 1986 Sep;44(9):708–13.
14. Liu B, Yu SF, Li TJ. Multinucleated giant cells in various forms of giant cell containing lesions of the jaws express features of osteoclasts. J Oral Pathol Med. 2003 July;32(6):367–75.
15. Eckardt A, Pogrel MA, Kaban LB, Chew K, Mayall BH. Central giant cell granulomas of the jaws. Nuclear DNA analysis using image cytometry. Int J Oral Maxillofac Surg. 1989 Feb;18(1):3–6.
16. Ficarra G, Kaban LB, Hansen LS. Central giant cell lesions of the mandible and maxilla: a clinicopathologic and cytometric study. Oral Surg Oral Med Oral Pathol. 1987 July;64(1):44–9.

17. O'Malley M, Pogrel MA, Stewart JC, Silva RG, Regezi JA. Central giant cell granulomas of the jaws: phenotype and proliferation-associated markers. J Oral Pathol Med. 1997 April;26(4):159–63.
18. Whitaker SB, Waldron CA. Central giant cell lesions of the jaws. A clinical, radiologic, and histopathologic study. Oral Surg Oral Med Oral Pathol. 1993 Feb;75(2):199–208.
19. Nogueira RL, Teixeira RC, Cavalcante RB, Ribeiro RA, Rabenhosrt SH. Intralesional injection of triamcinolone hexacetonide as an alternative treatment for central giant-cell granuloma in 21 cases. Int J Oral Maxillofac Surg. 2010 Dec;39(12):1204–10.
20. Terry BC, Jacoway JR. Management of central giant cell lesions: an alternative to surgical therapy. Oral Maxillofac Clin North Am. 1994;6:579.
21. de Lange J, van den Akker HP, Veldhuijzen van Zanten GO, Engelshove HA, van den Berg H, Klip H. Calcitonin therapy in central giant cell granuloma of the jaw: a randomized double-blind placebo-controlled study. Int J Oral Maxillofac Surg. 2006 Sep;35(9):791–5.
22. Pogrel MA. Calcitonin therapy for central giant cell granuloma. J Oral Maxillofac Surg. 2003 June;61(6):649–53; discussion 53–4.
23. Vered M, Shohat I, Buchner A, Dayan D, Taicher S. Calcitonin nasal spray for treatment of central giant cell granuloma: clinical, radiological, and histological findings and immunohistochemical expression of calcitonin and glucocorticoid receptors. Oral Surg Oral Med Oral Pathol Oral Radiol Endod. 2007 Aug;104(2):226–39.
24. Nicholson GC, Horton MA, Sexton PM, et al. Calcitonin receptors of human osteoclastoma. Horm Metab Res. 1987 Nov;19(11):585–9.
25. Abukawa H, Kaban LB, Williams WB, Terada S, Vacanti JP, Troulis MJ. Effect of interferon-alpha-2b on porcine mesenchymal stem cells. J Oral Maxillofac Surg. 2006 Aug;64(8):1214–20.
26. Takayanagi H, Kim S, Matsuo K, et al. RANKL maintains bone homeostasis through c-Fos-dependent induction of interferon-beta. Nature. 2002 April 18;416(6882):744–9.
27. Jaffe HL. Giant-cell reparative granuloma, traumatic bone cyst, and fibrous (fibro-oseous) dysplasia of the jawbones. Oral Surg Oral Med Oral Pathol. 1953 Jan;6(1):159–75.

Nasal Glioma

22

Frank W. Virgin and Reza Rahbar

Introduction

Nasal gliomas are rare congenital nasal masses that predominantly appear in the pediatric population. These lesions are part of a larger group of benign nasal and anterior skull base masses that include entities such as dermoids, encephaloceles, and hemangiomas.

These lesions typically present early in life with nasal obstruction, difficulty feeding, or cosmetic deformity. More importantly, these lesions can be foci of infection. Given the occurrence of intracranial communication, these lesions can put patients at high risk of developing intracranial complications.

Biology and Epidemiology

Congenital nasal masses are rare and are encountered in approximately 1 in every 20,000–40,000 live births [1]. These lesions are often noted at birth, but some are not noticed until later in childhood or adulthood. The differential diagnosis includes dermoid, hemangioma, glioma, and encphalocele. Nasal glioma was first described by Reid in 1852 [2]. Schmidt was the first to present a comprehensive description of this entity and coined the term glioma in 1900 [3].

Pathophysiology

- Embryology of the nasofrontal region.
  - Fonticulus frontalis: located between the paired nasal bones.
  - Prenasal space: located between nasal capsule and nasal bone.
- Second month of gestation a diverticulum of dura extends through the prenasal space and contacts superficial exoderm.
- The nasal processes of the frontal bone grow and surround the dural projection and form the foramen cecum [4].
- In normal development, the dural projection involutes.
- Nasal glioma results from a failure of involution of this dural projection.
- Encephaloceles are differentiated from glioma by presence of intracranial contents into the dural diverticulum.
- Gliomas form when the connection to brain parenchyma is obliterated leaving glial tissue trapped in this mass [5, 6].

Molecular/Genetic Pathology

Incidence and Prevalence

- Rare condition with only 250 cases reported in the English literature

Age Distribution

- Present in the pediatric patient population
- Average age of presentation in one series was 9 months [7]

Sex Predilection

- Male to female ratio of 3:2

R. Rahbar (✉)
Department of Otolaryngology, Boston Children's Hospital, Harvard Medical School, Boston, MA, USA
e-mail: reza.rahbar@childrens.harvard.edu

F. W. Virgin
Department of Otolaryngology Head and Neck Surgery, Monroe Carell Jr. Children's Hospital at Vanderbilt, Nashville, TN, USA

R. Rahbar et al. (eds.), *Pediatric Head and Neck Tumors*,
DOI 10.1007/978-1-4614-8755-5_22, © Springer Science+Business Media New York 2014

Geographic Distribution

- None

Risk Factors

- Rare condition with no known definite risk factors

Relationships to Other Disease States, Syndromes

- Close relationship to encephalcele
- No known relationship to syndromes

Presentation

Nasal gliomas typically present early in childhood as a nasal mass or pit that causes some degree of cosmetic deformity. However, smaller lesions may not present themselves until later in childhood or even adulthood. Recently, a case report described prenatal diagnosis of a nasal glioma with ultrasound followed by magnetic resonance imaging (MRI) [8]. Nasal gliomas may manifest as an extranasal (60%), an intranasal (10%), or a combined lesion (10%) [9, 10].

Differential Diagnosis

Nasal gliomas fall into the category of congenital midline nasal masses.

- Encephalocele
- Dermoid
- Hemangioma

Diagnosis and Evaluation

Physical Examination

- Extranasal gliomas.
  - Firm, noncompressible, smooth masses that may appear any where from the nasal tip to the nasal glabella.
- Widened nasal bridge.
- Intranasal gliomas.
  - Pale mass within the nasal cavity or protruding from the nostril (Fig. 22.1).
  - Nasal congestion.
- No pulsation or expansion of lesion with crying, coughing, or straining.

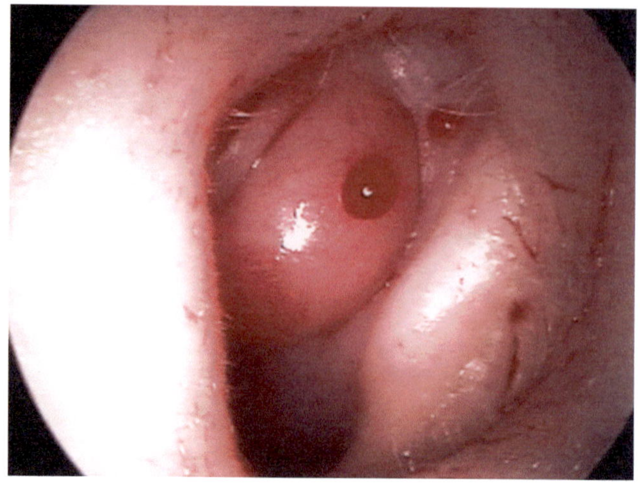

Fig. 22.1 Anterior rhinoscopy demonstrating a pale mass obstructing the nasal cavity

- Compression of the ipsilateral jugular vein does not result in expansion or pulsation of the mass (negative Furstenberg test).

Laboratory Data

Patients with nasal glioma typically do not have other underlying conditions. Routine lab workup including CBC, electrolytes, and coagulation studies are expected to be normal. However, presentation of these lesions is often in the setting of infection in which case there may be an elevated white blood cell count.

Imaging Evaluation

Imaging of these lesions is one of the most critical aspects of the workup. Approximately 10–20% of nasal gliomas may appear with a fibrous stalk extending toward the base of skull with an underlying bony defect [5]. Cross-sectional imaging through the area of interest provides information regarding the masses' size, location, and contents. Computerized tomography (CT) with contrast is the imaging study of choice to initially evaluate these lesions (Fig. 22.2). The images should be fine cuts and reformatted in the axial, coronal, and sagittal planes. CT provides some soft tissue detail, but is ideally suited to evaluate the bony anatomy and the presence of a defect in the anterior skull base (Fig. 22.3). However, in young infants, the anterior skull base is either not ossified or only partially ossified; additionally, CT only provides minimal information of soft tissue extent. Therefore, thin-section, high-resolution MRI is indicated in the workup of all of these patients. These images give additional information regarding the soft tissue

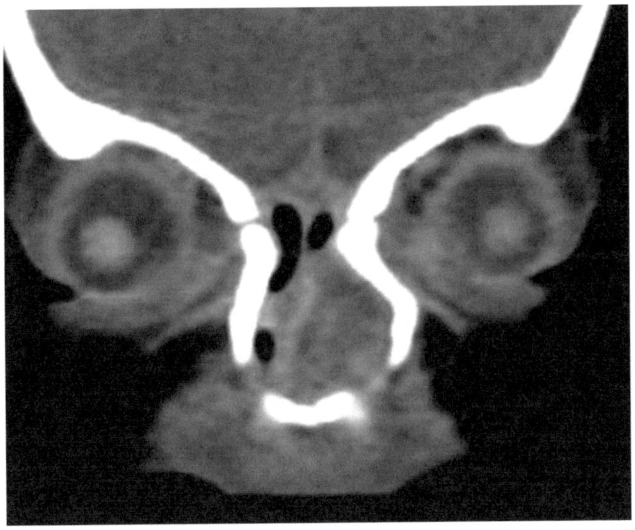

Fig. 22.2 Coronal CT scan demonstrating nasal glioma involving the left nasal cavity with extension toward the skull base

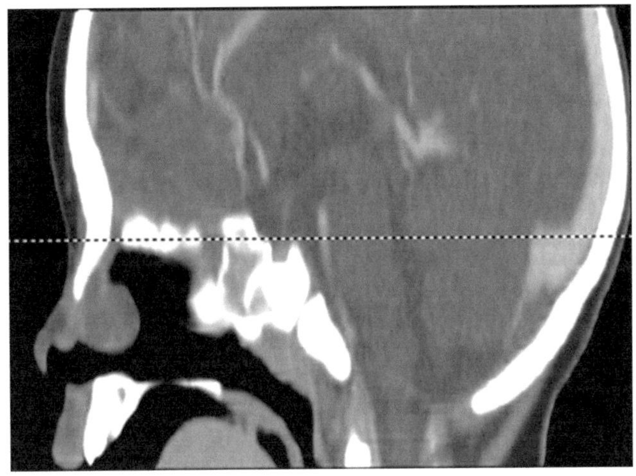

Fig. 22.3 Sagittal CT scan demonstrating nasal glioma with bony defect in the anterior cranial fossa. MRI would be needed to further characterize the soft tissue and intracranial extension

contents of the mass and the presence of intracranial extension.

Pathology

Gliomas and encephaloceles are very difficult to distinguish on pathology alone. On histopathological examination, glial tissue may be the exclusive or predominant component in both lesions. Occasionally ependymal tissue will be identified in encephaloceles and can make the diagnosis of encephalocele more likely [7] (Fig. 22.4). Separation of the two entities is dependent largely on clinicopathologic correlation.

Treatment

Treatment of nasal glioma can be complex and requires a multidisciplinary approach that includes otolaryngology, neurosurgery, plastic surgery, and neuroradiology. Full evaluation of the patient to exclude other congenital abnormalities is important. Characterization of the mass on physical exam, including nasal endoscopy, is essential in diagnosis and treatment planning. Imaging can provide additional details regarding size and extent of the mass. Biopsy of midline nasal masses should be avoided due to the risk of intracranial connection, bleeding, or cerebrospinal fluid leak. Surgical removal of the mass is the treatment of choice.

Medical

Occasionally midline nasal masses, including gliomas, can become infected. This is often the presenting symptom. Because of the potential for intracranial connection, treatment of the infection with antibiotics is of utmost importance. There is no medical treatment for resolution of nasal glioma.

Surgical

Surgical excision is the treatment of choice for nasal gliomas. The surgical approach used should be based on the location and size of the mass, associated cartilage or bone deformity, and the experience of the surgeon.

- Extranasal glioma
  - External rhinoplasty approach
  - Midline nasal incision
  - Lateral rhinotomy
  - Bi-coronal incision
  - Osteotomies may be required in the setting of intracranial extension
- Intranasal glioma
  - Transnasal endoscopic excision
  - Use of intraoperative image guidance
- Intracranial extension
  - Frontal craniotomy may be required to completely excise lesion
    - Prevent CSF rhinorrhea
    - Minimize intracranial infections complications

Complications

- Bleeding
- Infection
- Cosmetic deformity from surgical approach
- CSF rhinorrhea
- Intracranial infection: meningitis, abscess

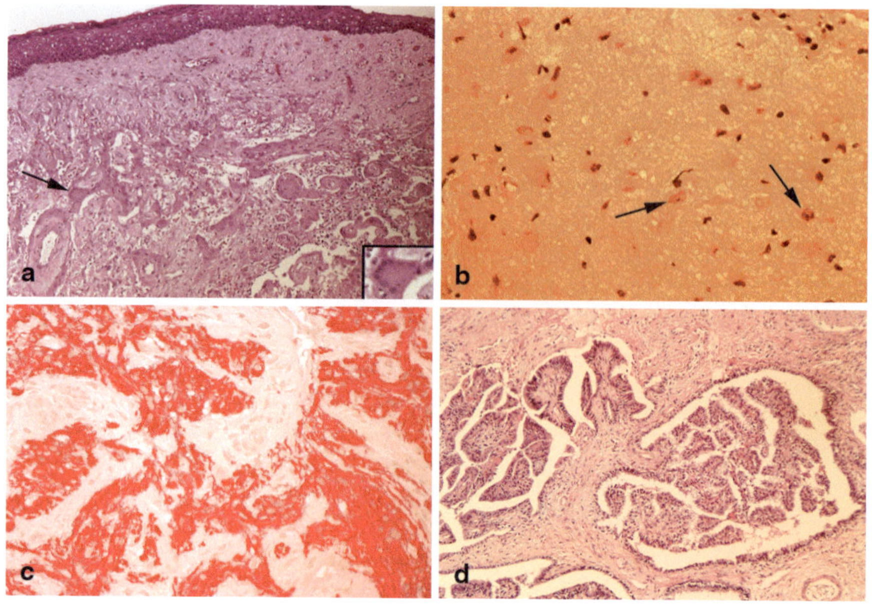

Fig. 22.4 Nasal glioma, light microscopy. **a** Meningothelial and glial tissue beneath squamous mucosa. A giant multinucleated meningothelial cell, indicated by an *arrow*, is seen at higher magnification in the inset. **b** Matured disorganized brain tissue with abundant glial component and occasional neurons (*arrows*). **c** Immunohistochemistry showing strong immunoreactivity of neuroglial tissue for glial fibrillary acidic protein (GFAP) is seen in *red*. **d** Cystic papillary structures in a background of neuroglial tissue represent choroid plexus

Outcomes

Overall, recurrence rates are reported to be anywhere from 4–10%. One series had no recurrence after excision with an average of 3.5 year follow-up [6, 7].

Follow-up

Nasal gliomas are lesions with no malignant potential that can be effectively removed surgically with low risk of recurrence. Patients should have follow-up in the immediate postoperative period at 6 months and then yearly. Physical examination and nasal endoscopy are sufficient for evaluation with repeat imaging reserved for select cases and when there is concern on physical exam for recurrence.

Conclusion

Nasal gliomas are rare congenital midline nasal masses. These are encountered early in life, but can present later in childhood and into adulthood. Physical examination and imaging studies are critical to initial evaluation. These lesions can be surgically excised, by a variety of approaches, with very low recurrence rates.

References

1. Hughes GB, Sharpino G, Hunt W, Tucker HM. Management of the congenital midline nasal mass: a review. Head Neck Surg. 1980;2(3):222–33.
2. Reid F. Uber angeborene hirnbrucke in den Stirn und Nasengegend. Illus Med. 1852;1:133.
3. Schmidt MB. Uber seltene Spaltbildungen im Bereiche des mittleren Stirnforsatzes. Virchows Arch Pathol Anat. 1900;162:340–70.
4. Sessions RB. Nasal dermal sinuses—new concepts and explanations. Laryngoscope. 1982;92(8 Pt 2 Suppl 29):1–28.
5. Patterson K, Kapur S, Chandra RS. "Nasal gliomas" and related brain heterotopias: a pathologist's perspective. Pediatr Pathol. 1986;5(3–4):353–62.
6. Puppala B, Mangurten HH, McFadden J, Lygizos N, Taxy J, Pellettiere E. Nasal glioma. Presenting as neonatal respiratory distress. Definition of the tumor mass by MRI. Clin Pediatr (Phila). 1990;29(1):49–52.
7. Rahbar R, Resto VA, Robson CD, Perez-Atayde AR, Goumnerova LC, McGill TJ, Healy GB. Nasal glioma and encephalocele: diagnosis and management. Laryngoscope. 2003;113(12):2069–77.
8. Grzegorczyk V, Brasseur-Daudruy M, Labadie G, Cellier C, Verspyck E. Prenatal diagnosis of a nasal glioma. Pediatr Radiol. 2010;40(10):1706–9.
9. Jaffe BF. Classification and management of anomalies of the nose. Otolaryngol Clin North Am. 1981;14(4):989–1004.
10. Pensler JM, Ivescu AS, Ciletti SJ, Yokoo KM, Byrd SE. Craniofacial gliomas. Plast Reconstr Surg. 1996;98(1):27–30.

Hamartomas

23

Kenneth R. Whittemore, Jr.

Introduction

A hamartoma is a nonneoplastic heterotopia composed of an overgrowth of cytologically normal, mature cells in an abnormal, disorganized architectural pattern. The term "hamartoma" was coined by Albrecht in 1904 [1] and comes from the Greek *hamartia,* meaning "error." Hamartomas can present either as a single lesion or as multiple lesions. They may arise from any of the germ layers and do not metastasize. Though there is the potential for presentation in any area of the body, hamartomas of the head and neck are relatively rare [1]. They have been found throughout the head and neck region, e.g., endotracheal, endobronchial, hypothalamic, dermal, lingual, and laryngeal. Figures 23.1, 23.2, 23.3, 23.4, and 23.5 show examples of the disorganized architecture seen in hamartomas. The figures are indicative of the histologic variability seen with this type of tumor.

Biology and Epidemiology

Pathophysiology

- The clinical presentation of hamartomas will depend upon the area of involvement.
- Hypothalamic hamartomas (HH) are associated with seizure activity and/or central precocious puberty (CPP).
  - Estimated that 14–58% of CPP cases are caused by HH; HHs are the most common cause of CPP [2].
  - Gelastic seizures are common and notoriously intractable.
    - The hypothalamic hamartoma is intrinsically epileptogenic.

K. R. Whittemore Jr. (✉)
Department of Otolaryngology and Communication Enhancement, Boston Children's Hospital, Harvard Medical School, Boston, MA, USA
e-mail: kenneth.whittemore@childrens.harvard.edu

Molecular/Genetic Pathology

- A molecular pathway to hamartoma formation can be seen in the disorder tuberous sclerosis, in which subependymal giant cell astrocytomas form [3]:
  - Caused by mutation in either of two tumor suppressor genes, TSC1 or TSC2.
  - The products may be involved in the inhibition of tumor formation.
    - Hamartin may regulate cellular adhesion by ezrin-radixin-moiesin family proteins and the GTP-binding protein Rho [4].
    - Tuberin may inhibit the G1/S transition and promote entry to the G0 phase by inhibiting rap1 or other small GTP-binding proteins [5].
- The inheritance pattern of hamartomas is dependent upon the specific tumor and area of involvement.
  - Tuberous sclerosis is autosomal dominantly inherited [3].
  - Nasal chondromesenchymal hamartomas (NCMH) may have a genetic basis with partial penetrance dependent upon environment [6].

Incidence and Prevalence

- Pediatric hamartomas are rare.
  - Fewer than 15 cases of lingual hamartomas exist in the literature [7].
  - Eleven reported cases of laryngeal hamartomas [8].
  - Two reported cases of pediatric tracheal hamartomas [9].
  - Three reported cases in the middle ear [10].
- Hamartomas are the second most common benign pediatric pulmonary tumor of the lung, though bronchial tumors in general are rare [11].

R. Rahbar et al. (eds.), *Pediatric Head and Neck Tumors,*
DOI 10.1007/978-1-4614-8755-5_23, © Springer Science+Business Media New York 2014

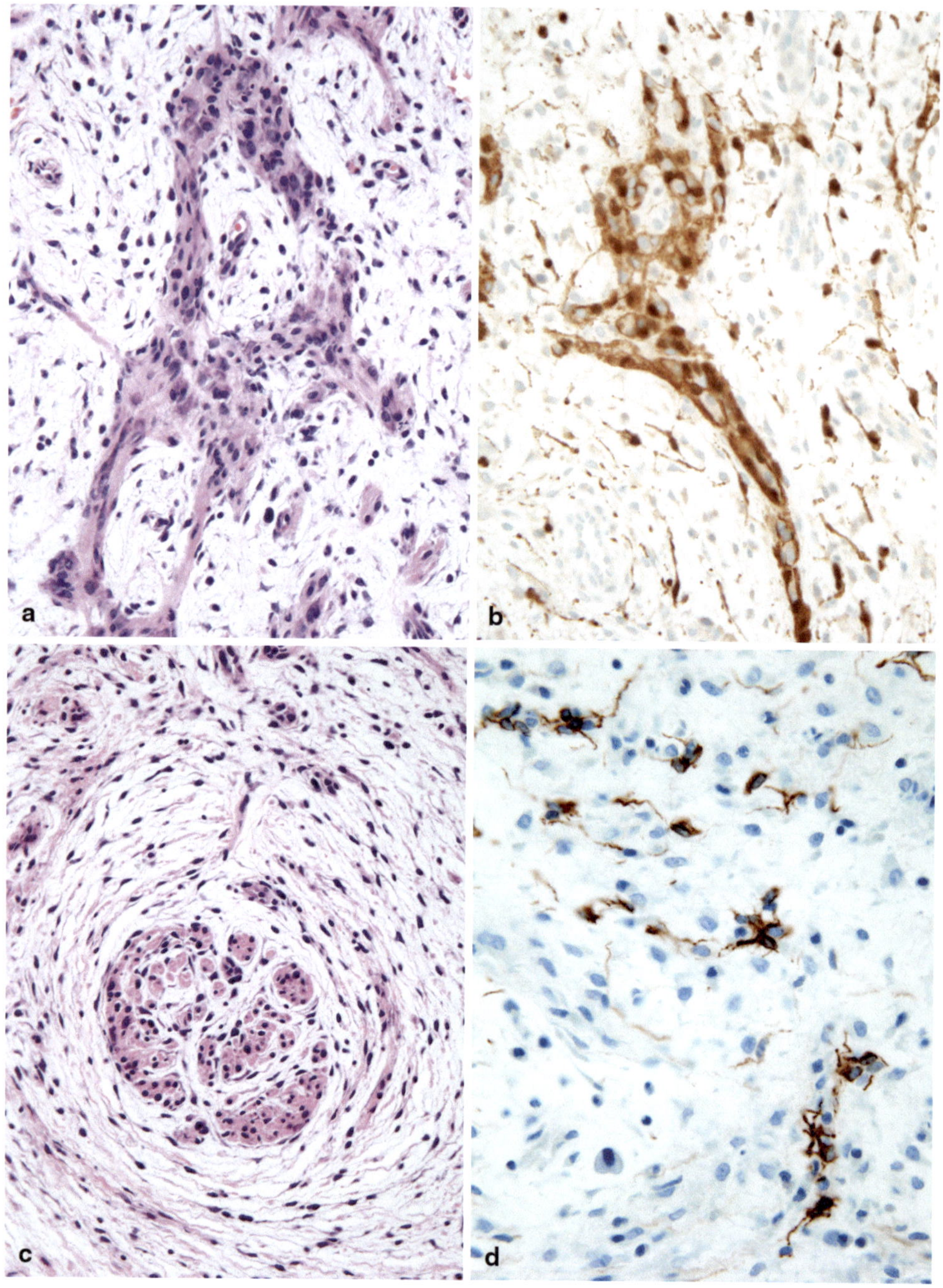

Fig. 23.1 Light microscopy of neuroglial hamartoma. **a** Mature neuroglial tissue with ribbons of ganglionic elements. **b** Immunohistochemically, ganglion cells with neuritic and axonal processes are strongly immunoreactive for S100 protein. **c** Nerve structure surrounded by concentrically arranged perineurial cells. **d** Neuroglial component immunoreactive for glial fibrillary acidic protein (GFAP)

Age Distribution

- Laryngeal hamartomas manifest most commonly in children younger than 10 years of age, or adults in their sixth decade of life [1].
- Nasal chondromesenchymal hamartoma occurs most often in those younger than 1 year of age [6].

Sex Predilection

- Two-thirds of laryngeal hamartoma patients are male [1].
- Male infants are more commonly affected in nasal chondromesenchymal hamartoma [6].
- Fibrous hamartoma of infancy also occurs primarily in male patients [12].

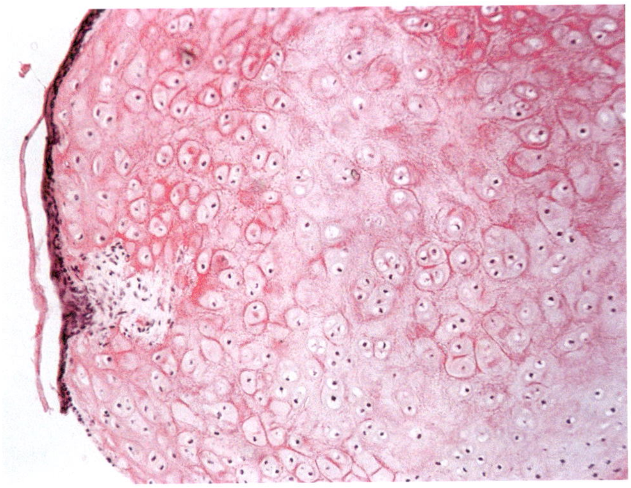

Fig. 23.2 Light microscopy of external ear canal hamartoma. Cartilaginous nodule partially covered by attenuated squamous epithelium

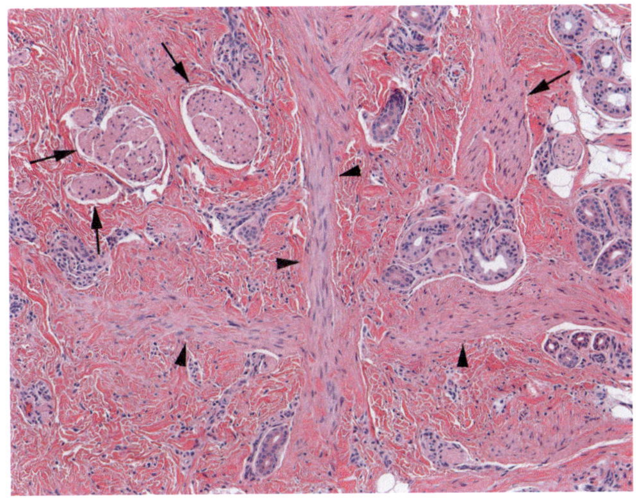

Fig. 23.4 Light microscopy of dermal hamartoma. Abnormal dermal tissue with enlarged erectory pili (*arrows*), thick bands of smooth muscle (*arrowheads*) and disorganized adnexa

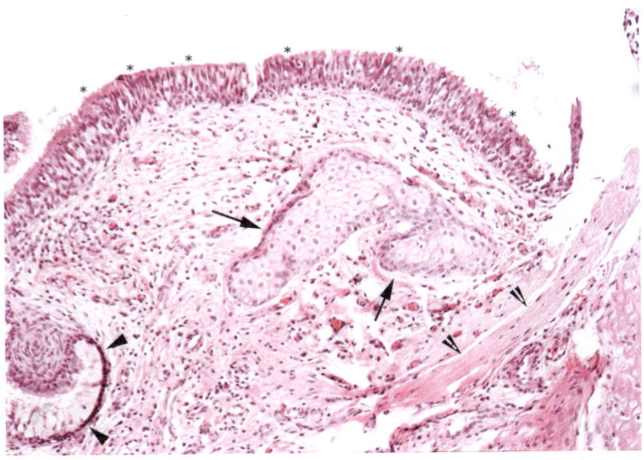

Fig. 23.3 Light microscopy of middle ear hamartoma. Connective tissue with sebaceous glands (*arrows*) and bundles of smooth muscle (*clefted arrowheads*) is covered by respiratory type ciliated epithelium (*asterisks*) and foci of mucous cells (*arrowheads*)

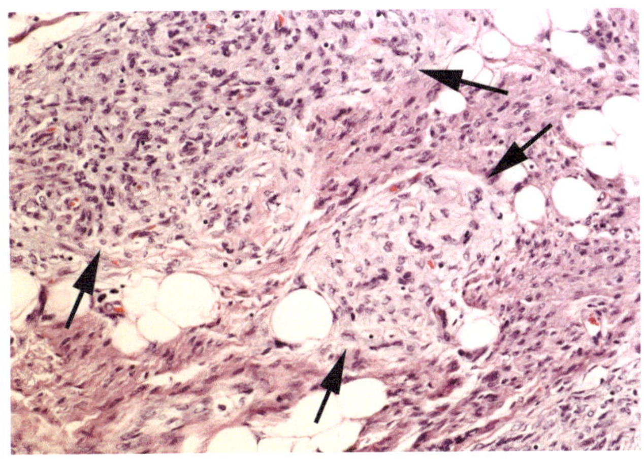

Fig. 23.5 Fibrous hamartoma of infancy. The lesion is composed of a mixture of mature adipose tissue, fibrocollagenous bands and islands of primitive mesenchyme (arrows). Fibrous hamartoma of infancy of the head and neck is usually located in the scalp

Relationships to Other Disease States, Syndromes

- Tuberous sclerosis may be associated with West Syndrome [3].

Presentation

Presentation depends on area of involvement:

Laryngeal hamartoma [1, 8]:

- Stridor
- Dysphagia
- Dysphonia
- Dyspnea
- Earache
- Aspiration

Nasal [13] or nasal chondromesenchymal hamartoma (NCMH) [6, 14]:

- Nasal obstruction
- Respiratory and feeding difficulties in infants
- Epistaxis
- Rhinorrhea
- Serous otitis media
- If orbital involvement: proptosis, enophthalmos, ophthalmoplegia, ptosis, or hypotropia
- If intracranial expansion: hydrocephalus or with oculomotor disturbances

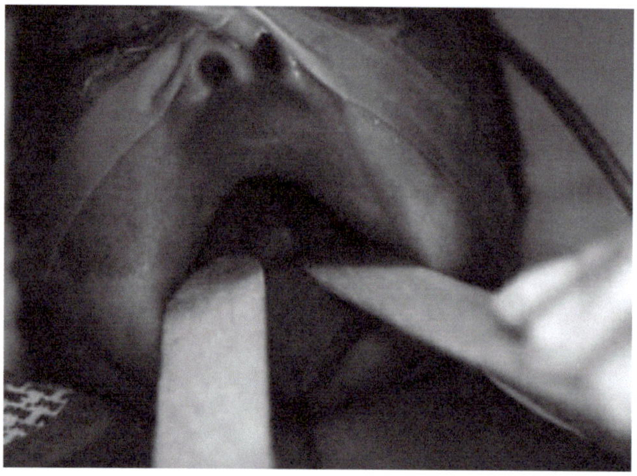

Fig. 23.6 An anterior, polypoid tongue mass that proved to be a hamartoma upon histological examination. (Reprinted from Horn et al. [8], with permission of SAGE Publications)

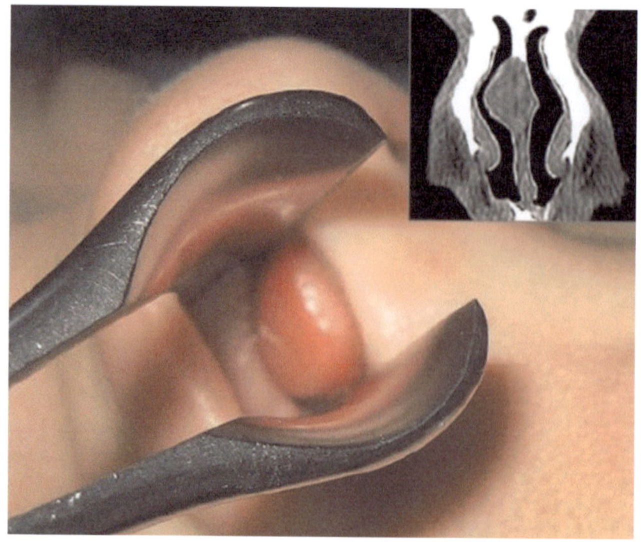

Fig. 23.7 A gross image of a nasal hamartoma that filled the right nasal meatus of a child, with the computed tomography (CT) scan revealing the right nasal mass adjacent to the nasal septum. (Reprinted from Gajda et al. [13])

Figure 23.6 shows a gross example of a nasal mass.

Tongue lesions [7]:

- Airway obstruction
- Oral bleeding
- Cosmetic concern
- Dysphagia
- Dysarthria
- Respiratory distress, especially if in posterior tongue

Figure 23.7 shows a gross example of a tongue lesion.

Tracheal [9]:

- Similar to intractable asthma or obstructive airway disease
- Expiratory wheezing
- Biphasic stridor

Fibrous hamartoma of infancy (FHI) [12, 15, 16]:

- Solitary mobile and firm mass, gradually enlarging
  - Most are 2.5–5 cm in diameter
- Can occur on neck
- Occasional skin change, such as pigmentation changes or eccrine gland hyperplasia

Hypothalamic hamartomas [17, 18]:

- Central precocious puberty
- Seizures, typically gelastic
- Intellectual disability
- Behavioral problems

Tuberous sclerosis [3]:

- Epilepsy
- Intellectual disability
- Autism
- Attention deficit hyperactivity disorder

Striated muscle hamartoma [19]:

- Solitary, firm, flesh-colored, and nontender lesion

Differential Diagnosis

Differential diagnosis depends on site of tumor.

- Laryngeal hamartoma: neoplastic lesions, e.g., hemangioma, rhabdomyosarcoma, neurofibroma [8].
- Nasal hamartoma: foreign body, antrochoanal polyp, dermoid, nasal polyp, papilloma, glioma, encephalocele, hemangioma, and olfactory neuroblastoma [20].
  - NCMH: hemangioma, angiofibroma, inverted papilloma, nasal glioma, giant cell reparative granuloma, ossifying fibroma, aneurismal bone cyst, chondro-osseous respiratory adenomatoid hamartoma, rhabdomyosarcoma, esthesioneuroblastoma, and chondro-sarcoma [14, 21]. If calcifications are present, possibilities are narrowed to ossifying fibroma, chondro-osseous respiratory adenomatoid hamartoma, and chondroid tumor [6].
  - Respiratory adenomatoid hamartoma of the anterior nasal septum (REAH): inverted schneiderian papilloma and adenocarcinoma [13].
- Thyroid gland: Lymphangiomas, hemangiomas, and teratomas [12, 22] may also mimic any of the thyroid carcinomas.
- Endobronchial chondromatous hamartomas: aspirated foreign bodies, cysts, ectopic thyroid tissue, mucosal webs, and other tumors [11].
- Hypothalamic hamartoma: craniopharyngioma and optic-hypothalamic gliomas (though these often show contrast

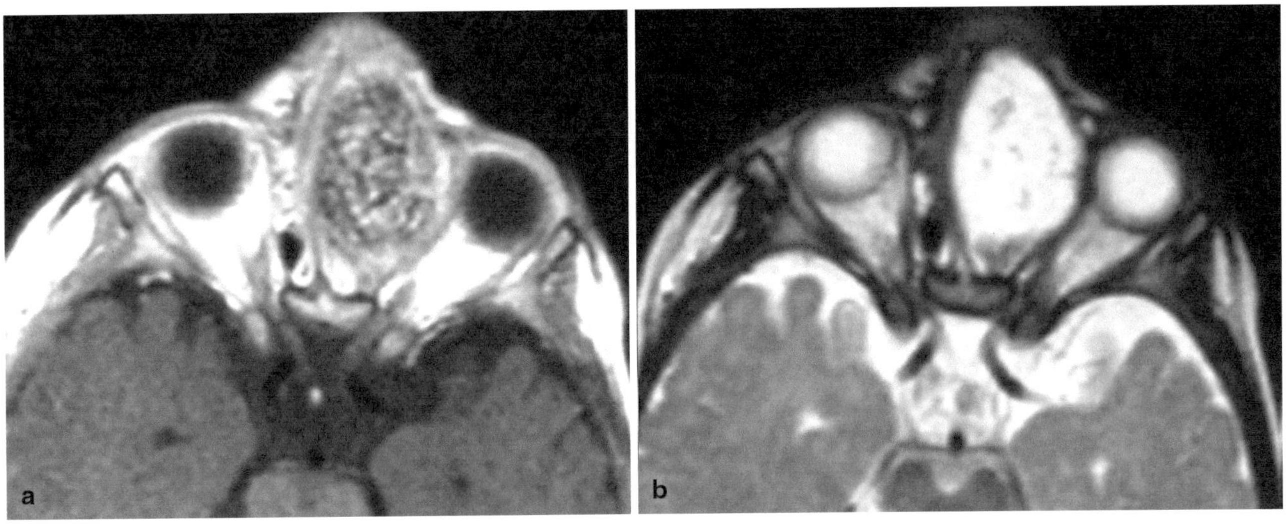

Fig. 23.8 **a** MRI of a nasal chondromesenchymal hamartoma. Axial contrast-enhanced T1-weighted images revealed a heterogeneously enhancing mass in the left nasal cavity. **b** Axial T2-weighted MRI scan revealed a diffuse high signal. (Reprinted from Finitsis et al. [14], with permission from Springer Science + Business Media)

enhancement, whereas hypothalamic hamartomas do not) [2].

- Tracheal hamartomas: bronchogenic cysts and teratomas [9] as well as neoplasms of the trachea.

Diagnosis and Evaluation

Evaluation

Evaluation for hamartomas includes a physical examination, with or without endoscopy depending on location [21]. A diagnostic laryngoscopy and bronchoscopy with biopsy may be required for tracheal and endobronchial lesions. If tuberous sclerosis is suspect, a genetics evaluation should be performed to check for mutations in either the TSC1 or TSC2 genes [3].

HHs can be diagnosed on the basis of location in the tuber cinereum, lack of enhancement upon contrast administration, isointensity to normal brain, and lack of change in size upon follow-up imaging [2]. When young children present with CPP, endocrine testing should be performed. Hormone levels of luteinizing hormone (LH), follicular stimulating hormone (FSH), and either estradiol or testosterone may be at pubertal levels. Additionally, bone age may be beyond the true age of the child.

Imaging Evaluation

CT with intravenous contrast should be used in most cases when a mass is seen upon endoscopic or visual examination. This will allow for the assessment of the extent and involvement of the tumor and should be performed, for example, when laryngeal [1], nasal [6, 14, 20, 23], middle ear [10], and tracheal [9] tumors are suspected. Figure 23.6 shows an example of a CT of a nasal mass.

If HH is suspected (either CPP or intractable seizures are present), magnetic resonance imaging (MRI) with contrast should be taken; HH will be found at the tuber cinereum, isointense with normal brain tissue, and will not enhance upon contrast medium administration [2]. Additionally, upon follow-up MRI, there should not be a change in the size or morphology of the mass.

In NCMH, the tumor may appear to be malignant because of the possibility for bony remodeling [14]. It typically appears as a nonencapsulated and poorly defined mass, frequently with cystic components and calcifications [6]. Figure 23.8 shows an example of an MRI of a NCMH.

CT can show calcified nodules in tuberous sclerosis [3].

Pathology

Histopathological results of a biopsy or total resection of a lesion will make a definitive diagnosis. Cytologically, the cells in a hamartoma will be similar to surrounding tissue, but architecturally, they will be arranged in an abnormal pattern; the types of cells present in the hamartoma will depend upon the area of the lesion. For instance, endobronchial chondromatous hamartomas typically are composed of an abundance of cartilage and glandular tissues [11], whereas NCMHs are characterized by mesenchymal components with islands of hyaline cartilage and occasionally binucleated chondrocytes [21]. FHI is characterized by an admixture of bundles of dense, uniform, fibrous connective tissue in fat, primitive mesenchyme, concentric whorls or bands, and mature adipose tissue [15].

Special stains generally are not necessary; hematoxylin and eosin should be sufficient [15]. Mesenchymal hamartomas are more common than either epithelial or glandular hamartomas [1].

Treatment

The treatment of choice for hamartomas is complete excision when possible; if total resection is achieved, it is curative. If remnants of the hamartoma remain, there is the possibility for regrowth of the tumor. However, if a choice must be made, function should be preserved over resecting the entire tumor, as there is the chance growth will cease spontaneously [1]. There is very little support for adjuvant therapies if the tumor is not excised in whole. Instead, follow-up imaging should be performed to assess any regrowth, with the potential for further resection.

Treatment of HHs may not necessitate surgery, as it is not an aggressive tumor [17]. If the only symptom is CPP, gonadotrophin-releasing hormone (GnRH) analogue treatment until puberty should be sufficient by effecting the regression of early pubertal development [2]. If the symptoms include seizures, antiepileptic drugs (AEDs) should be tried, though gelastic seizures tend to be refractory to AED regimens [17]. If the seizures are severe enough, surgery may be required [17]. Surgical resection in HH patients with refractory seizures leads to seizure freedom in 50 % of patients [24], although resection is difficult [18]. It may also help control behavioral issues related to poor frustration tolerance in children with HH. Ng et al. found that 88 % of families described an improvement in functioning following surgical resection [25]. Even in cases where seizures are relatively infrequent, if the behavioral problems are sufficiently severe, resection may be advised.

Outcomes

Typically, a complete resection is curative, and the recurrence rate is low [16]. If complete resection is impossible, regular follow-up radiographic imaging should be performed to assess further growth. Recurrence is possible if there has been an incomplete resection [6]. Risks of surgery depend upon the area of the hamartoma. For instance, with lingual hamartomas, surgery to an anterior region of the tongue involves minimal risk, but a posterior lesion resection may interfere with function [7]. Issues can also arise if sufficient treatment is not given in a timely fashion. If HH-associated CPP is not diagnosed quickly enough, and treatment with a GnRH agonist is not administered, potential for adult height might be reduced [26]; however, timely treatment will preserve growth potential [18]. Generally, though, the prognosis is good, as there is the strong chance growth will spontaneously cease [1].

Acknowledgments I would like to thank Jenna M. Dargie, BS for helping research, prepare, and edit this manuscript, as well as Antonio R. Perez-Atayde, MD for preparing the histology slides.

References

1. Windfuhr JP. Laryngeal hamartoma. Acta Otolaryngol. 2004;124:301–8.
2. Kizilkilic O, Yalcin O, Yildirim T, Sener L, Parmaksiz G, Erdogan B. Hypotahlamic hamartoma associated with a craniopharyngeal canal. Am J Neuroradiol. 2005;26:65–7.
3. Mizuguchi M, Takashima S. Neuropathology of tuberous sclerosis. Brain Dev. 2001;23:508–15.
4. Lamb RF, Roy C, Diefenbach TJ, Vinters HV, Johnson MW, Jay DG, et al. The TSC1 tumor suppressor hamartin regulates cell adhesion through ERM proteins and the GTPase Rho. Nat Cell Biol. 2000;2:281–7.
5. Wienecke R, Konig A, DeClue JE. Identification of tuberin, the tuberous sclerosis-2 product. Tubern possesses specific Rap1GAP activity. J Biol Chem. 1995;270:16409–14.
6. Kim JE, Kim HJ, Kim JH, Ko YH, Chung SK. Nasal chondromesenchymal hamartoma: CT and MR imaging findings. Korean J Radiol. 2009;10:416–9.
7. Horn C, Thaker HM, Tampakopoulou DA, De Serres LM, Keller JL, Haddad J. Tongue lesions in the pediatric population. Otolaryngol Head Neck Surg. 2001;124:164–9.
8. Jakubikova J, Harustiak S, Galbavy S, Chebenova M. Laryngeal hamartoma: surgical management. Int J Pediatr Otorhi. 1999;50:145–9.
9. Gross E, Chen MK, Hollabaugh RS, Joyner RE. Tracheal hamartoma: report of a child with a neck mass. J Pediatr Surg. 1996;31:1584–5.
10. Baget S, Francois A, Andrieu-Guitrancourt J, Marie JP, Dehesdin D. Hamartoma of the middle ear: a case study. Int J Pediatr Otorhi. 2003;67:287–91.
11. Abdulhamid I, Rabah R. Endobronchial chondromatous hamartoma in an infant. Pediatr Pulmonol. 2003;35:67–9.
12. Weinberger MS, Pransky SM, Krous HF. Fibrous hamartoma of infancy presenting as a perspiring neck mass. Int J Pediatr Otorhi. 1993;26:173–6.
13. Gajda M, Zagolski O, Jasztal A, Lis GJ, Pyka-Fosciak G, Litwin JA. Respiratory epithelial adenomatoid hamartoma of the anterior nasal septum a rare localization of an unusual tumour in a child: a case report. Cases J. 2009;2:8151.
14 Finitsis S, Giavroglou C, Potsi S, Constantinidis I, Mpaltatzidis A, Rachovitsas D, Tzioufa V. Nasal chondromesenchymal hamartoma in a child. Cardiovasc Intervent Radiol. 2009;32:593–7.
15 Dickey GE, Sotelo-Avila C. Fibrous hamartoma of infancy: current review. Pediat Devel Path. 1999;2:236–43.
16 Agrawal CS, Agrawal S, Sinha A. Fibrous hamartoma of infancy: a case report. Acta Derm Venereol. 2004;85:276–7.
17 Kramer U, Spector S, Nasser W, Siomin V, Fried I, Constantini S. Surgical treatment of hypothalamic hamartoma and refractory seizures. Pediatr Neurosurg. 2001;34:40–2.
18 Debeneix C, Bourgeois M, Trivin C, Sainte-Rose C, Brauner R. Hypothalamic hamartoma: comparison of clinical presentation and magnetic resonance images. Horm Res. 2001;56:12–8.

19 Fannon EM, Pride H. Asymptomatic plaque on the chin of a 10-year-old girl. Arch Dermatol. 2000;136:1263–8.
20. Terris MH, Billman GF, Pransky SM. Nasal hamartoma: case report and review of the literature. Int J Pediatr Otorhi. 1993;28:83–8.
21 . Johnson C, Nagaraj U, Esguerra J, Wasdahl D, Wurzbach D. Nasal chondromesenchymal hamartoma: radiographic and histopathologic analysis of a rare pediatric tumor. Pediatr Radiol. 2007;37:101–4.
22. Zachariou Z, Beiler HA, Roth H, Daum R. A rare case of an antenatally diagnosed tumor of the neck—a hamartoma of the thyroid gland. Journal Pediatr Surg. 1996;31:1294–6.
23. Olnes SQ, Schwartz RH, Bahadori RS. Diagnosis and management of the newborn and young infant who have nasal obstruction. Pediatr Rev. 2000;21:416–20.
24. Chapman KE, Kim DY, Rho JM, Ng YT, Kerrigan JF. Ketogenic diet in the treatment of seizures associated with hypothalamic hamartomas. Epilepsy Res. 2011;94:218–21.
25. Ng YT, Hastriter EV, Wethe J, Chaman KE, Prenger EC, Prigatano GP, Oppenheim T, Varland M, Rekate HL, Kerrigan JF. Surgical resection of hypothalamic hamartomas for severe behavioral symptoms. Epilepsy Behav. 2011;20:75–8.
26. Arisaka O, Negishi M, Numata M, Hoshi M, Kanazawa S, Oyama M, Nitta A, Suzumuara H, Kuribayashi T, Nakayama Y. Precocious puberty resulting from congenital hypothalamic hamartoma: persistent darkened areolae after birth as the hallmark of estrogen excess. Clin Pediatr. 2001;40:163–7.

Hemangiomas

24

Rafael A. Couto and Arin K. Greene

Introduction

Most vascular tumors of childhood are benign. The most common types are infantile hemangioma (IH), congenital hemangioma (CH), kaposiform hemangioendothelioma (KHE), and pyogenic granuloma (PG) (see Fig. 24.1). Although vascular tumors may look similar, they are managed differently. Vascular tumors must be differentiated from vascular malformations.

Key Points

- Vascular tumors of childhood are typically benign.
- Most pediatric vascular tumors can be diagnosed by history and physical examination.
- IH is the most common tumor of infancy; most do not require treatment.
- Pharmacotherapy is usually the first-line therapy for problematic IH and KHE.

Biology and Epidemiology

Vascular tumors are distinguished by endothelial cell proliferation, whereas vascular malformations result from dysmorphogenesis [1].

Pathophysiology

- The precursor cell for IH may be a multipotent hemangioma-derived-stem cell (HemSC) [2]. HemSCs express CD90, a mesenchymal cell marker, and can differentiate into multiple cell lineages. They produce human GLUT1-positive microvessels after clonal expansion in immunodeficient mice [2]. Hemangioma endothelial cells share similarities with placental endothelium, and it has been postulated that the precursor cell for IH might have embolized from the placenta [3, 4].
- Several mechanisms may contribute to the rapid enlargement of IH. Hypoxia might recruit circulating hemangioma-derived endothelial progenitor cell (HemEPCs) to the tumor [5]. Hemangioma endothelial cells have defective nuclear factor of activated T-cells (NFAT) activity that stimulates endothelial proliferation [6]. Local factors, such as a reduction in antiangiogenic proteins, also may potentiate tumor growth [7].

Incidence and Prevalence

- IH is the most common tumor of infancy. It affects 4–5 % of Caucasians and is rare in dark-skinned individuals [8].
- IH is the most frequent vascular tumor referred to a vascular anomalies center (85.9 %), followed by KHE (7.8 %), CH (5.4 %), and PG (0.9 %) [9].

Age Distribution

- The median age of appearance of IH is 2 weeks; subcutaneous lesions may not be noted until 3–4 months of age [10].
- CH is present at birth [11–13].
- Half of KHEs are present at birth, but can develop during infancy (58 %), between 1–10 years of age (32 %), or after 11 years of age (10 %) [14].
- The mean age of onset of PG is 6.7 years; only 12.4 % develop during the first year of life [15].

A. K. Greene (✉) · R. A. Couto
Department of Plastic and Oral Surgery, Boston Children's Hospital, Harvard Medical School, Boston, MA 02115, USA
e-mail: arin.greene@childrens.harvard.edu

R. Rahbar et al. (eds.), *Pediatric Head and Neck Tumors*,
DOI 10.1007/978-1-4614-8755-5_24,

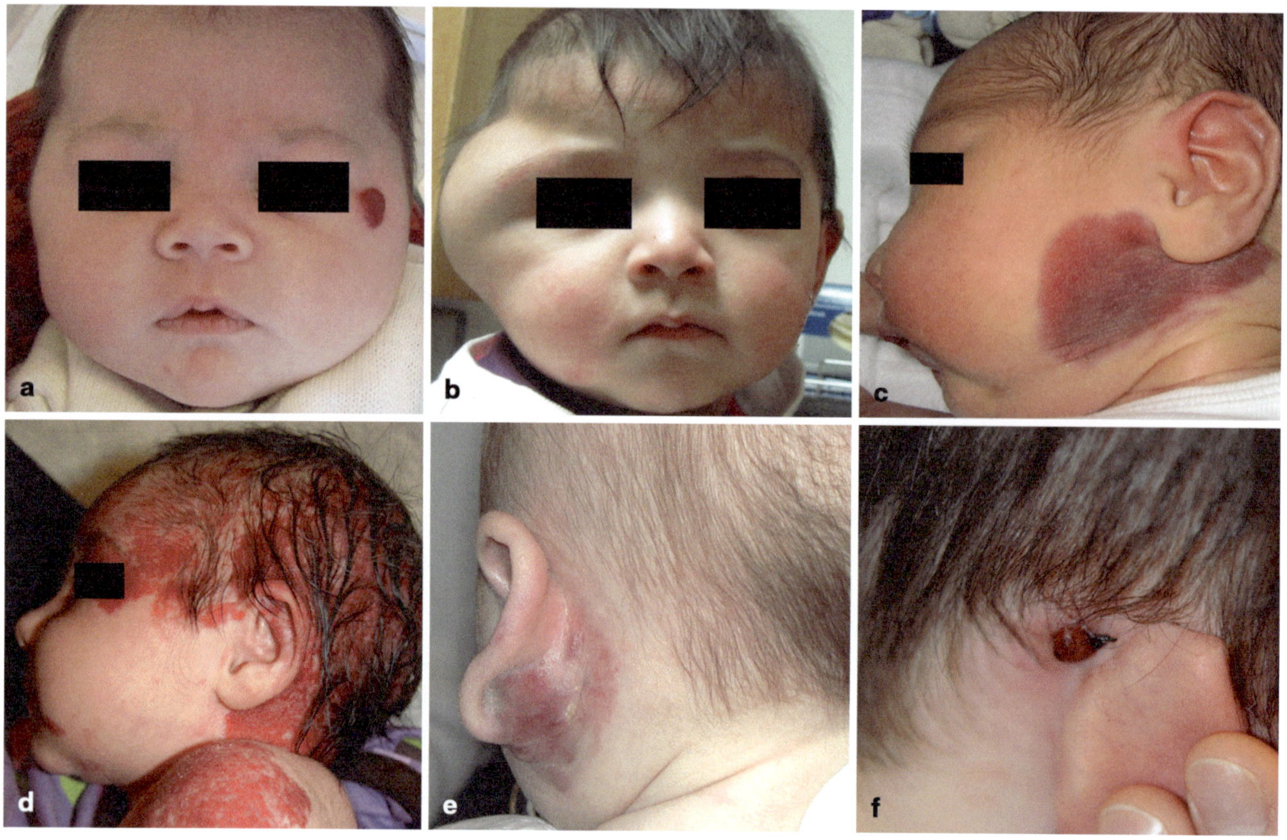

Fig. 24.1 Types of vascular tumors. **a** Two-month-old female child with a superficial infantile hemangioma (IH) of the cheek. **b** Five-month-old female child with a deep IH without overlying skin changes. **c** One-week-old male child with a congenital hemangioma (CH) (rapidly involuting CH) of the neck. **d** One-month-old female child with PHACE association (Posterior fossa brain malformation, Hemangioma, Arterial cerebrovascular anomalies, Coarctation of the aorta and cardiac defects, Eye/endocrine abnormalities). **e** Three-month-old female child with a kaposiform hemangioendothelioma. **f** Five-year-old male child with a pyogenic granuloma

Sex Predilection

- IH is more frequent in females (3:1 to 5:1) [9, 16].
- CH and KHE have equal sex distribution [14].

Risk Factors

- Risk factors for IH include Caucasian race, female sex, and preterm birth [8, 16, 17].

Relationships to Other Disease States, Syndromes

- A total of 16% of children with ≥5, small, domed-like lesions (hemangiomatosis) have a hepatic IH [18, 19].
- PHACE association consists of a plaque-like IH in a segmental/trigeminal distribution with at least one of the following anomalies: *P*osterior fossa brain malformations, *H*emangioma, *A*rterial cerebrovascular anomalies, *C*oarctation of the aorta and cardiac defects, and *E*ye/*E*ndocrine abnormalities (see Fig. 24.1d) [20]. If ventral developmental defects (*S*ternal clefting and *S*upraumbilical raphe) are present, the condition is termed PHACES association [20]. Eight percent of patients suffer a stroke during infancy, and 42% have a structural brain anomaly [21].

Presentation

Infantile Hemangioma

- IH grows faster than the rate of the child during the first 9 months of life (proliferating phase); 80% of its size is achieved by 5 months [22]. After this age the tumor begins to shrink (involuting phase). Regression stops in most children by 4 years of age (involuted phase).
- IHs are located on the head/neck (66.5%), trunk (16.9%), extremities (9.8%), or viscera (6.8%) [9].
- Approximately 10% of IH are problematic during the proliferating phase [10].
- Complications:
  - Alopecia

  - IHs in the scalp or eyebrow can injure hair follicles.
- Obstruction
  - IHs involving the external auditory canal may cause otitis externa; sensorineural hearing loss does not occur if the contralateral canal is patent [10].
  - Periorbital IHs can cause obstructive or astigmatic amblyopia [10].
  - Nasal or subglottic lesions can cause airway obstruction [10].
- Ulceration
  - Approximately 16 % of proliferating IHs will ulcerate at a median age of 4 months; anogenital, labial, and neck tumors are most likely to develop a wound [23].
- Deformity
  - Following involution, 50 % of patients will have anetoderma from loss of elastic fibers, destruction of anatomical structures, fibrofatty residuum, redundant skin, residual telangiectasias, or scarring [10, 18].

Congenital Hemangioma

- Unlike IH, CH is fully grown at birth and does not grow postnatally [11–13].
- Rapidly involuting congenital hemangioma (RICH) regresses immediately after birth; lesions fully involute by 14 months of age [11–13]. Noninvoluting congenital hemangioma (NICH) does not regress [12].
- The most common sites of RICHs are the extremities (52 %), followed by the head/neck (42 %), and trunk (6 %) [11, 13]. NICHs affect the head/neck (43 %), limbs (38 %), or trunk (19 %) [12]. After involution, a RICH may leave behind atrophic tissue and/or residual telangiectasia [10].
- Most NICHs are nonproblematic, but may cause a deformity [10].

Kaposiform Hemangioendothelioma

- KHE is a locally aggressive tumor that does not metastasize [24, 25].
- KHE is solitary, and involves the trunk (34.8 %), extremities (34.1 %), head/neck (20.5 %), or viscera (10.6 %) [10].
- The tumor enlarges in early childhood, and then undergoes partial regression after 2 years of age; lesions typically persist causing chronic pain and stiffness [26].
- A total of 50 % of patients have Kasabach Merritt phenomenon (KMP) (thrombocytopenia $<25{,}000/mm^3$, petechiae, and bleeding) [27, 28].

Pyogenic Granuloma

- The average age of onset is 6.7 years; 72.5 % occur before 10 years of age [15].
- Involves the head/neck (80.0 %), trunk (13.3 %), and extremities (6.7 %) [15].
- The skin (88.2 %) or mucous membranes (11.8 %) are affected [15].
- History of trauma or an underlying cutaneous condition (e.g., capillary malformation) is present in 25 % of patients [15].
- The most common complications are bleeding (64.2 %) and ulceration (36.3 %) [15].

Differential Diagnosis for Hemangiomas

Arteriovenous malformation (AVM)
Capillary malformation (CM)
Infantile fibrosarcoma
Infantile myofibromatosis
Kaposiform Hemangioendothelioma (KHE)
Lymphatic malformation (LM)
Pyogenic Granuloma (PG)
Venous malformation (VM)

Diagnosis and Evaluation

Physical Examination

Infantile Hemangioma

- Findings:
  - IH is red when it involves the superficial dermis. Subcutaneous lesions may appear bluish or have normal overlying skin.
  - Unlike CH, IH is not present at birth and undergoes rapid postnatal growth.
  - Hand-held Doppler examination showing fast-flow can facilitate the diagnosis [10].

Congenital Hemangioma

- Findings:
  - CH is red-violaceous with coarse telangiectasias, central pallor, and a peripheral pale halo [11–13].
  - Lesions are solitary with an average diameter of 5 cm [11–13].
  - CH is fully grown at birth and does not exhibit postnatal growth [11–13].
  - The tumor either regresses immediately after birth (RICH) or remains unchanged (NICH).
  - A hand-held Doppler can exclude slow-flow lesions [10].

Kaposiform Hemangioendothelioma

- Findings:
  - Lesions are flat, reddish-purple, and edematous [28].
  - The tumor is usually greater than 5 cm in diameter [25].

Pyogenic Granuloma

- Findings:
  - Appears as a solitary, red, pedunculated lesion with an average size of 6.5 mm; it is smaller than IH, CH, or KHE [10, 15].
  - Unlike IH, CH, or KHE, PG rarely presents within the first month of life.

Laboratory Data

- A total of 50 % of patients with KHE have thrombocytopenia <25,000/mm^3. Fibrinogen is low and fibrin split products (D-dimers) are elevated [27, 28].

Imaging Evaluation

Ultrasonography (US) The first-line confirmatory study for hemangiomas when history and physical examination is unclear [10]. Proliferating IH exhibits a soft tissue mass with fast-flow, decreased arterial resistance, and increased venous drainage [29].

Magnetic Resonance Imaging (MRI) It is rarely used for IH, CH, or PG. However, MRI is indicated if KHE is suspected to confirm the diagnosis and define the extent of the lesion. KHE has small vessels, poorly defined margins, and invades adjacent tissues; lesions are T2 hyperintense and enhance with contrast [25, 30, 31].

Pathology

Infantile Hemangioma Biopsy is indicated only if malignancy is suspected or if the diagnosis remains unclear following imaging studies. Proliferating IH shows disorganized capillary-sized vessels composed of plump, immature endothelial cells [32]. The intervascular stroma is comprised of scattered fibroblasts, mast, and mononuclear cells (see Fig. 24.2) [32]. Tumors in the involuted phase are characterized by fibrofatty tissue, loss of dermal elastic fibers, and small residual capillaries (see Fig. 24.3) [32]. Immunostaining for erythrocyte glucose transporter (GLUT1) can differentiate IH from other tumors and malformations (see Fig. 24.3c) [33].

Congenital Hemangioma Biopsy is rarely indicated. Unlike IH, CH is immunonegative for GLUT1. CH shows an accumulation of dermal and subcutaneous lobular capillaries, surrounded by fibrotic tissue (see Fig. 24.4) [32]. Unlike NICHs, the center of most RICHs exhibit involuting features (e.g., fibrotic tissue, residual draining veins, and a lack of capillaries) [32].

Kaposiform Hemangioendothelioma KHE shows infiltrating sheets or nodules of endothelial cells lining capillaries [24, 34]. Hemosiderin-filled slit-like vascular spaces, as well as thrombi and platelet aggregates within the vessels, are present [32]. Nuclear atypia and mitotic activity is rarely observed [32].

Pyogenic Granuloma On low magnification, PG appears as an exophytic mass attached to a narrow stalk. The superficial lesion demonstrates immature capillaries with fibroblastic, granulation-like tissue [15, 35]. The deeper component contains proliferating lobular capillaries extending to the reticular dermis, with a dense, fibrous stroma [15, 35].

Treatments and Outcomes

Nonoperative Management

Infantile Hemangioma Most IHs are managed by observation because 90 % are small, localized, and nonproblematic [10]. To reduce the risk of ulceration, proliferating IHs are kept moist with hydrated petroleum to minimize desiccation and accidental shearing of the skin [10]. If ulceration occurs, it will almost always heal with local wound care; if not, intralesional or systemic corticosteroid may be necessary [10].

First-line treatment for small, localized, problematic IH is intralesional corticosteroid (triamcinolone 3 mg/kg) [10]. Topical corticosteroid is less effective than intralesional delivery, because it only treats the superficial component [10, 36, 37]. Corticosteroid injections stabilize the growth of IH in at least 95 % of patients, and decrease the size of 75 % of tumors (see Fig. 24.5a, b) [38]. The drug lasts 4–6 weeks; patients may require additional injections during the proliferative phase.

Systemic corticosteroid is reserved for problematic, proliferating tumors that are too large to inject. The child is given 3.0 mg/kg/day of oral prednisolone (Orapred®) for 1 month, followed by a 0.5 ml taper every 2–4 weeks until it is discontinued between 9–10 months of age when the tumor is no longer proliferating [39]. The drug is administered once daily in the morning to facilitate compliance and reduce adrenal suppression [39]. Using this protocol all tumors will respond; 88 % will become smaller and 12 % will stop grow-

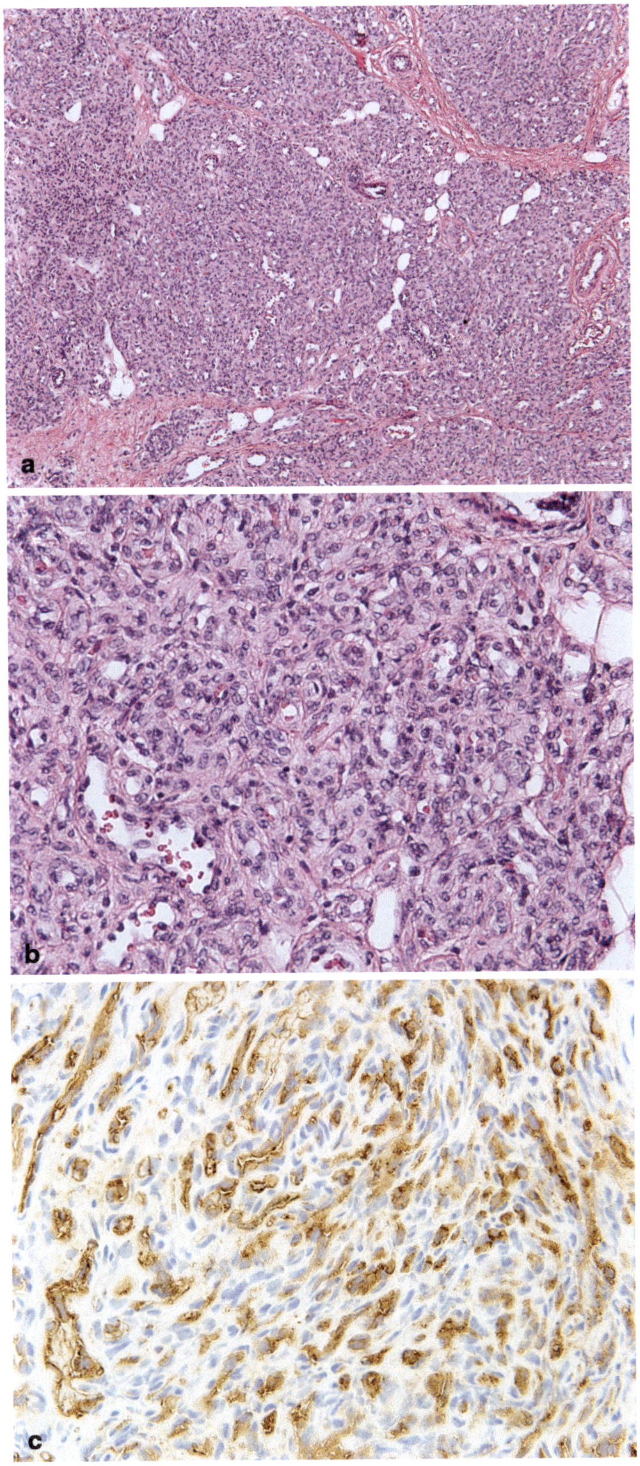

Fig. 24.2 Infantile hemangioma (IH) proliferating phase. **a** Lobules of capillaries are densely cellular and infiltrating soft tissue. **b** At higher magnification, capillaries are back to back with little intervening tissue, plump endothelial cells, and difficult to visualized lumens. Mitoses are frequently observed. **c** Endothelial immunoreactivity for Glut-1 is characteristic of IH

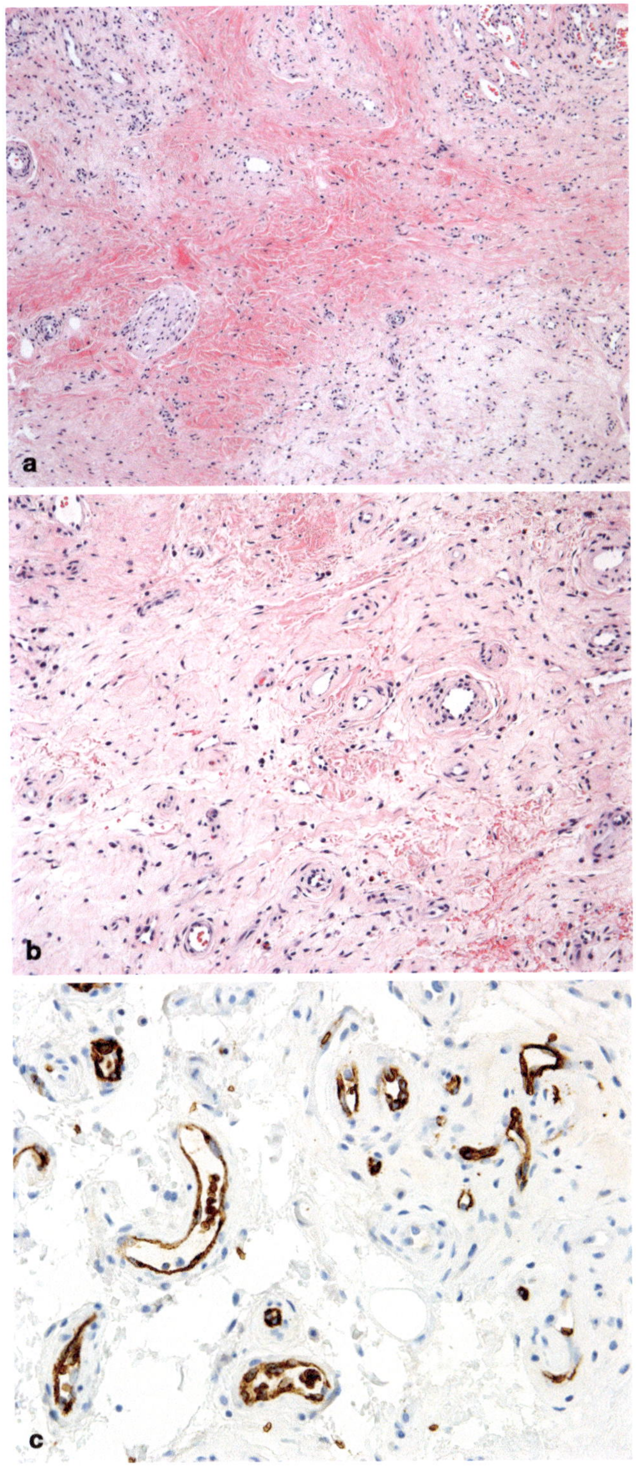

Fig. 24.3 Infantile hemangioma involuting phase. **a** Capillary lobules are less cellular and vastly replaced by loose fibrous tissue. **b** Vessels are separated from each other by fibrous tissue and appear larger, and ectatic with thickened walls. **c** Strong endothelial Glut-1 immunoreactivity persists

ing (see Fig. 24.5c–e) [39]. Twenty percent of patients will have a temporary cushingoid response that resolves when the steroid is weaned [39]. Approximately 12–33 % of infants exhibit decreased gain in height, but return to their pretreatment growth curve by 24 months of age [40, 41].

Complications from corticosteroid (e.g., adverse neurodevelopment, aseptic necrosis of the femoral head, diabetes,

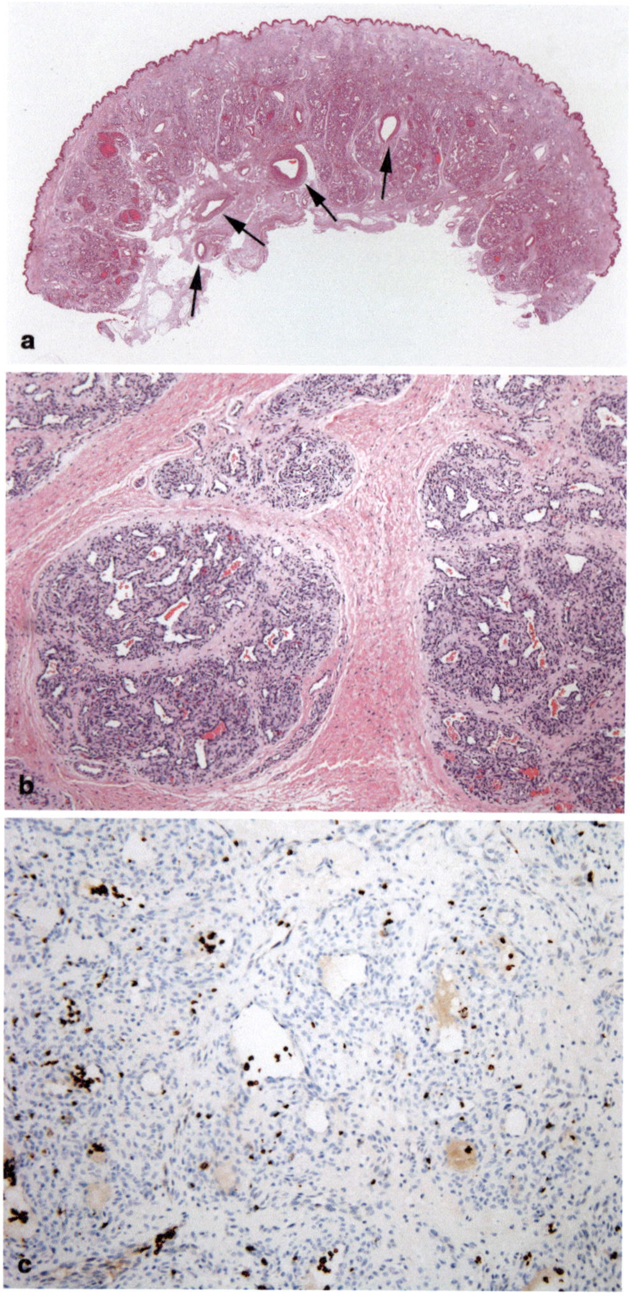

Fig. 24.4 Congenital hemangioma (CH) of the scalp. **a** CH expanding diffusely into the dermis. Large feeding vessels are present at the base (*arrows*). **b** The hemangioma has a distinct lobular pattern of growth. Small vascular channels form the lobules, which are centered by larger channels containing blood. **c** In contrast to infantile hemangioma, immunohistochemistry for Glut-1 is negative in endothelial cells. Circulating red blood cells are immunoreactive for Glut-1 (*dark brown staining cells*)

osteoporosis, adrenal insufficiency, cataracts, and glaucoma) are associated with high-dose, long-term therapy [42, 43] and have not been observed in patients treated with corticosteroid for IH [39–41, 44]. Unlike individuals with hypercortisolism or receiving chronic corticosteroid, children with IH are only treated for several months [39]. In addition, the drug is rapidly weaned as (1) the infant gains weight and (2) the physician lowers the dose [39].

Propanolol has been described for the management of IH, but its efficacy and safety compared to corticosteroid has not been studied [39, 45, 46]. Some authors report that all IHs respond to propanolol [45, 46]; however, treatment failures have been described [47–49]. Furthermore, several complications have been reported in infants receiving propanolol for IH: bronchospasm [46, 48], bradycardia [50–53], hypotension [46, 51–54], hypoglycemia [50–53, 55, 56], seizures [52, 55], psoriatic-like rash [49], hyperkalemia [57], and diarrhea [58]. Hypoglycemia, hypotension, and seizures in infancy can result in permanent adverse neurological morbidity [59, 60].

Unlike patients managed with corticosteroid for IH, infants receiving propranolol require close monitoring for potential drug toxicity. Prior to the initiation of treatment, patients typically are evaluated with a baseline electrocardiogram and echocardiogram, vital signs, and blood glucose measurement; cardiology consultation usually is obtained [46, 49, 51, 60–62]. During the initiation of treatment, infants are either hospitalized or have their vital signs and blood glucose monitored at home [46, 48, 49, 60–62].

Compared to propranolol therapy, management of IH with corticosteroid is more comfortable for the infant, easier for the parents and physician, and less-expensive [39]. The parents and physician managing a child on corticosteroid also have less concern about an acute, life-threatening adverse drug event, compared to the infant receiving propanolol.

Congenital Hemangioma RICH may be complicated by congestive heart failure, which is typically controlled by corticosteroid as the lesion involutes. Unlike RICH, NICH does not respond to pharmacotherapy [10]. Rarely, RICH or NICH causing heart failure may require embolization.

Kaposiform Hemangioendothelioma Treatment depends on the size of the lesion and presence of KMP. Patients with KMP require intervention to prevent life-threatening complications. Children with large lesions without KMP also are treated to reduce fibrosis and subsequent long-term pain and stiffness [10]. The first-line treatment for KHE is vincristine; the response rate is 90 % [63]. KHE does not respond as well to second-line drugs such as interferon (50 %) or corticosteroid (10 %) [28, 63]. Platelet transfusion does not improve thrombocytopenia; platelets are trapped in the lesion worsening the swelling [10]. Platelet transfusion should be avoided unless there is active bleeding or a surgical procedure is indicated [28]. Heparin is contraindicated because it can promote tumor growth, aggravate platelet trapping, and worsen bleeding [28].

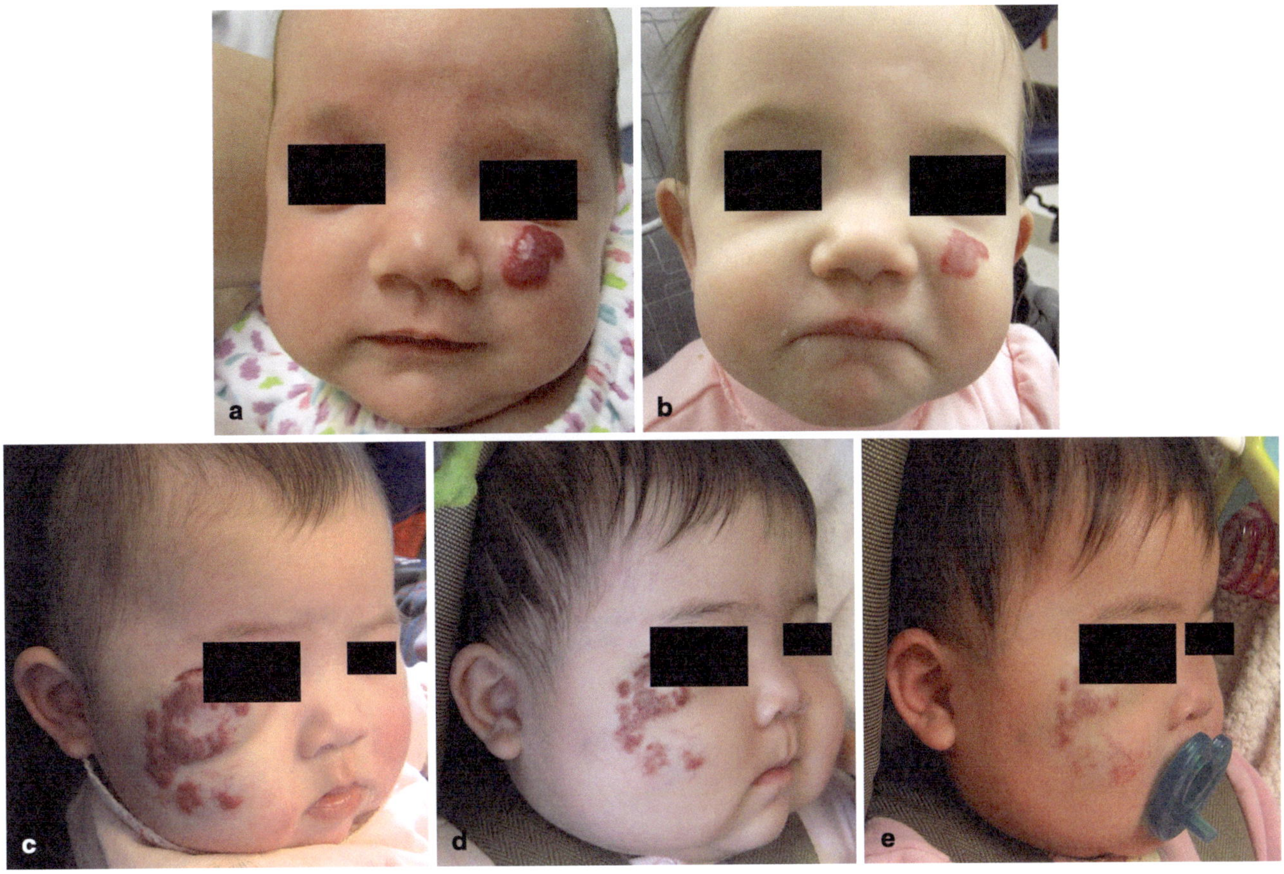

Fig. 24.5 Management of infantile hemangioma (IH) with intralesional or systemic corticosteroid. **a** Three-month-old female child treated with triamcinolone injection. **b** Accelerated involution at 12 months of age. **c** Four-month-old female child prior to initiation of oral corticosteroid. **d** After 1 month of drug treatment, the IH has regressed. **e** Age 12 months, after completing corticosteroid therapy

Operative Management

Infantile Hemangioma Surgical intervention during the proliferating phase is not recommended. Because the tumor is highly vascular, the risk for blood loss, iatrogenic injury, and a poor outcome is high [10, 39, 64]. Factors that lower the threshold for excision of a problematic, proliferating IH are: (1) failure or contraindication to corticosteroid, (2) localized lesion in a safe anatomical area, (3) complicated reconstruction is not necessary, and (4) resection will be required in the future and the scar will be the same [10, 18].

During the involuting phase the hemangioma is less-vascular and smaller; thus, resection is safer, less extensive, and the scar is shorter [10]. Excision should be considered during this period, rather than waiting for complete regression if: (1) reconstruction is inevitable (e.g., destroyed structures, expanded skin, postulceration scarring, and significant fibrofatty residuum), (2) the length of the scar would be similar, and (3) the scar is in a favorable location (see Fig. 24.6) [10]. Because long-term memory and personal identity begin to develop around 3.5 years of age, an advantage of intervening during this period is that psychosocial morbidity may be prevented [10].

Delaying the resection until the IH has fully involuted guarantees that the least amount of fibrofatty residuum and excess skin is resected, giving the smallest possible scar [10]. However, allowing the tumor to completely regress must be weighed against potential psychosocial morbidity. Permitting full involution is advocated when it is unclear if a surgical scar would leave a greater deformity than the appearance of the residual hemangioma [10]. IH acts as a tissue expander, and thus adequate skin usually enables linear closure of the wound. Circular lesions located in visible areas are best managed by circular excision and purse-string closure [65]. This technique takes advantage of the loose skin created by the tumor and reduces the length of the scar, as well as distortion of surrounding structures [65]. A lenticular excision of a circular IH results in a scar as long as 3 times the diameter of the lesion, whereas a 2-stage circular resection followed by a lenticular excision 6–12 months later leaves a scar approximately the same length as the diameter of the original tumor [65]. The disadvantage of circular excision and purse-string closure is that a second stage may be required, and the skin around the edges of the circular scar may not flatten for several weeks [65]. In the scalp, lenticular

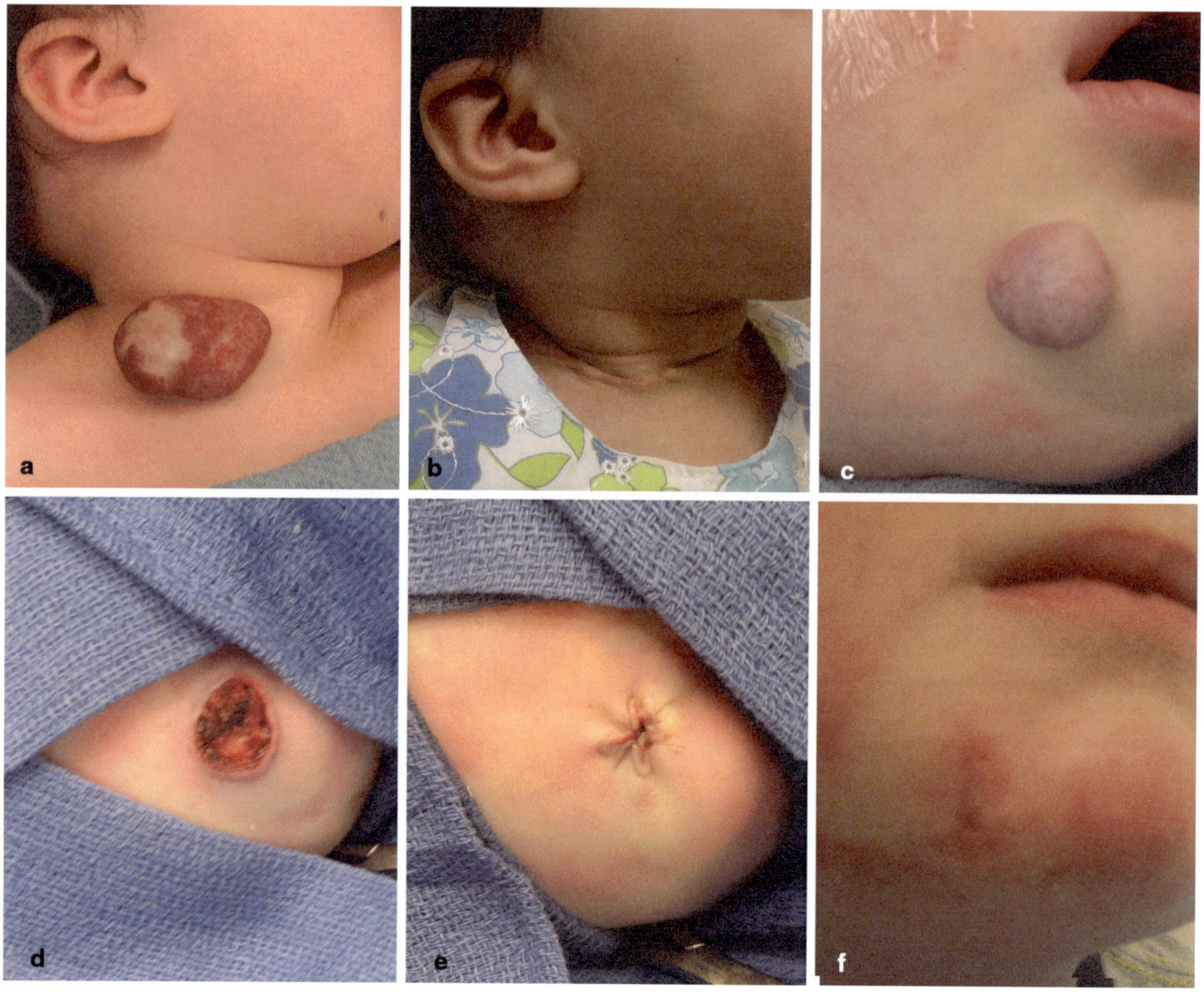

Fig. 24.6 Operative management of infantile hemangioma (IH). **a** A 2.5-year-old female patient with fibrofatty residuum. **b** A one-stage lenticular excision was performed because the length-to-width ratio favored linear closure, and the scar is placed in a relaxed skin tension line. **c–f** A 2.5-year-old male patient with a residual fibrofatty IH of the chin. Circular excision and purse-string closure was chosen to confine the scar length to the diameter of the original lesion. (Reprinted from [10], pp. 54–55, with permission from Elsevier)

excision and linear closure is preferred to circular resection and purse-string closure because: (1) the length of the scar is not critical because it is covered by hair, (2) it is a one-stage procedure, (3) the scalp lacks the skin redundancy necessary for purse-string closure, and (4) the circular scar may result in an area of alopecia requiring another procedure [10].

Pulsed-dye laser (PDL) treatment is contraindicated for a proliferating IH. The laser penetrates only 0.75–1.2 mm and thus, only treats the superficial portion of the tumor. Although lightening may happen, the subcutaneous component is not affected and accelerated involution does not occur [66, 67]. Patients have an increased risk of bleeding, hypopigmentation, pain, scarring, and skin atrophy [66–68]. However, PDL is indicated during the involuted phase to treat residual telangiectasias [10]. Unlike the PDL, a carbon dioxide laser may be used to treat a proliferating subglottic IH [69].

Congenital Hemangioma Because RICH undergoes accelerated postnatal regression, surgical intervention is not required during infancy; tumors are observed [10]. RICH can leave behind atrophic tissue that may be reconstructed with autologous grafts or acellular dermis [10]. Residual telangiectasias can be lightened with PDL [10].

Most NICHs are nonproblematic and do not cause significant deformity. However, the threshold for resection of a problematic NICH is lower than for IH, because NICHs do not involute or respond to pharmacotherapy [10]. PDL or resection may improve the appearance of the lesion [10].

Kaposiform Hemangioendothelioma KHE typically involves multiple tissue planes and important structures, making the tumor difficult to resect [10]. Excision may be indicated for symptomatic patients with localized tumors or for lesions that have failed chemotherapy [10]. Reconstruction for secondary deformities caused by the tumor (e.g. contractures) may be necessary. Because KHE is benign, resection of an asymptomatic lesion is unnecessary.

Pyogenic Granuloma PG should be treated after diagnosis to prevent ulceration and bleeding. Numerous interventions have been described: curettage, shave excision, laser therapy, or full-thickness resection [15, 70]. Because lesions involve the reticular dermis, PDL, cautery, or shave excision may not treat the entire lesion; the recurrence rate for these modalities is 43.5% [15]. Definitive treatment of PG is full-thickness skin excision.

References

1. Mulliken JB, Glowacki J. Hemangiomas and vascular malformations in infants and children: a classification based on endothelial characteristics. Plast Reconstr Surg. 1982;69:412–22.
2. Khan ZA, Boscolo E, Picard A, et al. Multipotential stem cells recapitulate human infantile hemangioma in immunodeficient mice. J Clin Invest. 2008;118:2592–9.
3. North PE, Waner M, Mizeracki A, et al. A unique microvascular phenotype shared by juvenile hemangiomas and human placenta. Arch Dermatol. 2002;137:559–70.
4. Barnes CM, Huang S, Kaipainen A, et al. Evidence of molecular profiling for a placental origin of infantile hemangioma. Proc Natl Acad Sci USA. 2005;102:19097–102.
5. Boscolo E, Bischoff J. Vasculogenesis in infantile hemangioma. Angiogenesis. 2009;12:197–207.
6. Jinnin M, Medici D, Park L, et al. Suppressed NFAT-dependent VEGFR1 expression and constitutive VEGFR2 signaling in infantile hemangioma. Nat Med. 2008;14:1236–46.
7. Bielenberg DR, Bucana CD, Sanchez R, et al. Progressive growth of infantile cutaneous hemangiomas is directly correlated with hyperplasia and angiogenesis of adjacent epidermis and inversely correlated with expression of the endogenous angiogenesis inhibitor, IFN-beta. Int J Oncol. 1999;14:401–8.
8. Kilcline C, Frieden IJ. Infantile hemangiomas: how common are they? A systematic review of the medical literature. Pediatr Dermatol. 2008;25:168–73.
9. Greene AK, Liu AS, Mulliken JB, et al. Vascular anomalies in 5621 patients: guidelines for referral. J Peditr Surg. 2011;46(9):1784–9.
10. Greene AK. Management of hemangiomas and other vascular tumors. Clin Plast Surg. 2011;38(1):45–63.
11. Boon LM, Burrows PE, Paltiel HJ, et al. Hepatic vascular anomalies in infancy: a twenty-seven-year experience. J Pediatr. 1996;129:346–54.
12. Enjolras O, Mulliken JB, Boon LM, et al. Noninvoluting congenital hemangioma: a rare cutaneous vascular anomaly. Plast Reconstr Surg. 2001;107:1647–54.
13. Berenguer B, Mulliken JB, Enjolras O, et al. Rapidly involuting congenital hemangioma: clinical and histopathologic features. Pediatr Dev Pathol. 2003;6:495–510.
14. Lyons LL, North PE, Mac-Moune Lai F, et al. Kaposiform hemangioendothelioma: a study of 33 cases emphasizing its pathologic, immunophenotypic, and biologic uniqueness from juvenile hemangioma. Am J Surg Pathol. 2004;28:559–68.
15. Patrice SJ, Wiss K, Mulliken JB. Pyogenic granuloma (lobular capillary hemangioma): a clinicopathologic study of 178 cases. Pediatr Dermatol. 1991;8:267–76.
16. Amir J, Metzker A, Krikler R, et al. Strawberry hemangioma in preterm infants. Pediatr Dermatol. 1986;3:331–2.
17. Haggstrom AN, Drolet BA, Baselga E, et al. Prospective study of infantile hemangiomas: demographic, prenatal, and perinatal characteristics. J Pediatr. 2007;150:291–4.
18. Mulliken JB, Fishman SJ, Burrows PE. Vascular Anomalies. Curr Prob Surg. 2000;37:517–84.
19. Horii KA, Drolet BA, Frieden IJ. Prospective study of the frequency of hepatic hemangiomas in infants with multiple cutaneous infantile hemangiomas. Pediatr Dermatol. 2011;28:245–53.
20. Frieden IJ, Reese V, Cohen D. PHACE syndrome. The association of posterior fossa brain malformations, hemangiomas, arterial anomalies, coarctation of the aorta and cardiac defects and eye abnormalities. Arch Dermatol. 1996;132:307–11.
21. Metry DW, Garzon MC, Drolet BA, et al. PHACE syndrome: current knowledge, future directions. Ped Derm. 2009;26:381–98.
22. Chang LC, Haggstrom AN, Drolet BA, et al. Growth characteristics of infantile hemangiomas: implications for management. Pediatrics. 2008;122:360–7.
23. Chamlin SL, Haggstrom AN, Drolet BA, et al. Multicenter prospective study of ulcerated hemangiomas. J Pediatr. 2007;151:684–9.
24. Zukerberg LR, Nikoloff BJ, Weiss SW. Kaposiform hemangioendothelioma of infancy and childhood: an aggressive neoplasm associated with Kasabach-Merritt syndrome and lymphangiomatosis. Am J Surg Pathol. 1993;17:321–8.
25. Sarkar M, Mulliken JB, Kozakewich HP, et al. Thrombocytopenic coagulopathy (Kasabach-Merritt phenomenon) is associated with kaposiform hemangioendothelioma and not with common infantile hemangioma. Plast Reconstr Surg. 1997;100:1377–86.
26. Enjolras O, Mulliken JB, Wassef M, et al. Residual lesions after Kasabach-Merritt phenomenon in 41 patients. J Am Acad Dermatol. 2000;42:225–35.
27. Enjolras O, Gelbert F. Superficial hemangiomas: associations and management. Pediatr Dermatol. 1997;14:173–9.
28. Mulliken JB, Anupindi S, Ezekowitz RA, et al. Case 13–2004: a newborn girl with a large cutaneous lesion, thrombocytopenia, and anemia. New Engl J Med. 2004;350:1764–75.
29. Paltiel H, Burrows PE, Kozakewich HPW, et al. Soft-tissue vascular anomalies: utility of US for diagnosis. Radiology. 2000;214:747–54.
30. Burrows PE, Laor T, Paltiel H, et al. Diagnostic imaging in the evaluation of vascular birthmarks. Dermatol Clin. 1998;16:455–88.
31. Karnes JC, Lee BT, Phung T, et al. Adult-onset kaposiform hemangioendothelioma in a post-traumatic site. Ann Plast Surg. 2009;62:456–8.
32. Gupta A, Kozakewich H. Histopathological of vascular anomalies. Clin Plast Surg. 2011;38(1):31–44.
33. North PE, Waner M, Mizeracki A, et al. GLUT1. A newly discovered immunohistochemical marker for juvenile hemangiomas. Hum Path. 2000;31:11–22.
34. Mentzel T, Mazzoleni G, Dei Tos AP, et al. Kaposiform hemangioendothelioma in adults. Clinicopathologic and immunohistochemical analysis of three cases. Am J Clin Pathol. 1997;108:450–5.
35. Mills SE, Cooper PH, Fechner RE. Lobular capillary hemangioma: the underlying lesion of pyogenic granuloma. Am J Surg Pathol. 1980;4:470–9.
36. Cruz OA, Zarnegar SR, Myers SE. Treatment of periocular capillary hemangioma with topical clobetasol propionate. Ophthalmology. 1995;102:2012–5.
37. Garzon MC, Lucky AW, Hawrot A, et al. Ultrapotent topical corticosteroid treatment of hemangiomas of infancy. J Am Acad Dermatol. 2005;52:281–6.
38. Sloan GM, Renisch JF, Nichter LS, et al. Intralesional corticosteroid therapy for infantile hemangiomas. Plast Reconstr Surg. 1989;83:459–67.
39. Greene AK, Couto RA. Oral prednisolone for infantile hemangioma: efficacy and safety using standardized treatment protocol. Plast Reconstr Surg. 2011;128:743–52.

40. Boon LM, MacDonald DM, Mulliken JB. Complications of systemic corticosteroid therapy for problematic hemangiomas. Plast Reconstr Surg. 1999;104:1616–23.
41. Lomenick JP, Backeljauw PF, Lucky AW. Growth, bone mineral accretion, and adrenal function in glucocorticoid-treated infants with hemangiomas – a retrospective study. Pediatr Dermatol. 2006;23:169–74.
42. Seale JP, Compton MR. Side-effects of corticosteroid agents. Med J Aust. 1986;144:139–42.
43. Fardet L, Abdulrhaman K, Cabane J, et al. Corticosteroid-induced adverse events in adults: frequency, screening and prevention. Drug Saf. 2007;30:861–81.
44. Bennett ML, Fleischer AB, Chamlin SL, et al. Oral corticosteroid use is effective for cutaneous hemangiomas. Arch Dermatol. 2001;137:1208–13.
45. Leaute-Labreze C, Dumas delaRE, Hubiche T, et al. Propranolol for severe hemangiomas of infancy. N Engl J Med. 2008;358:2649–51.
46. Sans V, Dumas delaRE, Berge J, et al. Propranolol for severe infantile hemangiomas: follow-up report. Pediatrics. 2009;124:423–31.
47. Canadas KT, Baum ED, Lee S, et al. Case report: treatment failure using propranolol for treatment of focal subglottic hemangioma. Int J Pediatr Otorhinolaryngol. 2010;74:956–8.
48. Leboulanger N, Fayoux P, Teissier N, et al. Propranolol in the therapeutic strategy of infantile laryngotracheal hemangioma: a preliminary retrospective study of French experience. Int J Pediatr Otorhinolaryngol. 2010;74:1254–7.
49. Buckmiller LM, Munson PD, Dyamenahalli U, et al. Propranolol for infantile hemangiomas: early experience at a tertiary vascular anomalies center. Laryngoscope. 2010;120:676–81.
50. Frieden IL, Drolet BA. Propranolol for infantile hemangiomas: promise, peril, pathogenesis. Pediatr Dermatol. 2009;26:642–4.
51. Lawley LP, Siegfried E, Todd JL. Propranolol treatment for hemangioma of infancy: risks and recommendations. Pediatr Dermatol. 2009;26:610–4.
52. Holland KE, Frieden IJ, Frommelt PC, et al. Hypoglycemia in children taking propranolol for the treatment of infantile hemangioma. Arch Dermatol. 2010;146:775–8.
53. Rosbe KW, Suh KY, Meyer AK, et al. Propranolol in the management of airway infantile hemangiomas. Arch Otolaryngol Head Neck Surg. 2010;136:658–65.
54. Chik KK, Luk CK, Chan HB, et al. Use of propranolol in infantile haemangioma among chinese children. Hong Kong Med J. 2010;16:341–6.
55. Bonifazi E, Acquafredda A, Milano A, et al. Severe hypoglycemia during successful treatment of diffuse hemangiomatosis with propranolol. Pediatr Dermatol. 2010;27:195–6.
56. Breur J, Graaf M de, Breugem CC, et al. Hypoglycemia as a result of propranolol during treatment of infantile hemangioma: a case report. Pediatr Dermatol. 2010;27:1–3.
57. Pavlakovic H, Kietz S., Lauerer P, et al. Hyperkalemia complicating propranolol treatment of an infantile hemangioma. Pediatrics. 2010;126:e1589–93.
58. Abbott J, Parulekar M, Shahidullah H, et al. Diarrhea associated with propranolol treatment for hemangioma of infancy (HOI). Pediatr Dermatol. 2010;27:558.
59. Burns CM, Rutherford MA, Boardman JP, et al. Patterns of cerebral injury and neurodevelopmental outcomes after symptomatic neonatal hypoglycemia. Pediatrics. 2008;122:65–74.
60. Siegfried EC, Keenan WJ, Al-Jureidini S. More on propranolol for hemangiomas of infancy. N Engl J Med. 2008;359:2846–7.
61. Manunza F, Syed S, Laguda B, et al. Propranolol for complicated infantile hemangiomas: a case series of 30 infants. Br J Dermatol. 2010;162:466–8.
62. Truong MT, Perkins JA, Messner A, et al. Propranolol for the treatment of airway hemangiomas: a case series and treatment algorithm. Int J Pediatr Otorhinolaryngol. 2010;74:1043–8.
63. Haisley-Royster C, Enjolras O, Frieden IJ, et al. Kasabach-Merritt phenomenon: a retrospective study of treatment with vincristine. J Pediatr Hematol Oncol. 2002;24:459–62.
64. Greene AK, Rogers G, Mulliken JB. Management of parotid hemangioma in 100 children. Plast Reconstr Surg. 2004;113:53–60.
65. Mulliken JB, Rogers GF, Marler JJ. Circular excision of hemangioma and purse-string closure: the smallest possible scar. Plast Reconstr Surg. 2002;109:1544–54.
66. Scheepers JH, Quaba AA. Does the pulsed tunable dye laser have a role in the management of infantile hemangiomas: observations based on 3 years experience. Plast Reconstr Surg. 1995;95:305–12.
67. Batta K, Goodyear HM, Moss C, et al. Randomized controlled study of early pulsed dye laser treatment of uncomplicated childhood haemangiomas: results of a 1-year analysis. Lancet. 2002;360:521–7.
68. Witman PM, Wagner AM, Scherer K, et al. Complications following pulsed dye laser treatment of superficial hemangiomas. Lasers Surg Med. 2006;38:116–23.
69. Sie KC, McGill T, Healy GB. Subglottic hemangioma: ten years experience with carbon dioxide laser. Ann Otol Rhinol Laryngol. 1994;103:167–72.
70. Kirschner RE, Low DW. Treatment of pyogenic granuloma by shave excision and laser photocoagulation. Plast Reconstr Surg. 1999;104:1346–9.

25 Juvenile Nasopharyngeal Angiofibroma

Karen Watters, Trevor McGill and Reza Rahbar

Introduction

Juvenile nasopharyngeal angiofibroma (JNA) is a rare benign tumor occurring almost exclusively in the nasopharynx of adolescent and young adult males. The tumor is slow growing but is characterized by locally aggressive growth, high vascularization, and a tendency to persist and recur.

Epidemiology and Biology

The incidence of JNA is approximately 1 in 150,000, accounting for 0.05–0.5 % of all head and neck neoplasms [1]. Although the etiology of JNA is unknown, a variety of growth factors and hormones are thought to have a role in tumor biology. Androgen dependency is the strongest explanation for its exclusivity in young male patients [2]. A number of other theories of etiopathogenesis have been suggested including [2, 3]:

- Undifferentiated epithelioid nest cells
- Desmoplastic response of the nasopharyngeal periosteum
- Embryonic fibrocartilage between the basiocciput and the basisphenoid
- Nonchromaffin paraganglionic cells of the terminal branches of the maxillary artery

K. Watters (✉)
Otolaryngology and Communication Enhancement, Boston Children's Hospital, Harvard Medical School, Boston, MA, USA
e-mail: karen.watters@childrens.harvard.edu

T. McGill
Department of Otolaryngology and Communication Enhancement, Boston Children's Hospital, Harvard Medical School, Boston, MA, USA

R. Rahbar
Department of Otolaryngology, Boston Children's Hospital, Harvard Medical School, Boston, MA, USA

Origin and Spread of JNA

The site of origin of JNA remains controversial; however, it is thought to originate from the superior lip of the sphenopalatine foramen (posterolateral nasal wall) at the junction of the pterygoid process of the sphenoid bone and the sphenoid process of the palatine bone [4]. Other sites of origin have been described, including the pterygopalatine fossa, the nasopharynx at the base of the sphenoid bone, the sphenoid sinus, paranasal region, and the lacrimal sac [5–7].

The tumor grows in the submucosal plane, spreading medially into the nasal cavity and nasopharynx [8, 9]. The tumor characteristically grows laterally through the pterygopalatine fissure into the pterygomaxillary fossa. Tumor extension into the sphenoid, maxillary, and ethmoidal sinuses, orbit, parasellar region, and middle cranial fossa is common. Erosion of the posterior wall of the maxillary sinus is usually caused by direct extension of tumor from the infratemporal fossa. In approximately one third of cases, tumor grows into the orbit from the ethmoid labyrinth through the medial orbital wall or through the inferior orbital fissure [10]. This is characterized by displacement of the orbital tissues without tissue infiltration. Intracranial extension, which is usually extradural, occurs secondary to tumor extension through the roof of the infratemporal fossa or via the superior orbital fissure, with subsequent extension into the cavernous sinus (Table 25.1).

JNA, in most cases, spreads through the paranasal sinuses by "pushing" of bony walls without destruction. Intracranial involvement secondary to skull base invasion is caused by local bony destruction through relentless expansion rather than cellular infiltration [11].

Blood Supply

In most cases, JNA receives the majority of its blood supply from the ipsilateral internal maxillary artery, a terminal branch of the external carotid artery [12]. The ascending pharyngeal artery and vidian artery may also contribute to

R. Rahbar et al. (eds.), *Pediatric Head and Neck Tumors*,
DOI 10.1007/978-1-4614-8755-5_25,

Table 25.1 Sites and routes of spread of JNA

Site of spread	Route of spread
1. Nasal cavity and nasopharynx	Medially through sphenopalatine foramen
2. Infratemporal fossa	Laterally through pterygomaxillary fissure
3. Maxillary sinus	Anteriorly by destruction and dislocation of sinus walls
4. Pterygopalatine fossa	Through inferior orbital fissure
5. Orbit	Through inferior orbital fissure
	Through medial orbital wall from ethmoid labyrinth
6. Ethmoid and sphenoid sinuses	Through natural ostia
	By bony destruction
7. Middle cranial fossa	From infratemporal fossa
	Through foramina (rotundum, ovale, lacerum)
	By bony destruction of greater sphenoid wings and pterygoids process
	Through superior orbital fissure
	By destruction of wall of sphenoid sinus
8. Anterior cranial fossa	By destruction of ethmoid roof
9. Cavernous sinus and chiasmatic-sellar region	By destruction of boundaries of sphenoid sinus

the blood supply. In rare cases, the tumor is supplied by unnamed branches from the internal carotid artery. Bilateral vascular supply of a JNA is rare, but has been reported and its incidence in JNA may in fact be underappreciated [13].

Presentation

The classic presentation of JNA is an adolescent male patient (mean 15 years of age) with the following:

1. Nasal obstruction (painless)
2. Epistaxis (usually unilateral)
3. Nasopharyngeal mass

Onset of JNA is most commonly in the second decade, ranging from 7 to 21 years of age. Mean age at diagnosis is 15 years of age [14, 15]. It is rare in patients older than 25 years of age. Symptoms are typically present for at least 6 to 12 months before the patient attends for assessment [14].

Advanced Disease JNA is a slow growing tumor but extranasopharyngeal symptoms can manifest as a result of its locally destructive nature and local spread. Facial swelling, proptosis, headache, visual disturbance, and cranial nerve palsies may be signs of advanced disease [14, 15]. Rare presenting symptoms include hyponasal speech, hyposmia, hearing loss, dacrocystitis, and palatal swelling or deformity [16]. Patients with intracranial extension, secondary to tumor extension through the roof of the infratemporal fossa or via the superior orbital fissure with extension into the cavernous sinus, may present with the classic signs of superior orbital fissure syndrome, ptosis, paralysis of extraocular muscles, and exophthalmos. Intracranial spread is observed in approximately 10–20% of all patients with JNA [11].

Table 25.2 Differential diagnosis of JNA

Inflammatory	Antrochoanal nasal polyp
	Nasal polyposis
	Inverting papilloma
Congenital/developmental	Dermoid cyst
	Encephalocele
Neoplastic	Rhabdomyosarcoma
	Squamous cell carcinoma
	Lymphoma

Differential Diagnosis

All causes of a nasopharyngeal mass, epistaxis, and orbital swelling should be included in the differential diagnosis of a JNA (Table 25.2).

Diagnosis and Evaluation

Clinical history and presentation should raise suspicion for JNA. A comprehensive history and physical examination is essential in all patients.

Examination

Examination includes a thorough nasoendoscopy, which typically reveals a vascular lesion with prominent submucosal blood vessels arising along the posterolateral wall of the nasal cavity at the sphenopalatine foramen, and frequently spreading anteriorly into the nasal cavity and posteriorly into the nasopharynx. Grossly, JNA appears sessile, lobulated, rubbery, and red-pink in appearance. It may be polypoid or pedunculated (Fig. 25.1a, b).

Other clinical findings on examination may include serous otitis due to eustachian tube blockage, zygomatic swelling, and trismus, which may indicate tumor spread to the infratemporal fossa. Vision may also be decreased secondary to spread into the orbit or tenting of the optic nerve.

Imaging Evaluation

Advances in imaging techniques allow for accurate measurement of tumor, and evaluation of its localization and spread, all of which are essential to enable correct staging

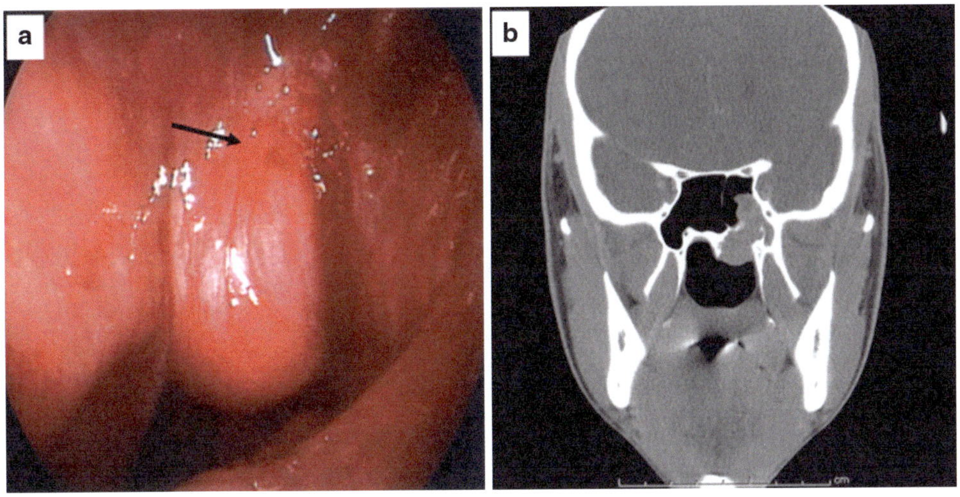

Fig. 25.1 Localized JNA. **a** Endoscopic image of a localized angiofibroma located at the sphenopalatine foramen in the left nasopharynx. The *black arrow* shows a site of pulsation consistent with the location of the sphenopalatine artery. **b** Coronal CT scan showing a soft tissue lesion centered on the left sphenopalatine foramen. It is extending into the left sphenoid sinus and left nasopharynx

and appropriate surgical planning. Plain radiography images of the sinuses may show opacification, but their usefulness has essentially been surpassed by newer radiographic modalities. Computed tomography (CT) and magnetic resonance imaging (MRI) with contrast enhancement are the two most commonly utilized modalities [5]. Due to the vascular nature of JNA, angiography is also important to identify the primary vessels that feed the tumor and allow for preoperative embolization to reduce intraoperative blood loss.

- **CT** scan is excellent for evaluation of bony erosion and extension of the tumor into the skull base. JNAs appear as hyperintense lesions on CT (Fig. 25.2a, b, c). Characteristic anterior bowing of the posterior wall of the maxillary sinus seen on CT, due to tumor in the pterygomaxillary space, is known as Holman-Miller's sign [11].
- **MRI** is indicated to delineate the extent of the tumor, especially in cases of intracranial involvement and extension into the cavernous sinus. MRI characteristics of JNA depend on the relative combination of vascular fibrous components and tissue edema. JNAs are markedly enhanced on contrast-enhanced T1-weighted MRI with multiple flow-related signal voids and have a lobulated appearance of variable signal intensity on T2-weighted MR images (Fig. 25.3a, b, c). MRI also enables the distinction between inssipated secretions in obstructed sinuses and tumor, which is important to prevent upstaging of the tumor.

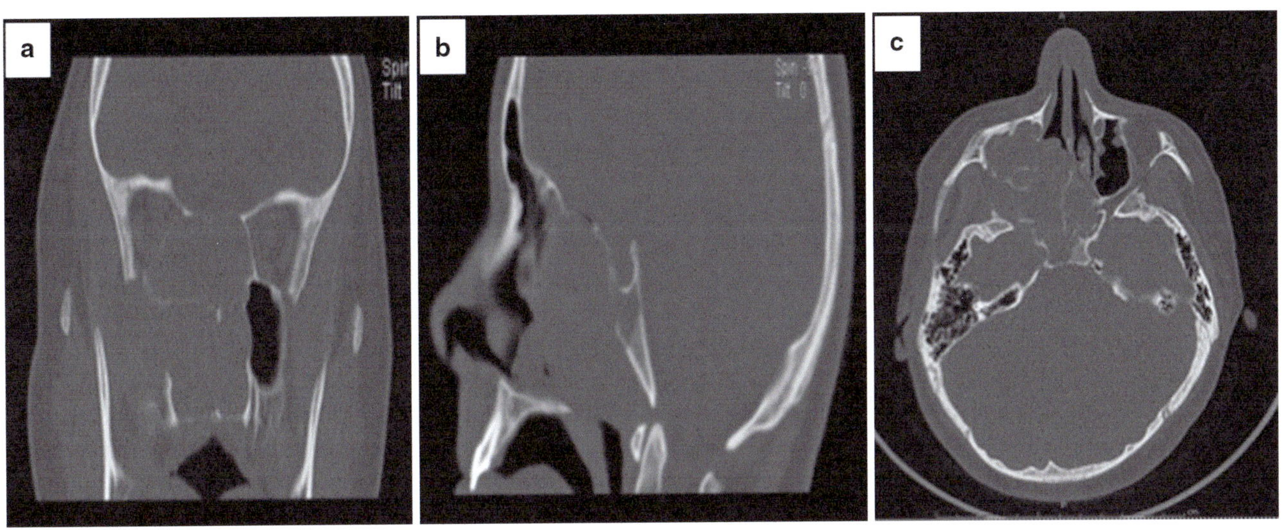

Fig. 25.2 Advanced JNA. Coronal (**a**), saggital (**b**), and axial (**c**) maxillofacial CT images showing a large right nasopharyngeal mass with a widened sphenopalatine foramen (**a**). The mass extends into the right pterygopalatine fossa with erosion of the right medial pterygoid plate (**c**). There is invasion of the clivus with erosion of the posterior wall of the clivus (**b**, **c**). There is erosion through the planum sphenoidale, with several foci of air at the site of cranial vault dehiscence (**b**)

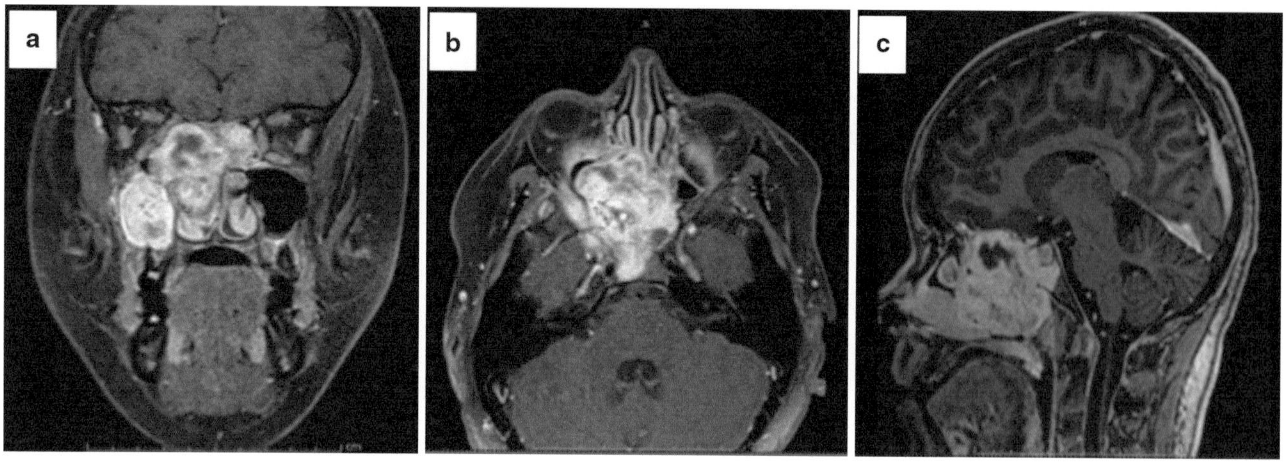

Fig. 25.3 Advanced JNA. Coronal (**a**), axial (**b**), and saggital (**c**) T1-weighted maxillofacial MRI images post contrast showing a large nasopharyngeal mass with multiple flow-related signal voids (**a**, **b**). Laterally the mass extends into the right maxillary antrum and right pterygopalatine fossa (**a**, **b**). The right medial and inferior recti muscles are displaced laterally by the mass, with convex remodeling of the right orbital floor (**a**). There is invasion of the clivus with erosion of the posterior wall of the clivus and through the planum sphenoidale (**b**, **c**). The mass erodes the anterior right carotid canal with possible invasion of the cavernous sinus (**c**). There is erosion of the right vidian canal and the right foramen rotundum is expanded (**b**)

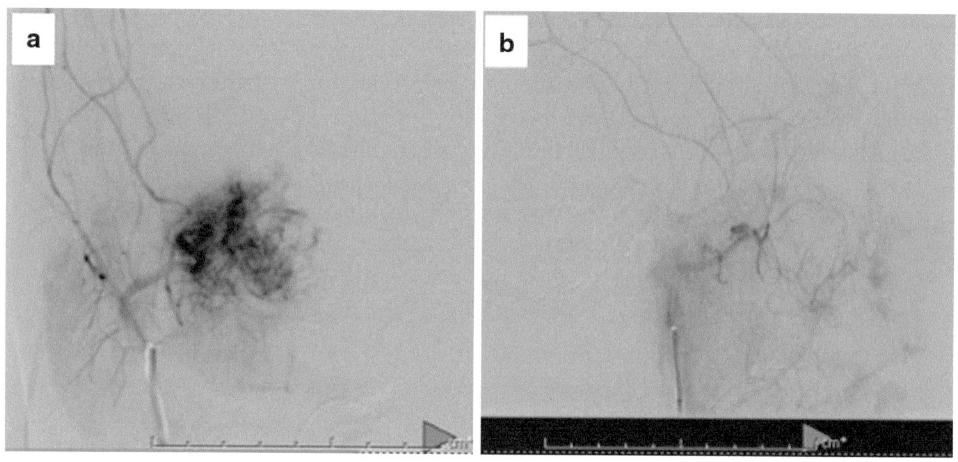

Fig. 25.4 Angiography and embolization of the right internal maxillary artery. Characteristic "tumor blush" seen in JNA following catheterization of right internal maxillary artery (**a**). Following selective embolization of distal right internal maxillary artery using PVA particles, there is virtually no residual tumor blush (**b**)

- **Angiography** should be routinely performed preoperatively. The characteristic "angiographic tumor blush" of JNA identifies the branches of the internal maxillary, ascending pharyngeal, and palatine arteries supplying the tumor (Fig. 25.4a, b).

Biopsy

Biopsy is almost never required prior to surgical intervention. In most cases it is avoided due to the vascular nature of JNA and the possibility of causing severe hemorrhage. The characteristic age of the patient, clinical presentation, and imaging features usually permit a confident preoperative diagnosis of JNA to be made without the need for tissue diagnosis. Key features of JNA, including the location in the nose and pterygopalatine fossa, prominent vascularity, and pattern of bony erosion posteriorly help to distinguish JNA from other tumors found in this site including rhabdomyosarcoma and lymphoma.

Staging

There is no consensus on the ideal staging system for JNA. Several staging systems have been proposed, including those of Sessions, Andrews, Chandler, and Radkowski [17–21]. The common feature of these systems is that staging is based on tumor spread, and sites of involvement, assessed radiologically by CT and MRI. Advanced lesions are those with skull base involvement and intracranial extension. A more recent staging system, UPMC staging system, was

Table 25.3 Staging systems for JNA

	Stage				
System	I	II	III	IV	V
Sessions et al. 1981	Ia: limited to nose and nasopharynx	IIa: minimal extension into pterygomaxillary fossa	Intracranial extension	NA	
	Ib: extension into $\geq$ 1 sinus	IIb: full occupation of pterygomaxillary fossas with or without orbital involvement			
		IIIc: extension into infratemporal fossa with or without cheek extension			
Chandler et al. 1984	Limited to nasopharynx	Extension into nasal cavity or sphenoid sinus	Extension into maxillary antrum, ethmoid sinus, pterygomaxillary fossa, infratemporal fossa, orbit, and/or cheek	Intracranial extension	
Andrews et al. 1989	Limited to nasopharynx; limited to sphenopalatine foramen; no bone destruction	Invading sphenoid, ethmoid, maxillary sinus or pterygopalatine fossa with bony destruction	Invading infratemporal fossa or orbit;	Intracranial, intradural extension;	
			IIIa: no intracranial extension	IVa: with cavernous sinus, pituitary or optic chiasm infiltration	
			IIIb: extradural extension	IVb: without cavernous sinus, pituitary or optic chiasm infiltration	
Radkowski et al. 1996	Ia: limited to nose or nasopharynx	IIa: extension through sphenopalatine foramen and into pterygomaxillary fossa	Erosion of skull base:	NA	
	Ib: extension into $\geq$ 1 sinus	IIb: fully occupying pterygomaxillary fossa, posterior maxillary wall displaced forward, orbit erosion	IIIa: minimal intracranial extension		
		IIc: extension to infratemporal fossa, cheek, posterior to prerygoid plates, sphenoid sinus or pterygopalatine fossa with bony destruction	IIIb: extensive intracranial extension $\pm$ cavernous sinus involvement		
University of Pittsburg Medical Center (UPMC) 2010	Nasal cavity, medial pterygopalatine fossa	Paranasal sinuses, lateral pterygopalatine fossa; no residual vascularity	Skull base erosion, orbit, infratemporal fossa; no residual vascularity	Skull base erosion, orbit, infratemporal fossa; residual vascularity	Intracranial extension, residual vascularity; medial extension (M), lateral extension (L)

proposed by Synderman et al. 2010, which accounts for two important prognostic factors, including tumor vascularity (the extent of vascular supply from the internal carotid artery) and route of skull base extension [22]. This newer staging system reflects changes in surgical approach, that is the increasing use of the endoscopic approach, and provides a better prediction of morbidity (blood loss) and tumor recurrence (Table 25.3).

Pathology

Histologically, JNA is a nonencapsulated tumor, consisting of both vascular and fibroblastic components (Fig. 25.5a, b). It is composed of an irregular network of blood vessels set in fibroblastic stroma. The abundant fibrous stroma has characteristic uniformly distributed irregular slit-like vascular channels lined by single endothelial cells. These chan-

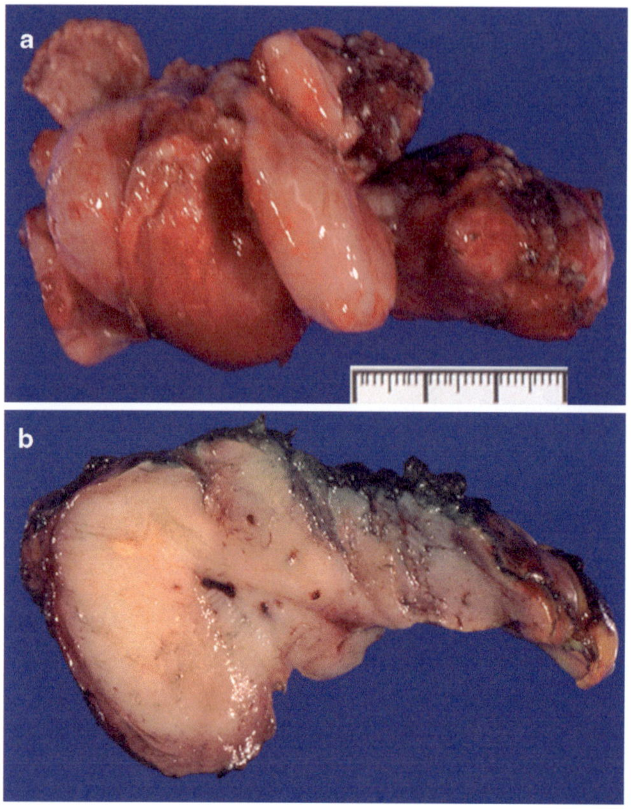

Fig. 25.5 Macroscopy of JNA. The tumor is multinodular and has a smooth shiny external surface (**a**). On cut section the tumor is firm, gray-white in color and appears solid and homogeneous (**b**)

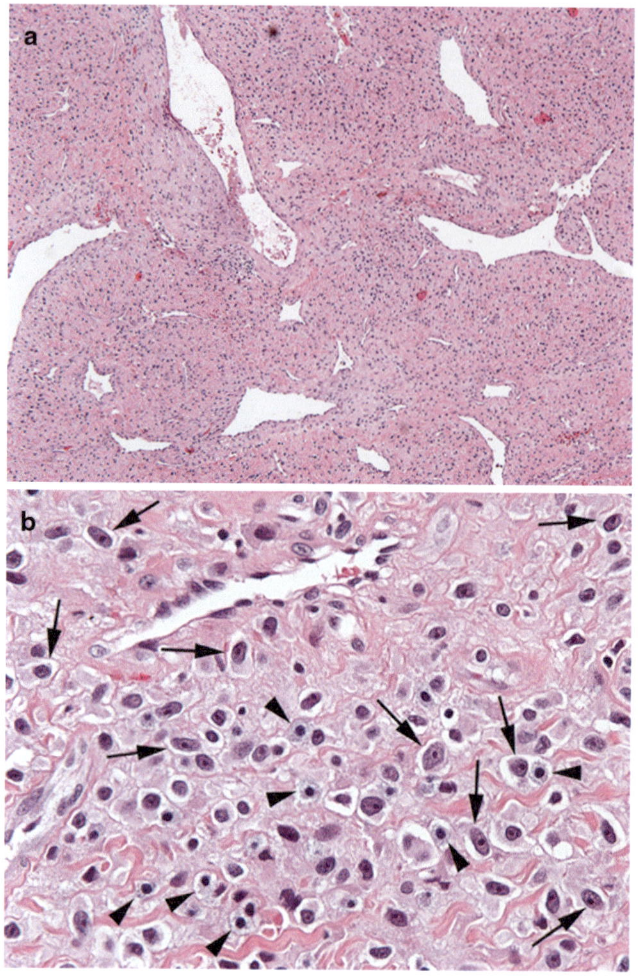

Fig. 25.6 Microscopy of JNA. Large stag horn-type vessels with thin walls and empty lumens are present throughout the field (**a**). Tumor cells are large with ovoid nuclei single prominent nucleolus and relatively abundant cytoplasm (*arrows*) (**b**). Infiltrating mast cells are frequently seen (*arrowheads*) (**b**)

nels are surrounded by a rich collagenous tissue network and have a "staghorn" appearance that lack contractile elements (Fig. 25.6a, b). The lack of a complete muscular layer explains why massive hemorrhage may often result following biopsy or manipulation of the tumor.

Treatment

Surgery is widely accepted as the primary modality of treatment for JNA.

Surgery

Multiple surgical approaches have been proposed for resection of JNA and are highly dependent on the stage of the tumor—size, location, and extent. Other factors that also need to be taken into account are the surgeon's experience with open versus endoscopic surgery, adequate visualization of the tumor, likelihood of achievement of hemostasis, absence of facial scars, and the influence on growth of facial skeleton [12].

Traditionally, open surgical approaches were used for all stages of JNA, with endoscopic approaches being reserved for stage I disease only. However, with advances in minimally invasive endoscopic techniques, the surgical management of JNAs has changed considerably [23]. Transnasal endoscopic resection is now a standard approach for early stage lesions (Fig. 25.7) and, along with endoscopic-assisted procedures (combination of endoscopic and open surgery), is being increasingly used for more advanced tumors with skull base and intracranial involvement [23–26].

Advanced JNA

Surgical management of JNA with intracranial extension is complex and requires an expert multidisciplinary team. Although craniofacial approaches appear to be the current standard of treatment, endoscopic resection or endoscopic-assisted resection of advanced tumors is being increasingly performed for resection of large tumors and is feasible in expert hands [23].

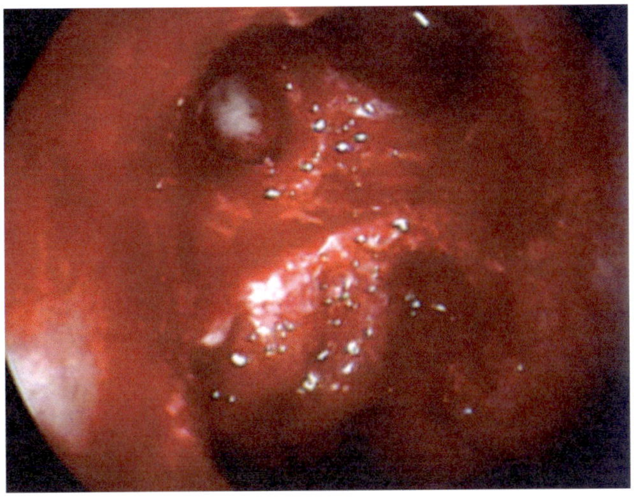

Fig. 25.7 Endoscopic resection of localized JNA. The lesion depicted in Fig. 25.1 following endoscopic resection. The sphenoid sinus has been opened and contents removed

The role and limitations of endoscopic approaches for advanced JNAs continue to be defined. Consensus regarding which approach is most appropriate with respect to morbidity and recurrence has not been reached. Studies analyzing the effectiveness and benefits of the endoscopic approach have been limited by low patient number, and outcome measures have been distorted by an aggregation of cases of different stage and a tendency for treating lower-stage disease with an endoscopic approach [14, 15].

Limitations of an endoscopic approach in advanced JNA may include intracranial involvement including extension into the cavernous sinus, orbit, growth around optic nerves, lateral growth into infratemporal fossa, and spreading behind the pterygoid process. In such cases, endoscopic resection alone is not recommended. Adequate visualization in the case of severe bleeding and the manipulation of endoscopic instruments in a confined space allowing complete tumor resection can be difficult with a pure endoscopic approach. In select cases, these difficulties may be circumvented by combining endoscopic techniques with traditional open approaches. It is generally agreed that endoscopic resection be reserved for limited stage III lesions and an extended transfacial approach, or a craniofacial resection is necessary for stage IV lesions [26, 27].

Endoscopic Approach

This approach has the advantage of not disrupting the facial skeleton and no scar. Hospital stay and recovery period are also significantly decreased. Removal of the middle turbinate or the vomer is usually necessary during an endoscopic approach to gain appropriate access to the tumor. Powered tools including the microdebrider and radiofrequency coblator are useful to assist in tumor debulking. Endoscopic drills can be used in sites where the tumor is adherent to bone, such as the root of the pterygoids or the face of the sphenoid. The sphenopalatine artery can frequently be identified at the sphenopalatine foramen and ligated with clips. Both monopolar and bipolar diathermy can also be used for hemostasis (Fig. 25.7).

Open Surgical Approach

These include transpalatal, lateral rhinotomy, midfacial degloving, and transcranial approaches (Fig. 25.8). The transpalatal approach is now infrequently performed, having been replaced by endoscopic techniques. A lateral rhinotomy allows for excellent exposure in patients with bulky stage II disease, but leaves a scar. Midfacial degloving is the most commonly performed open approach, providing excellent surgical exposure with the benefit of no facial incision. The pterygopalatine and infratemporal fossae can be accessed by removal of the posterior wall of the maxillary sinus. Craniofacial resection in conjunction with the neurosurgical team is required in cases of intracranial extension.

Embolization

Regardless of the approach, preoperative angiography with embolization of the tumor is recommended at least 24–72 h prior to surgical resection. Embolization has been shown to result in significantly reducing intraoperative blood loss and also facilitates resection of larger tumors by improving visualization [28, 29]. It is performed via a transarterial route using reabsorbable microparticulate substances such as gelfoam, polyvinyl alcohol, dextran microspheres, or nonabsorbable microparticulates such as Ivalon and Terbal (Fig. 25.8).

A concern that embolization may obscure tumor extensions intraoperatively thereby resulting in incomplete tumor removal has also been reported [30, 31]. Despite these reports, the risk of significant hemorrhage associated with resection of advanced JNA supports the routine recommendation of preoperative embolization. Loss of vision secondary to central retinal artery occlusion following embolization has been reported [32, 33].

Complications

Side effects from surgery are associated not only with the surgical approach performed but also with the stage of disease being resection. It is important that they are discussed in detail preoperatively. The most common complications are sinonasal and neurologic [14, 15]. Complications include blood loss, nasal crusting, epiphora, and nasolacrimal duct

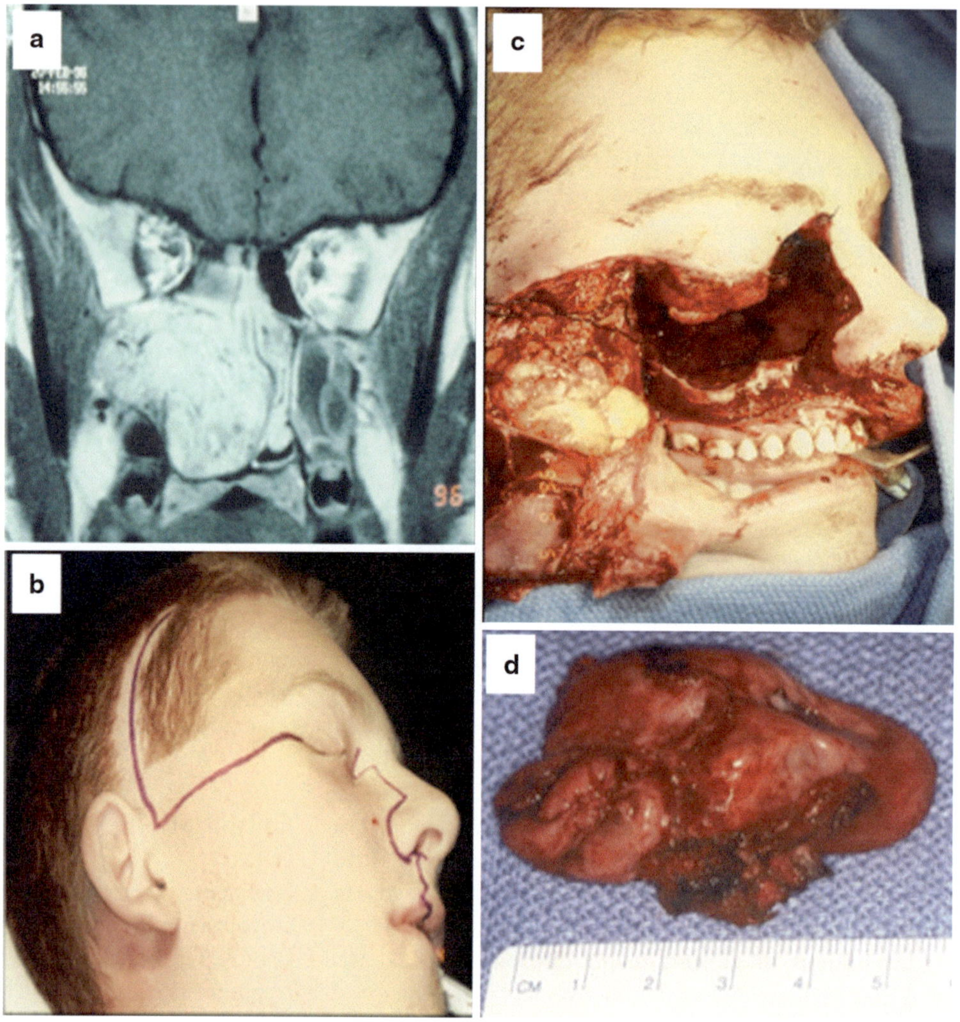

Fig. 25.8 Open resection of an advanced JNA. Coronal CT scan showing an advanced JNA (**a**). A Weber-Ferguson incision (**b**) allowed adequate access for en bloc tumor resection (**c**). The resected specimen is shown (**d**)

stenosis. Parathesia in the infraorbital nerve region, impaired growth of the facial skeleton, facial deformity and scar are primarily associated with open approaches. Anesthesia of the cheek is a frequent occurrence following a Weber-Ferguson incision. Trismus may be secondary to an infratemporal fossa approach. Meningitis and hemiparesis are rare but can occur following a transcranial approach. Ophthalmologic complications include ophthalmoplegia and blindness. Transient blindness may also be associated with embolization. Fistula of the palate at the junction of the soft and hard palate may occur with a transpalatal approach but is prevented by preservation of the greater palatine vessels during flap elevation.

Outcome

The likelihood of local control after surgery varies with tumor extent and the procedure that is performed. Recurrence is a prominent feature of the natural history of JNA. The overall recurrence rate is approximately 18 %, and long-term disease-free survival is 87 % [14, 15]. Recurrence rates as high as 30–50 % have been reported [26, 31]. Risk factors found associated with recurrence include advanced disease at diagnosis, the presence of tumor in the pterygoid fossa and basisphenoid, erosion of the clivus, intracranial extension, invasion of the sphenoid diploe through a widened pterygoid canal, and a younger age at diagnosis. Recurrence does not appear to be increased in the endoscopic approach, although studies are limited by the length of follow-up and criteria for selection in the endoscopic group [14, 15, 34].

Adjuvant Therapies

Radiation Therapy

Radiation therapy is typically reserved for extensive unresectable intracranial disease, and recurrent disease that is life threatening due to its location. Conventional radiation therapy is no longer recommended as a primary treatment due to the concern for complications including [35]:

- Radiation-induced malignancies

- Cataracts
- Keratopathy
- Impaired growth of facial skeleton
- Panhypopituitarism
- Transient neurological deficit
- Temporal lobe radionecrosis

Recent studies using radiation therapy as the definitive treatment of advanced JNAs have demonstrated impressive local control rates, varying from 78–85 %; however, significant side effects were also reported, making radiation a nonviable therapy in most cases [16, 36]. Recurrence rate among patients who underwent isolated radiation therapy were 20–33 %. Newer radiation techniques, such as intensity modulated radiotherapy (IMRT) and stereotactic radiotherapy (Cyberknife) may decrease radiation-induced complications, but clinical experience remains limited in this respect [36].

Interferon

Interferon is used in select cases that are not amenable to surgical resection or have extensive intracranial involvement. Reports of its use are limited.

Flutamide

Treatment with Flutamide, a nonsteroidal antiandrogen (testosterone receptor blocker), administered orally, has been reported to induce tumor regression, although clinical experience remains limited [37]. Flutamide has been shown to reduce stage I and II tumor volume by 44 %, but has not shown any significant improvement over surgical resection alone of tumors of this stage. In the largest case series of 20 patients, it was noted that postpubertal male patients were most likely to respond compared to prepubertal; and in those that had a greater than 25 % tumor regression, the final surgical approach that was undertaken was more conservative than the approach planned at initial presentation [38]. The only reported side effect was that of breast tenderness. Flutamide may have a future role to play as a neoadjuvant treatment in extensive JNAs; however, at present further studies are warranted.

Spontaneous Regression

Spontaneous regression of JNA has been reported in some patients at the age of 20–25 years of age. This has been particularly noted in patients with residual tumor following resection [39–41].

Follow-Up

MRI with contrast enhancement is recommended at least 6 months after initial resection to detect residual or recurrent disease. Tissue suggestive of recurrent or residual tumor on MRI should be biopsied. A watchful waiting approach with interval imaging in asymptomatic patients with residual disease that is surgically unresectable is a reasonable option in some cases.

References

1. Lund VJ, Stammberger H, Nicolai P, Castelnuovo P, Beal T, Beham A, Bernal-Sprekelsen M, Braun H, Cappabianca P, Carrau R, Cavallo L, Clarici G, Draf W, Esposito F, Fernandez-Miranda J, Fokkens W, Gardner P, Gellner V, Hellquist H, Hermann P, Hosemann W, Howard D, Jones N, Jorissen M, Kassam A, Kelly D, Kurschel-Lackner S, Leong S, McLaughlin N, Maroldi R, Minovi A, Mokry M, Onerci M, Ong YK, Prevedello D, Saleh H, Sehti DS, Simmen D, Snyderman C, Solares A, Spittle M, Stamm A, Tomazic P, Trimarchi M, Unger F, Wormald PJ, Zanation A, European rhinologic society advisory board on endoscopic techniques in the management of nose, paranasal sinus and skull base tumours. European position paper on endoscopic management of tumours of the nose, paranasal sinuses and skull base. Rhinol Suppl. 2010;2010(22):1–143.
2. Coutinho-Camilo CM, Brentani MM, Nagai MA. Genetic alterations in juvenile nasopharyngeal angiofibromas. Head Neck. 2008;30:390–400.
3. Tewfik TL, Tan AK, al Noury K, Chowdhury K, Tampieri D, Raymond J, Vuong T. Juvenile nasopharyngeal angiofibroma. J Otolaryngol. 1999;28:145–51.
4. Neel 3rd HB, Whicker JH, Devine KD, et al. Juvenile angiofibroma. Review of 120 cases. Am J Surg. 1973;126:547–56.
5. Lloyd G, Howard D, Lund VJ, Savy L. Imaging for juvenile angiofibroma. J Laryngol Otol. 2000;114:727–30.
6. Ferreira LM, Gomes EF, Azevedo JF, Souza RF, Araujo R, Rios AS. Endoscopic surgery of nasopharyngeal angiofibroma. Rev Bras Otorrinolaryngol. 2006;72(4):475–80.
7. Moschos M, Demetra A, Kontogeorgos G. Juvenile nasopharyngeal angiofibroma—a rare case of primary orbital development. Acta Ophthalmol Scand. 1998;78:506–8.
8. Banhiran W, Casiano RR. Endoscopic sinus surgery for benign and malignant nasal and sinus neoplasm. Curr Opin Otolaryngol Head Neck Surg. 2005;13:50–4.
9. Cansiz H, Güvenç MG, Sekercioğlu N. Surgical approaches to juvenile nasopharyngeal angiofibroma. J Craniomaxillofac Surg. 2006;34(1):3–8.
10. Cruz AAV, Atique JMC, Melo-Filho FV, Elias J. Orbital involvement in juvenile nasopharyngeal angiofibroma: prevalence and treatment. Ophth Plast Reconstr Surg. 2004;4:296–300.
11. Bales C, Kotapka M, Loevner LA, Al-Rawi M, Weinstein G, Hurst R, Weber RS. Craniofacial resection of advance juvenile nasopharyngeal angiofibroma. Arch Otolaryngol Head Neck Surg. 2002;128:1071–8.
12. Marshall AH, Bradley PJ. Management dilemmas in the treatment and follow-up of advanced juvenile nasopharyngeal angiofibroma. ORL. 2006;28:273–8.
13. Wu AW, Mowry SE, Vinuela F, Abemayor E, Wang MB. Bilateral vascular supply in juvenile nasopharyngeal angiofibromas. Laryngoscope. 2011;121(3):639–43.

14. Leong SC. A systematic review of surgical outcomes for advanced juvenile nasopharyngeal angiofibroma with intracranial involvement. Laryngoscope. 2013;123(5):1125–31.
15. Boghani Z, Husain Q, Kanumuri VV, Khan MN, Sangvhi S, Liu JK, Eloy JA. Juvenile nasopharyngeal angiofibroma: a systematic review and comparison of endoscopic, endoscopic-assisted, and open resection in 1047 cases. Laryngoscope. 2013;123(4):859–69.
16. Cherekaev VA, Golbin DA, Kapitanov DN, Roginsky VV, Yakovlev SB, Arustamian SR. Advanced craniofacial juvenile nasopharyngeal angiofibroma. Description of surgical series, case report, and review of literature. Acta Neurochir. 2011;153:499–508.
17. Sessions RB, Bryan RN, Naclerio RM, Alford BR. Radiographic staging of juvenile angiofibroma. Head Neck Surg. 1981;3:279–83.
18. Fisch U. The infratemporal fossa approach for nasopharyngeal tumors. Laryngoscope. 1983;93:36–44.
19. Andrews JC, Fisch U, Valavanis A, Aeppli U, Makek MS. The surgical management of extensive nasopharyngeal angiofibromas with the infra-temporal fossa approach. Laryngoscope. 1989;99:429–37.
20. Chandler JR, Goulding R, Moskowitz L, Quencer RM. Nasopharyngeal angiofibromas: staging and management. Ann Otol Rhinol Laryngol. 1984;93:322–9.
21. Radkowski D, McGill T, Healy GB, Ohlms L, Jones DT. Angiofibroma: changes in staging and treatment. Arch Otolaryngol Head Neck Surg. 1996;122:122–9.
22. Snyderman CH, Pant H, Carrau RL, Gardner P. A new endoscopic staging system for angiofibromas. Arch Otolaryngol Head Neck Surg. 2010;136:588–94.
23. Renkonen S, Hagstrom J, Vuola J, Niemelä M, Porras M, Kivivuori SM, Leivo I, Mäkitie AA. The changing surgical management of juvenile nasopharyngeal angiofibroma. Eur Arch Otorhinolaryngol. 2011;268:599–607.
24. Hackman T, Snyderman CH, Carrau R, Vescan A, Kassam A. Juvenile nasopharyngeal angiofibroma: the expanded endonasal approach. Am J Rhinol Allergy. 2009;23:95–9.
25. Pryor SG, Moore EJ, Kasperbauer JL. Endoscopic versus traditional approaches for excision of juvenile nasopharyngeal angiofibroma. Laryngoscope. 2005;115:1201–7.
26. Gullane PJ, Davidson J, O'Dwyer T, Forte V. Juvenile angiofibroma: a review of the literature and a case series report. Laryngoscope. 1992;102:928–33.
27. Douglas R, Wormald PJ. Endoscopic surgery for juvenile nasopharyngeal angiofibroma: where are the limits? Curr Opin Otolaryngol Head Neck Surg. 2006;14(1):1–5.
28. Moulin G, Chagnaud C, Gras R, Gueguen E, Dessi P, Gaubert JY, Bartoli JM, Zanaret M, Botti G, Cannoni M. Juvenile nasopharyngeal angiofibroma: comparison of blood loss during removal in embolized group versus nonembolized group. Cardiovasc Intervent Radiol. 1995;18:158–61.
29. Li JR, Qian J, Shan XZ, Wang L. Evaluation of the effectiveness of preoperative embolization in surgery for nasopharyngeal angiofibroma. Eur Arch Otorhinolaryngol. 1998;255:430–2.
30. Mann WJ, Jecker P, Amedee RG. Juvenile angiofibromas: changing surgical concept over the last 20 years. Laryngoscope. 2004;114:291–3.
31. McCombe A, Lund VJ, Howard DJ. Recurrence in juvenile angiofibroma. Rhinology. 1990;28:97–102.
32. Onerci M, Gumus K, Cil B, Eldem B. A rare complication of embolization in juvenile nasopharyngeal angiofibroma. Int J Pediatr Otorhinolaryngol. 2005;69:423–8.
33. Ramezani A, Haghighatkhah H, Moghadasi H, Taheri MS, Parsafar H. A case of central retinal artery occlusion following embolization procedure for juvenile nasopharyngeal angiofibroma. Indian J Ophthalmol. 2010;58:419–21.
34. Hyun DW, Ryu JH, Kim YS, Kim KB, Kim WS, Kim CH, Yoon JH. Treatment outcomes of juvenile nasopharyngeal angiofibroma according to surgical approach. Int J Pediatr Otorhinolaryngol. 2011;75(1):69–73.
35. Chakraborty S, Ghoshal S, Patil VM, Oinam AS, Sharma SC. Conformal radiotherapy in the treatment of advanced juvenile nasopharyngeal angiofibroma with intracranial extension: an institutional experience. Int J Radiat Oncol Biol Phys. 2011;80:1398–404.
36. Roche PH, Paris J, Regis J, Moulin G, Zanaret M, Thomassin JM, Pellet W. Management of invasive juvenile nasopharyngeal angiofibromas: the role of a multimodality approach. Neurosurgery. 2007;61:768–77.
37. Labra A, Chavolla-Magaña R, Lopez-Ugalde A, Alanis-Calderon J, Huerta-Delgado A. Flutamide as a preoperative treatment in juvenile angiofibroma (JA) with intracranial invasion: report of 7 cases. Otolaryngol Head Neck Surg. 2004;130(4):466–9.
38. Thakar A, Gupta G, Bhalla AS, Jain V, Sharma SC, Sharma R, Bahadur S, Deka RC. Adjuvant therapy with flutamide for presurgical volume reduction in juvenile nasopharyngeal angiofibroma. Head Neck. 2011;33(12):1747–53.
39. Tosun F, Onerci M, Durmaz A, Ugurel S. Spontaneous involution of nasopharyngeal angiofibroma. J Craniofac Surg. 2008;19(6):1686–9.
40. Weprin LS, Siemers PT. Spontaneous regression of juvenile nasopharyngeal angiofibroma. Arch Otolaryngol Head Neck Surg. 1991;117(7):796–9.
41. Dohar JE, Duvall AJ 3rd. Spontaneous regression of juvenile nasopharyngeal angiofibroma. Ann Otol Rhinol Laryngol. 1992;101(6):469–71.

Langerhans Cell Histiocytosis

26

Adam L. Green and Carlos Rodriguez-Galindo

Introduction

Langerhans cell histiocytosis (LCH) is a disease characterized by clonal proliferation of histiocytes, so named because the involved cells resemble, both morphologically and immunophenotypically, dendritic cells in the skin known as Langerhans cells. Recent studies have shown that the cells of origin in LCH, however, are distinct from Langerhans cells. Head and neck involvement is common, ranging from 55 to 80% in various series [1], with involvement of the head and neck alone occurring in approximately one-third of patients [2]. The most common affected sites of the head and neck in children are the bones, skin, lymph nodes, and brain. It is a highly heterogeneous disease, ranging from single-site involvement curable by resection alone, to life-threatening multisystem disease requiring multimodality treatment. Treatment of LCH is risk-adapted; patients with single lesions may respond well to local treatment, whereas patients with multisystem disease and risk-organ involvement (hematopoietic, liver, spleen) require more intensive therapy. While survival for patients without organ dysfunction is excellent, mortality rates for patients with organ dysfunction may reach 30–40%. While cure is almost universal for patients with low-risk disease, the reactivation rate is in excess of 30%.

Key Points

- LCH affects children of all ages, although infants more often present with multisystem disease.
- The disease can affect many tissues and organs of the head and neck. Bony lesions are most common, but skin, lymph nodes, and brain can also be involved.
- LCH should be confirmed pathologically. Workup at diagnosis should generally be broad in terms of laboratory and imaging, since disease of one organ system often portends involvement of other organs.
- Patients with involvement of only one organ system can often be treated with surgery alone and have excellent outcomes. On the other hand, patients with multisystem disease, especially with risk-organ involvement, need multimodality treatment and have variable prognoses.

Biology and Epidemiology

The cells involved in LCH are myeloid histiocyte-like cells that express the same antigens as Langerhans cells in the skin, but gene expression data differentiate these groups [3, 4]. The disease is rare and tends to affect toddlers more commonly and severely, although it can occur at any age. In adults, LCH may present with more severe bone and skin involvement; systemic disease with involvement of risk organs is much less frequent. Isolated pulmonary disease may develop in adult smokers; this form of LCH appears to have a different pathogenesis, with lack of clonality, and is responsive to smoking cessation.

Pathophysiology

- Pathologic Langerhans cells activate other immunologic cells, including dendritic cells, leading to cytokine release and inflammation. This leads to a characteristic inflammatory reaction and mass effect that define the histopathology of the lesion.
- These cells also activate regulatory T cells (T-regs), which induce tolerance to the disease by inhibiting active T cells [5].

C. Rodriguez-Galindo (✉)
Department of Pediatric Oncology, Dana-Farber/Boston Children's Hospital Cancer and Blood Disorders Center, Harvard Medical School, 450 Brookline Avenue D3-133, Boston, MA 02215, USA
e-mail: carlos_rodriguez-galindo@dfci.harvard.edu

A. L. Green
Pediatric Oncology, Dana-Farber Cancer Institute, 450 Brookline Avenue, Dana 3, Boston, MA 02458, USA

R. Rahbar et al. (eds.), *Pediatric Head and Neck Tumors*,
DOI 10.1007/978-1-4614-8755-5_26, © Springer Science+Business Media New York 2014

Molecular/Genetic Pathology

- There has long been debate as to whether LCH is a reactive or neoplastic condition. Increased cytokine levels, activation of T-regs, and occasional spontaneous remissions in patients support a reactive process.
- On the other hand, the recent finding of mutations in the oncogene *BRAF V600E* in two-thirds of the cases, as well as uniform phosphorylation of BRAF targets MEK and ERK [6], argues that LCH is a neoplasm. The disease's clonality and response to chemotherapy support this assertion; LCH is currently considered a myeloid malignancy.
- There are no consistent cytogenetic abnormalities in LCH.

Incidence and Prevalence

- LCH is likely underdiagnosed given its broad spectrum of manifestations at presentation, but the reported incidence is 3–5 per million children [7, 8].
- The disease occurs in all age-groups but is most common in children ages 1–3 years.

Age Distribution

- Younger patients tend more commonly to have involvement of risk organs (liver, spleen, and bone marrow) and rapid disease development and dissemination, leading to a worse prognosis in patients under 2 years of age. This effect on prognosis disappears when cases are controlled for risk-organ involvement [2].

Geographic/Racial Distribution

- The disease appears to be more common in Caucasians than African-Americans.

Risk Factors—Environmental, Lifestyle

- LCH does not seem to be associated with environmental factors. However, one epidemiologic study suggested correlations of the disease with solvent exposure in parents and perinatal infections [9].

Relationships to Other Disease States, Syndromes

- LCH rarely occurs in twins or siblings. There have been rare cases in patients with concomitant histiocytic disorders, including Erdheim–Chester disease and Rosai–Dorfman disease [10, 11].

Presentation

LCH is limited to a single organ system at presentation in 55 % of patients, with multisystem disease in the remainder. Head and neck organs are some of the most commonly involved organs in LCH; bone involvement is present in up to 77 % of the cases, followed by skin (39 %), lymph nodes (19 %), oral mucosa (13 %), and central nervous system (CNS) (6 %).

Since the majority of LCH patients have bony involvement, pain and tumor formation in a localized area of bone is a very common presentation. The skull is the most commonly involved bone [12], and the lesions are usually soft and tender to touch. Skull lesions may include a soft tissue mass pressing on the dura, but severe intracranial extension is rare. When vertebrae are involved, the cervical region is most commonly affected [13]. Involvement of the skull base is also very common in LCH; typical locations include the bones of the orbit or the temporal bone (typically the mastoid). The temporal bone(s) is involved in 17 % of patients, with unilateral disease (70 %) more common than bilateral (30 %). A temporal bone mass is most common (70 %), with otitis media or externa also common (60 %) [14]. Presenting symptoms related to ear involvement include aural discharge, pain, hearing loss, and vertigo; discharge that does not resolve with treatment of otitis media or externa should raise suspicion for LCH [2].

CNS LCH most often presents with diabetes insipidus (DI) due to involvement of the pituitary stalk; this complication occurs in approximately 25 % of cases, usually after therapy. LCH is also a common diagnosis in patients with DI of unknown etiology, and almost all patients with DI due to LCH have involvement of other organs concurrently or subsequently [15]. Mass lesions of the gray or white matter are less frequent (1 %). Recognition of skull base involvement is important since it has been associated with a higher risk for the development of late neurodegeneration, an inflammatory phenomenon of unclear pathogenesis that is characterized by cerebellar dysfunction and neurocognitive deficits. Involvement of the sphenoid, orbital, ethmoid, zygomatic, or temporal bones confers a higher (25 % overall) risk for CNS involvement, including intracranial extension of these lesions.

Other presenting symptoms related to the head and neck include swelling, cervical lymphadenopathy, rhinorrhea, proptosis, cranial nerve palsy, jaw pain, and loose teeth [16]. Dyspnea may be a sign of thymic or mediastinal node enlargement causing airway compression. Patients with lung involvement, usually infants, may also present with cough, fever, weight loss, or spontaneous pneumothorax.

Skin involvement of the head and neck areas is also common. Infants may present with brown or purple papules, known as Hashimoto–Pritzker disease, which resolve spontaneously during the first year of life [17, 18]. The most typical presentation of cutaneous LCH involvement is a rash that resembles eczema or Candida infection, usually in intertriginous areas such as the neck folds. In the scalp, this rash may have more inflammatory characteristics, with patchy areas of desquamation, resembling cradle cap (Fig. 26.1). All patients with skin lesions should undergo thorough evaluation

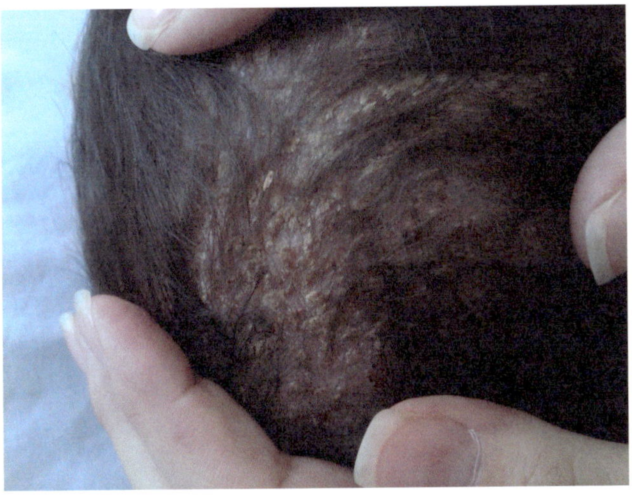

Fig. 26.1 Typical involvement of the scalp by LCH in a young child, showing an erythematous plaque with significant desquamation and scaling

for involvement of other organs, since multiple studies have shown that the majority of these patients have multisystem disease [19–21].

Children under 3 years of age are more likely to present with acute disseminated disease, usually involving bones and skin, and risk organs such as liver, spleen, and the hematopoietic system. In older children, the presentation tends to be more indolent, usually involving bones only, and indeed, patients may go for years without a diagnosis.

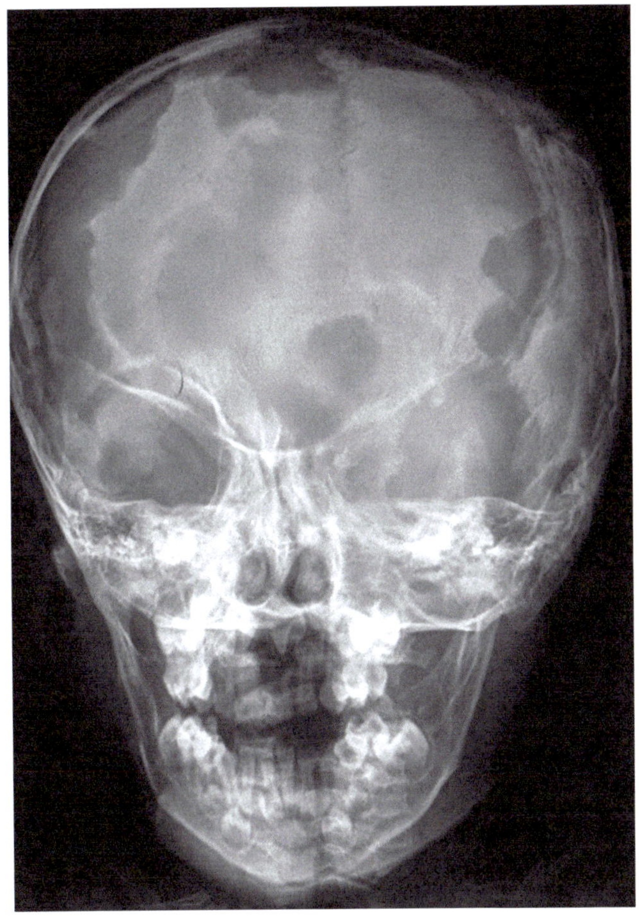

Fig. 26.2 Plain X-ray of a child with severe involvement of the skull with multiple lytic lesions

Differential Diagnosis

LCH can be a challenging diagnosis to make, since the disease has such heterogeneous presentations, may affect many different organs, and can emulate the appearance of many other diseases (infectious, inflammatory, and neoplastic). The following Table 26.1 lists diagnoses, by type, in the differential diagnosis for common presentations of head and neck LCH in children.

Diagnosis and Evaluation

Physical Examination

- Bony lesions usually manifest as a tender, raised, soft mass.
- Cervical lymph nodes are most often soft and matted on palpation, and are usually associated with bone involvement.
- Thorough skin examination is necessary to look for cutaneous manifestations [14].

Laboratory Data

- Complete blood count (CBC) with differential; bone marrow aspirate and biopsy should be performed as well if there are signs of hematopoietic dysfunction [22].
- Electrolytes, liver function tests, renal function tests, and protein and albumin.
- If DI is suspected, a water restriction test should be performed.

Imaging Evaluation

- A "punched-out" osteolytic lesion, with indistinct margins, is typical [14]; there is sometimes an accompanying mass (Fig. 26.2).
- CT of the head and neck to further characterize involvement of these tissues.
- MRI with contrast for all patients with DI or other signs and symptoms suggestive of CNS involvement or risk

Table 26.1 Differential diagnosis of head and neck LCH in children

Histiocytoses	Malignancies	Other
Erdheim–Chester disease	Lymphoma	Eczema
Hemophagocytic lymphohistiocytosis/macrophage activation syndrome	Germinoma	Vasculitis
Rosai–Dorfman disease	Glioma	Otitis media/externa
Juvenile xanthogranuloma	Primitive neuroectodermal tumor	
	Rhabdomyosarcoma	

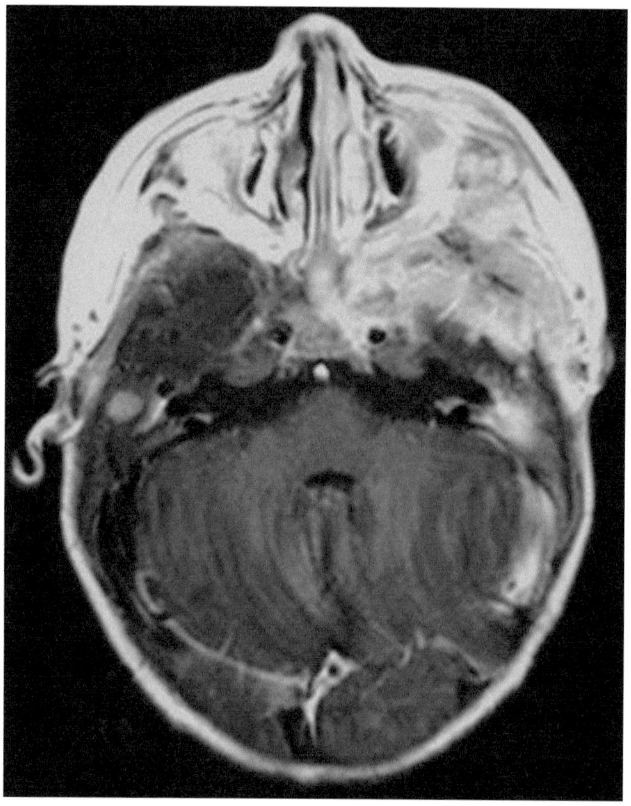

Fig. 26.3 MRI performed at the time of diagnosis in a child with severe involvement of the skull base with intracranial extension

(multisystem disease and/or involvement of the sphenoid, orbital, ethmoid, zygomatic, or temporal bones at diagnosis) [23] (Fig. 26.3).
  - Pituitary involvement classically manifests as loss of the posterior bright spot and thickening of the pituitary stalk [24–26] (Fig. 26.4).
- Middle ear erosion extending to the posterior and lateral semicircular canals is a typical CT finding of temporal LCH [14].
- LCH generally appears iso- or hypointense on T1, with marked contrast enhancement, and hyperintense on T2 images [27].
- A full skeletal screening should be performed to investigate other sites of bone involvement. A skeletal survey is recommended, along a nuclear medicine scan (PET or bone scan).

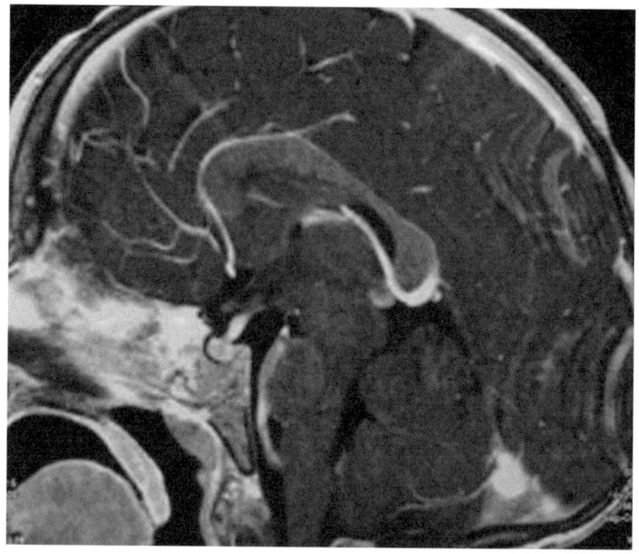

Fig. 26.4 MRI performed at the time of development of diabetes insipidus in a child followed with history of LCH. The pituitary stalk is shown thickened

Pathology

Since pathologic Langerhans cells activate other immunologic cells, microscopic examination of diseased tissue shows eosinophils, neutrophils, lymphocytes, and histiocytes in addition to Langerhans cells; this appearance is what has been traditionally described as eosinophilic granuloma. Abscesses and necrosis may be present. Pathologic Langerhans cells are large, oval in shape, and mononuclear, with a prominent nucleus and eosinophilic cytoplasm. They do not have dendritic cell processes like cutaneous Langerhans cells. They stain positive for protein S-100, CD1a, and CD207 (langerin) and contain cytoplasmic rod-shaped inclusions called Birbeck granules as revealed by electron microscopy. A diagnosis of LCH is done by the characteristic histopathology and immunoreactivity for CD1a or CD207 in the large mononuclear cells (Fig. 26.5).

Treatment

The treatment of LCH over the years has reflected the changing concepts of the disease process. Indeed, the difficulties in developing more effective therapies are linked to the

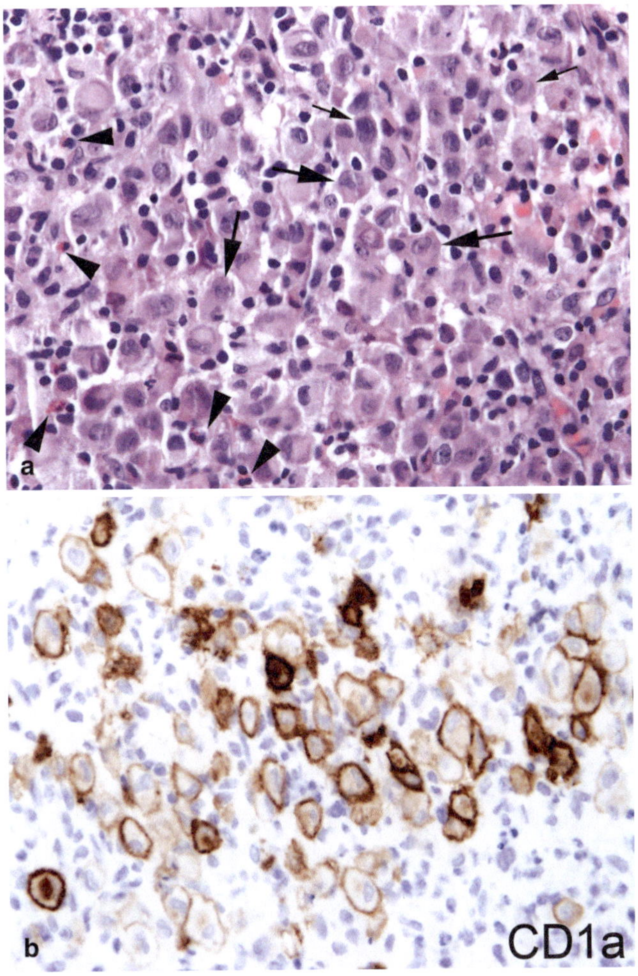

Fig. 26.5 **a** Characteristic histopathology with an infiltrate of mixed inflammatory cells including lymphocytes, plasma cells, eosinophils (*arrowhead*), and large histiocyte-like Langerhans cells with prominent cleaved nuclei, single nucleolus, and abundant eosinophilic cytoplasm (*arrows*). **b** CD1a membranous and Golgi immunoreactivity highlights the Langerhans cells

deficiencies in the understanding of the pathogenesis of LCH. Treatment for patients with LCH is currently risk-adapted.

Patients with single-system disease confined to a single site usually require only local therapy or observation. Patients with more extensive disease (multiple bone lesions or multiple lymph nodes) usually require systemic therapy. The best therapeutic option in these cases has not been defined, and responses have been observed with short courses of steroids with or without the addition of chemotherapeutic agents. The treatment recommended by the Histiocyte Society for this group of patients includes a 6-week induction with prednisone and vinblastine, followed by continuation treatment with pulses of the same agents every 3 weeks. The prognosis for this group of patients is usually excellent, although approximately 30 % of the patients will experience disease reactivations that continue to respond to treatment.

For patients with multisystem disease, the treatment currently recommended by the Histiocyte Society is a 12-month regimen with prednisone and vinblastine, with an early switch to more intensive nucleoside analog-based regimen in patients with slow response. Involvement of the risk organs carries the worst prognosis. This high-risk group of patients is characterized by early age at presentation (usually <2 years), and different degrees of liver, spleen, hematopoietic, and lung involvement. Patients respond poorly to treatment, and mortality rate is approximately 40 %. Thrombocytopenia and hypoalbuminemia are particularly poor prognostic signs, conferring a 5-year survival rate of less than 20 % [28].

Surgical Therapy

- Curettage alone is considered curative in patients with single skull lesions of the frontal, occipital, or parietal bones [29]. Complete resection of a unifocal bone lesion may not be necessary and may lead to deformity [30]. Injection of intratumoral methylprednisolone may be useful as an adjunct [31, 32].
- Surgical removal only is also the standard of care for patients with single lymph node involvement.
- For patients with involvement of the sphenoid, orbital, ethmoid, zygomatic, or temporal bones, skin, or more than one lymph node, surgical resection is usually not recommended, and patients should be treated with systemic chemotherapy. Importantly, chemotherapy in these patients usually achieves long-term control, and additional surgery or radiation therapy are not required.
- For CNS LCH with mass lesion, resection is usually not indicated; these patients are also treated with chemotherapy, usually with agents that cross the blood–brain barrier, such as cytarabine or cladribine.
- Surgical resection is the standard for single skin lesions, but in the case where full resection would be mutilating, topical treatment with steroids or chemotherapy is possible [30].

Complications

- Vertebra plana can occur in affected vertebrae, although this is rare with treatment.
- Cholesteatoma can be a late occurrence in patients treated for head and neck LCH [14].
- Conductive hearing loss occurs in 7.4 % of patients with middle ear involvement [33].

Radiation Therapy

- Radiation therapy is generally avoided in LCH due to its known side effects and the favorable prognosis of this entity.

- Radiation therapy has been used in the past for the treatment of CNS mass lesions, although its benefit is unclear and currently it is not recommended [34].
- Radiation could be considered in patients with vertebral disease causing risk of collapse, as the response rate is high at 90 % in children [35–38], and pain usually improves. Low doses of radiation, typically less than 12–15 Gy are usually sufficient to induce a response.

Outcomes

Outcome After Surgery

- Patients with single site disease who qualify for surgical treatment alone have excellent outcomes. However, disease reactivation (usually at other sites) occurs in approximately 30 % of the cases.

Outcome After Nonsurgical Treatments

- Induction chemotherapy with vinblastine and prednisolone is generally administered for 6 weeks in all LCH patients requiring chemotherapy [39]. The response to treatment after 6 weeks is important and helps determine subsequent therapy. Evaluation at this stage should include MRI and PET.
- The most recent clinical trials suggest that lower recurrence rates can be achieved by extending subsequent maintenance chemotherapy to a total treatment duration of 12 months. Patients without risk-organ involvement can continue on vinblastine and prednisolone; patients with risk-organ involvement likely benefit from the addition of mercaptopurine to the maintenance regimen [40].
- The use of cladribine for DI caused by LCH involvement of the pituitary has not been shown to reverse the DI [24].
- Patients with LCH causing DI have a 54 % 10-year risk of growth hormone deficiency and a 76 % 5-year risk of radiologic neurodegeneration; these also do not resolve with treatment, but chemotherapy in patients with DI alone may prevent progression to these conditions [30].
- Cladribine has also been shown to achieve partial responses or stabilization of CNS LCH manifesting as mass lesions.
- Patients with LCH may have a higher rate of other cancers unrelated to their treatment, including retinoblastoma, brain tumors, and Ewing sarcoma [41, 42].
- The probability of recurrence at 5 years from diagnosis in a large series of patients with multisystem LCH who achieved remission was 46 % [43].
- Patients with low-risk disease who experience recurrence are generally salvageable with chemotherapy [43, 44].
- Patients with relapsed or refractory high-risk LCH generally require alternative chemotherapeutic agents and have poorer response rates [45, 46].

Follow-Up

Frequency of Office Visits

- The Histiocyte Society recommends that patients with no evidence of disease or a continuous response to treatment be assessed at least every 6 weeks while on treatment, then every 3 months for 2 years, every 6 months for 2 subsequent years, and then yearly.

Frequency of Imaging

- Imaging of affected organs should be done with visits as described earlier.
- Patients who have had CNS involvement, or involvement of CNS-risk bones (sphenoid, orbital, ethmoid, or temporal), should undergo brain MRI every 1–2 years for 10 years from diagnosis to look for new CNS disease and evidence of neurodegeneration [47].
- BAERs should also be performed regularly [48].

References

1. Buchmann L, Emami A, Wei JL. Primary head and neck Langerhans cell histiocytosis in children. Otolaryngol Head Neck Surg. 2006;135(2):312–7.
2. Nicollas R, Rome A, Belaich H, Roman S, Volk M, Gentet JC, et al. Head and neck manifestation and prognosis of Langerhans' cell histiocytosis in children. Int J Pediatr Otorhinolaryngol. 2010;74(6):669–73.
3. Willman CL, Busque L, Griffith BB, Favara BE, McClain KL, Duncan MH, et al. Langerhans'-cell histiocytosis (histiocytosis X)—a clonal proliferative disease. N Engl J Med. 1994;331(3):154–60.
4. Yu RC, Chu C, Buluwela L, Chu AC. Clonal proliferation of Langerhans cells in Langerhans cell histiocytosis. Lancet. 1994;343(8900):767–8.
5. Senechal B, Elain G, Jeziorski E, Grondin V, Patey-Mariaud de SN, Jaubert F, et al. Expansion of regulatory T cells in patients with Langerhans cell histiocytosis. PLoS Med. 2007;4(8):e253.
6. Badalian-Very G, Vergilio JA, Degar BA, MacConaill LE, Brandner B, Calicchio ML, et al. Recurrent BRAF mutations in Langerhans cell histiocytosis. Blood. 2010;116(11):1919–23.
7. Carstensen H, Ornvold K. The epidemiology of LCH in children in Denmark, 1975–89. Med Pediatr Oncol. 1993;21:387–8.
8. Baumgartner I, von Hochstetter A, Baumert B, Luetolf U, Follath F. Langerhans'-cell histiocytosis in adults. Med Pediatr Oncol. 1997;28(1):9–14.
9. Nicholson HS, Egeler RM, Nesbit ME. The epidemiology of Langerhans cell histiocytosis. Hematol Oncol Clin North Am. 1998;12(2):379–84.
10. Pineles SL, Liu GT, Acebes X, Arruga J, Nasta S, Glaser R, et al. Presence of Erdheim-Chester disease and Langerhans cell histiocytosis in the same patient: a report of 2 cases. J Neuroophthalmol. 2011;31(3):217–23.
11. Wang KH, Cheng CJ, Hu CH, Lee WR. Coexistence of localized Langerhans cell histiocytosis and cutaneous Rosai-Dorfman disease. Br J Dermatol. 2002;147(4):770–4.
12. Slater JM, Swarm OJ. Eosinophilic granuloma of bone. Med Pediatr Oncol. 1980;8(2):151–64.
13. Garg S, Mehta S, Dormans JP. Langerhans cell histiocytosis of the spine in children. Long-term follow-up. J Bone Joint Surg Am. 2004;86-A(8):1740–50.

14. Saliba I, Sidani K, El Fata F, Arcand P, Quintal MC, Abela A. Langerhans' cell histiocytosis of the temporal bone in children. Int J Pediatr Otorhinolaryngol. 2008;72(6):775–86.
15. Howarth DM, Gilchrist GS, Mullan BP, Wiseman GA, Edmonson JH, Schomberg PJ. Langerhans cell histiocytosis: diagnosis, natural history, management, and outcome. Cancer. 1999;85(10):2278–90.
16. D'Ambrosio N, Soohoo S, Warshall C, Johnson A, Karimi S. Craniofacial and intracranial manifestations of langerhans cell histiocytosis: report of findings in 100 patients. AJR Am J Roentgenol. 2008;191(2):589–97.
17. Munn S, Chu AC. Langerhans cell histiocytosis of the skin. Hematol Oncol Clin North Am. 1998;12(2):269–86.
18. Kapur P, Erickson C, Rakheja D, Carder KR, Hoang MP. Congenital self-healing reticulohistiocytosis (Hashimoto-Pritzker disease): ten-year experience at Dallas Children's Medical Center. J Am Acad Dermatol. 2007;56(2):290–4.
19. Minkov M, Prosch H, Steiner M, Grois N, Potschger U, Kaatsch P, et al. Langerhans cell histiocytosis in neonates. Pediatr Blood Cancer. 2005;45(6):802–7.
20. Lau L, Krafchik B, Trebo MM, Weitzman S. Cutaneous Langerhans cell histiocytosis in children 2 one year. Pediatr Blood Cancer. 2006;46(1):66–71.
21. Stein SL, Paller AS, Haut PR, Mancini AJ. Langerhans cell histiocytosis presenting in the neonatal period: a retrospective case series. Arch Pediatr Adolesc Med. 2001;155(7):778–83.
22. Minkov M, Potschger U, Grois N, Gadner H, Dworzak MN. Bone marrow assessment in Langerhans cell histiocytosis. Pediatr Blood Cancer. 2007;49(5):694–8.
23. Grois N, Potschger U, Prosch H, Minkov M, Arico M, Braier J, et al. Risk factors for diabetes insipidus in langerhans cell histiocytosis. Pediatr Blood Cancer. 2006;46(2):228–33.
24. Kaltsas GA, Powles TB, Evanson J, Plowman PN, Drinkwater JE, Jenkins PJ, et al. Hypothalamo-pituitary abnormalities in adult patients with langerhans cell histiocytosis: clinical, endocrinological, and radiological features and response to treatment. J Clin Endocrinol Metab. 2000;85(4):1370–6.
25. Maghnie M, Bossi G, Klersy C, Cosi G, Genovese E, Arico M. Dynamic endocrine testing and magnetic resonance imaging in the long-term follow-up of childhood langerhans cell histiocytosis. J Clin Endocrinol Metab. 1998;83(9):3089–94.
26. Grois N, Prayer D, Prosch H, Minkov M, Potschger U, Gadner H. Course and clinical impact of magnetic resonance imaging findings in diabetes insipidus associated with Langerhans cell histiocytosis. Pediatr Blood Cancer. 2004;43(1):59–65.
27. Fernandez-Latorre F, Menor-Serrano F, Alonso-Charterina S, Arenas-Jimenez J. Langerhans' cell histiocytosis of the temporal bone in pediatric patients: imaging and follow-up. AJR Am J Roentgenol. 2000;174(1):217–21.
28. Braier JL, Rosso D, Latella A, Chantada G, Ozuna B, Ripoli M, et al. Importance of multi-lineage hematologic involvement and hypoalbuminemia at diagnosis in patients with "risk-organ" multisystem Langerhans cell histiocytosis. J Pediatr Hematol Oncol. 2010;32(4):e122–5.
29. Nauert C, Zornoza J, Ayala A, Harle TS. Eosinophilic granuloma of bone: diagnosis and management. Skeletal Radiol. 1983;10(4):227–35.
30. Abla O, Egeler RM, Weitzman S. Langerhans cell histiocytosis: current concepts and treatments. Cancer Treat Rev. 2010;36(4):354–9.
31. Chu T. Langerhans cell histiocytosis. Australas J Dermatol. 2001;42(4):237–42.
32. Lallemant B, Fayoux P, Nelken B, Leroy X, Vaneecloo FM. Management of head and neck Langerhan's cell histiocytosis in children. Ann Otolaryngol Chir Cervicofac. 2003;120(1):30–9.
33. Pollono D, Rey G, Latella A, Rosso D, Chantada G, Braier J. Reactivation and risk of sequelae in Langerhans cell histiocytosis. Pediatr Blood Cancer. 2007;48(7):696–9.
34. Kasper EM, Aguirre-Padilla DH, Alter RY, Anderson M. Histiocytosis X: characteristics, behavior, and treatments as illustrated in a case series. Surg Neurol Int. 2011;2:57.
35. Willis B, Ablin A, Weinberg V, Zoger S, Wara WM, Matthay KK. Disease course and late sequelae of Langerhans' cell histiocytosis: 25-year experience at the University of California, San Francisco. J Clin Oncol. 1996;14(7):2073–82.
36. Selch MT, Parker RG. Radiation therapy in the management of Langerhans cell histiocytosis. Med Pediatr Oncol. 1990;18(2):97–102.
37. el-Sayed S, Brewin TB. Histiocytosis X: does radiotherapy still have a role? Clin Oncol. 1992;4(1):27–31.
38. Greenberger JS, Cassady JR, Jaffe N, Vawter G, Crocker AC. Radiation therapy in patients with histiocytosis: management of diabetes insipidus and bone lesions. Int J Radiat Oncol Biol Phys. 1979;5(10):1749–55.
39. Gadner H, Grois N, Potschger U, Minkov M, Arico M, Braier J, et al. Improved outcome in multisystem Langerhans cell histiocytosis is associated with therapy intensification. Blood. 2008;111(5):2556–62.
40. Gadner H, Heitger A, Grois N, Gatterer-Menz I, Ladisch S. Treatment strategy for disseminated Langerhans cell histiocytosis. DAL HX-83 study group. Med Pediatr Oncol. 1994;23(2):72–80.
41. Egeler RM, Neglia JP, Arico M, Favara BE, Heitger A, Nesbit ME, et al. The relation of Langerhans cell histiocytosis to acute leukemia, lymphomas, and other solid tumors. The LCH-malignancy study group of the histiocyte society. Hematol Oncol Clin North Am. 1998;12(2):369–78.
42. Egeler RM, Neglia JP, Puccetti DM, Brennan CA, Nesbit ME. Association of Langerhans cell histiocytosis with malignant neoplasms. Cancer. 1993;71(3):865–73.
43. Minkov M, Steiner M, Potschger U, Arico M, Braier J, Donadieu J, et al. Reactivations in multisystem Langerhans cell histiocytosis: data of the international LCH registry. J Pediatr. 2008;153(5):700–5, 705.e1–2.
44. Weitzman S, Braier J, Donadieu J, Egeler RM, Grois N, Ladisch S, et al. 2′-Chlorodeoxyadenosine (2-CdA) as salvage therapy for Langerhans cell histiocytosis (LCH). results of the LCH-S-98 protocol of the Histiocyte Society. Pediatr Blood Cancer. 2009;53(7):1271–6.
45. Bernard F, Thomas C, Bertrand Y, Munzer M, Landman Parker J, Ouache M, et al. Multi-centre pilot study of 2-chlorodeoxyadenosine and cytosine arabinoside combined chemotherapy in refractory Langerhans cell histiocytosis with haematological dysfunction. Eur J Cancer. 2005;41(17):2682–9.
46. Apollonsky N, Lipton JM. Treatment of refractory Langerhans cell histiocytosis (LCH) with a combination of 2-chlorodeoxyadenosine and cytosine arabinoside. J Pediatr Hematol Oncol. 2009;31(1):53–6.
47. Wnorowski M, Prosch H, Prayer D, Janssen G, Gadner H, Grois N. Pattern and course of neurodegeneration in Langerhans cell histiocytosis. J Pediatr. 2008;153(1):127–32.
48. Allen CE, Flores R, Rauch R, Dauser R, Murray JC, Puccetti D, et al. Neurodegenerative central nervous system Langerhans cell histiocytosis and coincident hydrocephalus treated with vincristine/cytosine arabinoside. Pediatr Blood Cancer. 2010;54(3):416–23.

Leukemia and Lymphoma

27

Natasha M. Archer and Lynda M. Vrooman

Introduction

Hematologic malignancies are the most common malignancies of childhood. They represent a diverse population of malignant diseases subdivided into leukemia and lymphoma based on percentage of blast cells in the bone marrow at diagnosis. While the majority of pediatric leukemias fall into one of two categories, lymphoid or myeloid, lymphoma is further subdivided into Hodgkin lymphoma (HL) and Non-Hodgkin lymphoma (NHL), with Burkitt lymphoma, large B-cell lymphoma, lymphoblastic B- or T-cell lymphoma, and anaplastic large-cell lymphoma as the most common NHLs in the pediatric population.

While pediatric leukemia and lymphoma most frequently present with fatigue, anemia, and/or bruising, both can present with head and neck lesions. The most common presentation of HL and NHL is cervical lymphadenopathy [1]. Primary and secondary central nervous system (CNS) lymphoma can present with lymphomatous meningitis and/or CNS masses. In addition, pediatric lymphoblastic leukemia can present with CNS involvement. Leukemia cutis, the cutaneous manifestations of leukemia, is most often myeloid in origin; however, scalp lesions have been reported in lymphoblastic leukemia as well [2]. Granulocytic sarcoma, also known as myeloid sarcoma, extramedullary leukemia, or chloroma, is a mass of immature myeloid cells that can occur in up to 10% of patients with acute myeloid leukemia (AML).

Key Points

- Both leukemia and lymphoma can present with head and neck lesions.
- The most common presentation of HL and NHL is cervical lymphadenopathy.
- Leukemia and lymphoma can present with CNS involvement.
- Granulocytic sarcoma can occur in up to 10% of patients with AML [3].

Biology and Epidemiology

Hematologic malignancies account for nearly 45% of childhood cancers. They are primarily derived from either myeloid or lymphoid cell lines and typically affect the blood, bone marrow, and lymph nodes.

Molecular/Genetic Pathology

- Several chromosomal abnormalities have been identified as having prognostic significance in pediatric patients with acute lymphoblastic leukemia (ALL). Those associated with a poor outcome include rearrangements of the MLL gene located at 11q23, (q.34;q11), t(9;22), also known as BCR/ABL1 translocation and hypodiploidy (less than 45 chromosomes). Those associated with a favorable outcome include t(12;21), (p13;q22) also known as ETV6/RUNX1, and hyperdiploidy (between 54 and 58 chromosomes) [4].
- The most frequent genetic abnormality seen in children with AML is the balanced translocation t(8;21)(q22;q22), RUNX1-RUNX1T1 (formerly known as AML. ETO rearrangement). This translocation is associated with a more favorable prognosis except in the presence of c-KIT mutations [5].

N. M. Archer (✉) · L. M. Vrooman
Department of Pediatric Hematology-Oncology, Dana-Farber/Boston Children's Cancer and Blood Disorders Center, Boston, MA, USA
e-mail: Natasha.Archer@childrens.harvard.edu

R. Rahbar et al. (eds.), *Pediatric Head and Neck Tumors*,
DOI 10.1007/978-1-4614-8755-5_27, © Springer Science+Business Media New York 2014

- There is an association between orbital granulocytic sarcoma and AML with t(8;21)(q22;q22) [6–8].
- Translocation t(15;17)(q24.1;q21.1), PML-RARA, is highly specific for acute promyelocytic leukemia (APL), a subtype of AML treated differently than other subtypes. Early mortality can occur as a consequence of coagulopathy and bleeding complications. If managed with rapid initiation of treatment and supportive care, APL is, however, associated with an overall favorable outcome [9].
- Mutations in (FLT3/ITD) (FMS-like tyrosine kinase 3 gene-producing internal transmembrane duplications) and constitutive activation of the FLT3 receptor tyrosine kinase is associated with poorer survival in children with AML [10].
- The c-MYC gene encodes proteins that control cell growth, differentiation, and apoptosis. Translocations involving the site of the c-MYC gene (8q24) are associated with Burkitt lymphoma. t(8;14)(q24;q32) is the most common translocation; it is found in nearly 80 % of Burkitt lymphomas [11].
- Anaplastic lymphoma kinase (ALK)-positive anaplastic large cell lymphoma is the most common mature T-cell neoplasm in the pediatric and adolescent population [12].

Incidence and Prevalence

- In the United States, acute leukemia accounts for 30 % of malignancies in children less than 20 years of age while HL and NHL account for 15 % of malignancies in children less than 20 years of age [11].

Geographic Distribution

- Endemic Burkitt has an increased incidence in equatorial Africa. This form is largely found in Africa, often associated with Epstein–Barr virus (EBV), and characteristically involves the jaw or other facial bones in children between 4 and 7 years of age [13].

Risk Factors—Environmental, Life Style

- Hematologic malignancies are not clearly associated with environmental or constitutional factors.
- EBV has been found in all three clinical forms of Burkitt lymphoma, but the role of EBV infection in its development is poorly understood. Malaria has also been implicated given such high incidence in areas where the disease is endemic. Mechanisms proposed include malaria-induced polyclonal activation of B cells which increases the chances of c-MYC translocation as well as decreased anti-EBV immunity as a result of generalized immunosuppression [14].
- EBV is also associated with HL [15].

Relationships to Other Disease States, Syndromes

- Congenital and acquired immunodeficiency syndromes including common variable immunodeficiency, Wiskott–Aldrich syndrome, ataxia telangiectasia, and X-linked lymphoproliferative syndrome have been associated with malignancy, including NHL [16].

Presentation

HL and NHL both frequently present with cervical lymphadenopathy [1]. In a study of 311 pediatric and adult patients, 76 with HL and 235 with NHL, cervical lymphadenopathy was the most common presentation with 24 % of patients with HL and 33 % with NHL presenting with an enlarged cervical node [1]. Mediastinal lymphadenopathy can also be seen at presentation in some types of lymphoma and in T-cell ALL. Patients with a mediastinal mass may present with superior vena cava syndrome, obstruction of the superior vena cava resulting in dyspnea, presyncope, headache, venous distention in the neck or chest, and facial or arm swelling.

Lymphoblastic leukemia and lymphoma most often present with fever, bleeding symptoms, bone pain and/or lymphadenopathy. Lymphadenopathy is usually nontender and fixed. While it is often cervical, it can present with enlargement of any lymph node.

In addition to lymphadenopathy, face and scalp lesions also occur. In a study of pediatric patients less than 18 years of age with ALL (1259 patients) and lymphoblastic lymphoma (LBL, 100 patients), 24 were found to have cutaneous involvement. Twenty-one of the 24 patients had at least one skin lesion located on the face or the scalp [17].

Acute megakaryocytic leukemia, in addition to pancytopenia, can present with bony lesions and hypercalcemia [18].

Granulocytic sarcomas typically present as firm, rapidly growing masses (Table 27.1). In a retrospective study looking at pediatric patients age less than 1 month to 21 years of age enrolled in Children's Cancer Group AML trials between March 1983 and April 1995, 199 patients (10.9 %) were found to have extramedullary leukemia at diagnosis. The most common site was skin (5.9 %), followed by the orbital, and head and neck regions. Of the 23 patients with non-skin extramedullary disease, 12 had orbital disease, 5 had head and neck disease, 3 CNS or spine disease, and 3 with multiple sites of disease suggesting a tendency to arise

Table 27.1 Location of granulocytic sarcoma and associated symptoms

Location	Associated symptoms
Orbital	Diplopia with cranial nerve palsy
	Proptosis
Gingival	Gingival hypertrophy
	Gum bleeding
Parotid gland	Facial nerve palsy [19]
Nasal cavity	Epistaxis, nasal airway obstruction
Temporal bone	Facial paralysis [20], otalgia, postauricular swelling, conductive hearing loss, tinnitus [21]
Middle ear	Otitis media, Bell's palsy [22]

adjacent to cranial and facial bones [3]. In this group, the presentation of disease is largely dependent on the location from which the masses arise.

Differential Diagnosis

Hematologic malignancies should be included in the differential diagnosis of head and neck tumors in children, particularly when systemic symptoms are present (Table 27.2).

Diagnosis and Evaluation

Physical Examination

- Patients with hematologic malignancies can present with hemodynamic instability including tachycardia and hypotension often secondary to infection. Patients are immunosuppressed and infections should be treated with aggressive resuscitation and broad-spectrum antibiotics.
- Assess for signs of respiratory distress including increased respiratory rate, stridor, wheezing, and retractions which can result from cervicothoracic masses.
- Nasal cavity and oropharynx should be assessed for lesions including mucosal ulceration and granulocytic sarcomas.
- Patients presenting with the endemic form of Burkitt lymphoma may present with large masses in the craniofacial bones, most typically the jaw or maxillary bones.
- Skin should also be assessed for granulocytic sarcomas as well as for signs of anemia, i.e., pallor and thrombocytopenia including petechiae and excessive bruising.
- The patient should have a complete lymph node exam and abdominal exam to assess for lymphadenopathy and hepatosplenomegaly.

Laboratory Data

- Standard laboratory studies include a complete blood count (CBC) with differential, coagulation studies (PT/PTT), and type and cross for blood bank. The presence of alterations in the CBC, even in the presence of enlarged lymph nodes, suggests bone marrow involvement and should lead to a bone marrow aspirate and biopsy as diagnostic procedures.
- A lumbar puncture for evaluation of cerebrospinal fluid (CSF) cytology is performed for staging and therapeutic purpose in acute leukemia and also in some cases of NHL, such as Burkitt lymphoma and LBL. In the setting of a diagnosis of leukemia, intrathecal chemotherapy is administered at the time of the diagnostic procedure, for treatment of the CNS and to avoid contamination of the CSF by leukemic cells.
- Tumor lysis labs including potassium, calcium, phosphate, uric acid, creatinine, and LDH should be checked especially in patients with rapidly dividing tumors and large masses, as is the case with some of the NHLs, and in patients with leukemia with high presenting white blood cell count.

Table 27.2 Differential diagnosis

Presentation	Inflammatory	Infectious	Neoplastic
Systemic symptoms	Rheumatoid arthritis	Tuberculosis EBV Cytomegalovirus (CMV)	Nasopharyngeal carcinoma Small round blue cell tumors (Ewing sarcoma, neuroblastoma, rhabdomyosarcoma) Rhabdoid tumor
Head and neck mass		Cat scratch disease EBV CMV Tuberculosis Mycobacterium Bacterial lymphadenitis	Nasopharyngeal carcinoma Small round blue cell tumors (Ewing sarcoma, neuroblastoma, rhabdomyosarcoma) Rhabdoid tumor
Skin Lesions		Lipoma	Langerhans cell histiocytosis Melanoma Neuroblastoma

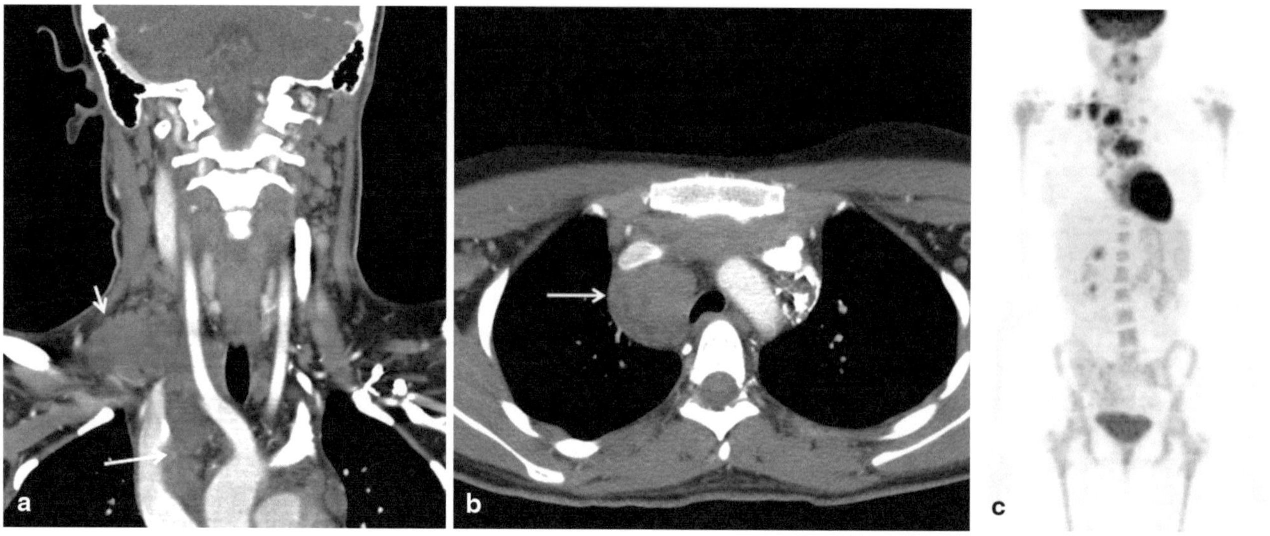

Fig. 27.1 Hodgkin lymphoma (HL). Sixteen-year-old girl with right neck and supraclavicular mass. CT scan (**a** and **b**) shows a nodal conglomerate extending from neck into the mediastinum (*arrows*). PET scan (**c**) shows increased fludeoxyglucose (FDG) avidity in the right supraclavicular region, anterior mediastinum, and right paratracheal region. Final diagnosis was stage IIA HL

Imaging Evaluation

- While most head and neck masses will not cause significant respiratory distress, mediastinal masses can. A chest radiograph (posteroanterior and lateral), specifically looking for a mediastinal mass, should be obtained on all patients that present with leukemia or lymphoma prior to any sedation.
- Evaluation with ultrasound can be considered for cervical masses or skin lesions, in the absence of signs of leukemia or lymphoma in the peripheral blood.
- Lymphoma staging generally includes a positron emission tomography (PET) scan to assess for other sites of disease in addition to ultrasound, CT, or MRI of lymphadenopathy or masses (Fig. 27.1).

Pathology

When leukemia is suspected, bone marrow aspirates and biopsy (usually from the posterior iliac crest) should be performed. Samples should be obtained for morphologic evaluation as well as for flow cytometry, cytogenetic studies, and molecular studies as indicated. In patients with AML presenting with chloroma, a biopsy of the lesion may be diagnostic (Fig. 27.2). Bone marrow studies are also performed in the staging work-up of HL and NHL.

In cases of lymphoma where a biopsy of a lymph node is required, an excisional biopsy is preferred over a needle biopsy, since it is important to evaluate the entire architecture of the lymph node for a proper diagnosis.

Both T-cell and B-cell ALL contain lymphoblasts, small- to medium-size uniform cells with little cytoplasm. Flow cytometry and antibody staining confirm the diagnosis and help distinguish between the two types of ALL. Lymphoblasts are almost always deoxynucleotidyl transferase (TdT) and CD34 positive. B-cell markers include CD19, CD20, CD22, CD79a, and PAX5. T-cell markers are CD2, CD3, CD5, and CD7 [23].

Classical HL is divided into four histologic subtypes: nodular sclerosis, mixed cellularity, lymphocyte rich, and lymphocyte depleted (Fig. 27.3). Nodular sclerosis HL is the most common subtype. As its name suggests, it is characterized by nodules and fibrous bands (sclerosis) separating the nodules. The classic Reed–Sternberg cells, large binucleated cells with abundant cytoplasm, and prominent eosinophilic nucleoli accompanied by a mixed inflammatory background including eosinophils, are rare. Multilobated nuclei in an abundant pale cytoplasm, aptly named lacunar cells, are more common. Mixed cellularity, the second most common subtype, also demonstrates a nodular growth pattern but without sclerosis. Reed–Sternberg cells are more common. The lymphocyte rich subtype is distinguished from the two above by a background infiltrate consisting predominantly of B lymphocytes, as opposed to T lymphocytes, and eosinophils, histiocytes and neutrophils. The lymphocyte depleted subtype has very few inflammatory cells but large numbers of Reed–Sternberg cells in a fibrotic background [23].

Nodular lymphocyte-predominant Hodgkin lymphoma (NLPHL) is a rare variant of classical HL distinguished by an atypical Reed–Sternberg cell called the lymphocytic and histiocytic (L&H) cell or the "popcorn cell" because of its

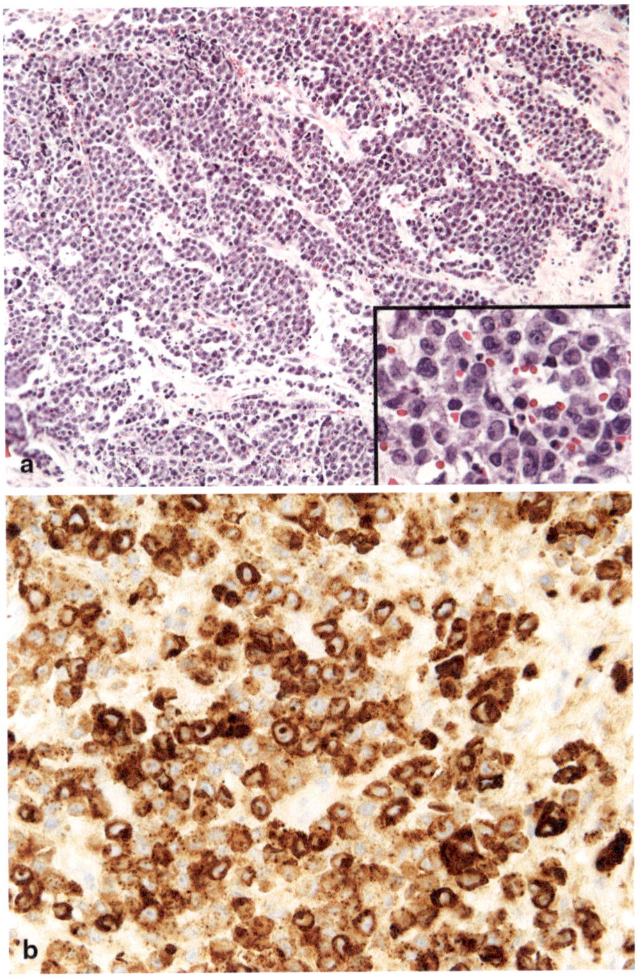

Fig. 27.2 Chloroma (myeloblastic sarcoma). **a** Profuse soft tissue infiltrate of medium-sized tumor cells. *Inset*: tumor cells at higher magnification showing relatively abundant cytoplasm, high nuclear cytoplasmic ratio, and reniform, clefted nuclei with prominent eosinophilic single nucleoli. **b** Tumor cells show diffuse strong cytoplasmic immunoreactivity for myeloperoxidase

appearance. While Reed–Sternberg cells are typically CD30 and CD15 positive and CD45 and CD20 negative, L&H cells are the opposite, CD30 and CD15 negative and CD45 and CD20 positive [23].

As mentioned earlier, NHL consists of a heterogeneous population of diseases. LBL pathology is very similar to that of lymphoblastic leukemia (Fig. 27.4). Three other common NHLs in children with distinct pathology are Burkitt lymphoma, large B-cell lymphoma, and anaplastic large cell lymphoma.

Burkitt lymphoma is the most common mature B-cell neoplasm in children. The tumor is comprised of a homogeneous population of medium-size cells with multiple prominent nucleoli and lipid-filled basophilic cytoplasm, intermixed with

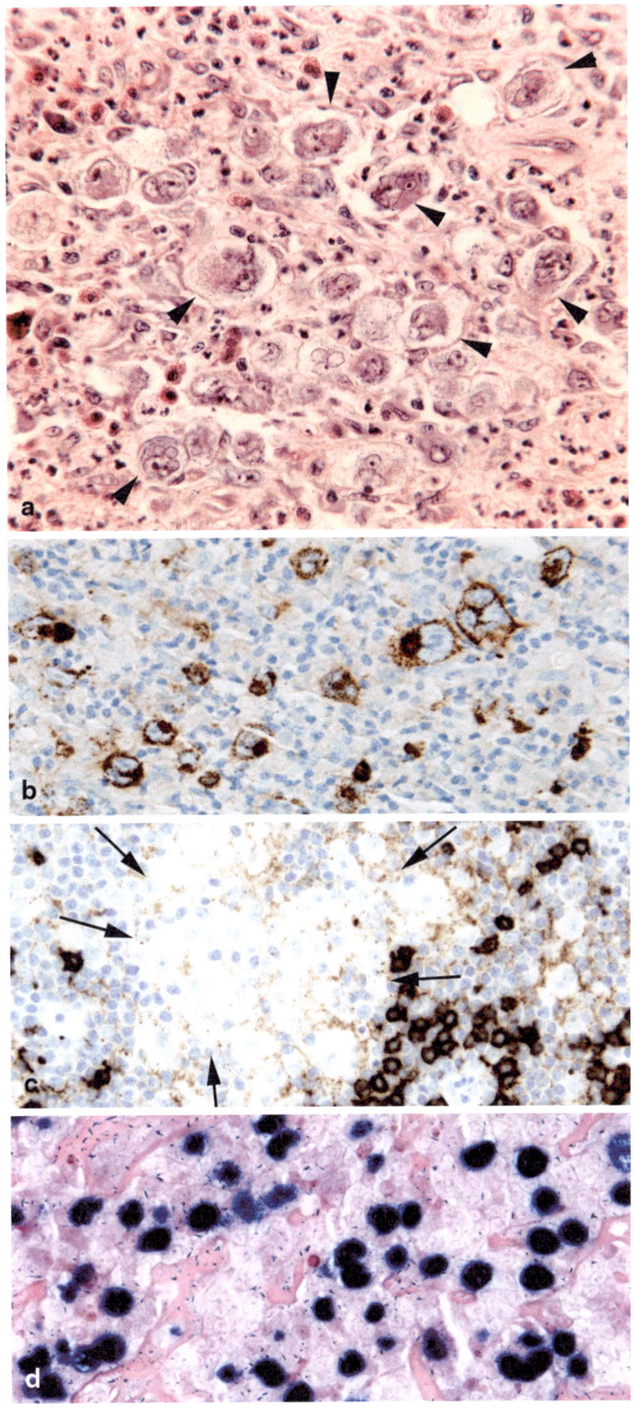

Fig. 27.3 Hodgkin lymphoma (HL). **a** Numerous large pleomorphic tumor cells with the characteristics of Hodgkin and Reed–Sternberg cells (*arrowheads*) are surrounded by a nonneoplastic mixed inflammatory background including numerous eosinophils. **b** Membranous and Golgi immunoreactivity for CD15 is present in large, neoplastic cells. **c** Large, neoplastic cells (between *arrows*) are negative for the B-cell marker CD20. Scattered nonneoplastic B lymphocytes (dark staining cells) are also present. **d** EBV EBER in-situ hybridization showing strong nuclear reactivity (*dark blue* nuclei) in all large, neoplastic cells

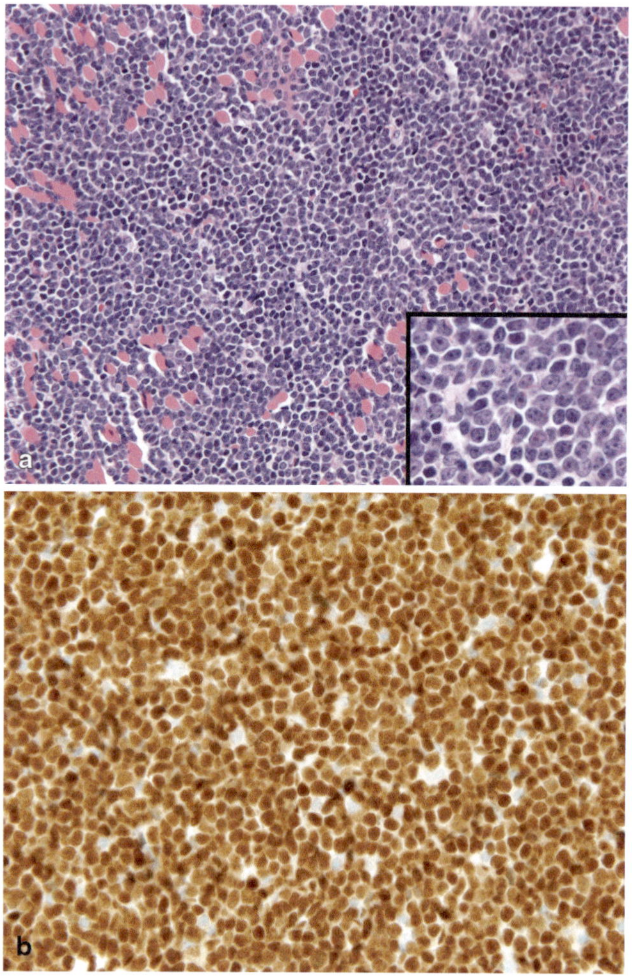

Fig. 27.4 Lymphoblastic lymphoma. **a** Diffuse, proliferation of monotonous small-sized tumor cells infiltrating skeletal muscle. *Inset*: small- to medium-sized tumor cells at higher magnification showing scant cytoplasm, irregular nuclear envelopes, finely dispersed chromatin, and small nucleoli. Muscle cells are the large eosinophilic cells interspersed throughout. **b** Diffuse, strong nuclear immunoreactivity for terminal TdT

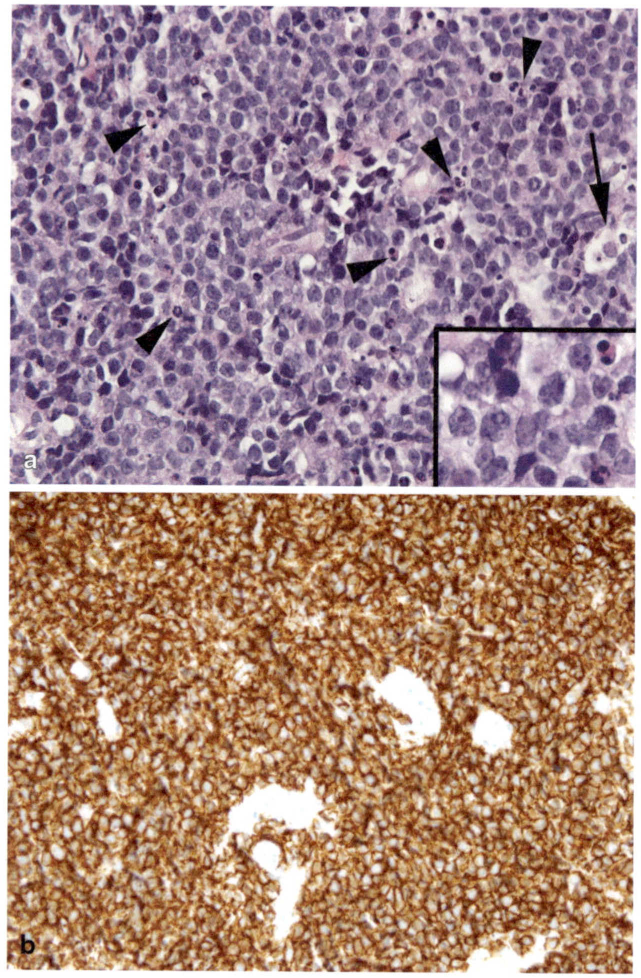

Fig. 27.5 Burkitt lymphoma. **a** Cellular infiltrate of undifferentiated, small- to medium-sized noncleaved lymphoblasts and numerous apoptotic tumor cells (*arrowheads*). A macrophage with cytoplasmic tingible bodies is indicated by *arrow*. *Inset*: higher magnification of tumor cells showing high nuclear cytoplasmic ratio, mild pleomorphism, single to multiple readily seen nucleoli, and scant cytoplasm. Apoptotic tumor cells are also seen. **b** Diffuse, strong immunoreactivity for CD20 a marker of B lymphocytes

macrophages full of debris from turnover of rapidly dividing and apoptotic tumor cells. Together they create the classic starry-sky appearance (Fig. 27.5). The tumor cells express B-cell antigens such as CD19 and CD20 and lack immature markers including TdT and CD34. Ninety percent will have a MYC gene translocation.

Pediatric diffuse large B-cell lymphoma (DLBCL) has a germinal center B-cell phenotype and is thus a BCL6 gene product and CD10 positive. It rarely demonstrates the t(14;18) translocation as in adult DLBCL. DLBCL cases with an IRF4 translocation are significantly more frequent in children than adults (15% vs. 2%) [24].

Anaplastic large cell lymphoma, the most common mature T-cell neoplasm in children, characteristically demonstrates large, pleomorphic cells that express one of the T-cell specific markers, i.e., CD2, CD3, or CD5. Few express the nonspecific CD43 antigen which is termed the null cell phenotype. The tumor cells in anaplastic large-cell lymphoma (ALCL) all strongly express CD30 [23]. Most pediatric cases also express ALK protein and have very characteristic cells with horseshoe- or kidney-shaped nuclei and eosinophilic cytoplasm (Fig. 27.6) [12].

Staging

In childhood ALL and AML risk groups have been and are being established to determine the optimal approach to treatment. In ALL, risk groups are based on factors such as age at diagnosis, presenting white blood cell count, cytogenetics/ploidy, and CNS involvement. AML risk assessment is

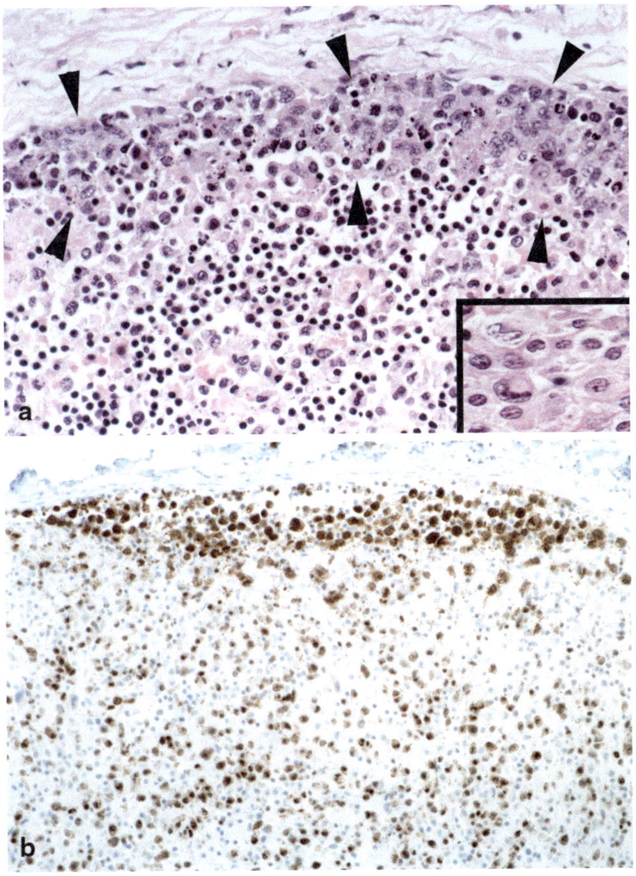

Fig. 27.6 Anaplastic large-cell lymphoma. **a** Densely cellular neoplastic infiltrate is occupying the distended subcapsular sinus of a lymph node (between *arrowheads*). *Inset*: Characteristic cytology with hallmark cells with abundant pale amphophilic cytoplasm and large kidney-shaped nuclei. **b** Tumor cells show strong nuclear and cytoplasmic immunoreactivity for ALK-1

mostly based on cytogenetics, as that has proven most predictive of outcome. Response to therapy is also being incorporated into risk assessment in childhood ALL and AML.

Lymphomas are typically staged using one of two staging systems; the Ann Arbor staging system is generally used for HL and the St. Jude/Murphy staging system is used for NHL (Tables 27.3 and 27.4) [25, 26].

Treatment

Chemotherapy

Chemotherapy is the standard therapy for hematology malignancies. Children with ALL require 2 years of therapy which includes induction, during which children are induced into remission, consolidation, and maintenance. While chemotherapy regimens differ, they almost always include treatment with corticosteroid, methotrexate, vincristine, mercaptopurine, asparaginase, and anthracycline (such as doxorubicin). AML includes an intensive 6 months of therapy and possible hematopoietic stem cell transplant depending on risk factors. Most regimens include high-dose cytarabine and an anthracycline. Treatment of APL, a sub-type of AML, includes all-trans retinoic acid (ATRA).

Lymphoma therapies vary greatly depending on the type of lymphoma and the staging evaluation, but all contain some form of combination therapy, which often includes steroids, anthracyclines, antimetabolites, and alkylating agents.

Surgical Therapy

Surgical lymph node removal is the most common diagnostic procedure in lymphoma, while leukemia is diagnosed via bone marrow biopsy. Both procedures are very rarely associated with complications.

Radiation Therapy

As stated above, standard therapy for hematologic malignancies is chemotherapy, which is necessary to achieve cure. However, radiation therapy can play an important role in some types of lymphoma and in leukemias with involvement of the CNS.

Complications

- General complications associated with radiation therapy include fatigue, nausea and vomiting, as well as skin

Table 27.3 Ann Arbor staging system for HL

Stage	
I	Involvement of a single-lymph node region or of a single-extranodal organ or site (I_E)
II	Involvement of two or more lymph node regions on the same side of the diaphragm, or localized involvement of an extranodal site or organ (II_E) and one or more lymph node regions on the same side of the diaphragm
III	Involvement of lymph node regions on both sides of the diaphragm, which may also be accompanied by localized involvement of an extranodal organ or site (III_E) or spleen (III_S) or both (III_{SE})
IV	Diffuse or disseminated involvement of one or more distant extranodal sites

B symptoms include fever >38 °C, night sweats, weight loss >10 % of body weight in the 6 months preceding, and are denoted by the suffix B. Patients without these symptoms are denoted by the suffix A

Table 27.4 St. Jude/Murphy staging system for NHL

Stage	
I	Involvement of a single-lymph node region or of a single-extranodal organ, excluding the mediastinum or abdomen
II	Involvement of a single tumor with regional node involvement, two or more tumors or nodal areas involved on one side of the diaphragm, or a primary gastrointestinal tract tumor (completely resected) with or without regional node involvement
III	Involvement of tumors or involved lymph node areas that occur on both sides of the diaphragm, any primary intrathoracic (mediastinal, pleural, or thymic) disease, extensive primary intraabdominal disease, or any paraspinal or epidural tumors
IV	Involvement of bone marrow and/or central nervous system (CNS), regardless of other sites of involvement

and mucosal changes in the area affected. Somnolence syndrome, excessive sleep, drowsiness, lethargy, and anorexia, can occur as early as 3 weeks following cranial radiotherapy.

- In addition, and of particular relevance in the head and neck region, is the impairment of soft-tissue and bone growth.
- Long-term side effects include a risk of second malignancies in the radiation field. Chest radiation increases the risk for the development of secondary breast cancers as well as cardiac complications [27, 28].

Outcomes

Overall survival of children with acute leukemia has improved dramatically over the last 40 years. Over 80% of children and adolescents presenting with ALL are expected to achieve long-term cure. Cure rates for AML are lower at 55–65% but risk-adapted protocols are hoped to improve prognosis. Childhood lymphoma has similarly high 5-year survival rates. Both HL and NHL survival rates are greater than 80% for all children less than 20 years of age. Given such high cure rates, newer risk-adapted treatment strategies are being investigated in order to minimize long-term secondary effects [29–31].

Follow-up

After cancer-directed therapy is complete, patients continue to be followed by their oncologists. The focus of follow-up is initially for close monitoring for disease recurrence. Follow-up visits include careful history, physical examination, and laboratory evaluation. In patients with a history of lymphoma, imaging evaluation (such as CT imaging or chest radiography) may also be incorporated into follow-up. Over time, the focus of follow-up shifts to screening and assessing for the development of late effects of therapy.

References

1. Urquhart A, Berg R. Hodgkin's and Non-Hodgkin's lymphoma of the head and neck. Laryngoscope. 2001;111:1565–9.
2. Anderson PC, Stotland MA, Dinulos JG, Perry AE. Acute lymphocytic leukemia presenting as an isolated scalp nodule in an infant. Ann Plast Surg. 2010;64:251–3.
3. Dusenbery KE, Howells WB, Arthur DC, Alonzo T, Lee JW, Kobrinsky N, Barnard DR, Wells RJ, Buckley JD, Lange BJ, Woods WG. Extramedullary leukemia in children with newly diagnosed acute myeloid leukemia: a report from the Children's Cancer Group. J Pediatr Hematol Oncol. 2003;25:760–8.
4. Schultz KR, Pullen DJ, Sather HN, Shuster JJ, Devidas M, Borowitz MJ, Carroll AJ, Heerema NA, Rubnitz JE, Loh ML, Raetz EA, Winick NJ, Hunger SP, Carroll WL, Gaynon PS, Camitta BM. Risk- and response-based classification of childhood B-precursor acute lymphoblastic leukemia: a combined analysis of prognostic markers from the Pediatric Oncology Group (POG) and Children's Cancer Group (CCG). Blood. 2007;109:926–35.
5. Shimada AT, Taki T, Tabuchi K, et al. KIT mutations, and not FLT3 internal tandem duplication, are strongly associated with a poor prognosis in pediatric acute myeloid leukemia with t(8;21); a study of the Japanese Childhood AML Cooperative Study Group. Blood. 2006;107:1806–9.
6. Tallman MS, Hakimian D, Shaw JM, Lissner GS, Russell EJ, Variakojis D. Granulocytic sarcoma is associated with the 8;21 translocation in acute myeloid leukemia. J Clin Oncol. 1993;11:690–7.
7. Schwyzer R, Sherman GG, Cohn RJ, Poole JE, Willem P. Granulocytic sarcoma in children with acute myeloblastic leukemia and t(8;21). Med Pediatr Oncol. 1998;31:144–9.
8. Johnston DL, Alonzo TA, Gerbing RB, Lange BJ, Woods WG. Superior outcome of pediatric acute myeloid leukemia patients with orbital and CNS myeloid sarcoma: a report from the Children's Oncology Group. Pediatr Blood Cancer. 2012;58:519–24.
9. De Botton S, Dombret H, Sanz M, et al. Incidence, clinical features, and outcome of all transretinoic acid syndrome in 413 cases of newly diagnosed acute promyelocytic leukemia. The European APL Group. Blood. 1998;92:2712–8.
10. Zwaan CM, Meshinchi S, Radich JP, et al. FLT3 internal tandem duplication in 234 children with acute myeloid leukemia: prognostic significance and relation to cellular drug resistance. Blood. 2003;102:2387–94.
11. Gross TG, Perkins SL. Malignant non-Hodgkin lymphomas in children. In: Pizzo PA, Poplack DG, editors. Principles and practice of pediatric oncology. 6th ed. Philadelphia: Lippincott Williams & Wilkins; 2011.
12. Stein H, Foss HD, Durkop H, Marafioti T, Desol G, Pulford K, Pilieri S, Falini B. CD30 + anaplastic large cell lymphoma: a review of its histopathologic, genetic, and clinical features. Blood. 2000;96:3681–95.
13. Magrath IT. African Burkitt's lymphoma: history, biology, clinical features, and treatment. Am J Pediatr Hematol Oncol. 1991;13:222–46.
14. Magrath I. Epidemiology: clues to the pathogenesis of Burkitt lymphoma. Br J Haematol. 2012;156:744–56.
15. Flavell KJ, Murray PG. Hodgkin's disease and the Epstein–Barr virus. Mol Pathol. 2000;53:262–9.
16. Salavoura K, Kolialexi A, Tsangaris G, Mavrou A. Development of cancer in patients with primary immunodeficiencies. Anticancer Res. 2008;28:1263–9.

17. Millot F, Robert A, Bertrand Y, Mechinaud F, Laureys G, Ferster A, Brock P, Rohrlich P, Mazingue F, Plantaz D, Plouvier E, Pacquement H, Behar C, Rialland X, Chantraine JM, Guilhot F, Otten J. Cutaneous involvement in children with acute lymphoblastic leukemia or lymphoblastic lymphoma. The Children's Leukemia Cooperative Group of the European Organization of Research and Treatment of Cancer (EORTC). Pediatrics. 1997;100:60–4.
18. Muler JH, Valdez R, Hayes C, Kaminski MS. Acute megakaryocytic leukemia presenting as hypercalcemia with skeletal lytic lesions. Eur J Haematol. 2002;68:392–6.
19. Sood BR, Sharma B, Kumar S, Gupta D, Sharma A. Facial palsy as first presentation of acute myeloid leukemia. Am J Hematol. 2003;74:200–1.
20. Cankaya H, Ugras S, Dilek I. Head and neck granulocytic sarcoma with acute myeloid leukemia: three rare cases. Ear Nose Throat J. 2001;80:224–6, 228–9.
21. Almadori G, Del Ninno M, Cadoni G, Di Mario A, Ottaviani F. Facial nerve paralysis in acute otomastoiditis as presenting symptom of FAB M2, T8;21 leukemic relapse. Case report and review of the literature. Int J Pediatr Otorhinolaryngol. 1996;36:45–52.
22. Manning D, Palacios E, Neitzschman H. Recurrent pre-B-cell acute lymphoblastic leukemia in the middle ear: a form of granulocytic sarcoma. Ear Nose Throat J. 2012;91:272–4.
23. Heerema-McKenney A, Cleary M, Arber DA. Pathology and molecular diagnosis of leukemias and lymphoma. In: Pizzo PA, Poplack DG, editors Principles and practice of pediatric oncology. 6th ed. Philadelphia: Lippincott Williams & Wilkins 2011.
24. Salaverria I, Philipp C, Oschlies I, et al. Translocations activating IRF4 identify a subtype of germinal center-derived B-cell lymphoma affecting predominantly children and young adults. Blood. 2011;118:139–47.
25. Carbone PP, Kaplan HS, Musshoff K, et al. Report of the Committee on Hodgkin's Disease Staging Classification. Cancer Res. 1971;31:1860–1861.
26. Murphy SB. Classification, staging and end results of treatment of childhood non-Hodgkin's lymphomas: dissimilarities from lymphomas in adults. Semin Oncol. 1980;7:332–339.
27. Cooke R, Jones ME, Cunningham D, Falk SJ, Gilson D, Hancock BW, Harris SJ, Horwich A, Hoskin PJ, Illidge T, Linch DC, Lister TA, Lucraft HH, Radford JA, Stevens AM, Syndikus I, Williams MV, England and Wales Hodgkin Lymphoma Follow-up Group, Swerdlow AJ. Breast cancer risk following Hodgkin lymphoma radiotherapy in relation to menstrual and reproductive factors. Br J Cancer. 2013;108:2399–406.
28. Adams MJ, Lipsitz SR, Colan SD, Tarbell NJ, Treves ST, Diller L, Greenbaum N, Mauch P, Lipshultz SE. Cardiovascular status in long-term survivors of Hodgkin's disease treated with chest radiotherapy. J Clin Oncol 2004;22:3139–48.
29. Mauz-Körholz C, Hasenclever D, Dörffel W, Ruschke K, Pelz T, Voigt A, Stiefel M, Winkler M, Vilser C, Dieckmann K, Karlén J, Bergsträsser E, Fosså A, Mann G, Hummel M, Klapper W, Stein H, Vordermark D, Kluge R, Körholz D. Procarbazine-free OEPA-COPDAC chemotherapy in boys and standard OPPA-COPP in girls have comparable effectiveness in pediatric Hodgkin's lymphoma: the GPOH-HD-2002 study. J Clin Oncol. 2010;28(23):3680–6.
30. Metzger ML, Weinstein HJ, Hudson MM, Billett AL, Larsen EC, Friedmann A, Howard SC, Donaldson SS, Krasin MJ, Kun LE, Marcus KJ, Yock TI, Tarbell N, Billups CA, Wu J, Link MP. Association between radiotherapy vs no radiotherapy based on early response to VAMP chemotherapy and survival among children with favorable-risk Hodgkin lymphoma. JAMA. 2012;307:2609–16.
31. Meyer RM, Gospodarowicz MK, Connors JM, Pearcey RG, Wells WA, Winter JN, Horning SJ, Dar AR, Shustik C, Stewart DA, Crump M, Djurfeldt MS, Chen BE, Shepherd LE, NCIC Clinical Trials Group, Eastern Cooperative Oncology Group. ABVD alone versus radiation-based therapy in limited-stage Hodgkin's lymphoma. N Engl J Med. 2012;366:399–408.

Lymphatic Malformations

28

Karen Watters, Raja Shaikh, Horacio M. Padua and Reza Rahbar

Introduction

Lymphatic malformations (LMs), initially described by Wernher in 1843, are slow-flow vascular anomalies, most commonly presenting in the head and neck of children. They continue to be a challenging management entity to this day.

Epidemiology

The incidence of LMs ranges between 1 in 2,000–4,000 live births [1, 2]. LMs typically occur in the first decade of life. 50 % of all LMs are detectable at birth, and as many as 90 % are diagnosed by the end of the 2nd year of life owing to clinical symptoms [3]. LMs account for approximately 5 % of all benign tumors in children. 75 % of all LMs occur in the head and neck region [4]. LMs are not race specific and both sexes are equally affected.

Classification

Previously, confusing terminology without pathologic basis surrounded the diagnosis of LMs, including that of "cystic hygroma" or watery tumor of the neck. This terminology has often led to delay in diagnosis, incorrect diagnoses, and incorrect treatments. In 1996, The International Society for the Study of Vascular Anomalies (ISSVA) proposed a binary classification of vascular anomalies based on clinical behavior and cellular kinetics [5, 6]. As part of this system, LAs are classified as slow-flow vascular malformations that exhibit normal endothelial cell turnover (Table 28.1).

LMs have also been categorized according to *histologic appearance, cyst size,* and *anatomical relationship to the mylohyoid muscle* [7, 8] (Type 1 and 2, see Table 28.2).

- *Type 1 lesions* are located below the mylohyoid muscle, and involve the anterior and posterior triangles of the neck. These lesions tend to be *macrocystic* (cysts >1 cm) and carry a more favorable prognosis (Fig. 28.1a).
- *Type 2 lesions* are found above the level of the mylohyoid muscle and frequently involve tongue, cheek, parotid, supraglottis, floor of mouth, oropharynx, and lip. These lesions tend to be *microcystic* (cysts <1 cm) and carry a less favorable prognosis (Fig. 28.1b).

Embryology

The lymphatic system develops at week 5 of gestation as endothelial outgrowths from the venous system. These outgrowths then develop into six lymphatic sacs that develop into the lymphatic system in a process of "sprouting" and branching. By the 9th week, the right and left thoracic ducts then connect with the venous system again at the junction of the internal jugular and subclavian veins. Although, the molecular mechanism underlying the formation of LMs remain unclear, it is thought to be the result of *lymphatic dysmorphogenesis* [9, 10].

K. Watters (✉)
Department of Otolaryngology and Communication Enhancement, Boston Children's Hospital, Harvard Medical School, Boston, MA, USA
e-mail: Karen.Watters@childrens.harvard.edu

R. Shaikh
Department of Interventional Radiology, Boston Children's Hospital, Harvard Medical School, Boston, MA, USA

H. M. Padua
Department of Radiology, Boston Children's Hospital, Harvard Medical School, Boston, MA, USA

R. Rahbar
Department of Otolaryngology and Communication Enhancement, Boston Children's Hospital, Harvard Medical School, Boston, MA, USA

R. Rahbar et al. (eds.), *Pediatric Head and Neck Tumors*,
DOI 10.1007/978-1-4614-8755-5_28, © Springer Science+Business Media New York 2014

Table 28.1 Binary classification of vascular anomalies [5, 6]

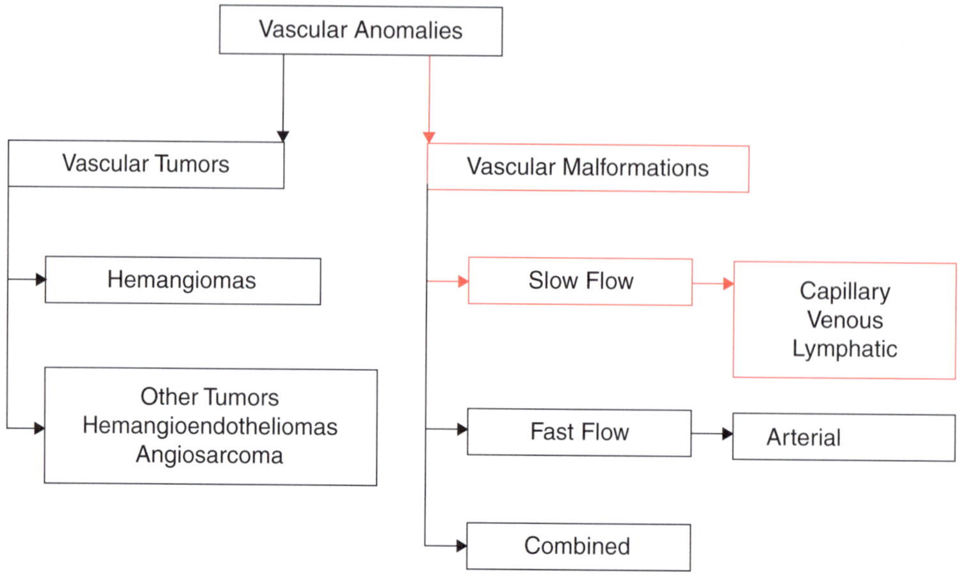

Table 28.2 LM types

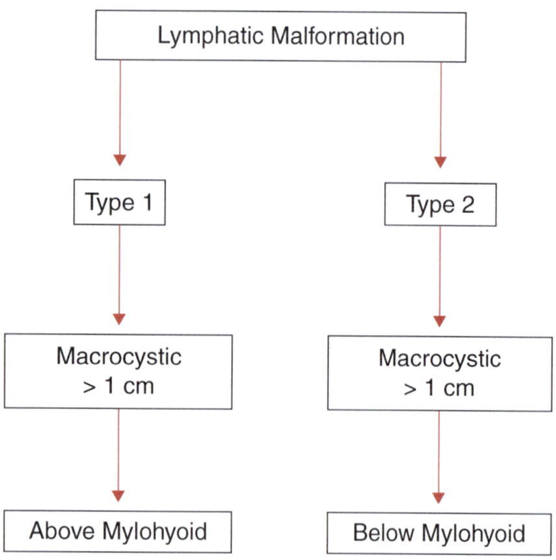

Pathogenesis

The majority of LMs are thought to form from parts of the lymph sac that fail to establish connections with the main lymphatic system or venous channels. Theories of LM development include:

1. Failure of the lymphatic system to adequately separate or connect to the venous system, giving rise to cyst formation and lymphatic accumulation.
2. Abnormal sequestration of lymphatic tissue in embryogenesis.
3. Anomalous budding or "sprouting" of lymphatic structures from the cardinal vein. This theory of "centrifugal" development, hypothesizes that lymphatic endothelium derives from venous endothelium and undergoes centrifugal sprouting to the periphery, and through the expression of factors like vascular endothelial growth factor receptor 3 (VEGFR-3) and prospero homeobox protein (Prox-1) develops into lymphatics [11]. Conditions that result in the inappropriate expression of lymphatic-specific molecules may cause or contribute to embryologic LM development. Further understanding of the possible influence of molecular markers on the development and growth of LMs may allow the development of lymphatic-specific therapeutic strategies that alter the clinical course of patients with LM [9–13].

Histopathology

In contrast to vascular tumors (hemangiomas), LMs generally have normal levels of endothelial turnover. Histologic evaluations of LMs show no evidence of cellular proliferation, but rather a progressive dilatation of vessels of abnormal structure.

LMs are composed of vascular spaces filled with eosinophilic and protein-rich fluid. Multiple dilated lymphatic channels are lined by a single layer of flattened quiescent endothelium that lies on a thin single laminar basement membrane (Fig. 28.2a). The fibrovascular vessel walls are of variable thickness containing both smooth and striated muscle elements. Nodular clusters of lymphocytes are commonly seen within the cystic structure. Hemorrhage within the cystic spaces is also common, which may indicate recent trauma or spontaneous intralesional bleeding.

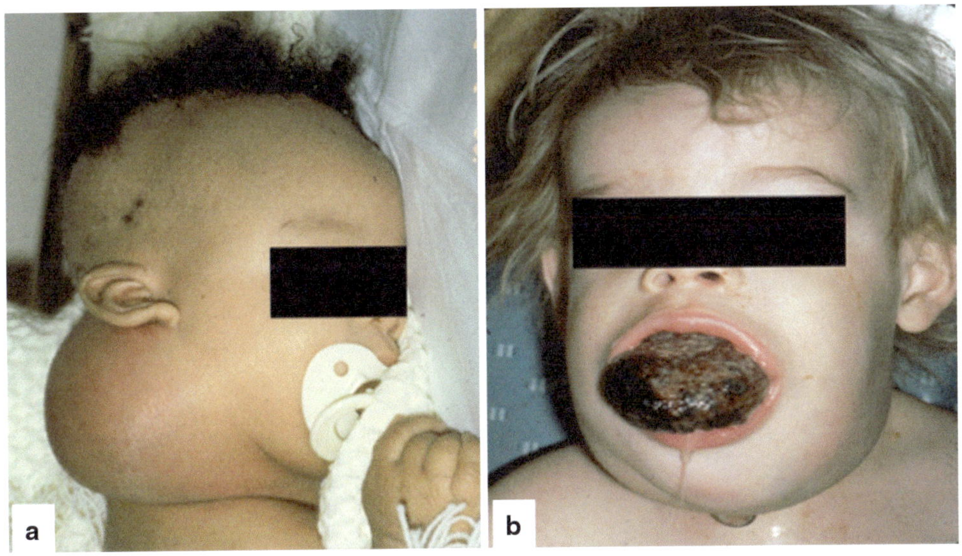

Fig. 28.1 Types of LM. **a** Type 1—macrocystic, typically below the mylohyoid muscle. **b** Type 2—microcystic, typically above the mylohyoid muscle

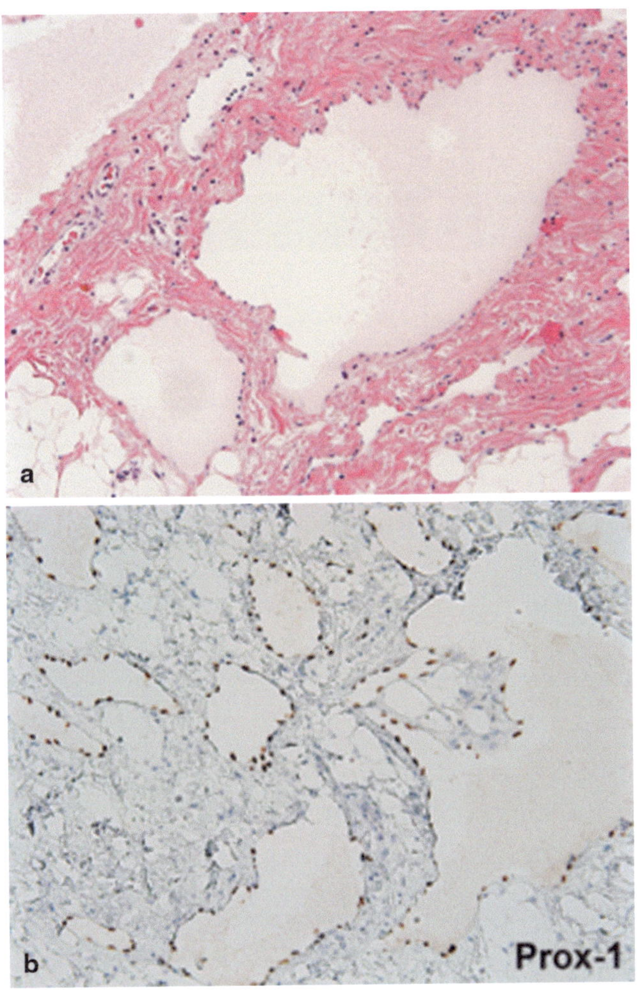

Fig. 28.2 Lymphatic malformation, soft tissue neck. **a** Thin-walled channels lined by flattened lymphothelium. **b** Lymphatic endothelial cells showing strong nuclear Prox-1 immunoreactivity, characteristic of lymphatic lineage

LMs express several common endothelial cell surface markers such as VEGFR-3, lymphatic vessel endothelial hyaluronan receptor 1 (LYVE-1) and nuclear Prox-1 immunoreactivity characteristic of lymphatic lineage (Fig. 28.2b). LMs, however, do not express the biologic markers associated with vascular tumors (glucose transporter 1 (GLUT 1), merosin, and Lewis Y antigen) [5, 6].

Clinical Presentation

Natural History

By definition, LMs are present at birth. Almost all LMs have presenting symptoms within the first 2 years of life. LMs grow commensurately with the child, with symptoms generally determined by the size and location of the malformation and to the perturbation of the adjacent tissues. Sudden enlargement may be seen secondary to infection or trauma, which may cause intralesional bleeding. LMs have also been reported as enlarging during increased hormonal stages, such as puberty [3]. LMs do not typically spontaneously regress, however, there have been reports of spontaneous regression following infection [7, 14].

Associated Disorders

Posterior cervical lesions that arise in the perinatal period have been associated with Turner's syndrome, as well as other syndromes such as Down's syndrome [15]. In these situations, there is an associated high prenatal mortality rate secondary to hydrops and diffuse lymphedema. Therefore,

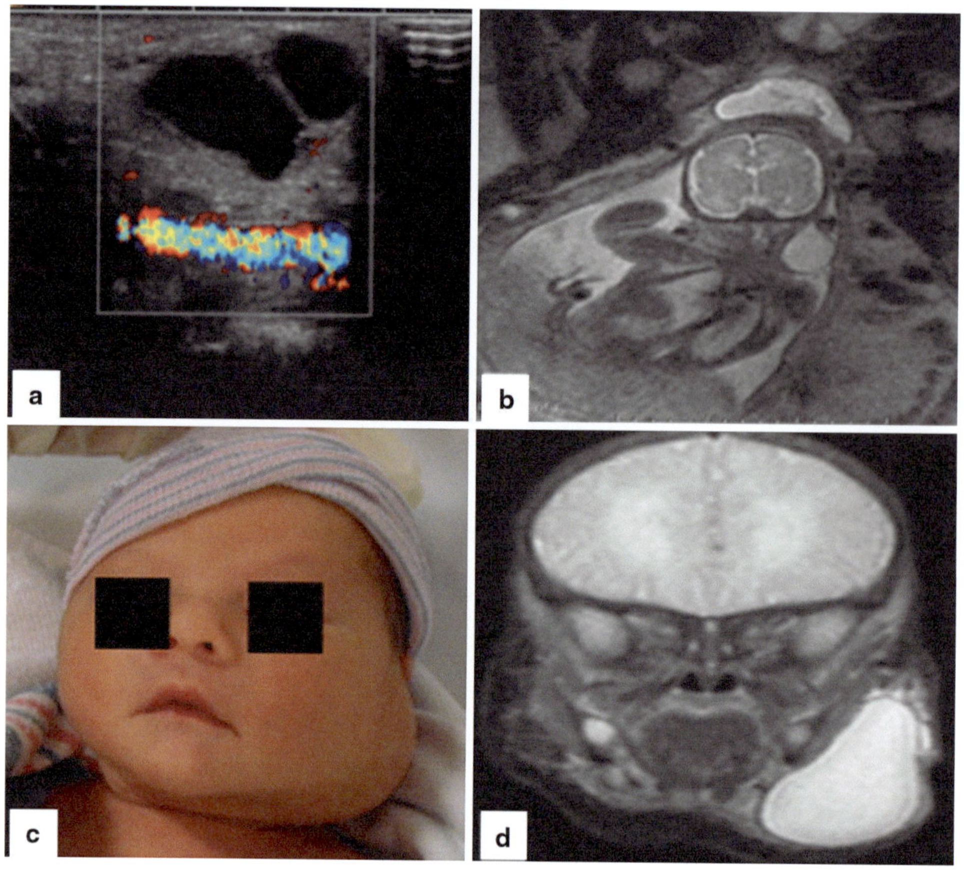

Fig. 28.3 Prenatal imaging of LM. **a** Prenatal US performed at 24 weeks gestation, showing a cystic lesion next to the carotid artery, consistent with an LM. **b** Fetal MRI at 24 weeks gestation of the same patient in **a**, showing the left cystic neck lesion. **c** The patient at delivery at 38 weeks, left neck swelling is visible. **d** Postnatal coronal MRI showing cystic left neck swelling

amniocentesis with chromosomal analysis and genetic counseling is recommended. Lymphatic malformations that present after birth are generally not associated with chromosomal abnormalities.

Prenatal Diagnosis

Antenatal diagnosis of LM can be made as early as 10–16 weeks gestation. The rate of antenatal detection has increased along with the increased widespread complementary use of prenatal fetal ultrasound (US) and fetal magnetic resonance imaging (MRI) [16] (Fig. 28.3).

The prenatal diagnosis of a large cervicofacial LM can have significant clinical implications, as it may be associated with significant airway obstruction, influencing the type, timing, and place of delivery [17, 18] (Fig. 28.4). Large cervicofacial LMs may require immediate airway intervention at the time of delivery. Such deliveries should be carefully planned at a tertiary referral center with a multidisciplinary team, including obstetrics, maternal fetal medicine, otolaryngology, pediatric surgery, neonatal medicine, and both obstetric and pediatric anesthesia. In some cases an ex-utero intrapartum treatment (EXIT) procedure may be required.

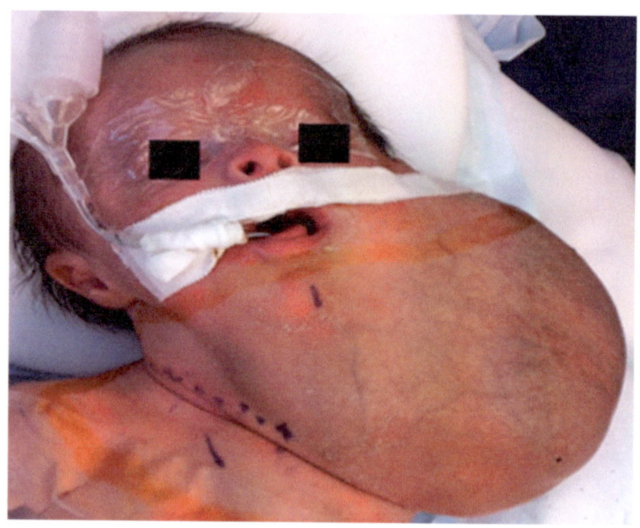

Fig. 28.4 EXIT Procedure. Newborn infant with a large, left cervicofacial LM, with associated airway compression. This patient was delivered via an EXIT procedure and was intubated by direct laryngoscopy on placental circulation

Diagnosis and Evaluation

In most cases, the diagnosis of an LM can be made by correlating a complete clinical history and physical examination. Key parts of the patient's history include:

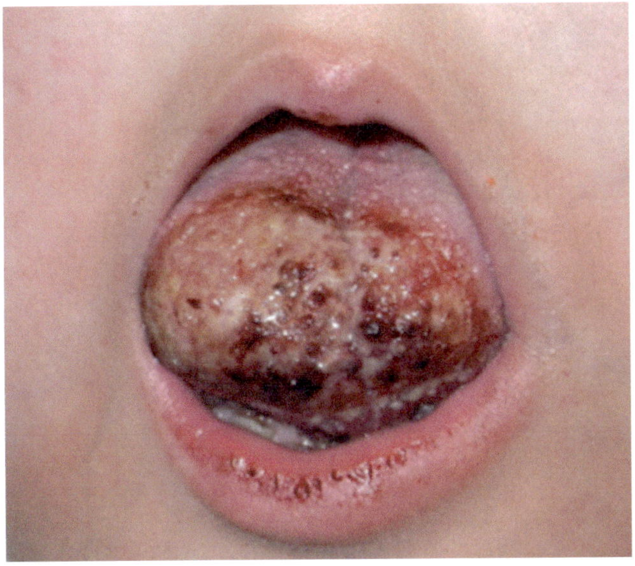

Fig. 28.5 Superficial dermal involvement in a tongue LM. Multiple tiny vesicles, which bleed easily, are present

1. Age at which the lesion was initially noticed.
2. Overall rate of growth of the lesion as well as recent changes in the size of the lesion.
3. Acute changes in the size of the lesion related to upper respiratory tract infections, trauma, and hormonal changes.

Salient features on physical examination include the color, temperature, compressibility, pulsatility, and configuration of the lesion, as well as its relationship to surrounding anatomic structures. LMs are typically soft and cystic. Transillumination may identify cystic lesions, although this is not helpful if hemorrhage has occurred into the cysts [19].

Microcystic lesions are commonly found above the level of the mylohyoid muscle, and involve the oral cavity, cheek, tongue, lip, supraglottis, floor of mouth, and parotid gland. Intraoral LMs are nearly always of the mixed or microcystic classification. These lesions are poorly defined and infiltrate into surrounding tissue, obscuring muscle and fatty planes. Tiny vesicles, which represent small lymph-filled cysts and macroscopically resemble fish eggs, may be present, indicating superficial dermal involvement. These vesicles, may develop a purple color secondary to intracystic hemorrhage and can bleed or ulcerate (Fig. 28.5). Tongue lesions may cause bleeding, halitosis, dysphagia, dysarthria, and airway obstruction.

Macrocystic lesions are usually found below the level of the mylohyoid muscle, in the anterior and posterior triangles of the neck. They are typically multilocular structures consisting of numerous cysts that vary in size and shape.

Although LMs are benign, they can continue to expand and may undergo rapid enlargement secondary to infection, hemorrhage, or trauma, including operative intervention. Rapid growth of cervicofacial LMs may lead to significant clinical sequelae including:

1. *Airway obstruction:* Infiltrative LMs that involve the floor of mouth, tongue, and oropharynx may frequently cause upper airway obstruction [20]. This may be sudden if there is a rapid increase in the LM secondary to infection, trauma, or hemorrhage, demanding immediate attention. Emergency orotracheal intubation is optimally performed under general anesthesia, allowing for full assessment of the extent of the lesion once the airway is secured. Tracheostomy may be required in cases of significant supraglottic or oropharyngeal involvement.
2. *Functional issues:* Dysphagia, speech impairment and dental problems, may all be caused by involvement of the LM in the oropharynx and upper airway. A gastrostomy tube may be required for feeding. Gross involvement of the tongue may cause macroglossia, tongue protrusion, and impair speech. Neuropathy secondary to compression by large lesions can cause pain and parathesia.
3. *Deformity:* Enlargement of LMs may cause gross cosmetic deformity, including macroglossia, prognathism, macrototia, and significant cervicofacial asymmetry, secondary to distortion of the craniofacial skeleton caused by bony hypertrophy. This in turn may lead to significant social ramifications and psychologic distress as the child becomes older.
4. *Hemorrhage and infection:* A rapid increase in the size of a LM may be associated with hemorrhage or infection. Hemorrhage into a cervical LM may be associated with acute respiratory distress and airway obstruction. Infection may cause increased macroglossia and oropharyngeal cellulitis. If severe, admission to hospital with close airway monitoring and intravenous antibiotics are required. Chylothorax and chylopericardium have been reported in large cervicomediastinal lesions.

Differential Diagnosis

An accurate clinical history and examination should distinguish between an LM from a vascular tumor (hemangiomas) and can usually exclude other neck lesions including branchial, cleft cyst, lipoma, etc. In cases where the LM may be a mixed lesion with a venous complement, imaging studies, such as US, computed tomography (CT), and MRI, can aid diagnosis.

Imaging Evaluation

Although LMs are primarily diagnosed on clinical history and examination, the role of imaging plays an important role in not only confirming the diagnosis, but also determining

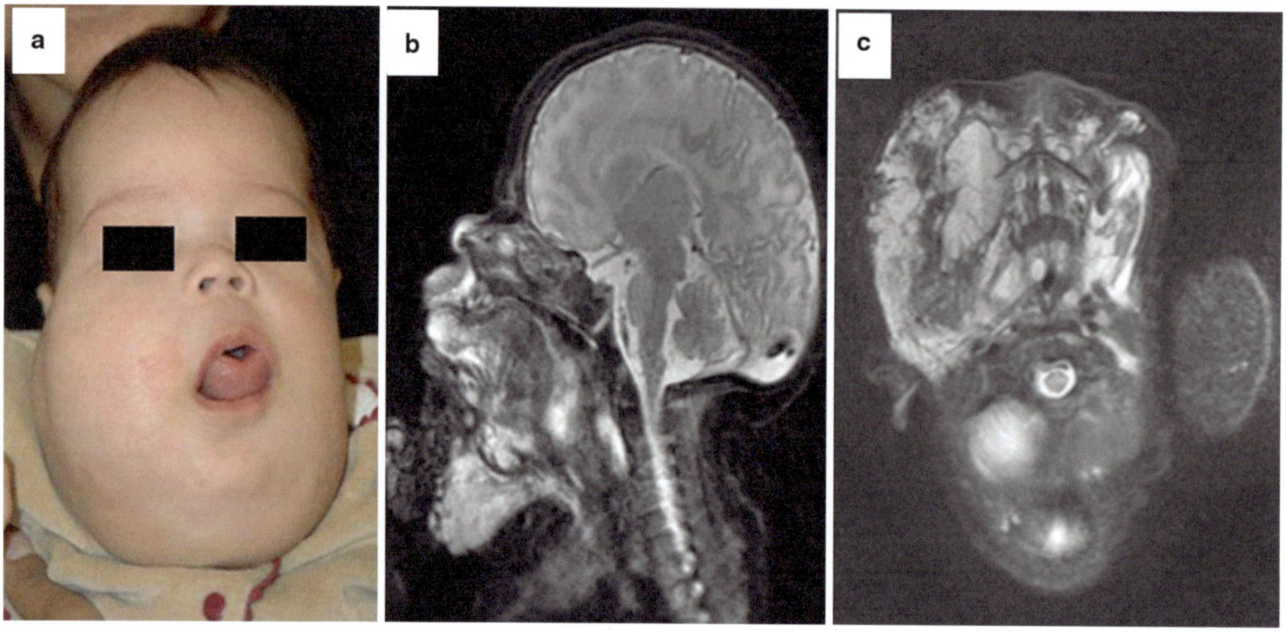

Fig. 28.6 **a** A large microcystic and macrocystic cervicofacial and tongue LM with microcystic and macrocystic components causing significant airway obstruction. **b** Saggital MRI scan. **c** Axial MRI showing the microcystic and macrocystic components of the LM and the relationship to surrounding structures

the extent, and type of the lesion (microcystic vs. macrocystic), and its anatomic relationship to surrounding tissue planes, muscles, and vascular structures. Imaging is essential for preoperative planning, if surgery is considered. Primary imaging modalities include US, CT, and MRI with gadolinium. MRI with contrast is the study of choice (Fig. 28.6).

Treatment

LMs of the head and neck are challenging management problems. The principal goal of management is restoration or preservation of function. Treatment depends on the clinical presentation, the size of the lesion, the anatomic location, and the complications. If symptoms are life threatening, then immediate intervention is warranted. In the absence of a significant functional deficit, there is a role for observation of the lesion until it "declares itself" as such and its growth pattern has become evident. Treatment can often be delayed well past infancy into preschool years—the timing relative to the age of the patient remains debatable. Careful treatment planning with multidisciplinary input is essential for all extensive cervicofacial LMs.

The main treatment modalities for LMs are observation, sclerotherapy, and surgical resection [21]. While macrocystic lesions are often amenable to sclerotherapy and surgery, the infiltrative nature of microcystic lesions makes total surgical excision not possible without causing unacceptable loss of function. Subtotal resection is complicated by a high recurrence rate [22].

1. Sclerotherapy

Sclerotherapy is a widely accepted minimally invasive approach to treat LMs. It is used extensively both as primary treatment as well as an alternative to surgery in patients where surgical resection is not possible. Sclerotherapy can also be used to treat residual or recurrent disease following resection. The procedure involves injection of a pharmacological agent that elicits an avid inflammatory response and induces endothelial damage, which leads to fibrosis and shrinkage of the lesions. Among the LMs, the macrocystic variety typically responds well to sclerotherapy. The microcystic lesions are technically difficult to treat and show a poor response to sclerotherapy.

Injection of a sclerosing agent is painful and therefore, in children, is typically done under general anesthesia under image guidance by an experienced interventional radiologist. Sedation with ketamine can also be used for small lesions and short procedures [23]. 20–23 gauge needles or angiocatheters are used for the percutaneous access. Image guidance, like US and real time fluoroscopy are frequently employed to gain safe access into the lymphatic macrocysts and study them with a radiological contrast agent [23, 24] (Figs. 28.7 and 28.8). This is very beneficial in complex macrocystic LMs as frequently there are arteries and veins traversing randomly into the lesion mass, and also often there is the neurovascular bundle coursing in the vicinity or ensheathing the cystic mass (Fig. 28.7).

Sclerosants reported for use in treating macrocystic LMs include ethanol, doxycycline, bleomycin, sodium sotradecol,

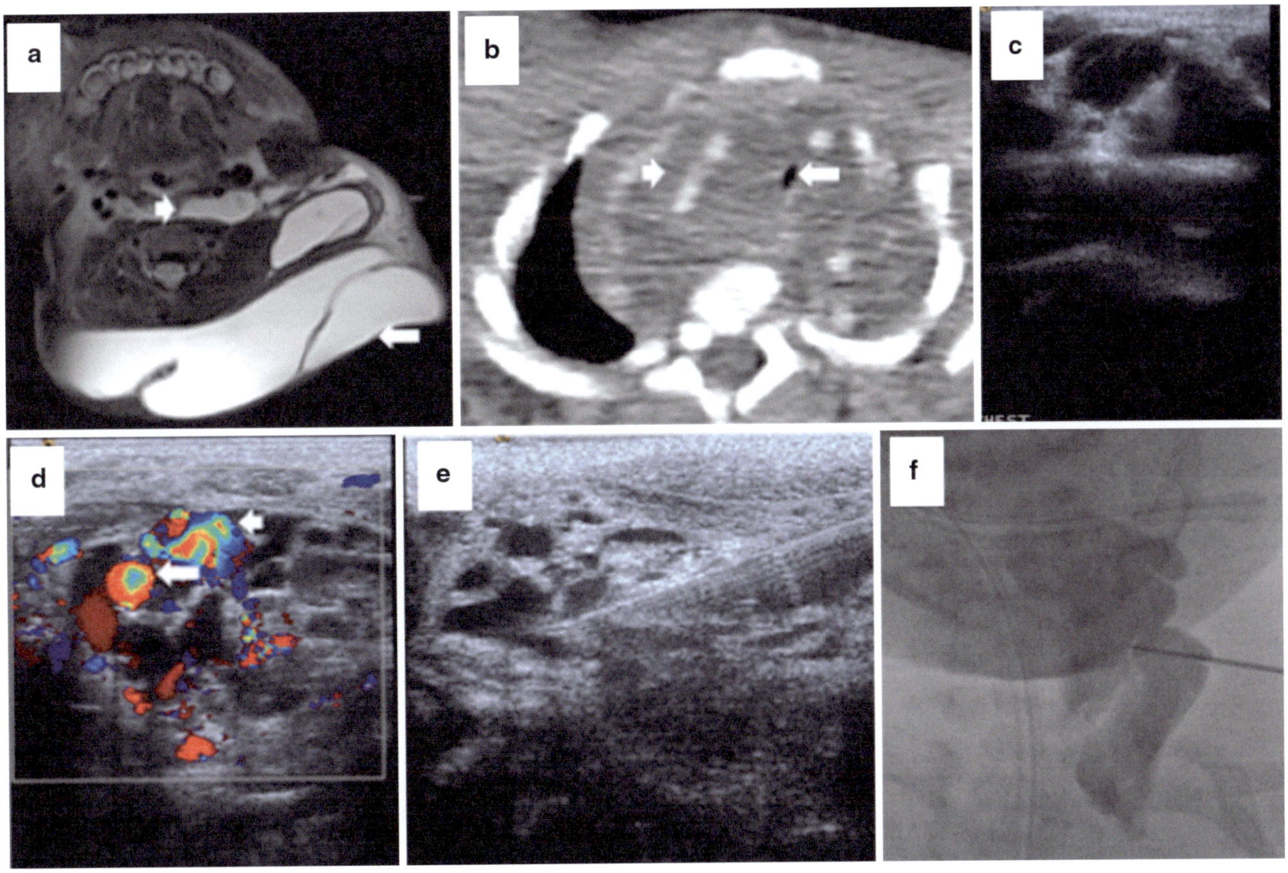

Fig. 28.7 **a** Axial T2-weighted image with inversion recovery MR image of the neck in a 5-month-old boy with a large macrocystic LM on his back (*long arrow*); invaginating into the deeper structures of the neck and around the airway (*short arrow*). **b** Contrast-enhanced CT of the superior mediastinum demonstrating mediastinal extension of the LM causing compression on the trachea, which appears slit-like (*long arrow*). There is separation of vessels with disease infiltrating into the vascular plane (*short arrow*). **c** Real time US image of the macrocysts. **d** Color duplex image demonstrating the carotid artery (*long arrow*) and the internal jugular vein (*short arrow*) coursing through the macrocysts. **e** Real time US guidance for safe needle access of the macrocysts. **f** Frontal fluoroscopic image during percutaneous sclerotherapy of the macrocyst with opacified doxycycline delineating intralesional dispersion of the sclerosant

Ethibloc, and OK-432; at our institution we prefer doxycycline at a concentration of 10 mg/ml as the first-line agent. It can be used in patients of all ages, including newborns. The sclerosant is usually reconstituted with a contrast agent, either water soluble, lipophilic (such as ethiodol), or negative contrast (air or carbon dioxide) to allow fluoroscopic and US monitoring of the injection [23]. For larger cysts, a pigtail catheter aspiration of the contents and volume measurement is made, followed by injection and drainage of the cyst with the sclerosant. The sclerosant is allowed to dwell in the cyst for about 3–4 h and then drained out. The procedure is repeated sequentially on days 2 and 3, through the indwelling catheters. It is important to disrupt the internal septations to increase the contact of the sclerosants within different compartments.

Cyst involution can be assessed approximately 6 weeks after the procedure. In extensive lesions, as the macrocysts start to shrink, more of the microcystic disease surfaces on follow-up imaging (Fig. 28.8). Swelling and perilesional edema following sclerotherapy is common. For lesions involving the tongue, buccal surfaces, soft palate, or airway, marked post-procedural edema can cause transient dysphagia and respiratory difficulties. Malformations that have extensive involvement in the neck and the superior mediastinum can cause tracheal compression (Fig. 28.7). Many such patients have a tracheostomy placed before commencing the procedure. The patients and anesthesia team are apprised of the likelihood of an extended intensive care unit (ICU) stay in advance. Nevertheless, pre-sclerotherapy steroids are imperative when sclerosing peri-airway LMs.

We routinely use bleomycin, an antibiotic with cytotoxic properties, around the airway lesions, because of significantly less post-treatment edema. Although pulmonary fibrosis is associated with chemotherapeutic doses of bleomycin, doses used for sclerotherapy are much smaller and have not demonstrated this adverse effect [25]. However, we routinely follow a bleomycin protocol that includes a chest radiograph and pulmonary function test prior to the procedure followed

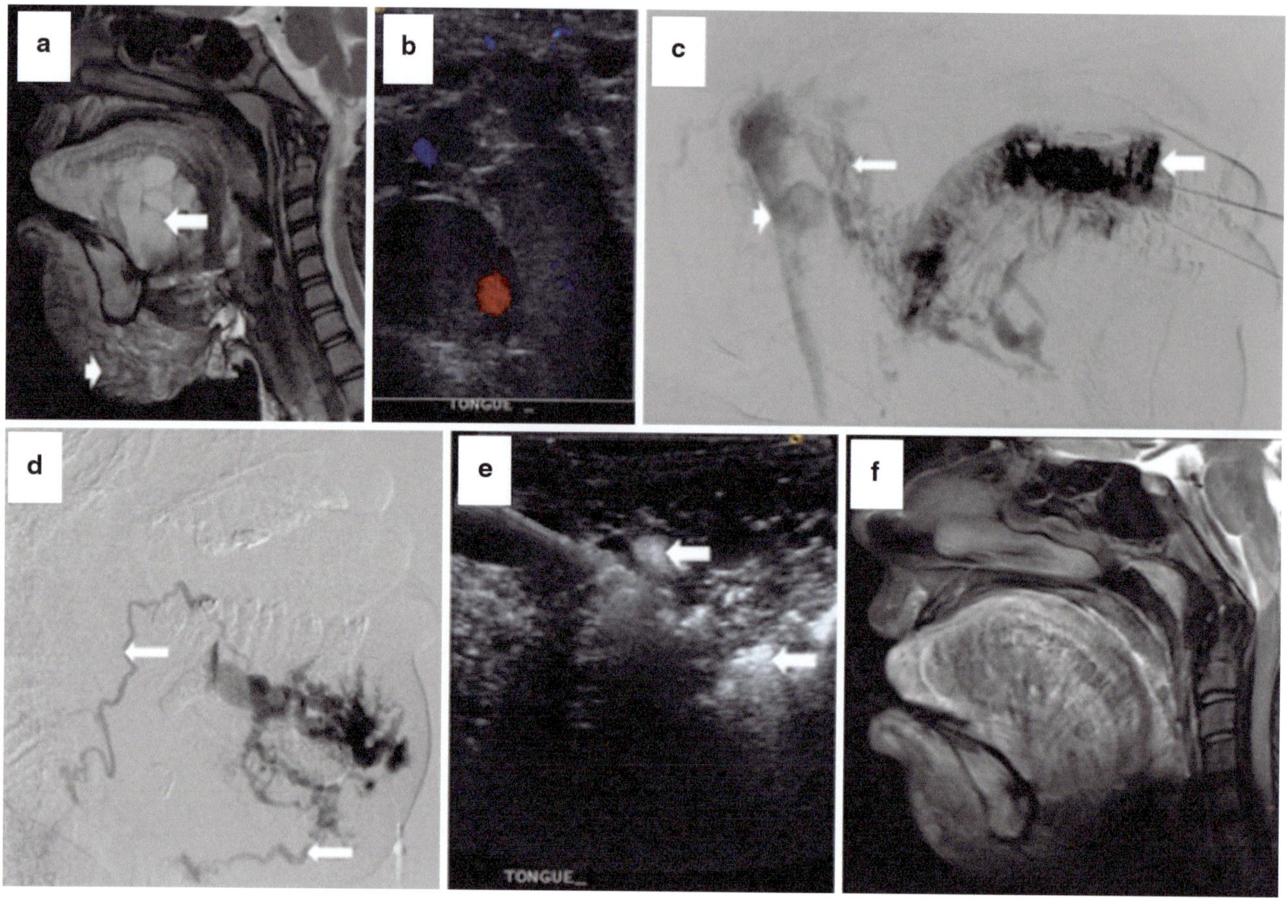

Fig. 28.8 **a** Sagittal T2-weighted inversion recovery image of the face in a 14-year-old boy demonstrating significant macrocystic disease in the tongue (*long arrow*) and combined disease in the cervico facial area (*short arrow*). **b** Color duplex demonstrating large cysts with echogenic lymph within the cysts. Few vessels are seen coursing through the cystic mass. **c** Digital subtraction contrast study demonstrating filling of the macrocysts which drain into the internal jugular veins (*short arrow*) and **d** via several aberrant veins (*thin arrows*). **e** Ultrasound guidance used to gain safe access into the lesion with injection of sclerosant foam into the cyst seen as echogenic curvilinear artifacts (*arrows*). **f** Sagittal T2-weighted inversion recovery image following serial-staged sclerotherapy over 2 years showed significant obliteration of the macrocystic disease

by another pulmonary function test in 6 months and annual chest radiographs thereafter for the next 10 years. Other less common adverse effects of sclerotherapy include blistering and, in rare occurrences, skin necrosis with permanent scarring. This can happen particularly when the lesion has a more superficial component. Very rarely, muscle atrophy and contracture can result if excessive sclerosant infiltrates the tissues [23]. Given the risks of extravasation, with consequent local soft tissue injury or inadvertent embolization of sclerosant into the systemic venous drainage, it is highly recommended to perform sclerotherapy using image guidance.

Following the procedure, the puncture sites are covered with antibiotic dressing. Post procedure pain is managed with analgesics. Routinely the patients are observed in the recovery for 3–4 h post procedure and then discharged home the same day with prescription analgesics. There is acute inflammation and swelling of the treated area, which peaks over the next 3–5 days. The parents or guardians are made aware of this before the discharge. Maintaining a scheduled dosing of analgesics helps to control the pain and anxiety during this event. Other than for the smallest of lesions, multiple treatment sessions are usually needed to achieve a satisfactory result; we typically space the sessions by approximately 4–6 weeks to allow for initial fibrosis formation. Continued injections can continue so long as imaging demonstrates an accessible, contained lymphatic space. Recurrence or emergence of new macrocysts following initial sclerotherapy can happen and is not a contraindication to reinjection. Complication rates with doxycycline sclerotherapy are low, with major and minor complication rates of 2 % and 10 %, respectively [26]. Overall, percutaneous sclerotherapy, when performed using optimal image guidance and experience provides a safe and effective, minimally invasive first- or second-line nonoperative option to treat LMs.

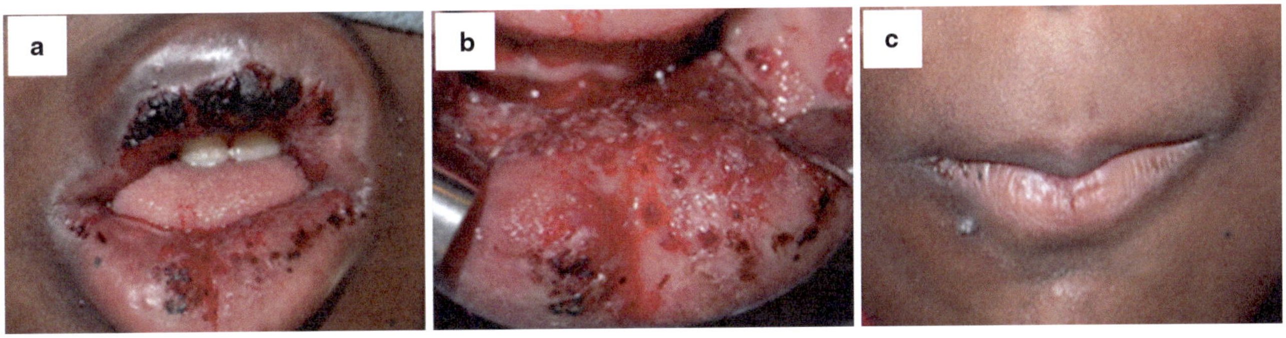

Fig. 28.9 Radiofrequency coblation of an oral LM with lip involvement. **a** Preoperative. Superficial vesicles are present causing recurrent bleeding. **b** Intraoperative coblation. **c** The patient seen 6 months following radiofrequency coblation

2. Surgical Resection

Although complete excision of the lesion is desired, this is often impossible. The surgical approach must take into account that LM is a benign process and vital structures need to be preserved. Surgery can be difficult due to scarring and fibrosis from sclerotherapy or infection, and anatomic distortion. Due to the infiltrative nature of LM and often extensive involvement of local neurovascular structures makes complete excision of the lesion difficult to achieve without a high rate of morbidity [27, 28]. The marginal mandibular nerve is the most frequently injured nerve intra-operatively. Parotid lesions can also be intimately associated with the facial nerve. Nerve monitoring is essential in most surgical cases [29]. Repeated procedures are often necessary. Subtotal resection is complicated by a high recurrence rate. *Macrocystic lesions* are more suited to surgical excision, and isolated cervical lesions can frequently be removed in a single procedure with an excellent prognosis. Aspiration, incision, and drainage of large cysts are a temporizing measure and are not recommended. *Microcystic lesions* are more difficult to manage surgically, because no distinct tissue planes exist between the malformation and normal structures. Partial glossectomy and tongue reduction is often required for lesions causing severe macroglossia.

Adjunctive Treatment Modalities

- *Radiofrequency coblation* is useful in symptomatic relief of ulcerated microcystic lesions of the tongue or oral mucosa that cause persistent irritation and bleeding. Radiofrequency energy is applied to the mucosal surface of the lesion only, destroying tissue with minimal damage to adjacent tissues, and dramatically reducing symptoms of bleeding, pain, infection, and vesicle formation [30] (Fig. 28.9).
- *Laser* can also be helpful in symptomatic relief of lesions involving the oral cavity, tongue, lip, and supraglottis. The CO_2 laser can help reduce bleeding and ulceration [31]. Recently, its use has been superseded by radiofrequency coblation.
- *Rapamycin* or *"Sirolimus"* is a mammalian target of rapamycin inhibitor, which has been found to be overexpressed in vascular malformations. Sirolimus also has antiangiogenesis and antiproliferative activity in tumors by impairing production of vascular endothelial growth factor (VEGF). Despite this, it has appeared to work well in small studies on lymphatic malformations, challenging the classic view of LMs, which are thought of as nonproliferative malformations. Sirolimus is commonly used for immunosuppression following renal transplantation in the pediatric population and is well tolerated. It is now being used in prospective clinical trials for patients with unresectable, life-threatening LMs. Preliminary results have been encouraging, however, further clinical studies are indicated to determine its role in the management of LMs [32, 33].

Multidisciplinary Approach

All extensive cervicofacial LMs should be managed by a multidisciplinary team, including otolaryngology, nutrition and growth, dental surgery, plastic surgery, interventional radiology, psychology and speech and language. Interventions such as tracheostomy for airway obstruction and gastrostomy tubes for feeding are frequently required. A multimodal staged treatment approach, involving both sclerotherapy and surgery, is frequently used based on the individual patient and the extent of their disease.

References

1. Brooks JE. Cystic hygroma of the neck. Laryngoscope. 1973;83:117–28.
2. de Serres LM , Sie KC, Richardson MA. Lymphatic malformations of the head and neck. A proposal for staging. Arch Otolaryngol Head Neck Surg. 1995;121:577–82.

3. Fageeh N, Manoukian J, Tewfik T, Schloss M, Williams HB, Gaskin D. Management of head and neck lymphatic malformations in children. J Otolaryngol. 1997;26(4):253–8.
4. Azizkhan RG, Rutter MJ, Cotton RT, Lim LH, Cohen AP, Mason JL. Lymphatic malformations of the tongue base. J Pediatr Surg. 2006;41(7):1279–84.
5. Mulliken JB, Glowacki J. Hemangiomas and vascular malformations in infants and children: a classification based on endothelial characteristics. Plast Reconst Surg. 1982;69:412.
6. Enjolras O, Mulliken JB. Vascualr tumors and vascular malformations (new issues). Adv Dermatol. 1997;13:375–423.
7. Kennedy TL. Cystic hygroma-lymphangioma: a rare and still unclear entity. Laryngoscope. 1989;99(suppl 49):1–10.
8. Perkins JA, Manning SC, Tempero RM, Cunningham MJ, Edmonds JL, Hoffer FA, Egbert MA. Lymphatic malformations: current cellular and clinical investigations. Otolaryngology Head and Neck Surg. 2010;142:789–94.
9. Sabin FR. The lymphatic system in human embryos, with a consideration of the morphology of the system as a whole. Am J Anat. 1909;9:43–91.
10. Wiegand S, Eivazi B, Barth PJ, et al. Pathogenesis of lymphangiomas. Virchows Arch. 2008;453:1–8.
11. Karkkainen MJ, Haiko P, Sainio K, et al. Vascular endothelial growth factor C is required for sprouting of the first lymphatic vessels from embryonic veins. Nat Immunol. 2004;5:74–80.
12. Bloom DC, Perkins JA, Manning SC. Management of lymphatic malformations. Curr Opin Otolaryngol Head Neck Surg. 2004;12:500–4.
13. Perkins JA, Manning SC, Tempero RM, Cunningham MJ, Edmonds JL, Hoffer FA, Egbert MA. Lymphatic malformations: review of current treatment. Otolaryngol Head Neck Surg. 2010;142:795–803.
14. Perkins JA, Maniglia C, Magit A, Sidhu M, Manning SC, Chen EY. Clinical and radiographic findings in children with spontaneous lymphatic malformation regression. Otolaryngol Head Neck Surg. 2008;138(6):772–7.
15. Garzon MC, Huang JT, Enjolras O, et al. Vascular malformations: part I. J Am Acad Dermatol. 2007;56:353–70.
16. Gallagher PG, Mahoney MJ, Gosche JR. Cystic hygroma in the fetus and newborn. Semin Perinatol. 1999;23:341–56.
17. Gedikbasi A, Gul A, Sargin A, et al. Cystic hygroma and lymphangioma: associated findings, perinatal outcome and prognostic factors in live-born infants. Arch Gynecol Obstet. 2007;276:491–8.
18. Steigman SA, Nemes L, Barnewolt CE, Estroff JA, Valima C, Jennings RW, Fauza DO. Differential risk for neonatal surgical airway intervention in prenatally diagnosed neck masses. J Pediatric Surg. 2009;44:76–9.
19. Makkar HS, Frieden IJ. Transillumination of a cystic lymphatic malformation. N Engl J Med. 2003;(19):349.
20. Hartl DM, Roger G, Denoyelle F, et al. Extensive lymphangioma presenting with upper airway obstruction. Arch Otolaryngol Head Neck Surg. 2000;126:1378–82.
21. Boardman SJ, Cochrane LA, Derek Roebuck R, Elliott M, Hartley BEJ. Multimodality treatment of pediatric lymphatic malformations of the head and neck using surgery and sclerotherapy. Arch Otolaryngol Head Neck Surg. 2010;136(3):270–6.
22. Renton J, Richard JH. Smith RJH. Current treatment paradigms in the management of lymphatic malformations. Laryngoscope. 2011;121:56–9.
23. Choi DJ, Alomari AI, Chaudry G, Orbach DB. Neurointerventional management of low-flow vascular malformations of the head and neck. Neuroimaging Clin N Am. 2009;19(2):199–218.
24. Donnelly LF, Bissett GS 3rd, Adams DM. Combined sonographic and fluoroscopic guidance: a modified technique for percutaneous sclerosis of low-flow vascular malformations. AJR Am J Roentgenol. 1999;173:655–7.
25. Choi DJ, Alomari AI, Chaudry G, Orbach DB. Neurointerventional management of low-flow vascular malformations of the head and neck. Neuroimaging Clin N Am. 2009;19(2):199–218.
26. Burrows PE, Mitri RK, Alomari A, Padua HM, Lord DJ, Sylvia MB, Fishman SJ, Mulliken JB. Percutaneous sclerotherapy of lymphatic malformations with doxycycline. Lymphat Res Biol. 2008;6(3–4):209–16.
27. Dasguptaa R, Adamsb D, Elluru R, Wentzela MS, Richard G. Noninterventional treatment of selected head and neck lymphatic malformations. J Pediatr Surg. 2008;43:869–73.
28. Emery PJ, Bailey CM, Evans JN. Cystic hygroma of the head and neck: a review of 37 cases. J Laryngol Otol. 1984;98(6):613–9.
29. Chiara J, Kinney G, Slimp J, Lee GS, Oliaei S, Perkins JA. Facial nerve mapping and monitoring in lymphatic malformation surgery. Int J Pediatr Otorhinolaryngol. 2009;73:1348–52.
30. Grimmer F, Mulliken JB, Burrows PE, Rahbar R. Radiofrequency ablation of microcystic lymphatic malformation in the oral cavity. Arch Otolaryngol Head Neck Surg. 2006;32:1251–6.
31. Glade RS, Buckmiller LM. CO2 laser resurfacing of intraoral lymphatic malformations: a 10-year experience. Int J Pediatr Otorhinolaryngol. 2009;73:1358–61.
32. Reinglas J, Ramphal R, Bromwich M. The successful management of diffuse lymphangiomatosis using sirolimus: a case report. Laryngoscope. 2011 Sep;121(9):1851–4.
33. Hammill AM, Wentzel M, Gupta A, Nelson S, Lucky A, Elluru R, Dasgupta R, Azizkhan RG, Adams DM. Sirolimus for the treatment of complicated vascular anomalies in children. Pediatr Blood Cancer. 2011;57(6):1018–24.

Melanoma

29

Adam L. Green and Carlos Rodriguez-Galindo

Introduction

Melanoma is a cancer of melanocytes, which are pigment-containing cells in the skin and related tissues. Although melanoma remains an uncommon malignancy in children, the incidence has been steadily increasing over the past 30 years.

Key Points

- Pediatric melanoma is associated with several genetic syndromes, most often in early childhood, and then increasingly with ultraviolet light exposure in adolescents.
- Differences in presentation and pathology versus adult disease can make childhood melanoma difficult to diagnose, so often children present with advanced disease.
- Surgical resection remains the primary treatment, although immunotherapy and, less often, chemotherapy are now being used in children with high risk of recurrence.

Biology and Epidemiology

Melanoma is associated with multiple mutations in the mitogen-activated protein kinase (MAPK) pathway that is important in melanocyte growth and survival. Melanoma in children is rare, with an incidence of 1 per million under 15 years of age [1]. The incidence of melanoma is higher in adolescents, representing 7 % of all cancers in this age group. Pediatric melanoma, however, accounts for only 1.3 % of all melanoma cases in the USA. Disturbingly, though, its incidence has been rising approximately 3 % per year since the 1970s. Incidence rates are highest in adolescent female patients. Disease in sun-exposed areas of both boys (trunk, face) and girls (leg, hips) is increasing [2].

Pathophysiology

- Melanocytes are pigment-containing cells that produce melanin and determine eye, hair, and skin color. They are derived from neural crest cells.
- *BRAF V600E* mutations are very common in both melanoma and benign melanocytic nevi; evidence suggests that these mutations help lead to malignant transformation, invasion, and progression but are not sufficient to cause malignant transformation alone [3].

Molecular/Genetic Pathology

- The MAPK pathway, which ordinarily promotes cellular growth through ligand binding to a transmembrane receptor, is activated in almost all cases of melanoma.
- Various components of the MAPK (more notably *BRAF* and *NRAS*) pathway are mutated in various subtypes of melanoma, often leading to constitutive activation of the pathway.
- Other commonly altered genes include *C-KIT* (particularly in acral and mucosal melanomas), *PTEN*, and *AKT3*.

Incidence and Prevalence

- There are approximately 300–420 new cases of pediatric melanoma diagnosed each year in the United States [4].

C. Rodriguez-Galindo (✉)
Department of Pediatric Oncology, Dana-Farber/Boston Childrens Hospital Cancer and Blood Disorders Center, Harvard Medical School, Boston, MA, USA
e-mail: carlos_rodriguez-galindo@dfci.harvard.edu

A. L. Green
Department of Pediatric Oncology, Dana-Farber Cancer Institute, Boston, MA, USA

R. Rahbar et al. (eds.), *Pediatric Head and Neck Tumors*,
DOI 10.1007/978-1-4614-8755-5_29, © Springer Science+Business Media New York 2014

- Approximately 10–25 % of these are located on the head and neck.

Age Distribution

- Pediatric melanoma incidence is seven times higher in the second decade than the first [5]; in children, there is a 46 % increase in incidence per year with advancing age [4].
- Congenital melanoma is extremely rare, although the development of transplacental metastasis from maternal disease has been reported [5].
- Head and neck are the most common sites in children 1–4 years; truncal disease is more common in adolescents.
- Presence of pubertal changes is a key risk factor for death from melanoma; the mortality rate among patients 15–19 years old is 8–18 times higher than in younger age groups.

Sex Predilection

- Boys have a higher incidence of melanoma in toddlers at a ratio of approximately 1.7:1 [5], but in adolescence, female patients outnumber male patients at a ratio of 1.6:1. Male patients may still predominate in head and neck disease, however [6].

Geographic and Racial Distribution

- Melanoma occurs more frequently in Caucasians than in other races, and the number of patients of color decreases with age [5].

Risk Factors—Environmental, Life Style

- Intermittent intense sun exposure is a risk factor, especially in patients with a tendency to sunburn or freckle, those with fair skin, blue or green eyes, and blond or red hair [5].

Relationships to Other Disease States, Syndromes

- About half of patients have known risk factors such as family history of melanoma, large congenital nevi, numerous nevi, and sun-sensitive phenotype [1]. The presence of family history of melanoma is estimated to increase the risk of melanoma in a child by a factor of 2.
- Familial melanoma has an autosomal dominant inheritance with incomplete penetration; *CDKN2A* and *CDK4* mutations have been found in 25–50 % of these families. These cases account for 5–10 % of melanomas and correlate with a lower age of onset and a higher chance of multiple primary lesions [7]. However, *CDKN2A* mutations are found in less than 2 % of children with melanoma.
- Polymorphisms and mutations in the melanocortin-1 receptor (MC1R) have also been associated with a 2–10-fold increase in the risk of melanoma.
- Xeroderma pigmentosum is an autosomal recessive disorder caused by an inability to repair sun UV-induced DNA damage; it leads to an overall melanoma incidence of 5 %, mostly of the head and neck, with a median age of 19 years [7].
- Approximately 12 % of childhood melanoma cases progress from a congenital melanocytic nevus (CMN), with about a third of these arising from giant CMN, although only 2 % of patients with giant CMN develop melanoma, mostly before age 5 [1]. However, this equates to a several hundredfold increased risk of melanoma [8]. The risk of melanoma increases with the size of the CMN, from 1–2 % in small (<1.5 cm) lesions to >10 % in giant (>20 cm) CMN. This risk seems to be higher during puberty. Excision of the CMN does not always prevent development of melanoma. Patients with 3 or more CMN or a large CMN in a paravertebral location are at risk for neurocutaneous melanosis, which affects the meninges, causes neurologic manifestations, often progresses to central nervous system (CNS) melanoma, and has a poor prognosis [5].
- Dysplastic nevi are potential precursors of melanoma (at the nevus site and elsewhere on the body) that can be sporadic or inherited as part of the autosomal dominant dysplastic nevus syndrome. Dysplastic nevi are distinguished by large size, irregular borders, and variable coloration [9]. In one series, half of pediatric melanoma patients had sporadic dysplastic nevi, and 9 % had dysplastic nevus syndrome [10].
- Children with more than 100 noncongenital nevi or more than 10 large nevi have a much greater risk of melanoma. About half of pediatric melanomas arise at the site of a benign nevus [11].
- Children on immunosuppression or with a history of cancer have a several-fold increased chance of developing melanoma.

Presentation

Presentation of melanoma in children has both important similarities and important differences from presentation in adults. Keeping the diagnosis in the differential, especially

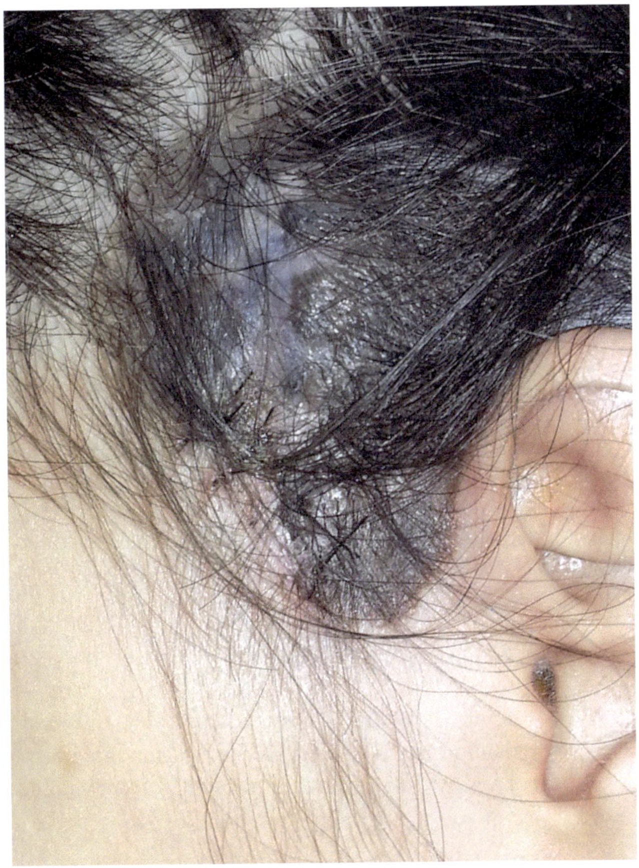

Fig. 29.1 Melanoma of the scalp in a 5-year-old girl

for patients in at-risk populations, allows cases to be diagnosed earlier. The following elements are important to consider in the evaluation of melanocytic lesions and in the diagnosis of melanoma:

- Key elements in the diagnosis are usually highlighted by the ABCDE acronym: *A*symmetry, *B*order (irregular), *C*olor *c*hange, *D*iameter (growth), and *E*volution over time (rapid changes) (Fig. 29.1). In addition, signs of malignant transformation include bleeding, itching, ulceration, pain, and palpable adenopathy. Unfortunately, pediatric melanoma is misdiagnosed in up to 50 % of the cases.
- However, the presentation of pediatric melanoma can be nonspecific, mimicking a benign or dysplastic nevus, a hemangioma, a Spitz nevus, a pyogenic granuloma, or a verruca. Also importantly, compared with adult melanoma, pediatric melanoma is often amelanotic or raised [12], and often the above symptoms are absent [13].
- Seven percent of melanomas that develop in an existing nevus are asymptomatic [14].
- The scalp and neck are the most common head and neck areas involved [15], although other tissues, including the mucus membranes or eyes, can be involved.

Table 29.1 Differential diagnosis of melanoma

Spitz nevus
Traumatized common congenital/acquired nevus
Pyogenic granuloma
Dysplastic nevus
Traumatized verrucae
Blue nevi
Hemangioma
Angiokeratoma
Thrombosed lymphangioma
Keloid
Seborrheic keratosis
Pigmented basal cell carcinoma

Patterns of Evolution

- The low incidence and differences in presentations from adult disease make pediatric melanoma difficult to diagnose and may result in late diagnosis and increased mortality in up to two-thirds of cases [16].

Evaluation at Presentation

- After complete characterization of the lesion by exam, punch biopsy should be performed. Punch biopsy is considered superior to shave biopsy because it offers more information on depth of invasion [13].

Differential Diagnosis

The differential diagnosis of melanoma is wide (Table 29.1), and thus proper referral and early biopsy should be done when melanoma is suspected. In early childhood, the diagnosis of Spitz nevus (also called spindle cell nevus or benign juvenile melanoma) should be considered. This entity usually presents during childhood, as uniformly pink, tan, or red-brown dome-shaped papules or nodules, in the face or lower extremities. Spitz nevus is usually well circumscribed and small (< 1 cm).

Diagnosis and Evaluation

Physical Examination

- The physical exam diagnostic criteria are similar to those used in adults:
  - Size greater than 10 mm

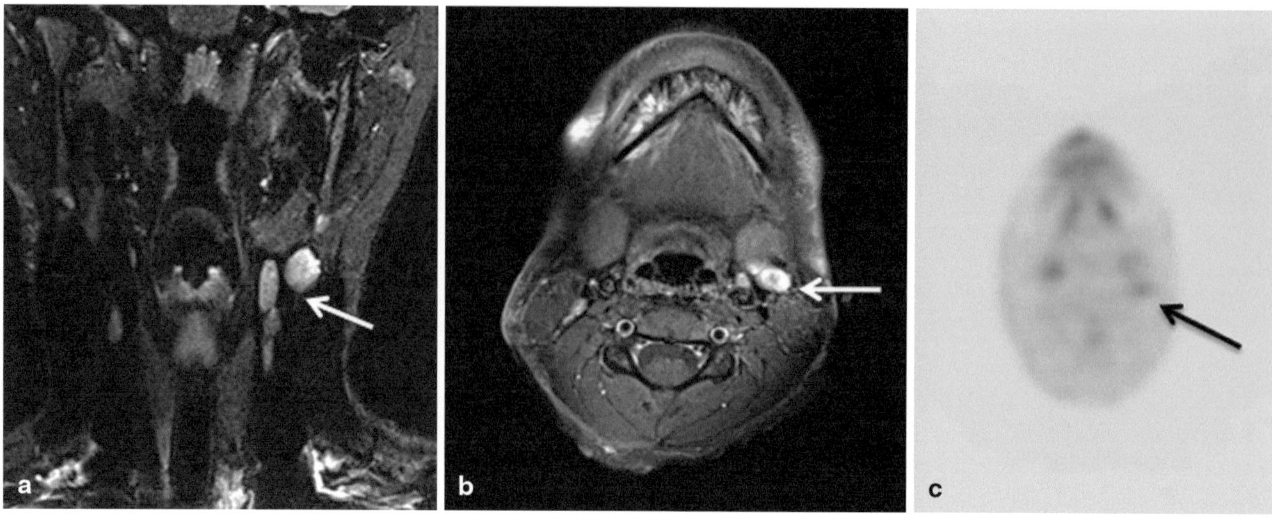

Fig. 29.2 Coronal (**a**) and axial (**b**) magnetic resonance imaging (MRI) images of the head and neck in a child with melanoma of the scalp showing multiple enlarged lymph nodes (*arrow*). Fluorodeoxyglucose positron emission tomography (FDG-PET) of the same patient shows FDG update in the involved nodes (*arrow*) (**c**)

  - Inconsistent color
  - Asymmetry
  - Poorly demarcated borders
  - Ulceration
- It should be noted, however, that some pediatric melanomas will not meet any of these criteria, so consideration of the diagnosis in other lesions is crucial for timely diagnosis.

Laboratory Data

- Sentinel lymph node (SLN) biopsy is well-tolerated and indicated for all melanomas greater than 1 mm thick, those with ulceration or Clark level III or IV, or with aggressive or uncertain pathology. If positive, a complete lymph node dissection should be undertaken [5]; if negative, patients are saved the morbidity of the complete dissection.
- SLN biopsy should include injection of both blue dye and radionucleotide lymphoscintigraphy to increase accuracy of sentinel node identification, especially in the head and neck, where there is great variability of lymphatic drainage. This procedure led to clearly identifiable SLNs in a series of seven pediatric head and neck melanoma cases, with excellent correlation between the two markers.
- SLN biopsy was definitive in differentiating melanoma from a benign lesion in this same case series [17], which can be difficult in children [18]. Results from this series also suggested that likelihood of positive sentinel node increased with primary lesion thickness, just as in adults [17].
- SLNs should be examined by hematoxylin and eosin (H&E) staining; if this is negative for melanoma, immunohistochemistry should be performed for melanoma-specific antigens.

Imaging Evaluation

- Imaging studies are usually recommended when nodal involvement is present. This should include imaging of the region to evaluate for nodal disease, as well as metastatic workup to evaluate for liver and lung involvement (Fig. 29.2). Although there are little data in children, PET imaging has been shown to be useful in the metastatic evaluation of adults with cutaneous melanoma, leading to a change in management in 35 % of patients and allowing a higher sensitivity than CT for occult metastases [19].

Pathology

On microscopic examination, the following features are suggestive of malignancy, though no one factor alone is diagnostic: prominent intraepidermal pagetoid of single cell spread, irregular intraepidermal tumor nests formation, atrophy or ulceration of the epidermis, extension into the dermis or subcutaneous tissue, expansive deep border, cellular atypia, deep or atypical mitoses, and absence of maturation [20]. Superficial spreading melanoma is easily the most common subtype in children, with the nodular subtype second. The lentigo maligna subtype, common in adults, appears to be very rare in pediatrics [15]. Amelanotic disease

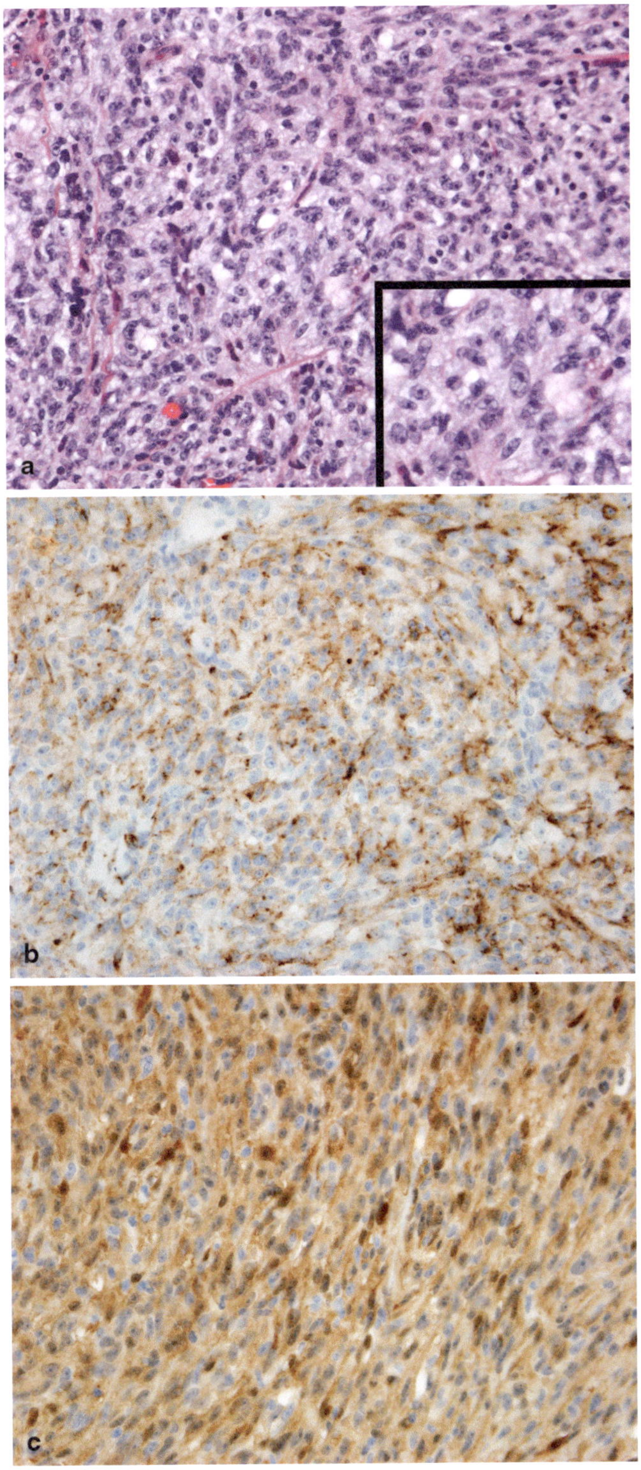

Fig. 29.3 **a** Undifferentiated tumor cells with a solid and vaguely nesting pattern of growth. Tumor cells have spindled and epithelioid morphology with large nuclei and prominent single, centrally located, eosinophilic nucleoli. *Inset* at higher magnification. **b** Tumor cells are diffusely immunoreactive for HMB45. **c** Strong immunoreactivity for S100 protein is also observed

is more common than in adults [5]. Spitzoid melanoma and nevoid melanoma often appear different pathologically and require awareness of these diagnoses to differentiate them from benign conditions. In the case of Spitz nevus, immunohistochemistry for HMB-45 and Ki-67 can help differentiate the condition from spitzoid melanoma. Mucosal melanoma is very rare and generally resembles cutaneous melanoma microscopically. About two-thirds of patients with Clark level IV–V or Breslow thickness greater than 1.5 mm have nodal disease, whereas nodal spread is unusual in thinner lesions [1]. The most common cytologic appearance and immunohistochemical characteristics of melanoma are shown in Fig. 29.3.

Treatment

Surgical excision is the cornerstone of treatment of melanoma in children. For patients with high risk of recurrence, including those with thick lesions and/or nodal spread, adjuvant treatment with high-dose interferon (IFN) is becoming the standard of care.

- IFN α2b is recommended as an adjuvant therapy for high-risk melanoma (thickness greater than 4 mm or presence of nodal disease) in adults [21]; in general, an intense induction month is followed by several months of lower-dose maintenance treatment. Children tolerate the treatment better than adults do [22]; the most common side effects are anxiety, agitation, and depression [13]. The efficacy in pediatrics, however, is unclear.
- For patients with unresectable, metastatic, or recurrent melanoma, systemic therapy is indicated. Standard chemotherapy has limited effect; DTIC, temozolomide, and taxanes are the most active agents, but responses are seen in only 20–30 % of patients, and usually do not last more than 4–6 months. High-dose IL-2 has also shown to be effective, and combinations of IL-2 with chemotherapy are often used.
- Melanoma is a very immunogenic neoplasm; in addition to IFN and IL-2, other immunological approaches have shown remarkable results for patients with advanced disease in recent years. Recently, the anti-CTLA4 monoclonal antibody ipilimumab demonstrated survival prolongation of several months in recurrent advanced melanoma [23]. In addition, treatment with autologous tumor-infiltrating lymphocytes achieved a durable remission over years in a substantial minority of patients with metastatic, mostly refractory disease [24].
- The documentation of the role of *BRAF* mutations in the development and progression of melanoma has led to the

use of specific *BRAF* inhibitors such as vemurafenib; these targeted agents have shown promising short-term results [25, 26], although patients invariably develop resistance [27].

Surgical Therapy

- Surgery is the mainstay of therapy for pediatric melanoma. Recommended margins depend on lesion depth:
  - 0.5 cm for in situ disease
  - 1 cm for thickness less than 1 mm
  - 1–2 cm for thickness 1–2 mm
  - 2 cm for thickness greater than 2 mm
- Wide excision accompanied by SLN biopsy can be accomplished by an experienced team in a mean of 3 h [17].
- Patients with at least one positive node on SLN biopsy should undergo therapeutic lymph node dissection (modified radical neck dissection for head and neck disease) [5].

Radiation Therapy

Radiation therapy is generally limited to unresectable disease, in patients with a high risk of regional recurrence [28], and in progressive melanoma to provide palliation in lesions causing pain or disfigurement [21].

Outcomes

- Major prognostic factors are similar to those in adults: thickness, stage, and presence or absence of ulceration [29].
- Prognoses are similar overall to those for adult melanoma. Stage is very important: 10-year survival in children with stage I–II disease is 90 %, but it decreases to 60 % for stage III and less than 30 % for stage IV.
- In one large series of pediatric head and neck melanoma, the median thickness for surviving patients was 1.2 mm, while the median thickness in patients who died was 2.3 mm [15].
- Presence of lymph node involvement does not seem to predict recurrence risk or prognosis [5].
- Early lymph node dissection does not clearly improve survival in children.
- Head and neck location has been inconsistently linked to worse prognosis in children; in adults, the linkage is clearer [30].
- Older age (greater than 10 years) appears to be a poor prognostic factor in pediatric head and neck melanoma [15, 31].
- Survival has improved 4 % per year over the last 30 years for all stages [4], but delayed diagnosis is still seen as a major obstacle to further gains.

Follow-up

Frequency of Office Visits

- Patients should be educated on the symptoms of recurrent melanoma. They should have a history and physical exam, including full skin exam and palpation of lymph nodes, yearly, or more often as indicated by symptoms or elevated recurrence risk (history of nodal disease, family history of melanoma, increased sun exposure, etc.).

Frequency of Imaging

- The utility of surveillance imaging in melanoma post-treatment follow-up, especially in children, is unclear. In high-risk (stage III or IV) disease, however, there is likely a role for routine PET/CT to diagnose treatable or curable recurrences and secondary malignancies.

References

1. Paradela S, Fonseca E, Prieto VG. Melanoma in children. Arch Pathol Lab Med. 2011;135(3):307–16.
2. Wong JR, Harris JK, Rodriguez-Galindo C, Johnson KJ. Incidence of childhood and adolescent melanoma in the United States: 1973–2009. Pediatrics. 2013;131(5):846–54.
3. Sullivan RJ, Flaherty KT. BRAF in melanoma: pathogenesis, diagnosis, inhibition, and resistance. J Skin Cancer. 2011;2011:423239.
4. Strouse JJ, Fears TR, Tucker MA, Wayne AS. Pediatric melanoma: risk factor and survival analysis of the surveillance, epidemiology and end results database. J Clin Oncol. 2005;23(21):4735–41.
5. Jen M, Murphy M, Grant-Kels JM. Childhood melanoma. Clin Dermatol. 2009;27(6):529–36.
6. Conti EM, Cercato MC, Gatta G, Ramazzotti V, Roscioni S, EUROCARE Working Group. Childhood melanoma in Europe since 1978: a population-based survival study. Eur J Cancer. 2001;37(6):780–4.
7. Berg P, Wennberg AM, Tuominen R, Sander B, Rozell BL, Platz A, et al. Germline CDKN2 A mutations are rare in child and adolescent cutaneous melanoma. Melanoma Res. 2004;14(4):251–5.
8. Krengel S, Hauschild A, Schafer T. Melanoma risk in congenital melanocytic naevi: a systematic review. Br J Dermatol. 2006;155(1):1–8.
9. Hoang MT, Friedlander SF. Rare cutaneous malignancies of childhood. Curr Opin Pediatr. 1999;11(5):464–70.
10. Paradela S, Fonseca E, Pita-Fernandez S, Kantrow SM, Diwan AH, Herzog C, et al. Prognostic factors for melanoma in children and adolescents: a clinicopathologic, single-center study of 137 patients. Cancer. 2010;116(18):4334–44.
11. Schmid-Wendtner MH, Berking C, Baumert J, Schmidt M, Sander CA, Plewig G, et al. Cutaneous melanoma in childhood and adolescence: an analysis of 36 patients. J Am Acad Dermatol. 2002;46(6):874–9.

12. Ferrari A, Bono A, Baldi M, Collini P, Casanova M, Pennacchioli E, et al. Does melanoma behave differently in younger children than in adults? A retrospective study of 33 cases of childhood melanoma from a single institution. Pediatrics. 2005;115(3):649–54.
13. French JC, Rowe MR, Lee TJ, Zwart JE. Pediatric melanoma of the head and neck: a single institutions experience. The Laryngoscope. 2006;116(12):2216–20.
14. Ruiz-Maldonado R, Orozco-Covarrubias ML. Malignant melanoma in children. A review. Arch Dermatol. 1997;133(3):363–71.
15. Tcheung WJ, Marcello JE, Puri PK, Abernethy AP, Nelson KC. Evaluation of 39 cases of pediatric cutaneous head and neck melanoma. J Am Acad Dermatol. 2011;65(2):e37–42.
16. Vandeweyer E, Sales F, Deraemaecker R. Cutaneous malignant melanoma in children. Eur J Pediatr. 2000;159(8):582–4.
17. Pacella SJ, Lowe L, Bradford C, Marcus BC, Johnson T, Rees R. The utility of sentinel lymph node biopsy in head and neck melanoma in the pediatric population. Plast Reconstr Surg. 2003;112(5):1257–65.
18. Zuckerman R, Maier JP, Guiney WB Jr, Huntsman WT, Mooney EK. Pediatric melanoma: confirming the diagnosis with sentinel node biopsy. Ann Plast Surg. 2001;46(4):394–9.
19. Brady MS, Akhurst T, Spanknebel K, Hilton S, Gonen M, Patel A, et al. Utility of preoperative [(18)]f fluorodeoxyglucose-positron emission tomography scanning in high-risk melanoma patients. Ann Surg Oncol. 2006;13(4):525–32.
20. Barnhill R. Pathology of melanocytic nevi and malignant melanoma. 2nd ed. New York: Springer; 2004.
21. Huynh PM, Grant-Kels JM, Grin CM. Childhood melanoma: update and treatment. Int J Dermatol. 2005;44(9):715–23.
22. Navid F, Furman WL, Fleming M, Rao BN, Kovach S, Billups CA, et al. The feasibility of adjuvant interferon alpha-2b in children with high-risk melanoma. Cancer. 2005;103(4):780–7.
23. Hodi FS, O'Day SJ, McDermott DF, Weber RW, Sosman JA, Haanen JB, et al. Improved survival with ipilimumab in patients with metastatic melanoma. N Engl J Med. 2010;363(8):711–23.
24. Rosenberg SA, Yang JC, Sherry RM, Kammula US, Hughes MS, Phan GQ, et al. Durable complete responses in heavily pretreated patients with metastatic melanoma using T-cell transfer immunotherapy. Clin Cancer Res. 2011;17(13):4550–7.
25. Patel SP, Lazar AJ, Papadopoulos NE, Liu P, Infante JR, Glass MR, et al. Clinical responses to selumetinib (AZD6244; ARRY-142886)-based combination therapy stratified by gene mutations in patients with metastatic melanoma. Cancer. 2013;119(4):799–805.
26. Infante JR, Fecher LA, Falchook GS, Nallapareddy S, Gordon MS, Becerra C, et al. Safety, pharmacokinetic, pharmacodynamic, and efficacy data for the oral MEK inhibitor trametinib: a phase 1 dose-escalation trial. Lancet Oncol. 2012;13(8):773–81.
27. Roumiantsev S, Shah NP, Gorre ME, Nicoll J, Brasher BB, Sawyers CL, et al. Clinical resistance to the kinase inhibitor STI-571 in chronic myeloid leukemia by mutation of Tyr-253 in the Abl kinase domain P-loop. Proc Natl Acad Sci U S A. 2002;99(16):10700–5.
28. Mack LA, McKinnon JG. Controversies in the management of metastatic melanoma to regional lymphatic basins. J Surg Oncol. 2004;86(4):189–99.
29. Hamre MR, Chuba P, Bakhshi S, Thomas R, Severson RK. Cutaneous melanoma in childhood and adolescence. Pediatr Hematol Oncol. 2002;19(5):309–17.
30. Lachiewicz AM, Berwick M, Wiggins CL, Thomas NE. Survival differences between patients with scalp or neck melanoma and those with melanoma of other sites in the Surveillance, Epidemiology, and End Results (SEER) program. Arch Dermatol. 2008;144(4):515–21.
31. Pappo AS. Melanoma in children and adolescents. Eur J Cancer. 2003;39(18):2651–61.

30 Nasopharyngeal Carcinoma

Carlos Rodriguez-Galindo

Introduction

Nasopharyngeal carcinoma (NPC) is very rare in children; only 1 % of all NPC occurs in patients less than 19 years of age [1]. In the USA, the incidence of NPC in children is approximately 1–1.5 cases per million per year. This represents approximately 1 % of all pediatric malignancies, but it accounts for 35–50 % of all nasopharyngeal malignancies. Pathology, biology, and clinical presentation are very similar to the endemic form of NPC, and treatment usually follows the same principles, with a combination of chemotherapy and radiation therapy.

Key Points

- Childhood NPC is a rare malignancy that usually presents in the second decade of life; patients usually have advanced disease at diagnosis.
- This malignancy is associated with Epstein–Barr virus (EBV); patients have positive EBV serology, and high-circulating EBV DNA levels are almost always detected in blood.
- Treatment includes chemotherapy and radiation therapy; surgery is seldom indicated.
- While outcomes are very good, patients are at high risk of long-term morbidities.

C. Rodriguez-Galindo (✉)
Department of Pediatric Oncology, Dana-Farber/Boston Children's Hospital Cancer and Blood Disorders Center, Harvard Medical School, Boston, MA, USA
e-mail: carlos_rodriguez-galindo@dfci.harvard.edu

Biology and Epidemiology

Nasopharyngeal carcinoma (NPC) is a tumor that originates from the surface epithelium and differs from other head and neck carcinomas by its very distinct histologic, epidemiologic and biologic characteristics. NPC is a rare disease, with an incidence of 0.5–2/100,000 persons per year. However, it has an endemic distribution among well-defined ethnic groups, such as inhabitants of some areas of Southeast Asia and in Alaskan Eskimos, where the incidence is 25–50 and 15–20/100,000 persons per year, respectively [2].

Three histologic subtypes of NPC are recognized: type I, or keratinizing squamous cell carcinoma, which is similar to carcinomas that arise from other sites of the head and neck; type II, or nonkeratinizing squamous cell carcinoma; and type III, or undifferentiated carcinoma (also called lymphoepithelioma), which is also the most common form of the disease. In the western world NPC occurs sporadically, it is usually type I, and is primarily related to the exposure to the classic head and neck cancer risk factors, such as alcohol and tobacco [3]. The endemic form, which occurs in areas of Southeast Asia, Mediterranean basin and in Alaskan Eskimos, is usually the type II or III histologic subtype. Unlike the type I sporadic form, the etiology of the endemic form includes virological and environmental risk factors, and genetic susceptibility. The Epstein–Barr virus (EBV) plays a key role in the pathogenesis of NPC. As a member of the herpes virus family, the EBV infects and establishes persistent infection in the host. Most human EBV infections initiate in the oropharynx. Among the EBV genes, the nuclear proteins (Epstein–Barr virus nuclear antigen (EBNA)) are involved in replication, and the latent membrane proteins (LMP) may stimulate cell growth. Increased levels of immunoglobulin G (IgG) and immunoglobulin A (IgA) against EBV are frequently observed in patients with NPC, particularly those with the undifferentiated type [4]. The anti-EBV serologic profile has been used in the screening and early diagnosis of NPC in high-incidence areas [5]. In addition to the serological evidence, there is also molecular evidence; EBV

R. Rahbar et al. (eds.), *Pediatric Head and Neck Tumors*,
DOI 10.1007/978-1-4614-8755-5_30,

DNA is present in the NPC tumor cells [6], and EBV DNA is detected in the serum of patients and its levels correlate with response to therapy and with recurrence [7]. Further, EBV DNA appears to be clonal, which indicates that EBV is present within the cell at the time of carcinogenic transformation, and suggests a role for the virus in the transformation event. Taken together, these data suggest that the etiology of NPC appears to follow a multistep process. A persistent EBV infection results in stimulation of growth of nasopharyngeal cells by the EBV LMP and NA genes. A secondary exposure to some environmental carcinogens, such as volatile nitrosamine or others, may induce the loss of a tumor suppressor gene that will eventually result in an uncontrolled proliferation and carcinogenic transformation [8].

The fact that EBV is found in *in situ* carcinoma lesions [9] and not in epithelial cells adjacent to NPC lesions suggests that EBV infection takes place before the expansion of the malignant cell clone occurs but probably does not represent the first step in the pathogenesis of NPC. The expression of the viral genome in EBV-positive NPC is consistent with the adoption of a restricted latency infection. *In situ* hybridization studies have demonstrated the presence of EBV-encoded small ribonucleic acid (EBER) [10]. EBNA-1 and LMP-1 are also detected at the protein level [11]. EBV has been detected in virtually all nonkeratinizing NPC, irrespective of geographic origin and, thus, appears to be a rate-limiting step in the pathogenesis of these tumors. By contrast, association of squamous NPC with EBV is much more controversial. EBV DNA is detected in a very small proportion of the cases [12].

In children, NPC presents in a form very reminiscent of the endemic NPC seen in adults, with an almost universal, type III histology and EBV positivity. In the USA, studies of pediatric NPC have shown a higher incidence in African-Americans and in children of Asian descent [1].

Presentation

Childhood NPC usually presents in the second decade of life (median age of 13–15 years) and with a strong male preponderance [1, 13–15]. In the USA, the incidence is higher among African-Americans [1].

The nasopharynx has a rich vascular supply and lymphatic drainage system. These characteristics define the route of tumor spread, symptoms, and treatment. Clinically, NPC has few early signs, such as nose bleeding, congestion, otitis media, or trismus. It spreads locally to adjacent areas of the oropharynx and may invade the skull base, resulting in cranial nerve paralysis as well. The drainage is usually through the internal jugular vein and posterior cervical and retropharyngeal chains, which results in early lymph node invasion, usually bilateral and bulky. Up to 80% of patients have lymph node involvement at diagnosis, and most patients have large, infiltrative tumors [1, 13, 14]. In comparison with adults, children present with more advanced disease, with larger primaries and higher nodal stage [1].

Table 30.1 Differential diagnosis of childhood nasopharyngeal carcinoma

Benign conditions	Infectious mononucleosis
	Atypical mycobacterial and other lymphadenitis
	Juvenile angiofibroma
Malignant conditions	NUT (nuclear protein in testis) midline carcinoma
	Sinonasal carcinoma
	Parameningeal rhabdomyosarcoma
	Esthesioneuroblastoma
	Lymphoma
	Cervical neuroblastoma
	Nonrhabdomyosarcoma soft tissue sarcoma

Differential Diagnosis

The differential diagnosis of NPC in children includes a variety of benign and malignant conditions (Table 30.1); early recognition is the key.

An important entity recently described, which should be included in the differential diagnosis of nasopharyngeal malignancies presenting with aggressive behavior and rapid progression, is NUT (nuclear protein in testis) midline carcinoma. This is a very rare and aggressive malignancy genetically defined by rearrangements of the gene, *NUT*. In the majority (75%) of cases, the *NUT* gene on chromosome 15q14 is fused with *BRD4* on chromosome 19p13, creating chimeric genes that encode the BRD-NUT fusion proteins. In the remaining cases, *NUT* is fused to *BRD3* on chromosome 9q34 or an unknown partner gene; these tumors are termed *NUT-variant* [16]. The tumors arise in midline epithelial structures, typically mediastinum and upper aerodigestive tract, and present as very aggressive undifferentiated carcinomas, with or without squamous differentiation [17]. Although the original description of this neoplasm was made in children and young adults, patients of all ages can be affected. The outcome is very poor, with an average chance of survival of less than 1 year. Preliminary data seem to indicate that *NUT-variant* tumors may have a more protracted course [17]. Preclinical studies have shown that NUT-BRD4 is associated with globally decreased histone acetylation and transcriptional repression and that this acetylation can be restored with histone deacetylase inhibitors, resulting in squamous differentiation, arrested growth in vitro, and growth inhibition in xenograft models. Response to vorinostat has been reported in a case of a child with refractory disease, thus suggesting a potential role for this class of agents in the treatment of this malignancy [18].

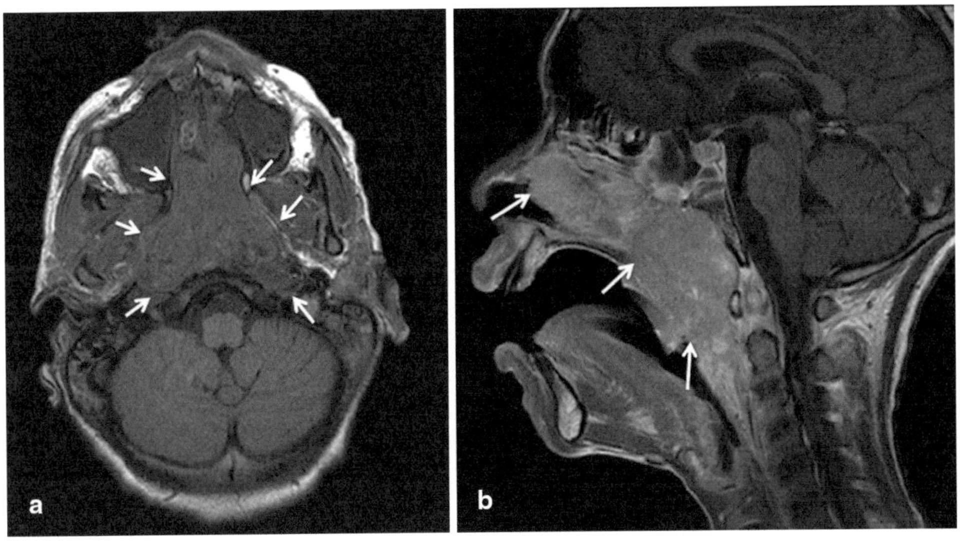

Fig. 30.1 Axial (**a**), and sagital (**b**) MRI images showing a large nasopharyngeal carcinoma in a 14-year-old African-American male patient

Diagnosis and Evaluation

NPC should always be suspected in an adolescent presenting with nasal congestion or epistaxis, headache, and a cervical mass. Most patients present with bilateral cervical metastases, and an asymptomatic cervical disease may be the presenting sign. Nasal endoscopy usually shows a nasopharyngeal mass, and a biopsy of the primary tumor is always recommended; however, a diagnosis can also be made with a biopsy of a cervical lymph node in the context of a suggestive nasopharyngeal mass. Imaging studies should include proper locoregional imaging and evaluation of metastatic sites. A magnetic resonance imaging (MRI) of the head and neck, extending to the supraclavicular fossa, is recommended, and a computed tomography (CT) may be performed to better define skull base erosion (Fig. 30.1). A CT scan of the chest is also recommended to evaluate the presence of parenchymal metastases as well as mediastinal nodal disease, which usually develops as an extension of the cervical metastases. While the role of a positron emission tomography (PET) scan is not clear at the time of diagnosis, it may facilitate the evaluation of response to therapy [19].

The keratinizing NPCs are conventional squamous cell carcinomas with readily seen keratinization and desmoplastic reaction. The nonkeratinizing carcinomas show minimal or absent keratinization mimicking urothelial transitional cell carcinomas. The undifferentiated type of NPC is the most frequent type seen in the pediatric age group. In this type, the neoplastic cells may have a diffuse, noncohesive growth pattern mimicking a lymphoma or may have a syncytial cohesive growth, forming nests. Characteristically, they lack keratinization. These tumors are associated with a prominent nonneoplastic lymphoid component. By immunohistochemistry, all types of NPC are immunoreactive with cytokeratin. EBV EBER in situ hybridization is positive in all undifferentiated NPCs and 100 % of the neoplastic cells contain the virus (Fig. 30.2).

Staging of NPC usually follows the TNM system, which has shown to be predictive of outcome and very helpful in defining therapy (Table 30.2) [20].

Treatment

NPC is considered to be unresectable due to the complex anatomical location. NPC is a very radiosensitive tumor, and radiation therapy is considered to be the primary treatment modality. High doses (>65 Gy) are usually required to achieve good locoregional control [13–15, 21, 22]. The regional lymph nodes in the entire head and neck area are irradiated, and the structures surrounding the nasopharynx and entire neck should be also included in the treatment. The disease control rates with radiation therapy are stage dependent, with survival rates of 65–85 % for patients with stage II and of less than 50 % for patients with stage IV disease [23]. The development of both locoregional and distant recurrence correlates with the size of the primary tumor and the nodal staging. Tumors of undifferentiated histology (World Health Organisation (WHO) type III) are more radiosensitive, and this correlates with better outcome [21].

Despite the progress in the delivery of radiation therapy and supportive care, a significant proportion of patients with locoregionally advanced disease fail treatment, and long-term survival rates are unsatisfactory. Unlike other head and neck cancers NPC is a very chemosensitive neoplasm, and the use of chemotherapy might thus provide benefit for patients with advanced disease. Among the drugs tested those with best single-agent activity include methotrexate, bleomycin, 5-fluorouracil (5-FU), cisplatin (CDDP), and carboplatin [13–15, 22]. The response rates in combination stud-

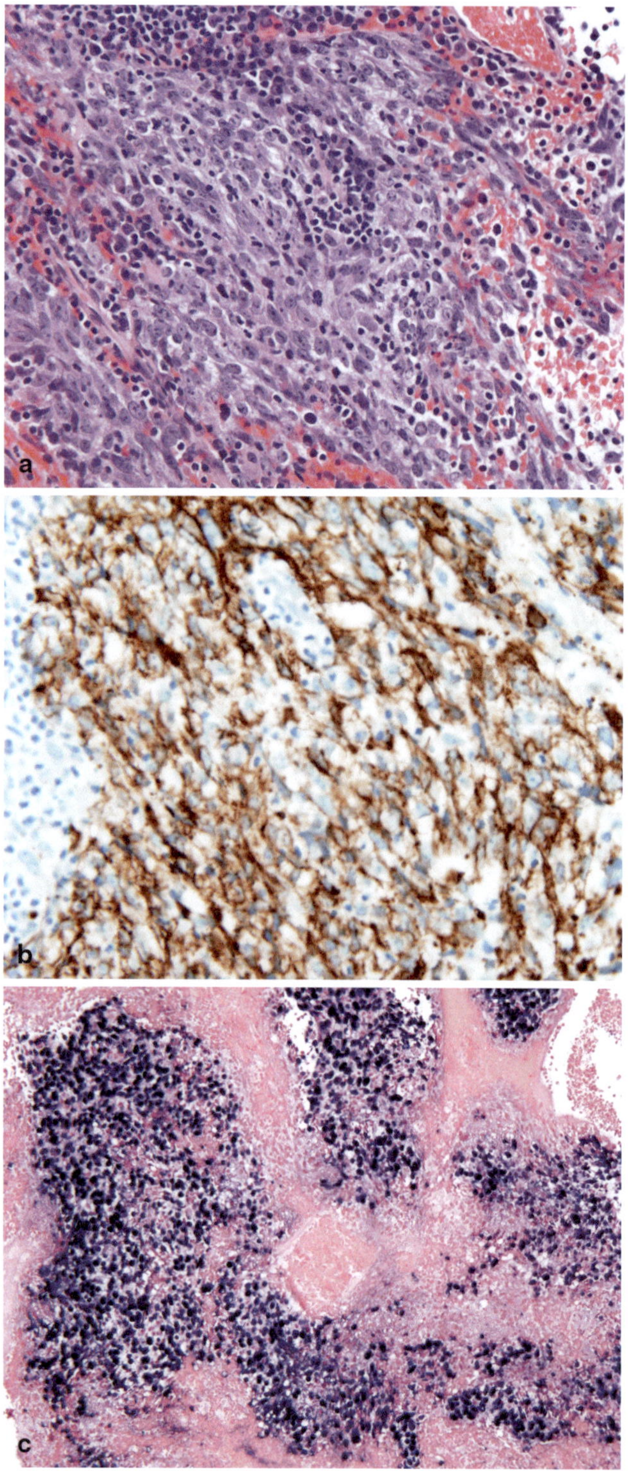

Fig. 30.2 **a** Undifferentiated type nasopharyngeal carcinoma (NPC) showing a large group of cohesive neoplastic cells with amphophilic cytoplasm and oval nuclei with single prominent eosinophilic nucleoli. Numerous, interspersed inflammatory cells (predominantly lymphocytes) are also present. **b** Tumor cells are strongly and diffusely immunoreactive for pancytokeratin AE1AE3. **c** EBV EBER in situ hybridization showing positive staining (*dark blue*) in the nuclei of all tumor cells

Table 30.2 AJCC (American Joint Committee on Cancer) staging system for nasopharyngeal carcinoma

Value	Definition		
T1	Tumor confined to the nasopharynx, or tumor extends to oropharynx and/or nasal cavity without parapharyngeal extension		
T2	Tumor with parapharyngeal extension		
T3	Tumor invades bony structures of skull base and/or paranasal sinuses		
T4	Tumor with intracranial extension and/or involvement of cranial nerves, hypopharynx, orbit, or with extension to the infratemporal fossa/masticator space.		
N0	No regional lymph node metastasis		
N1	Unilateral metastasis in cervical lymph node(s), ≤6 cm in greatest dimension, above the supraclavicular fossa, and/or unilateral or bilateral, retropharyngeal lymph nodes, ≤6 cm in greatest dimension		
N2	Bilateral metastasis in cervical lymph node(s), ≤6 cm in greatest dimension, above the supraclavicular fossa		
N3	Metastasis in a lymph node(s)[c] >6 cm and/or to supraclavicular fossa		
	N3a: >6 cm in dimension		
	N3b: Extension to the supraclavicular fossa		
M0	No distant metastasis		
M1	Distant metastasis		
Stage I	T1	N0	M0
Stage IIA	T2a	N0	M0
Stage IIB	T1	N1	M0
	T2	N0	M0
	T2	N1	M0
Stage III	T1	N2	M0
	T2	N2	M0
	T3	N0-2	M0
Stage IVA	T4	N0-2	M0
Stage IVB	Any T	N3	M0
Stage IVC	Any T	Any N	M1

ies range from 38–91 %, with CDDP-containing regimens showing clear advantage over non-CDDP containing regimens. Most of the information on the role of chemotherapy derives from studies performed in adult NPC [24]. Chemotherapy has been administered in the neoadjuvant, concurrent, and adjuvant settings. Considering the chemosensitivity of NPC, the administration of neoadjuvant chemotherapy has the advantage of inducing an immediate response and symptom alleviation, while allowing for more time for radiation planning. Cisplatin may enhance radiation toxicity by inhibiting the repair of sublethal damage, reoxygenation and recruitment of cells into a proliferative state, and radiosensitization of hypoxic cells [25]. Thus, the administration of cisplatin during radiation therapy (concurrent chemoradiation) has a strong rationale, and randomized studies have shown a survival advantage when compared with radiation alone [24]. Administration of chemotherapy after radiation therapy has also been explored; however, this sequence

Table 30.3 Treatment of advanced childhood nasopharyngeal carcinoma

Protocol	Neoadjuvant chemotherapy	Concurrent chemoradiotherapy	Radiation Dose
TREP [14]	CDDP 100 mg/m², d1	CDDP 30 mg/m²/wk x 7 doses	T: I-IIA 60 Gy IIB-IV 65 Gy
	5-FU 1000 mg/m², d1–5		N: N+65 Gy N-45 Gy
NPC-2003-GPOH [15]	CDDP 100 mg/m², d1	CDDP 20 mg/m² d1–3 x weeks 1 and 3 of RT	CR+: 54.4 Gy
	5-FU 1000 mg/m², d1–5		CR–: 59.4 Gy
	LV 25 mg/m² x 6 doses		
ARAR0331	CDDP 80 mg/m², d1	CDDP 100 mg/m² d1 x weeks 1 and 3 of RT	CR/PR: 61.2 Gy
	5-FU 1000 mg/m², d1–4		PD: 70.2 Gy

CDDP cisplatin, *5-FU* 5-fluorouracyl, *LV* leucovorin, *RT* radiation therapy, *CR* complete response, *PR* partial response, *PD* progressive disease, *d* days, *wk* week, *T* tumor, *N* nodes

seems to be much less tolerable, and compliance is lower [24]. In a meta-analysis evaluating randomized clinical trials that explored the role of neoadjuvant, concurrent, and adjuvant chemotherapy for NPC, the greatest survival advantage was associated with the use of concurrent chemoradiation, with a survival benefit of 20%. Neoadjuvant chemotherapy was also associated with improved survival, as result of a decrease in distant and local relapses [24]. Administration of chemotherapy in the adjuvant setting does not seem to be associated with any significant benefit, and was shown to be associated with more toxicity and lower compliance rates [24, 26]. Few studies have evaluated the impact of neoadjuvant chemotherapy followed by concurrent chemotherapy, but this seems to be an approach associated with reasonable toxicity and good outcomes in adult NPC [27].

In children, the use of neoadjuvant chemotherapy is consistently associated with remarkable initial responses, and most studies incorporate this approach followed by chemoradiotherapy [13–15, 22]. The German, Italian, and North American cooperative groups have used a similar approach combining neoadjuvant chemotherapy with cisplatin and 5-FU, followed by concurrent chemoradiation with cisplatin as single agent; using this approach, survival rates are 80–90% [14, 15] (Table 30.3). An important observation of recent studies is that for patients with good response to induction chemotherapy, the radiation therapy dose can be reduced to less than 55–60 Gy without compromising local control rates [15, 22].

Based on the strong role played by EBV in the pathogenesis of childhood NPC, the German group has incorporated interferon-beta for 6 months after completion of therapy in order to provide an added antiviral and antitumoral effect. The results of the German study NPC-2003-GPOH are the best reported to date, with a 30-month overall survival rate of 97% [15].

The prognosis for patients with recurrent disease is very poor [13]. Responses to taxanes and gemcitabine have been documented, and most salvage regimens incorporate those agents, often in combination with carboplatin or oxaliplatin [28, 29]. The use of cytotoxic T lymphocytes (CTL) against EBV has proven to induce durable responses, and patients with EBV + recurrent NPC should be considered for this type of therapy in combination with a taxane-containing salvage regimen [30].

Table 30.4 Late effects after the treatment of childhood nasopharyngeal carcinoma (NPC)

Category	Morbidity
Orodental	Xerostomia
	Trismus
	Osteonecrosis
	Dental decay
Endocrine	Hypothyroidism
	Panhypopituitarism
Auditory	Sensorineural hearing loss
	Chronic otitis media
Digestive	Esophageal stricture
	Swallowing dysfunction
Ocular	Xerophthalmia
	Cataracts
	Vision loss
Renal	Cisplatin tubulopathy
Other	Chronic sinusitis
	Cranial nerve palsy
Second malignancies	Skin carcinoma
	Salivary gland carcinoma
	Osteosarcoma

Outcome

With current therapies that combine neoadjuvant chemotherapy and concurrent chemoradiation, survival rates for children with NPC are greater than 80–85% [14, 15, 22]. These results appear to be superior to those reported for adults [1]. However, treatment is associated with severe late effects derived from the use of high doses of radiation therapy and intensive use of platinum agents, including neuroendocrine, dental, and ocular morbidities, as well as second malignancies [1, 13] (Table 30.4). The use of imaging-guided radiation therapy modalities such as conformal and intensity-modulated radiation therapy, as well as the use of proton therapy may eventually result in a decrease in the cumulative incidence of morbidities. Long-term survivors of childhood NPC should be followed by a multidisciplinary team to identify, prevent, and treat the treatment-related late effects.

References

1. Sultan I, Casanova M, Ferrari A, Rihani R, Rodriguez-Galindo C. Differential features of nasopharyngeal carcinoma in children and adults: a SEER study. Pediatr Blood Cancer. 2010;55:279–84.
2. Fandi A, Cvitkovic E. Biology and treatment of nasopharyngeal cancer. Curr Opin Oncol. 1995;7:255–63.
3. Vokes EE, Liebowitz DN, Weichselbaum RR. Nasopharyngeal carcinoma. Lancet. 1997;350:1087–91.
4. Zeng Y, Zhang LG, Wu YC, et al. Prospective studies on nasopharyngeal carcinoma in Epstein-Barr virus IgA/VCA antibody-positive persons in Wuzhou City, China. Int J Cancer. 1986;36:545–8.
5. de-Vathaire F, Sancho-Garnier H, de-The H, et al. Prognostic value of EBV markers in the clinical management of nasopharyngeal carcinoma (NPC): a multicenter follow-up study. Int J Cancer. 1988;42:176–81.
6. Pathmanathan R, Prasad U, Chandrika G, et al. Undifferentiated, nonkeratinizing, and squamous cell carcinoma of the nasopharynx: variants of Epstein-Barr virus-infected neoplasia. Am J Pathol. 1995;146:1355–67.
7. Lo YMD, Chan ATC, Chan LYS, et al. Molecular prognostication of nasopharyngeal carcinoma by quantitative analysis of circulating Epstein-Barr virus DNA. Cancer Res. 2000;60:6878–81.
8. Liebowitz D. Nasopharyngeal carcinoma: the Epstein-Barr virus association. Semin Oncol. 1994;21:376–81.
9. Sam CK, Brooks LA, Niedobitek G, et al. Analysis of Epstein-Barr virus infection in naospharyngeal biopsies from a group at high risk of nasopharyngeal carcinoma. Int J Cancer; 1993;53:957–62.
10. Wu TC, Mann RB, Epdtein JI, et al. Abundant expression of EBER1 small nuclear RNA in nasopharyngeal carcinoma: a morphologically distinctive target for detection of Epstein-Barr virus in formalin-fixed paraffin-embeded carcinoma specimens. Am J Pathol. 1991;138:1461–9.
11. Murray PG, Niedobitek G, Kremmer E, et al. In situ detection of the Epstein-Barr virus-encoded nuclear antigen 1 in oral hairy leukoplakia and virus-associated carcinomas. J Pathol; 1996;178:44–7.
12. Hording U, Nielsen HW, Albeck H, et al. Nasopharyngeal carcinoma—histopathological types and association with Epstein-Barr virus. Eur J Cancer B Oral Oncol. 1993;29B:137–9.
13. Cheuk DKL, Billups CA, Martin MG, et al. Prognostic factors and long-term outcomes of childhood nasopharyngeal carcinoma. Cancer. 2011;117:197–206.
14. Casanova M, Bisogno G, Gandola L, et al. A prospective protocol for nasopharyngeal carcinoma in children and adolescents. Cancer. 2012;118:2718–25.
15. Buehrlen M, Zwaan CM, Granzen B, et al. Multimodal treatment, including interferon beta, of nasopharyngeal carcinoma in children and young adults: preliminary results.from the prospective, multicenter study NPC-2003-GPOH/DCOG. Cancer. 2012;118:4892–900.
16. French CA. Pathogenesis of NUT midline carcinoma. Annu Rev Pathol. 2012;7:247–65.
17. Bauer DE, Mitchell CM, Strait KM, et al. Clinicopathologic features and long-term outcomes of NUT midline carcinoma. Clin Cancer Res. 2012;18:5773–9.
18. Schwartz BE, Hofer MD, Lemieux ME, et al. Differentiation of NUT midline carcinoma by epigenomic reprogramming. Cancer Res. 2011;71:2686–96.
19. Cheuk DK, Sabin ND, Hossain M, et al. PET/CT for staging and follow-up of pediatric nasopharyngeal carcinoma. Eur J Nucl Med Mol Imaging. 2012;39:1097–106.
20. Pharynx. In: Edge SB, Byrd DR, Compton CC et al., Editors. AJCC cancer staging manual. 7th ed. New York: Springer; 2010. pp. 41–56.
21. Sanguineti G, Geara FB, Garden AS, et al. Carcinoma of the nasopharynx treated by radiotherapy alone: determinants of local and regional control. Int J Radiat Oncol Biol Phys. 1997;37:985–96.
22. Orbach D, Brisse H, Helfre S, et al. Radiation and chemotherapy combination for nasopharyngeal carcinoma in children: radiotherapy dose adaptation after chemotherapy response to minimize late effects. Pediatr Blood Cancer. 2008;50:849–53.
23. Perez CA, Devineni VR, Marcial-vega V, Marks JE, Simpson JR, Kucik N. Carcinoma of the nasopharynx: factors affecting prognosis. Int J Radiat Oncol Biol Phys. 1992;23:271–80.
24. Langendijk JA, Leemans C, Buter J, Berkhof J. Slotman BJ. The additional value of chemotherapy to radiotherapy in locally advanced nasopharyngeal carcinoma: a meta-analysis of the published literature. J Clin Oncol. 2004;22:4604–12.
25. Dewit L. Combined treatment of radium and cis-diamminedichloroplatinum (II): a review of experimental and clinical data. Int J Radiat Oncol Biol Phys. 1987;13:403–26.
26. Chen L, Hu CS, Chen XZ, et al. Concurrent chemoradiotherapy plus adjuvant chemotherapy versus concurrent chemoradiotherapy alone in patients with locoregionally advanced nasopharyngeal carcinoma: a phase 3 multicentre randomised controlled trial. Lancet Oncol. 2012;13:163–71.
27. Rischin D, Corry J, Smith J, Stewart J, Hughes P, Peters L. Excellent disease control and survival in patients with advanced nasopharyngeal cancer treated with chemoradiation. J Clin Oncol;2002:1845–52.
28. Johnson FM, Garden A, Palmer JL, et al. A Phase II study of docetaxel and carboplatin as neoadjuvant therapy for nasopharyngeal carcinoma with early T status and advanced N status. Cancer. 2004;100:991–8.
29. Zhang L, Zhang Y, Huang PY, Xu F, Peng PJ, Guan ZZ. Phase II clinical study of gemcitabine in the treatment of patients with advanced nasopharyngeal carcinoma after the failure of platinum-based chemotherapy. Cancer Chemother Pharmacol. 2008;61:33–8.
30. Louis CU, Straathof K, Bollard CM, et al. Adoptive transfer of EBV-specific T cells results in sustained clinical responses in patients with locoregional nasopharyngeal carcinoma. J Immunother. 2010;33:983–90.

31 Neuroblastoma

Natasha M. Archer and Suzanne Shusterman

Introduction

Neuroblastoma (NB), a solid neoplasm of the sympathetic nervous system, is the third most common malignancy of childhood. Although it presents as an abdominal mass in 65% of cases, the tumor can develop anywhere along the sympathetic nervous system [1]. In approximately 50% of cases, it has spread to the bone, bone marrow, and/or other organ via the blood or lymphatic system at the time of presentation. As a result, head and neck lesions, primary or metastatic, are not uncommon. Although some forms of the disease spontaneously regress, treatment generally consists of local control and often systemic therapies in the form of neoadjuvant and adjuvant chemotherapy, autologous stem cell transplantation, and retinoic acid with monoclonal antibody.

Key Points

- NB is the third most common malignancy of childhood accounting for 8–10% of all cancers of childhood and 15% of all childhood cancer deaths [1].
- Approximately 2–5% of neuroblastic tumors occur primarily in the cervical region [2].
- Eight percent of patients with NB present with ocular signs and symptoms at diagnosis [3].
- Treatment of NB requires a multidisciplinary team approach as many modes of therapy are often required to provide a chance at cure.

N. M. Archer (✉) · S. Shusterman
Department of Pediatric Hematology-Oncology, Dana-Farber/Boston Children's Cancer and Blood Disorders Center, Boston, MA, USA
e-mail: Natasha.archer@childrens.harvard.edu

Biology and Epidemiology

Neuroblastic tumors develop from the neural crest, an ectodermal tissue with pluripotent differentiating capability. It belongs to a class of tumors that include NB, stroma-rich ganglioneuroblastoma and ganglioneuroma, a benign lesion composed of mature ganglion cells. Although NB of the head and neck is usually a secondary metastatic lesion, it can sometimes occur primarily at this site.

Pathophysiology

- The migration of neural crest cells during fetal development accounts for the diversity of tumor presentation sites.
- NB of the head and neck is usually a secondary metastatic lesion; however in the cervical region, NB most often develops from the sympathetic superior cervical ganglion or along the cervical plexus and nerve roots.
- Primary cervical NB may invade cranial nerves IX, XI, and XII and extend intracranially through the base of the skull, the jugular foramen, and carotid canal.

Molecular/Genetic Pathology

- Approximately 20% of NBs overexpress MYCN via amplification of the distal arm of chromosome 2 (2p24) [1]. The MYCN oncogene amplification is associated with advanced stage disease and a dismal prognosis [4].
- Loss of heterozygosity (LOH) at 1p (1p36) is associated with MYCN amplification and high risk disease [5].
- Segmental deletions of 11q (11q23) are rarely found in tumors with MYCN amplification, but are associated with other high risk factors such as advanced stage, older age at diagnosis, and unfavorable histopathology [6].

R. Rahbar et al. (eds.), *Pediatric Head and Neck Tumors*,
DOI 10.1007/978-1-4614-8755-5_31, © Springer Science+Business Media New York 2014

- In some studies, gain of chromosome 17q material conveys a poor prognosis, while others have failed to show such an association [7, 8].
- Anaplastic lymphoma kinase (ALK) gene mutations have been identified as a major cause of familial NB, while a small subset of familial NB associated with congenital central hypoventilation syndrome has been linked with germline mutations in paired-like homeobox 2B (PHOX2B), a transcription factor that plays a role in the development of the neural crest [9, 10].
- Somatic ALK gene mutations are found in 7–10% of sporadic tumors [11].
- Alpha thalassemia/mental retardation syndrome X-linked (ATRX) mutations are most often present in an older patient population with an indolent disease course and poor overall survival [12].

Incidence

- NB is the most common solid, extracranial malignancy of childhood. The incidence is approximately 10.4 per million per year in white children and 8.3 per million per year in black children less than 15 years of age in the USA. Approximately 800 new cases per year are diagnosed in the USA [1].
- It accounts for 8–10% of all childhood cancers in pediatric patients younger than 15 years of age and 15% of all childhood cancer deaths [1].
- Primary cervical NB is rare, accounting for approximately 2–5% of all NB cases. In a series of 617 localized NB cases, 4.2% were in the cervical region and an additional 2.7% were in the cervicothoracic region [2].
- Of the 50% of patients that present with metastasis, most have bony skull lesions.

Age Distribution

- Most NBs present in infancy or early childhood with a median age of presentation of 19 months [1]. Cervical NB tends to present at an even younger age.
- Only 10% of neuroblastic tumors occur in people above 5 years of age [13].

Geographic Distribution

- International reports indicate that the incidence of NB is higher among high-resource than low-resource settings, however, that may be due to underreporting in countries with limited health care infrastructure and thus an inability to appropriately diagnose the disease [14].

Risk Factors—Environmental, Lifestyle

- No environmental risk factors have been identified.

Relationships to Other Disease States, Syndromes

- Children with Beckwith–Wiedemann syndrome have an increased risk, estimated between 4 and 21%, of both benign and malignant tumors in the first decade of life [15, 16]. Although hepatoblastoma and Wilms tumor are more commonly observed, NB has also been reported [15, 17]. DeBaun et al. showed that the average annual incidence of cancer in children less than 4 years old with Beckwith–Wiedemann syndrome was 0.027 with a relative risk of 197 (CI 22–711), for NB compared to 0.019 expected in a control cohort without the syndrome [18].

Presentation

Symptoms

The clinical presentation of the disease is mostly dependent on mass effect on structures in the head and neck. In primary cervical NB, the most common symptoms are neck mass, ocular symptoms, and signs of respiratory distress. Metastatic lesions to the bony structures of the face and skull are often painful.

Ocular Symptoms

- Eight percent of all patients with NB present with ocular symptoms at diagnosis including Horner's syndrome, opsoclonus, and proptosis [3].
- Opsoclonus is defined as uncontrolled eye movements. Together with myoclonus, it is thought to be an immune-mediated paraneoplastic syndrome which occurs in 2–3% of patients with NB [19, 20]. In this syndrome, antibodies directed against tumor, cross-react with neural cells in the cerebellum.
- Horner syndrome is characterized by unilateral ptosis, miosis, and anhidrosis due to blockage of sympathetic feedback to the eye and face (Fig. 31.1). Heterochromia iridis can also occur in the ipsilateral eye.
- Bone is the most frequent site of metastasis in patients with NB, with the posteriolateral part of the bony orbits being one of the most frequent sites of clinical presentation. (Fig. 31.2) With bony or soft tissue metastasis around the eye, proptosis can occur. "Raccoon eyes," a dramatic presentation of the disease, is a result of metastatic hemorrhagic tumor in orbital bone and soft tissue.

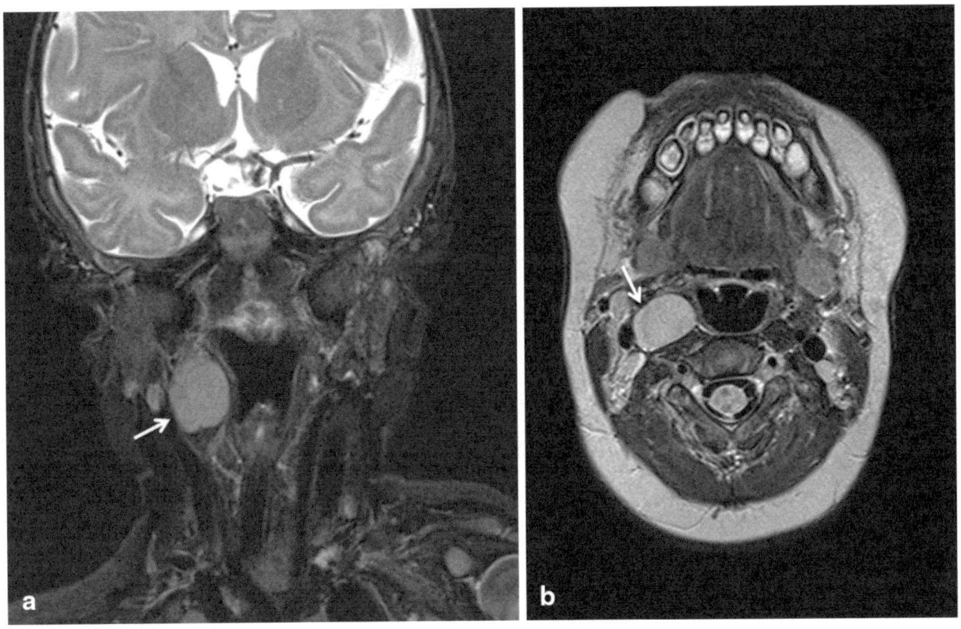

Fig. 31.1 MRI of a 4-month-old infant who presented with right Horner syndrome. T1 coronal (**a**) and T2 axial (**b**) images show a mass within the carotid space. Biopsy showed neuroblastoma

Respiratory and Gastrointestinal Issues

- Respiratory distress due to trachea compression can occur with large masses or masses that arise in the retropharyngeal space.
- Difficulty swallowing and vocal cord paralysis have also been reported [21].

Differential Diagnosis

Most patients will present with a mass; thus the differential diagnosis includes mostly a variety of neoplastic and few nonneoplastic conditions (Table 31.1).

Diagnosis and Evaluation

Physical Examination

Physical examination should include a detailed head and neck evaluation looking for fixed, hard cervical masses as well as common ocular presentations of the disease, including Horner's syndrome, opsoclonus, proptosis, and periorbital ecchymoses. Skull based metastatic lesions may also be palpable. The abdominal exam should aim to assess for the presence of hepatomegaly and/or a fixed, hard abdominal mass, as primary tumors arising from the adrenal gland are most common. Lastly, a detailed neurologic exam specifically looking for an evolving paralysis is essential in all patients with NB until paraspinal masses have been ruled out.

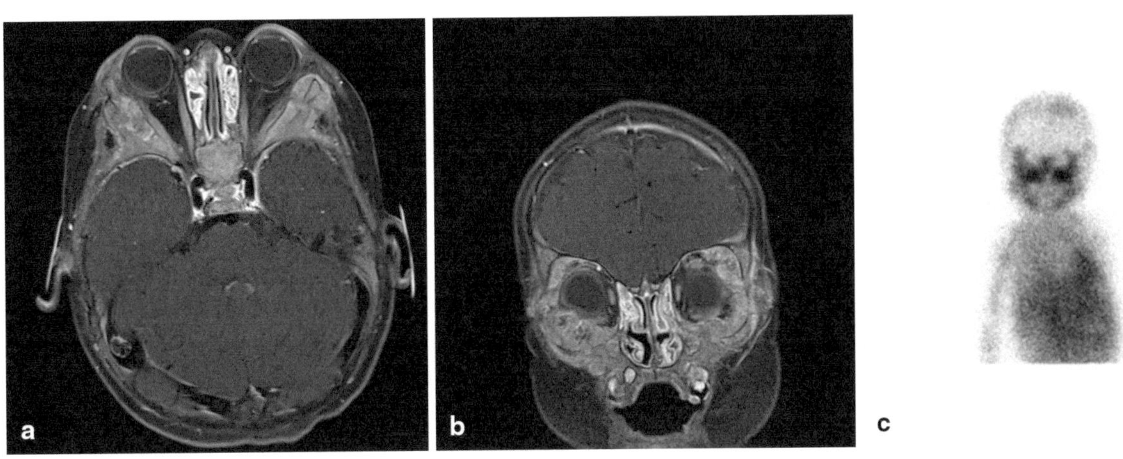

Fig. 31.2 Metastatic neuroblastoma. **a** Axial T1 MRI image showing diffuse expansile marrow infiltration involving the bilateral craniofacial bones. **b** Coronal T1 MRI image showing diffuse involvement of the orbital bones. **c** I-metaiodobenzylguanidine (MIBG) scan showing uptake in the involved structures

Table 31.1 Differential diagnosis of neuroblastoma

Primary site	Differential diagnosis
Abdomen	Wilms tumor
	Hepatoblastoma
	Rhabdomyosarcoma
	Lymphoma
Thorax and retroperitoneum	Lymphoma
	Germ cell tumor
Neck	Lymphoma
	Infection
Bone	Lymphoma
	Rhabdomyosarcoma
	Soft tissue sarcomas
	Langerhans cell histiocytosis
Bone marrow	Lymphoma
	Leukemia (especially megakaryoblastic leukemia)
Spinal canal	Desmoid tumor
	Epidermoid tumor
	Teratoma
	Astrocytoma
Skin	Dermoid cysts
	Subcutaneous fat necrosis
	Infantile fibrosarcoma
	Rhabdomyosarcoma
	Congenital leukemia

Laboratory Data

- Urinary catecholamine metabolites 4-hydroxy-3-methoxymandelic acid (VMA) and homovanillic acid (HVA) are elevated in greater than 90% of patients with NB.
- Standard preoperative laboratory studies (complete blood count (CBC) with differential, clotting times (PT/PTT), type and cross (T&C) for blood bank, chemistry panel (Chem 10)).

Imaging Evaluation

- Evaluation of the head and neck usually should include an MRI for better evaluation of extent of disease and compromise of vital structures (Figs. 31.1 and 31.2).
- As most cases of NB have a primary lesion in the abdomen either arising from the adrenal gland or somewhere along the sympathetic chain, CT and/or MRI will likely be needed to assess tumor burden in the abdomen.
- Chest radiograph (Posterior Anterior and lateral) is needed to assess for thoracic disease. If positive, CT of the chest should follow.
- Evaluation of the bony skeleton is necessary to assess for metatstatic lesions. I-metaiodobenzylguanidine (MIBG), an agent that concentrates in cells that receive sympathetic innervation, is taken up by 90% of NBs. As a result,

Table 31.2 International Neuroblastoma Pathology Classification. (Shimada index)

	Schwannian stroma	Age (years)	Grade of neuroblastic differentiation	MKI
Favorable	≥50%	All	GN of GNB, non-nodular	
	<50%	1.5–5	Differentiated	MKI<100
	<50%	<1.5		MKI<200
Unfavorable	≥50%	All	Nodular	
	<50%	>5		
	<50%	1.5–5	Undifferentiated	
	<50%	<1.5		MKI<200

MIBG scans are more sensitive and specific than a bone scan. The ^{123}I MIBG scan is thought to be a better diagnostic tool than the ^{131}I MIBG scan [22]. Most institutions will perform a bone scan and ^{123}I MIBG scan at presentation, but will then limit to ^{123}I MIBG scan if the scans are concordant (Fig. 31.2).

Pathology

The International Neuroblastoma Pathology Classification (INPC), established in 1999 and later revised in 2003, uses morphologic features including Schwannian stroma development, grade of neuroblastic differentiation, and mitosis-karyorrhexis index (MKI) to determine if neuroblastic tumors are of favorable or unfavorable histology (Table 31.2) [23, 24]. The INPC includes age at diagnosis as well, but the morphologic features alone have been found to be prognostic independent of age [25].

Undifferentiated and poorly differentiated NB are the most immature and aggressive of the neuroblastic tumors with no significant Schwannian stroma and composed of neuroblasts without or with neuropil, respectively (Fig. 31.3a). MKI can vary throughout the tumor cells. NB is one of the many small round blue cell tumors of childhood and when devoid of neuropil can be difficult to distinguish from other small round blue cell tumors such as lymphoma, osteosarcoma, rhabdomyosarcoma, and Ewing Sarcoma. Immunohistochemistry using antibodies that specifically interact with neural tissue such as synaptophysin and chromogranin, is often positive in NB. Ganglionic differentiation as well as the presence of significant Schwannian stroma in neuroblastic tumors are important in the histopathologic classification. In differentiating NB, more than 5% of tumor cells show ganglionic differentiation (Fig. 31.3b). Ganglioneuroma is benign and composed entirely of mature ganglion cells (Fig. 31.3c; a variant of ganglioneuroma, the maturing ganglioneuroma is also benign but some ganglion cells are small and not fully developed). Ganglioneuroblastomas are composite tumors

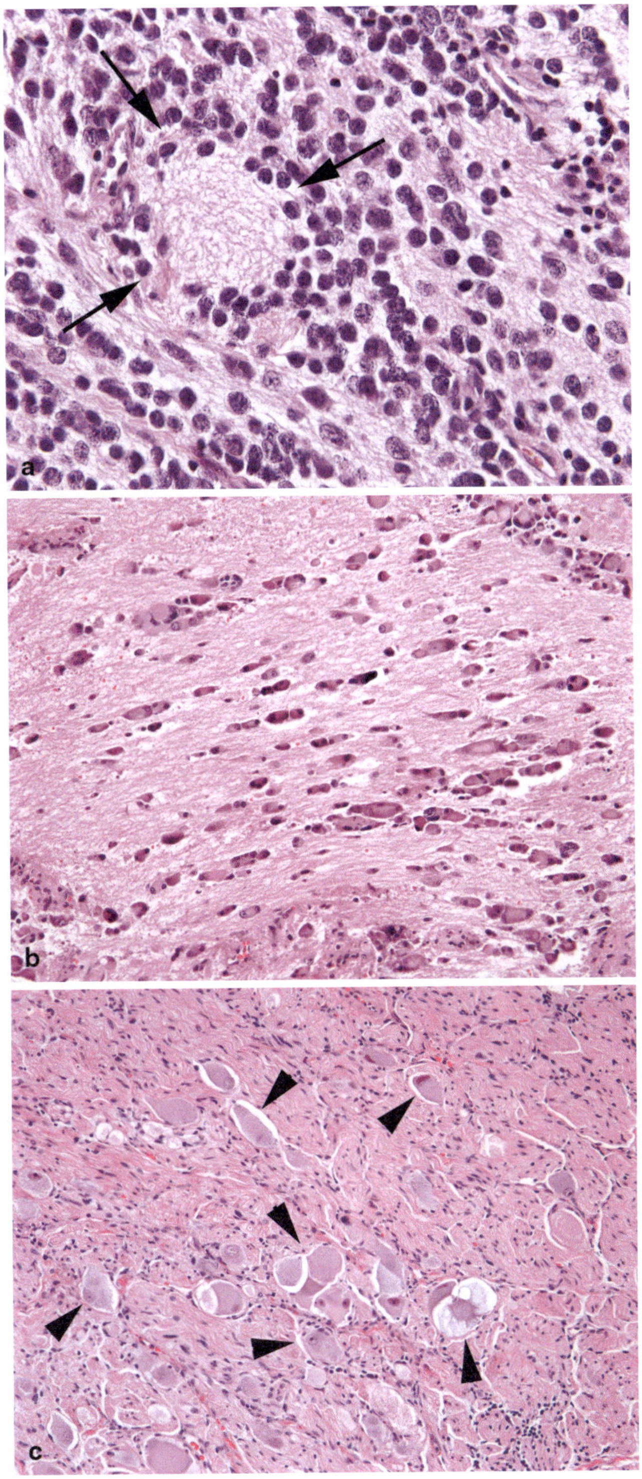

Fig. 31.3 **a** Poorly differentiated neuroblastoma. *Round blue* cells are immersed in a fibrillary background rich in neuropil. A characteristic rosette centered around neuropil is indicated by *arrows*. **b** Differentiating neuroblastoma. Ganglionic differentiation is present in most of the tumor cells, which are separated by abundant neuropil. **c** Ganglioneuroma. Tumor composed of numerous mature ganglion cells (*arrowheads*) and a bland neurofibroma-like stroma are shown.

made of NB and ganglioneuroma. There are two variants: the intermixed ganglioneuroblastoma in which poorly differentiated neuroblasts are dispersed within the ganglioneuroma and the nodular ganglioneuroblastoma in which the NB component form separate grossly visible nodules.

Pathologic review of the bone marrow aspirate and biopsy from bilateral iliac crests as well as the primary mass should be performed in the evaluation of NB. Approximately ten core needle biopsies of the mass should be obtained for histopathologic diagnosis.

Treatment

Surgical Therapy

Current International Neuroblastoma Risk Group (INRG) pretreatment risk stratification takes into account disease stage, patient age, histopathology classification, MYCN amplification status, ploidy and allelic loss of heterozygosity at 1p or 11q. It is this risk stratification that determines the next steps in NB treatment (Table 31.3) [26].

- Very low and low risk disease, like a localized cervical NB, often requires surgery alone. In the case of localized tumors without high risk features, the goal of surgery is to establish a definite diagnosis, determine the extent of tumor spread, excise tumor, and provide tissue for genetic studies all while minimizing damage to local structures. Surgical risk factors were developed for localized NB in an effort to better define the surgical approach to localized disease. In 2005, Cecchetto et al. as part of the LNESGI Study of the European International Society of Pediatric Oncology Neuroblastoma Group, validated certain risk factors as predictors of adverse surgical outcome (Table 31.4). These should be reviewed prior to making decisions regarding local control [27].
- Although the importance of surgery in the treatment of localized NB is clear, the precise role and timing of surgery in the management of advanced NB is still debated. Some studies have noted an improvement in outcome with aggressive surgery, while others have questioned its benefit [28, 29].
- In a cohort of 278 children aged 18 months or older with stage IV NB enrolled on the German prospective clinical trial NB97, the extent of first operation (prior to induction chemotherapy) and best operation (most extensive removal of primary tumor) had no impact on event-free survival (EFS), local progression-free survival (LPFS) and overall survival suggesting that surgical teams should accept incomplete resection to avoid serious complications [30].
- Proper clinical, histological, and biological characterization of cervical NB is important to adjust the intensity of

Table 31.3 International Neuroblastoma Risk Group (INRG) pretreatment risk stratification. [26]

INRG stage	Age (months)	Histological category	Grade of tumor differentiation	MYCN	11q aberration	Ploidy	Pretreatment risk group
L1/L2		GN maturing; GNB intermixed					Very low
L1		Any, except GN maturing or GNB intermixed		NA			Very low
				Amp			High
L2	< 18	Any, except GN maturing or GNB intermixed		NA	No		Low
					Yes		Intermediate
L2	≥ 18	GNB nodular; neuroblastoma	Differentiating	NA	No		Low
					Yes		Intermediate
			Poorly differentiated or undifferentiated	NA			Intermediate
				Amp			High
M	< 18			NA		Hyperdiploid	Low
	< 12			NA		Diploid	Intermediate
	12 to < 18			NA		Diploid	Intermediate
	< 18			Amp			High
	≥ 18						High
MS	< 18			NA	No		Very low
					Yes		High
				Amp			High

L1 localized tumor confined to one body compartment and with the absence of image-defined risk factors, *L2* locoregional tumor with the presence of one or more image-defined risk factors, *M* distant metastatic disease (except stage MS), *MS* metastatic disease confined to skin, liver, and/or bone marrow in children younger than 18months, *Amp* amplified, *NA* Non-amplified. *Blank* can be "any"

treatment. For low risk (biologically favorable) disease, a conservative surgical approach is indicated; residual disease may mature or regress with no additional therapy. For patients with skull-base and orbital metastases, treatment is directed at the systemic involvement, with no surgery indicated in the management of the metastatic sites.

Complications

- Complications can include intraoperative bleeding, intestinal obstruction, postoperative diarrhea and ascites after resection of lesions in the abdomen, postoperative local and systemic infections, tumor rupture, neurovascular injury, and nephrectomy.
- In the SFOP NB LNESGI study on localized NB, the detection of surgical risk factors is associated with an increased risk of surgery related complications [27].
- Despite the fact that surgical risk factors were created for localized NB and not metastatic NB in mind, they may be helpful when considering the resection of a primary tumor in patients with metastatic disease.

Radiation Therapy

Although NB is thought to be a radiosensitive disease, radiation therapy is rarely used to treat head and neck lesions due to likely side effects and the presence of micro-metastatic disease making radiation therapy alone unlikely curable.

Complications

- General complications associated with radiation therapy include fatigue, nausea and vomiting, as well as skin and mucosal changes in the area affected.
- In addition, and of particular relevance in the head and neck region, is the likely halting of bone growth.

Chemotherapy

Chemotherapy is the principle form of treatment for intermediate-risk and high-risk NB. For intermediate risk disease, a carboplatin-based regimen, usually including cyclophosphamide, etoposide, and doxorubicin, is the treatment of choice. This regimen results in rapid response, facilitating local control usually with surgery. For patients with high-risk and metastatic disease, a more intensive treatment is required. This approach usually includes an induction phase with multiagent chemotherapy, followed by local control of the primary tumor, and consolidation with high-dose chemotherapy and autologous hematopoietic stem cell transplant. Treatment of minimal residual disease is then added, which includes a differentiating agent such as cis-retinoic acid and more recently anti GD-2 monoclonal antibodies [31].

Table 31.4 Surgical risk factors related to tumor site. [27]

Tumor site	Type of surgical risk factor
Neck	Encasement of vertebral artery
	Involvement of other major vessels
	Encasement of the brachial plexus
	Crossing of the midline
	Thoracic extension
	Dumbbell tumor
	Tumor size
	Tumor fragility
Thoracic	Encasement of subclavian vessels
	Involvement of other major vessels
	Lower mediastinal tumor
	Abdominal extension
	Encasement of trachea and/or principal bronchi
	Dumbbell tumor
	Tumor size
	Tumor fragility
Abdomen	Encasement of celiac axis
	Encasement of superior mesenteric artery
	Encasement of aorta
	Encasement of inferior vena cava
	Encasement of iliac and/or hypogastric vessels
	Infiltration of renal pedicle(s)
	Infiltration of porta hepatis
	Compromise of kidney and/or ureter
	Pelvic tumor crossing the sciatic notch
	Muscular infiltration
	Dumbbell tumor
	Tumor size
	Tumor fragility

Outcomes

Localized cervical NB has a good overall prognosis likely due to its location [2, 21]. Metastatic NB, especially in children greater than 18 months and with high risk features including MYCN amplification and unfavorable histopathology classification, has a poor prognosis with overall survival rates of approximately 40–60 %.

References

1. Brodeur GM, HM, Mosse YP, Maris JM. Neuroblastoma. In: Pizzo PA, Poplack DG, editors. Principles and practice of pediatric oncology. 6th ed. Philadelphia: Lippincott Williams & Wilkins; 2011.
2. Haddad M, Triglia JM, Helardot P, Couanet D, Gauthier F, Neuenschwander S, Bourlière B, Bergeron C, Munzer C, Rubie H, Guys J. Localized cervical neuroblastoma: prevention of surgical complications. Int J Pediatr Otorhinolaryngol. 2003;67:1361–7.
3. D'Ambrosio N, Lyo J, Young R, Haque S, Karimi S. Common and unusual craniofacial manifestations of metastatic neuroblastoma. Neuroradiology. 2010;52:549–53.
4. Brodeur GM, Seeger RC, Schwab M, Varmus HE, Michael JB. Amplification of N-myc in untreated human neuroblastomas correlates with advanced disease stage. Science. 1984;224:1121–4.
5. Attiyeh EF, London WB, Mossé YP, Wang Q, Winter C, Khazi D, McGrady PW, Seeger RC, Look AT, Shimada H, Brodeur GM, Cohn SL, Matthay KK, Maris JM. Chromosome 1p and 11q deletions and outcome in neuroblastoma. N Engl J Med. 2005;353:2243–53.
6. Guo C, White PS, Weiss MJ, Hogarty MD, Thompson PM, Stram DO, Gerbing R, Matthay KK, Seeger RC, Brodeur GM, Maris JM. Allelic deletion at 11q23 is common in MYCN single copy neuroblastomas. Oncogene. 1999;18:4948–57.
7. Plantaz D, Mohapatra G, Matthay KK, Pellarin M, Seeger RC, Feuerstein BG. Gain of chromosome 17 is the most frequent abnormality detected in neuroblastoma by comparative genomic hybridization. Am J Pathol. 1997;150:81–9.
8. Spitz R, Hero B, Ernestus K, Berthold F. Gain of distal chromosome arm 17q is not associated with poor prognosis in neuroblastoma. Clin Cancer Res. 2003;9:4835–40.
9. Mossé YP, Laudenslager M, Longo L, Cole KA, Wood A, Attiyeh EF, Laquaglia MJ, Sennett R, Lynch JE, Perri P, Laureys G, Speleman F, Kim C, Hou C, Hakonarson H, Torkamani A, Schork NJ, Brodeur GM, Tonini GP, Rappaport E, Devoto M, Maris JM. Identification of ALK as a major familial neuroblastoma predisposition gene. Nature. 2008;455:930–5.
10. Mosse YP, Laudenslager M, Khazi D, Carlisle AJ, Winter CL, Rappaport E, Maris JM. Germline PHOX2B mutation in hereditary neuroblastoma. Am J Hum Genet. 2004;75:727–30.
11. Mossé YP, Lim MS, Voss SD, Wilner K, Ruffner K, Laliberte J, Rolland D, Balis FM, Maris JM, Weigel BJ, Ingle AM, Ahern C, Adamson PC, Blaney SM. Safety and activity of crizotinib for paediatric patients with refractory solid tumours or anaplastic large-cell lymphoma: a Children's Oncology Group phase 1 consortium study. Lancet Oncol. 2013;14:472–80.
12. Cheung NK, Zhang J, Lu C, Parker M, Bahrami A, Tickoo SK, Heguy A, Pappo AS, Federico S, Dalton J, Cheung IY, Ding L, Fulton R, Wang J, Chen X, Becksfort J, Wu J, Billups CA, Ellison D, Mardis ER, Wilson RK, Downing JR. Dyer MA, St Jude Children's Research Hospital–Washington University Pediatric Cancer Genome Project. Association of age at diagnosis and genetic mutations in patients with neuroblastoma. JAMA. 2012;307:1062–71.
13. Howman-Giles R, Shaw PJ, Uren RF, Chung DK. Neuroblastoma and other neuroendocrine tumors. Semin Nucl Med. 2007;37:286–302.
14. Parkin DM, Kramárová E, Draper GJ. International incidence of childhood cancer. IARC Scientific Publications; 1998.
15. Yoon G, Graham G, Weksberg R, Gaul HP, DeBaun MR, Coppes MJ. Neuroblastoma in a patient with the Beckwith-Wiedemann syndrome (BWS). Med Pediatr Oncol. 2002;38:193–9.
16. Sorrentino S, Conte M, Nozza P, Granata C, Capra V, Avanzini S, Garaventa A. Simultaneous occurrence of pancreatoblastoma and neuroblastoma in a newborn with Beckwith-Wiedemann syndrome. J Pediatr Hematol Oncol. 2010;32:e207–9.
17. Emery LG, Shields M, Shah NR, Garbes A. Neuroblastoma associated with Beckwith-Wiedemann syndrome. Cancer. 1983;52:176–9.
18. DeBaun MR, Tucker MA. Risk of cancer during the first four years of life in children from The Beckwith-Wiedemann Syndrome Registry. J Pediatr. 1998;132:398–400.
19. Pranzatelli MR. The neurobiology of the opsoclonus–myoclonus syndrome. Clin Neuropharmacol. 1992;15:186–228.
20. Rudnick E, Khakoo Y, Antunes NL, Seeger RC, Brodeur GM, Shimada H, Gerbing RB, Stram DO, Matthay KK. Opsoclonus-myoclonus-ataxia syndrome in neuroblastoma: clinical outcome and antineuronal antibodies-a report from the Children's Cancer Group Study. Med Pediatr Oncol. 2001;36:612–22.

21. Abramson SJ, Berdon WE, Ruzal-Shapiro C, Stolar C, Garvin J. Cervical neuroblastoma in eleven infants—a tumor with favorable prognosis. Clinical and radiologic (US, CT, MRI) findings. Pediatr Radiol. 1993;23:253–7.
22. Shulkin BL, Shapiro B. Current concepts on the diagnostic use of MIBG in children. J Nucl Med. 1998;39:679–88.
23. Shimada H, Ambros IM, Dehner LP, Hata J, Joshi VV, Roald B, Stram DO, Gerbing RB, Lukens JN, Matthay KK. Castleberry RP. The International Neuroblastoma Pathology Classification (the Shimada system). Cancer. 1999;86:364–72.
24. Peuchmaur M, d'Amore ES, Joshi VV, Hata J, Roald B, Dehner LP, Gerbing RB, Stram DO, Lukens JN, Matthay KK, Shimada H. Revision of the International Neuroblastoma Pathology Classification: confirmation of favorable and unfavorable prognostic subsets in ganglioneuroblastoma, nodular. Cancer. 2003;98:2274–81.
25. Sano H, Bonadio J, Gerbing RB, London WB, Matthay KK, Lukens JN, Shimada H. The international neuroblastoma pathology classification adds independent prognostic information beyond the prognostic contribution of age. Eur J Cancer. 2006;42:1113–9.
26. Cohn SL, Pearson AD, London WB, Monclair T, Ambros PF, Brodeur GM, Faldum A, Hero B, Iehara T, Machin D, Mosseri V, Simon T, Garaventa A, Castel V, Matthay KK, INRG Task Force. The International Neuroblastoma Risk Group (INRG) classification system: an INRG Task Force Report. J Clin Oncol. 2009;27:289–97.
27. Cecchetto G, Mosseri V, De Bernardi B, Helardot P, Monclair T, Costa E, Horcher E, Neuenschwander S, Toma P, Rizzo A, Michon J, Holmes K. Surgical risk factors in primary surgery for localized neuroblastoma: the LNESG1 study of the European International Society of Pediatric Oncology Neuroblastoma Group. J Clin Oncol. 2005;23:8483–9.
28. La Quaglia MP, Kushner BH, Su W, Heller G, Kramer K, Abramson S, Rosen N, Wolden S, Cheung NK. The impact of gross total resection on local control and survival in high-risk neuroblastoma. J Pediatr Surg. 2004;39:412–7.
29. Castel V, Tover JA, Costa E, Cuadros J, Ruiz A, Rollan V, Ruiz-Jimenez JI, Perez-Hernández R, Cañete A. The role of surgery in stage iv neuroblastoma. J Pediatr Surg. 2002;37:1574–8.
30. Simon T, Häberle B, Hero B, von Schweinitz D, Berthold F. Role of surgery in the treatment of patients with stage 4 neuroblastoma age 18 months or older at diagnosis. J Clin Oncol. 2013;31:752–8.
31. Yu AL, Gilman AL, Ozkaynak MF, London WB, Kreissman SG, Chen HX, Smith M, Anderson B, Villablanca JG, Matthay KK, Shimada H, Grupp SA, Seeger R, Reynolds CP, Buxton A, Reisfeld RA, Gillies SD, Cohn SL, Maris JM, Sondel PM, Children's Oncology Groups. Anti-GD2 antibody with GM-CSF. interleukin-2, and isotretinoin for neuroblastoma. N Engl J Med. 2010;363:1324–34.

32 Odontogenic Cysts

Sang Yoon Kim, Alfredo A. Dela Rosa and Bonnie Padwa

In children, the odontogenic cyst is often found incidentally during routine dental screening or preorthodontic evaluation; however some patients may present with signs and symptoms associated with cystic lesions of the jaw. Understanding the different types of cyst with their unique features in the oral and maxillofacial region will aid in developing the optimal treatment plan and help guide patient management.

A cyst is a sac-like structure containing luminal or semifluid substance [1]. A true cyst has an epithelial luminal lining [1, 2]. The odontogenic cysts are broadly divided into *inflammatory* and *developmental,* and the classification (Table 32.1) has been adopted from the World Health Organization (WHO) classification of cysts of the jaws in 1992 with one modification in 2005 (odontogenic keratocyst (OKC) to keratocystic odontogenic tumor (KCOT)) [3].

Odontogenic Cysts

Inflammatory Cysts

Radicular Cysts

Introduction The radicular cyst is an odontogenic cyst of inflammatory origin with a chronic periapical granuloma precursor that matures from the stimulation of cell rests of Malassez present in the periodontal membrane [3, 4]. Radicular cysts have different classifications by location:

- *Periapical cyst:* presents at the root apex.
- *Lateral radicular cyst:* presents at the opening of lateral accessory root canals of affected teeth.
- *Residual cyst:* remains after extraction of the affected tooth [2, 5].

Biology and Epidemiology An inflammatory process stimulates proliferation of the rest of Malassez, and the center of the lesion degenerates and liquefies to form a cyst [1, 2, 5, 6]. The lesion forms a fairly well-defined periapical radiolucency which continues to enlarge via cell break down and hyperosmotic gradient resulting in transudation of the fluid into the lumen of the lesion [2, 5, 6].

Presentation

- The most common cystic lesion in the jaw, comprising up to 60 % of odontogenic cysts [2, 5, 6].
- Clinical features: pain on palpation or percussion on decayed or traumatized teeth.
- Often asymptomatic if the lesion is chronic in nature [2].

Differential Diagnosis

- Odontogenic cyst: inflammatory (radicular cyst) vs. developmental (dentigerous cyst).
- Odontogenic tumor: keratocyst odontogenic tumor, ameloblastoma.
- Nonodontogenic bone lesions such as giant cell tumor.

Diagnosis and Evaluation

- Physical examination:
  - Tooth is often nonvital.
  - Tenderness to palpation or percussion of affected teeth.
- Imaging evaluation:
  - Periapical or panoramic radiographs: radiolucency around the apex of the involved tooth (Fig. 32.1).
  - Usually smaller than 1–2 cm in size but occasionally can be much larger [2, 7, 8].

B. Padwa (✉)
Department of Plastic and Oral Surgery, Boston Children's Hospital, Harvard Medical School, 300 Longwood Avenue, Boston, MA 02115, USA
e-mail: bonnie.padwa@childrens.harvard.edu

S. Y. Kim
Department of Oral and Maxillofacial Surgery, INOVA Fairfax Hospital, 361 Maple Ave, Suite 200, Vienna, VA 22180, USA

A. A. Dela Rosa
Department of Oral and Maxillofacial Surgery, University of the Pacific, School of Dentistry, 2155 Webster Street, San Francisco, CA 94115, USA

R. Rahbar et al. (eds.), *Pediatric Head and Neck Tumors,*
DOI 10.1007/978-1-4614-8755-5_32, © Springer Science+Business Media New York 2014

Table 32.1 Odontogenic cysts in pediatric population

Inflammatory
Radicular cyst (Apical, lateral, and residual cyst)
Paradental cyst (Inflammatory collateral, mandibular infected buccal, or buccal bifurcation)
Developmental
Dentigerous (follicular) cyst
Eruption cyst
Gingival cysts of infants (newborn)
Calcifying odontogenic cyst
Odontogenic keratocyst (primordial cyst)→ Keratocystic odontogenic tumor (2008)
Lateral periodontal cyst
Glandular odontogenic cyst: sialo-odontogenic cyst
Nonodontogenic cysts
Nasopalatine duct (Incisive canal) cyst
Nasolabial (Nasoalveolar) cyst

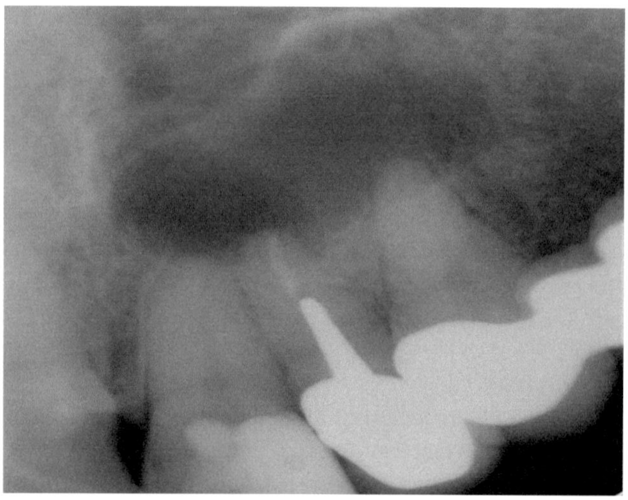

Fig. 32.1 Periapical radiograph showing periapical radiolucency involving previously root canal treated tooth

Pathology Histologic examination shows a connective tissue wall with various thicknesses and degrees of inflammatory cell infiltrates. There are nonkeratinized, stratified squamous cells [1, 2, 4–8].

Treatment The offending tooth is often nonvital and requires root canal therapy to remove the pulpal tissue and eliminate bacterial load.

- If the lesion is large, enucleation is required to eradicate the inflammatory cystic lesion and subsequent apicoectomy of the tooth with retrograde filling can be done.
- If the offending tooth is nonrestorable, removal of the tooth is another method to eliminate the source of infection.
- The *residual cyst* will require enucleation if it persists after extraction of the offending tooth.

Complications Rare.

- Squamous cell carcinoma or epidermoid carcinoma potentially can arise from the epithelial lining of a radicular cyst [2, 8].
- Secondary infections can occur which might require an additional incision and drainage procedure.
- If the cysts enlarge and perforate into the cortical bone, pathologic fracture of the mandible is also a potential risk [2, 7].

Buccal Bifurcation Cyst (BBC)

Introduction The BBC, also previously known as the mandibular infected buccal cyst described by Stoneman and Worth in 1983, is a type of paradental cyst based on the WHO classification [9]. It is a rare inflammatory cyst of odontogenic origin. It is easily misdiagnosed as radicular cyst because radicular cysts are more common lesions and have a similar presentation [2, 9–11].

Lesions with similar characteristics have been called other names, such as "circumferential dentigerous cysts" by Thoma in 1964. Thoma described a cyst that involved the mandibular second molar with cystic development of the enamel organ around the neck of the tooth interfering with its eruption. The "inflammatory collateral dental cyst" was described by Main in 1970. It is histologically identical to the inflammatory radicular cyst and is associated with vital mandibular third molars that have chronic periocoronitis. In 1976, Craig called the cyst "juvenile paradental cyst." He described the cyst around a vital third molar tooth and attachment to the buccal bifurcation [11].

Biology and Epidemiology The BBC is inflammatory rather than developmental in origin. It also has distinct clinical and radiographic features which distinguish it from other inflammatory paradental cysts [2, 10].

- The BBC develops on the buccal aspect of vital mandibular first molars and occasionally involves the second molars [9–11].
- Etiology: unknown but many speculate that the inflammatory response in the dental follicle during eruption may be the inciting factor. As the mesiobuccal cusp of the first molar penetrates through the oral epithelium, it induces an inflammatory reaction in the connective tissue, causing epithelial proliferation and cyst formation [2, 7–11]. Alternatively, it is also believed that the inflammatory response from pericoronitis may stimulate cyst formation [9–11].
- The BBC may be a variant of lateral periodontal cyst, and the cystic epithelium is derived from the cell rests of Serres, the cell rests of Malassez, the cells of the dental lamina, or the reduced enamel epithelium [9].
- Age distribution: seen in children with a range of 4–14 years.

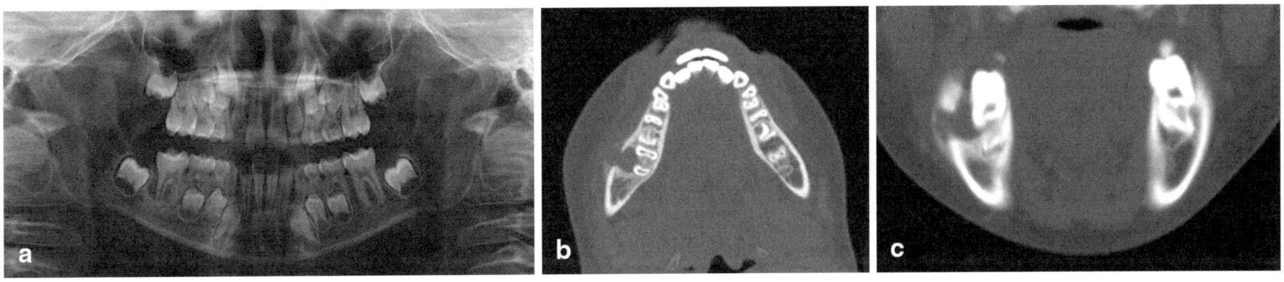

Fig. 32.2 **a** Panoramic radiograph demonstrating U-shaped radiolucency around the root of the lower, right first molar. Axial (**b**) and coronal (**c**) CT cuts show cortical perforation with a well-circumscribed lesion located on the buccal surface of the involved tooth

Presentation

- Site and age specific.
- Patients may present with swelling and/or pain associated with the lesion.
- They occur as a localized buccal swelling of the affected erupting molar [2, 8, 11].

Differential Diagnosis

- Odontogenic cysts (BBC, radicular cyst, or dentigerous cyst).
- Benign odontogenic tumors (ameloblastoma or keratocyst odontogenic tumor).
- Nonodontogenic tumors (giant cell tumor, myxoma, or vascular malformation).

Diagnosis and Evaluation

- Primarily based on the clinical and radiographic features.

Physical Examination

- Swelling and tenderness over the affected molar area (usually mandibular first molar) as Stoneman and Worth reported in 1983 under the term mandibular infected buccal cyst.
- Deep periodontal pocket on the buccal aspect of the involved vital tooth with an altered eruption pattern [6, 9–11].
- Crown often is tilted buccally [9–12].

Imaging Evaluation

- Panoramic or periapical radiograph supplemented by occlusal view radiograph are sufficient for diagnosis. The lesion appears as a U-shaped radiolucent lesion on the buccal aspect of the tooth covering the roots (Fig. 32.2). The periodontal ligament space (lamina dura) is intact and the cyst is unlikely to extend to the inferior border of the mandible. The buccal tilting of the tooth pushes the apices of the roots toward the lingual plate, and a buccal periosteal reaction is often evident. The lesion can be 1 cm in size [2, 9–13].
- Computerized tomography (CT) scan: In today's modern health care system, a CT scan is often used to better delineate the lesion (Fig. 32.2).

Pathology Histopathologic examination (Fig. 32.3) shows the cyst wall lined by nonkeratinizing, stratified, squamous epithelium and a fibrous stroma with chronic inflammation [9–11]. These findings are nonspecific, and are similar to those found in a radicular cyst. As a result, diagnosis cannot be made from the histopathologic features alone [9].

Treatment Surgical treatment is successful with low recurrence.

- Treatment options: curretage, marsupialization, enucleation, removal of the tooth.
- Nonsurgical approaches: periodontal probing or daily irrigation of the buccal periodontal pocket with saline have been reported [9].
- Some studies have suggested that these are self-resolving lesions because they are rarely seen in adults [2, 10, 13].

Developmental Cysts

Dentigerous (Follicular) Cyst

Introduction The dentigerous or follicular cyst is the second most common odontogenic cyst following the radicular cyst [1, 14–17]. The KCOT (previously known as odontogenic keratocyst) has similar clinical and radiographic appearances to the dentigerous cyst [2, 10, 13].

Biology and Epidemiology The dentigerous cyst originates from the dental follicle of an unerupted, developing tooth.

- Peak incidence: second to third decades of life.
- Male predilection (1.6:1) with prevalence in Caucasians.
- Occur more commonly in the posterior mandible often associated with the mandibular and maxillary third molars and maxillary canines [2, 14, 15].

Presentation/Diagnosis

- These cysts may be found incidentally on routine radiographs or they can cause painless expansion of the mandible/maxilla (Fig. 32.4).
- Often associated with a tooth that fails to erupt.

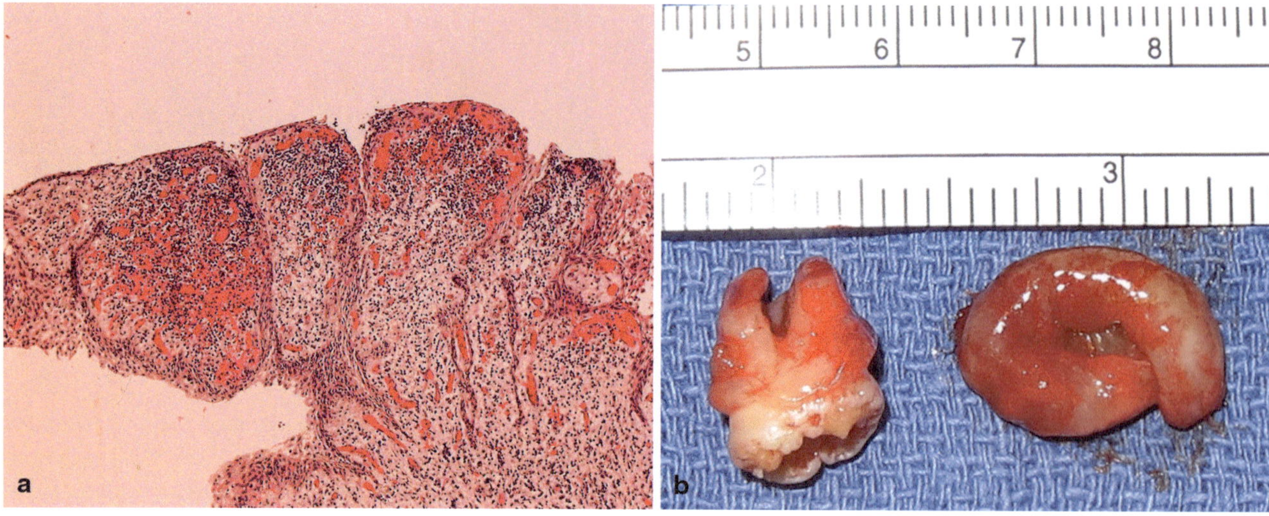

Fig. 32.3 **a** Histologic examination showing nonkeratinizing, stratified, squamous epithelium with spongiosis overlying chronically inflamed fibrous connective tissue. The specimen (**b**) shows the U-shaped lesion

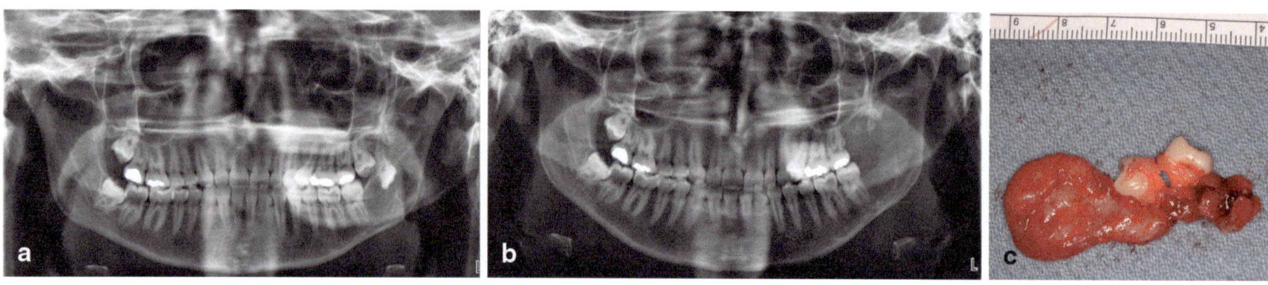

Fig. 32.4 **a** Panoramic radiographs demonstrating an impacted mandibular left third molar with associated radiolucency expanding from the cementoenamel junction (CEJ). **b** Postoperative panoramic radiograph and **c** specimen

Differential Diagnosis

- Odontogenic cysts (BBC, radicular cyst, or dentigerous cyst).
- Benign odontogenic tumors (ameloblastoma or keratocyst odontogenic tumor).
- Nonodontogenic tumors (giant cell tumor, myxoma, or vascular malformation).

Imaging

- Panoramic radiograph: well-circumscribed, unilocular radiolucency associated with the crown of an unerupted tooth. It is attached to the tooth at the CEJ (Fig. 32.4).
- The cysts can cause tooth displacement and root resorption of adjacent teeth.

Histopathology Lining of reduced enamel epithelium (2–3 rows of cuboidal or flattened epithelium) and there may be mucous cells [2, 7, 8, 14–17].

Treatment Enucleation of the cyst or removal of the affected tooth.

Prognosis Recurrence is rare.

Complications Rare.

- Can become large and can place the patient at risk for a pathologic jaw fracture [14–16].
- Neoplastic transformation to an ameloblastoma can occur if not treated.
- Dentigerous cyst epithelium can differentiate into ciliated and mucus-secreting epithelium. Untreated cysts can rarely develop into an intraosseous mucoepidermoid carcinoma or squamous cell carcinoma [17, 18].

Eruption cyst

Introduction The eruption cyst is a developmental cyst from the erupting primary or adult teeth [2, 7, 8, 19]. It is a benign cyst, and is the soft tissue counterpart of the dentigerous cyst [19–21].

Biology and Epidemiology The eruption cyst forms when epithelium separates from the enamel of the crown of a tooth.

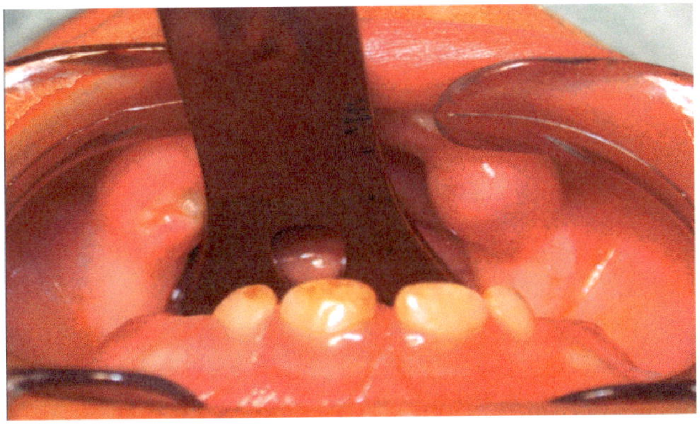

Fig. 32.5 Eruption cyst associated with unerupted mandibular, right primary molar

This occurs as the result of fluid accumulating in the dilated follicular space.

- Occurs in newborns with eruption of natal teeth up to 21 years of age with the eruption of the third molars.
- Approximately 11 % of children develop cysts during eruption of the incisors, and 30 % of children when the canines and molars erupt.
- Female predilection (2:1) [2, 8, 19–21].

Presentation/Diagnosis The cysts are typically painless although if secondarily infected they can be tender to palpation. They

- Size: usually less than 1 cm in diameter.
- Can be bluish in color.
- Dome-shaped appearance on the alveolar ridge [20] (Fig. 32.5).

Differential Diagnosis

- Eruption cyst
- Hematoma
- Amalgam tattoo
- Granuloma

Histopathology A thin layer of nonkeratinizing squamous epithelium with variable inflammatory cell infiltrate over the underlying lamina propria.

Treatment Treatment is not usually indicated as the cysts resolve on their own with eruption of the tooth.

- If the lesion is symptomatic or causes disturbance in eruption, surgical intervention including decompression of the cyst or excision of the overlying gingiva can be performed. These methods generally permit the eruption of the tooth [19, 21].

Gingival Cyst of the Newborn (Infants)

Introduction Gingival cysts of the newborn are multiple, small, superficial keratin-filled lesions found on the alveolar ridges of infants [2, 22].

- Arise from the remnants of the dental lamina.
- Usually smaller than 2–3 mm.
- Maxillary alveolus is more commonly involved than the mandible.

Differential Diagnosis

- Gingival cyst of the newborn
- Eruption cyst
- Congenital epulis of the newborn
- Fibroma

Treatment Treatment is not indicated for gingival cysts of the newborn, because the lesions spontaneously involute [2, 7, 8, 22].

Calcifying Odontogenic Cyst/Gorlin Cyst/ Dentinogenic Ghost Cell Tumor/Calcifyling Ghost Cell Odontogenic Cyst

Introduction In 1962, Gorlin et al. described the calcifying odontogenic cyst (COC) which is an uncommon, mostly intraosseous lesion with histopathologic diversity and variable clinical behavior [23, 24]. The COC represents less than 1 % of the jaw cysts. Some prefer to classify COC as a benign neoplasm since it can occasionally be aggressive and recur [23].

- Three variants: simple unicystic type, unicystic odontoma-associated type, and unicystic ameloblastomatous proliferating type [23].
- The neoplastic variant of COC: dentinogenic ghost cell tumor or epithelial odontogenic ghost cell tumor without cystic features [2, 23–27].

Biology and Epidemiology

- Most cases are diagnosed in the second and third decades of life with a mean age of 33 years [23, 26].
- COCs associated with an odontoma (20 %) tend to occur at a younger age with a mean age of 17 years.
- No gender predilection.
- Intra-osseous vs. extra-osseous: intra-osseous cysts are more common in the second decade of life. Extra-osseous forms accounting for 13–30 % of all COCs occur more commonly in the sixth decade of life.
- Both intra and extra-osseous lesions occur with equal frequency in both upper and lower jaws.
- Rare neoplastic variants (2–16 %) of COC appear in older patients [2, 7, 8, 23, 26].

Presentation The COC is incidentally found and patients are usually asymptomatic. The majority of cases are in the incisor or canine area.

Differential Diagnosis

- Adenomatoid odontogenic tumor
- Calcifying epithelial odontogenic tumor
- Ossifying fibroma
- Ameloblastoma
- Ameloblastic fibroma
- Ameloblastic fibro-odontoma
- Odontoma

Diagnosis and Evaluation

- Physical examination:
  - Palpable, firm, soft tissue mass measuring 2–4 cm in size with a range of 1–12 cm.
  - 32 % of COCs are associated with unerupted teeth.
- Imaging evaluation:
  - Panoramic radiograph: Usually unilocular, well defined radiolucency which can occasionally appear as a multilocular lesion. Radiopaque structures within the lesion can be due to irregular calcifications or tooth-like structures.
  - Calcifications may be seen radiographically with three radiographic patterns including "salt and pepper flecks," "fluffy cloud like pattern," and "crescent shape" [23, 24, 26, 27].
  - Sometimes, the lesion is associated with an unerupted tooth and root resorption or divergence of adjacent roots can also occur [23, 26].

Pathology The cystic (nonneoplastic) form comprises 86–98 % of COCs. Histopathologically, this lesion has a fibrous capsule, lined by odontogenic epithelium, 4–10 cells in thickness [23, 25]. Basal cells in the epithelial lining are cuboidal or columnar. The presence of variable ghost cells within the epithelial component is a unique histologic feature of this cyst, although these are also found in some odontogenic tumors (e.g., ameloblastoma, ameloblastic fibroma, ameloblastic fibro-odontoma, and odontoma) [26].

Treatment Enucleation with curettage is recommended for the cystic types of COC and is associated with a low recurrence rate.

- Some clinicians advocate a minimally invasive approach such as marsupilization or decompression to reduce the size of the lesion prior to excision [2, 23, 26].
- The solid neoplastic variant, the dentinogenic ghost cell tumor, can recur after the excision.

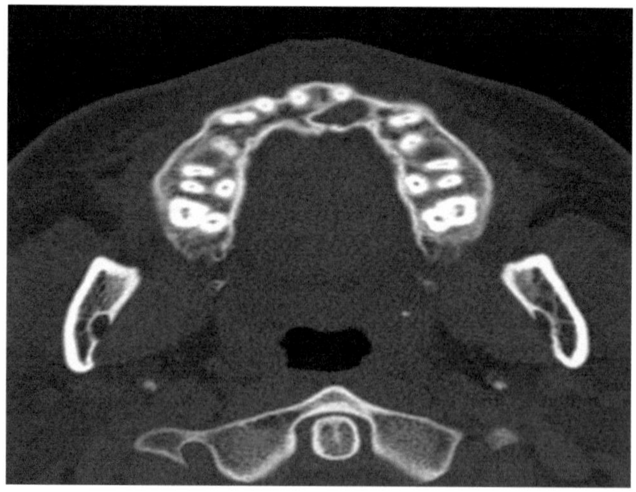

Fig. 32.6 Axial view of CT scan demonstrating well-corticated, round/ovoid lesion in the anterior maxilla

Nonodontogenic Cysts

Nasopalatine Duct Cyst (NPDC)

Introduction The NPDC is a nonodontogenic developmental cyst, also known as incisive canal cyst or nasopalatine canal cyst [2, 7, 8].

Biology and Epidemiology

- Prevalence: between 1 % and 11.6 % of all jaw cysts [28, 29].
- NPDC can occur at any age, but more frequently between the third and sixth decades of life.
- Male predilection.
- Etiology is due to proliferation of epithelial remnants of the embryologic nasopalatine duct [28, 30].

Presentation NPDC is usually found incidentally on routine radiographic examination.

- Pain and/or swelling on the anterior palate.
- If the cyst becomes secondarily infected, there may be a draining fistula.
- Average size: less than 20 mm. These lesions can get as large as 60 mm. The size and dimension of the cyst does not correlate with the presence of symptoms [30].

Imaging Evaluation

- Occlusal plain film radiograph: a midline heart-shaped unilocular radiolucency is seen.
- CT scan can be obtained to better delineate the lesion (Fig. 32.6). The cyst can cause displacement and/or resorption of the adjacent incisor roots. A small NPDC is hard to distinguish from normal incisive canal (normal canal $\leq$6 mm).

Pathology On histology, NPDC lesions show stratified squamous epithelium, pseudostratified columnar epithelium, or a combination of both. Respiratory (ciliated) epithelium is also seen in 28 % of lesions [8, 10].

Treatment The treatment is enucleation.

- Recurrence rate has been reported to be between 0–11 % depending on adequacy of enucleation.
- Malignant transformation is extremely rare [2, 8, 28–30].

Nasolabial Cyst (Nasoalveolar Cyst)

Introduction The nasolabial cyst is an uncommon lesion previously known as nasoalveolar cyst [2, 31]. It presents in the soft tissue adjacent to the alveolar process above the apices of the maxillary incisors.

Epidemiology/Presentation

- Etiology is unclear.
- Patients present with swelling of the upper lip with obliteration of the nasolabial fold and elevation of the alar base.
- Pain is uncommon, unless infected [2, 7, 8, 31].
- Age range: from early teens to the seventh decade of life.
- Strong predilection for women (3:1).

Imaging Evaluation

- Plain film: not diagnostic because these are extra-osseous lesions and there can be a bony deformity of the lateral or anterior edges of nasal floor and/or anterior nasal spine [2, 31, 32].
- CT scan or magnetic resonance imaging (MRI) is more useful in making the diagnosis and can clearly define the lesion.

Pathology The nasolabial cyst is a soft tissue lesion with a thick connective tissue capsule containing mucoid and serous fluid unless infected. The lining is pseudostratified squamous epithelium, stratified squamous epithelium, or cuboidal epithelium with goblet cells.

Treatment Excision is the treatment of choice.

References

1. Shear M. Developmental odontogenic cysts. An update. J Oral Pathol Med. 1994 Jan;23(1):1–11.
2. Neville BW, Damm DD, Allen CM, et al. Odontogenic cysts and tumors. 2nd ed. Philadelphia: Saunders; 2002. pp. 589–642.
3. Li TJ. The odontogenic keratocyst: a cyst, or a cystic neoplasm? J Dent Res. 2011 Feb;90(2):133–42.
4. Antoh M, Hasegawa H, Kawakami T, Kage T, Chino T, Eda S. Hyperkeratosis and atypical proliferation appearing in the lining epithelium of a radicular cyst. Report of a case. J Craniomaxillofac Surg. 1993 Jul;21(5):210–3.
5. Gardner DG. Residual cysts. Oral Surg Oral Med Oral Pathol Oral Radiol Endod. 1997 Aug;84(2):114–5.
6. Gardner DG, Sapp JP, Wysocki GP. Odontogenic and "fissural" cysts of the jaws. Pathol Annu. 1978;13(Pt 1):177–200.
7. Sapp JP, et al. Contemporary oral and maxillofacial pathology. St Louis: Mosby; 2004.
8. Marx RE, Stern DS, editors. Odontogenic and nonodontogenic cysts. In: Oral and Maxillofacial Pathology: a rationale for diagnosis and treatment. Chicago: Quintessence; 2003.
9. Corona-Rodriguez J, Torres-Labardini R, Velasco-Tizcareño M, Mora-Rincones O. Bilateral buccal bifurcation cyst: case report and literature review. J Oral Maxillofac Surg. 2011 Jun;69(6):1694–6.
10. Zadik Y, Yitschaky O, Neuman T, Nitzan DW. On the self-resolution nature of the buccal bifurcation cyst. J Oral Maxillofac Surg. 2011 Jul;69(7):e282–4.
11. Pompura JR, Sándor GK, Stoneman DW. The buccal bifurcation cyst: a prospective study of treatment outcomes in 44 sites. Oral Surg Oral Med Oral Pathol Oral Radiol Endod. 1997 Feb;83(2):215–21.
12. Stoneman DW, Worth HM. The mandibular infected buccal cyst–molar area. Dent Radiogr Photogr. 1983;56(1):1–14.
13. David LA, Sándor GK, Stoneman DW. The buccal bifurcation cyst: in non-surgical treatment an option? J Can Dent Assoc. 1998 Nov;64(10):712–6.
14. Zhang LL, et al. Dentigerous cyst: a retrospective clinicopathological analysis of 2082 dentigerous cysts in British Columbia, Canada. Int J Oral Maxillofac Surg. 2010 Sep;39(9):878–82.
15. Norris LH, Piccoli P, Papageorge MB. Multiple dentigerous cysts of the maxilla and mandible: report of a case. J Oral Maxillofac Surg. 1987 Aug;45(8):694–7.
16. Güven O, Keskin A, Akal UK. The incidence of cysts and tumors around impacted third molars. Int J Oral Maxillofac Surg. 2000 Apr;29(2):131–5.
17. Johnson LM, Sapp JP, McIntire DN. Squamous cell carcinoma arising in a dentigerous cyst. J Oral Maxillofac Surg. 1994 Sep;52(9):987–90.
18. Yasuoka T, Yonemoto K, Kato Y, Tatematsu N. Squamous cell carcinoma arising in a dentigerous cyst. J Oral Maxillofac Surg. 2000 Aug;58(8):900–5.
19. Seward MH, et al. Eruption cyst: an analysis of its clinical features. J Oral Surg. 1973 Jan;31:31–5.
20. Nagaveni NB, Umashankara KV, Radhika NB, Maj Satisha TS. Eruption cyst: a literature review and four case reports. Indian J Dent Res. 2011;22:148–51.
21. Anderson RA. Eruption cysts: a retrograde study. ASDC J Dent Child. 1990 Mar–Apr;57(2):124–7.
22. Cataldo E, Berkman MD. Cysts of the oral mucosa in newborns. Am J Dis Child. 1968 Jul;116(1):44–8.
23. Souza LN, Souza AC, Gomes CC, Loyola AM, Durighetto AF Jr, Gomez RS, Castro WH. Conservative treatment of calcifying odontogenic cyst: report of 3 cases. J Oral Maxillofac Surg. 2007 Nov;65(11):2353–6.
24. Gorlin RJ, Pindborg JJ, Odont, Clausen FP, Vickers RA. The calcifying odontogenic cyst—a possible analogue of the cutaneous calcifying epithelioma of Malherbe. An analysis of fifteen cases. Oral Surg Oral Med Oral Pathol. 1962 Oct;15:1235–43.
25. Idia S, et al. Calcifying odontogenic cyst: radiologic findings in 11 cases. Oral Surg Oral Med Oral Pathol Oral Radiol Endod. 2006;101(3):356–62.
26. Phillips MD, Closmann JJ, Baus MR, Torske KR, Williams SB. Hybrid odontogenic tumor with features of ameloblastic fibro-odontoma, calcifying odontogenic cyst, and adenomatoid odontogenic

tumor: a case report and review of the literature. J Oral Maxillofac Surg. 2010 Feb;68(2):470–4.

27. Buchner A. The central (intraosseous) calcifying odontogenic cyst: an analysis of 215 cases. J Oral Maxillofac Surg. 1991;49(4):330–9.
28. Swanson KS, Kaugars GE, Gunsolley JC. Nasopalatine duct cyst: an analysis of 334 cases. J Oral Maxillofac Surg. 1991 Mar;49(3):268–71.
29. Allard RH, van der Kwast WA, van der Waal I. Nasopalatine duct cyst. Review of the literature and report of 22 cases. Int J Oral Surg. 1981 Dec;10(6):447–61.
30. Suter VG, Sendi P, Reichart PA, Bornstein MM. The nasopalatine duct cyst: an analysis of the relation between clinical symptoms, cyst dimensions, and involvement of neighboring anatomical structures using cone beam computed tomography. J Oral Maxillofac Surg. 2011;69(10):2595–603.
31. Sumer AP, Celenk P, Sumer M, Telcioglu NT, Gunhan O. Nasolabial cyst: case report with CT and MRI findings. Oral Surg Oral Med Oral Pathol Oral Radiol Endod. 2010 Feb;109(2):e92–4.
32. Allard RH. Nasolabial cyst. Review of the literature and report of 7 cases. Int J Oral Surg. 1982 Dec;11(6):351–9.

Odontogenic Tumors

33

Alfredo A. Dela Rosa, Sang Yoon Kim and Bonnie Padwa

Introduction

While odontogenic cysts are common in children, odontogenic tumors are not seen as frequently. These tumors are broadly divided into three groups based on their histopathologic derivation: tumors derived from odontogenic epithelium, odontogenic mesenchyme, and mixed tumors composed of odontogenic epithelium and mesenchyme. The classification of odontogenic tumors (Table 33.1) has been set forth by the World Health Organization (WHO) [1].

Tumors of Odontogenic Epithelium

Ameloblastoma

Introduction Ameloblastoma is a tumor of odontogenic epithelial origin [1]. It is the second most common odontogenic tumor after the odontoma. There are three major types, solid or multicystic (86 % of all cases), unicystic (13 % of all cases), and peripheral (1 % of all cases), that have different treatments and prognosis [2].

Biology and Epidemiology Ameloblastoma arises from the rests of dental lamina. It is a benign tumor that is slow-growing but can be locally invasive.

- Unicystic type: most often seen in young patients, with 50 % diagnosed during the second decade of life. The mean age at presentation is 23 years [2] and there is no sex predilection. There are three histopathologic variants of the unicystic ameloblastoma (intraluminal, luminal, and mural) that have different treatments and prognosis [3]. The mural variant appears to be more aggressive than the intraluminal or luminal variants because of its presence outside the cyst wall and closer to the surrounding bone.
- Solid or multicystic type: occurs in patients over a wide age range. Though it is prevalent mainly during the third to seventh decades of life, it can be seen in the second decade. It is rare in children [2]. There is no sex predilection. It is benign but locally aggressive.
- Peripheral ameloblastomas: usually seen in middle age persons with average age of 52 years [2].
- There is an increase in frequency of ameloblastoma in children of African descent. Tumors in these children have a different site of predilection, being more common in the mandibular symphysis region. The morphologic type closely resembles the adult type and not the unicystic pattern [4]. It is not known whether there is a true racial difference, and the tumor incidence is not known.
- Ameloblastoma can exhibit malignant behavior with development of metastases and is therefore called metastasizing or malignant ameloblastoma. It occurs in less than 1 % of all ameloblastomas [2].

Presentation It can occur in either of the jaws, with asymptomatic swelling and/or expansion. Pain and paresthesia are uncommon.

- Unicystic ameloblastomas: most are associated with an impacted tooth and the mandibular third molar is the most common site.
- Solid and multicystic types: occur mostly in the mandible, usually in the posterior region [5].

B. Padwa (✉)
Department of Plastic and Oral Surgery, Boston Children's Hospital, Harvard Medical School, 300 Longwood Avenue, Boston, MA 02115, USA
e-mail: Bonnie.padwa@childrens.harvard.edu

A. A. Dela Rosa
Department of Oral and Maxillofacial Surgery, University of the Pacific, School of Dentistry, 2155 Webster Street, San Francisco, CA 94115, USA

S. Y. Kim
Department of Oral and Maxillofacial Surgery, INOVA Fairfax Hospital, 361 Maple Ave, Suite 200, Vienna, VA 22180, USA

R. Rahbar et al. (eds.), *Pediatric Head and Neck Tumors*,
DOI 10.1007/978-1-4614-8755-5_33, © Springer Science+Business Media New York 2014

Table 33.1 Odontogenic tumors in the pediatric population

Tumors of odontogenic epithelium
Ameloblastoma
Squamous odontogenic tumor
Adenomatoid odontogenic tumor
Keratocyst odontogenic tumor
Calcifying epithelial odontogenic tumor (Pindborg)
Clear cell odontogenic carcinoma
Intraosseous odontogenic carcinoma
Tumors of odontogenic mesenchyme
Odontogenic myxoma
Cementoblastoma
Odontogenic fibroma
Mixed odontogenic tumors
Ameloblastic fibroma
Ameloblastic fibro-odontoma/fibrodentinoma
Odontoma

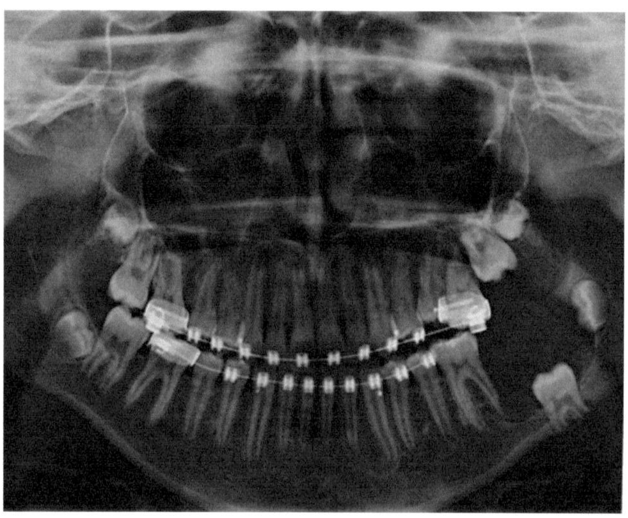

Fig. 33.1 Panoramic radiograph demontrates large, unilocular, radiolucent lesion in the left mandible associated with the crown of the impacted second mandibular molar, which is inferiorly displaced. The lesion extends from the first molar to mid ramus, with displacement of the third molar bud

Differential Diagnosis A variety of odontogenic and nonodontogenic lesions may have similar clinical and radiographic presentations.

- Dentigerous cyst
- Keratocystic odontogenic tumor
- Ameloblastoma
- Odontogenic myxoma
- Giant cell lesion
- Lymphoma
- Langerhans cell histiocytosis

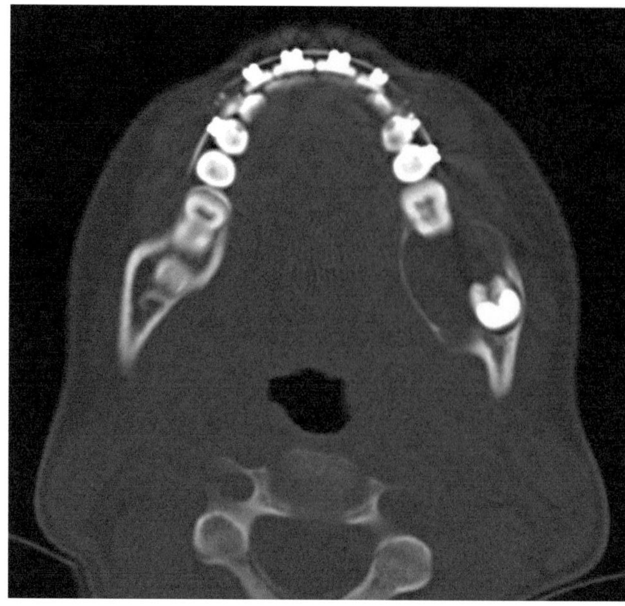

Fig. 33.2 Axial computed tomography (CT) scan demontrating unilocular lesion, with buccal and lingual cortical thinning and expansion, but no evidence of cortical perforation or soft tissue involvement

Diagnosis and Evaluation

Physical Examination

- Buccal and/or lingual cortical expansion is common
- Usually nontender
- Can cause root resorption and/or displacement
- Unicystic ameloblastoma: commonly associated with an unerupted mandibular third molar tooth

Imaging Evaluation Panoramic radiograph:

- Unicystic ameloblastoma: well circumscribed radiolucency, usually surrounding an unerupted mandibular third molar, often mimicking a dentigerous cyst (Figs. 33.1 and 33.2) [3].
- Multicystic ameloblastoma: multilocular radiolucent lesion, often described as "soap bubble" or "honeycombed." The radiolucent areas often have irregularly scalloped margins.
- Solid variant: unilocular radiolucent lesion is not typically associated with the crown of a tooth.

Pathology Three histologic variants of unicystic ameloblastoma are described in the literature (Figs. 33.3, 33.4a, b) [2, 3]. In the luminal unicystic ameloblastoma, the tumor is confined to the luminal surface of the cyst while the intraluminal unicystic ameloblastoma has tumor nodules that project from the cystic lining into the lumen of the cyst. In the mural unicystic ameloblastoma, the fibrous wall of the cyst is infiltrated with tumor nodules. The solid and multicystic variants also have several microscopic subsets. The follicular

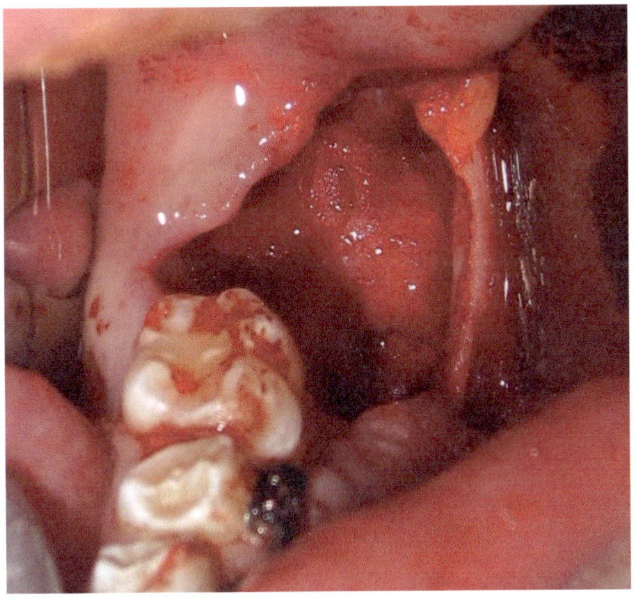

Fig. 33.3 Intraoperative photograph of the defect after enucleation and extraction of second and third molars

and plexiform patterns are the most common. Less common patterns include granular cell, desmoplastic, acanthomatous, and basal cell types. The follicular pattern shows islands of odontogenic epithelium within a fibrous stroma. The basal cells of these islands are tall, columnar, and hyperchromatic. The nuclei are displaced away from the basement membrane (reverse polarity). Mitotic activity is rare in all variants of ameloblastomas.

Treatment and Prognosis

- Luminal and intraluminal variants of unicystic ameloblastoma: enucleation and currettage with close follow-up [3, 6]. There is a less than 25% recurrence after enucleation and curettage [7]. Intraoperatively, frozen section should be obtained to properly subclassify the variant of unicystic ameloblastoma [3]. If there is evidence of extension into the fibrous capsule, the tumor becomes the mural variant and, then, a marginal resection with 1 cm margins should be performed.
- Solid and multicystic types: resection with 1–1.5 cm bony margins and one uninvolved anatomic barrier margin [8]. Enucleation and curettage is inadequate treatment for these types with a 50–60% recurrence rate [9] but only a 2–4.5% recurrence after wide resection [8, 9].
- It must be followed for at least 10 years because recurrence can occur late [10].

Squamous Odontogenic Tumor

Introduction Squamous odontogenic tumor is a rare benign epithelial odontogenic tumor. It was first described in 1975, and less than 50 cases have been reported in the literature [11, 12].

Biology and Epidemiology It arises from the neoplastic transformation of the rests of dental lamina or the epithelial rests of Malassez [11, 12].

- Occurs intraosseously within the periodontal ligament that is associated with the lateral root surface of an erupted tooth [11, 12].
- Found over a wide age range, from the second to the seventh decade with the incidence peaking in the third decade of life [12].
- No sex predilection [12].

Presentation

- The most common complaint is a local painful gingival swelling with mobility of the associated teeth although 25% of patients are asymptomatic [2].
- Mandible and maxilla are equally affected [13].

Differential Diagnosis

- Dentigerous cyst
- Radicular cyst
- Ameloblastoma
- Squamous cell carcinoma

Diagnosis and Evaluation

Physical Examination

- Most lesions are small; no greater than 1.5 cm in diameter [2] (Fig. 33.5).
- Swelling and tenderness along the gingiva with associated tooth mobility.

Imaging Evaluation

- Panoramic radiograph: the findings are variable and not diagnostic (Fig. 33.6). It can range from small to large in size and is irregularly shaped or has semicircular radiolucencies with smooth sclerotic borders. They are seen within the alveolar bone along the lateral surfaces of tooth roots [14].

Pathology These tumors are composed of numerous islands of well-differentiated squamous epithelium with focal areas of keratinization, calcification, and cystic degeneration scattered in mature fibrous connective tissue stroma [15]. It is similar to squamous metaplasia described in ameloblastomas, but it differs by the lack of peripheral columnar cells with palisading nuclei. No polarization of nuclei is seen in this lesion and the cells lack atypical mitosis which could differentiate it from a well-differentiated squamous cell carcinoma.

Treatment Enucleation and curettage [8].

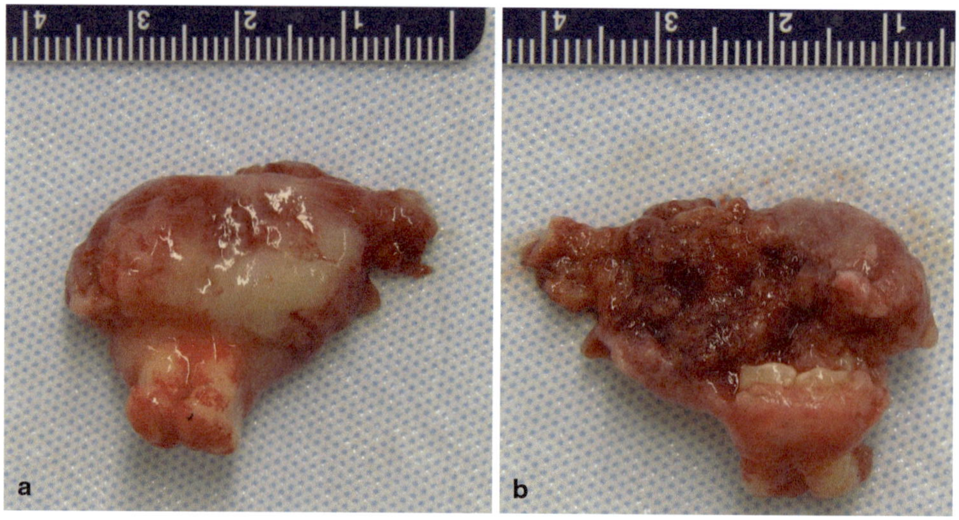

Fig. 33.4 Gross specimen of the outer surface of cyst (**a**); roots of second molar can be seen. The inside of the cyst is filled with projections (**b**)

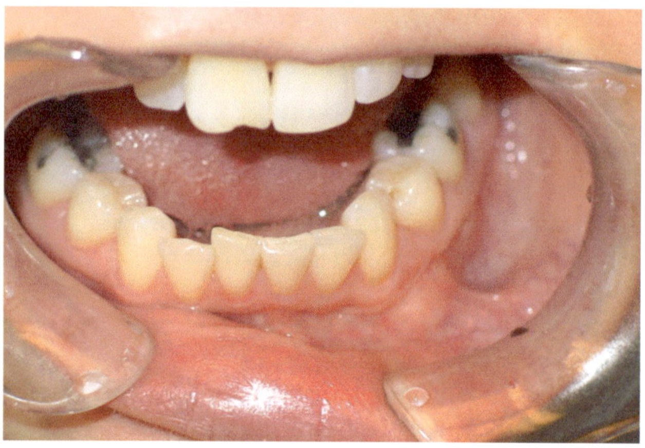

Fig. 33.5 Left buccal gingival swelling in a 35-year-old woman

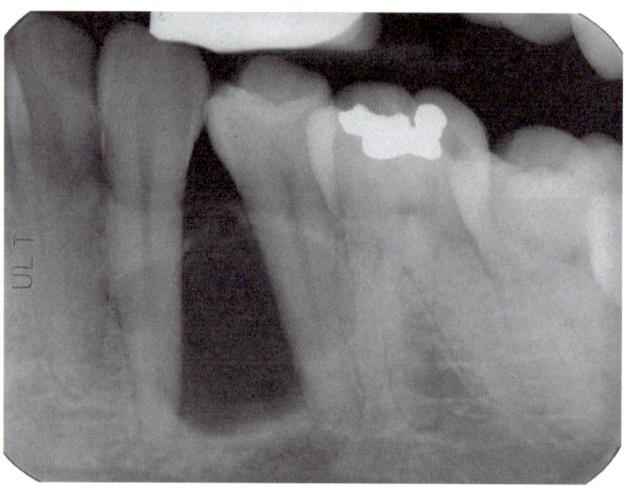

Fig. 33.6 Periapical dental radiograph demonstrates irregularly shaped, well-demarcated, radiolucent lesion in the alveolar bone between roots of adjacent teeth

Outcome Recurrences are rare and are likely due to incomplete removal. Further excision is usually curative. Twenty percent of patients can have new lesions at different locations [15].

Adenomatoid Odontogenic Tumor

Introduction Adenomatoid odontogenic tumor (AOT) is a benign hamartoma which was initially considered a variant of ameloblastoma [2, 16, 17]. However, its clinical features and biologic behavior are significantly different. The terminology, AOT, was introduced by Philipsen and Birn [16] and classified by the WHO in 1971 [16, 17].

Biology and Epidemiology AOT is a benign neoplasm and comprises only 3–7 % of all odontogenic tumors [2, 17]. The lesion arises from the remnants of dental lamina.

- Three variants: follicular, extrafollicular, and peripheral [16, 17]. The follicular type is the predominant form (75 %) with a central intraosseous lesion associated with an impacted tooth [2, 13, 16–18]. The extrafolicular type is also an intraosseous lesion, but is not associated with teeth. The peripheral type is very rare and is extraosseous.
- It affects young patients and is usually diagnosed in the second decade of life.
- It has a female predilection, with a 2:1 ratio.

Presentation These tumors are usually asymptomatic, found incidentally on radiographic examination for an unerupted tooth. AOT occurs more often in the anterior maxilla [2, 13, 16–18].

Differential Diagnosis

- Keratocystic odontogenic tumor
- Ameloblastoma

- Dentigerous cyst
- Calcifying odontogenic cyst
- Calcifying epithelial odontogenic tumor

Diagnosis and Evaluation

Physical Examination

- Size: usually less than 3 cm in diameter.
- Larger lesions can cause a tender bony expansion [2].

Imaging Evaluation

- Panoramic radiograph: appears as a well circumscribed, pear-shaped radiolucency. Seventy-five percent of the cases are associated with an unerupted tooth. Unlike dentigerous cysts that attach to the cementoenamel junction of an impacted tooth, the attachment of AOT to the impacted tooth occurs more apically onto the root surface [2, 13]. There may also be fine calcifications found within the radiolucent lesion.

Pathology They have a thick capsule with nodules and whorls of epithelium that may form rosette-like structures around a central space. There may also be small foci of calcification. The tubular or duct-like structures with a central space surrounded by a layer of columnar or cuboidal epithelial cells are the characteristic features [2, 13].

Treatment Treatment is enucleation, making sure the capsule is intact upon removal.

- Recurrence is rare.
- Because there is no documentation of aggressive behavior, it is important to distinguish AOT from ameloblastoma to avoid a more aggressive operation.

Keratocystic Odontogenic Tumor

Introduction Keratocystic odontogenic tumor (KCOT) is a benign intraossesous cystic tumor of odontogenic origin which can be locally destructive and has a high recurrence rate. This lesion had previously been called odontogenic keratocyst but it was renamed by the WHO in 2005 because the current name better reflects its behavior as a neoplasm [1, 19].

Biology and Epidemiology KCOT arises from the cell rests of the dental lamina [20]. Recent studies have also demonstrated that the PTCH gene plays a role in sporadic KCOT.

- Found in people over a wide age range, from the first to the ninth decades, with a peak in frequency in the second and third decades [21].
- Slight male predilection.
- If multiple KCOTs are present, the patient should be evaluated for other findings that make up the nevoid basal cell carcinoma (Gorlin) syndrome.

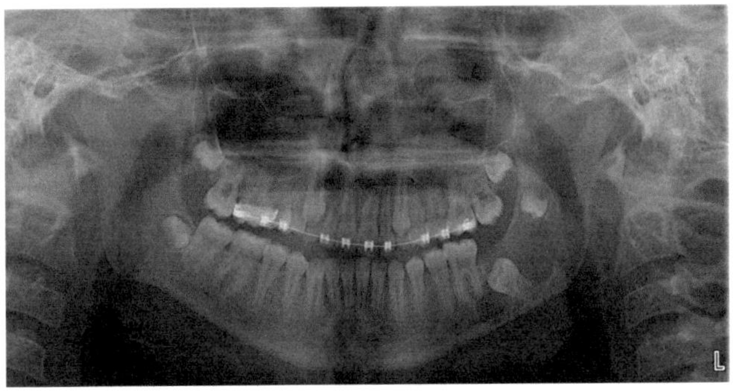

Fig. 33.7 Panoramic radiograph showing large left mandibular body and ramus radiolucent lesion associated with unerupted second molar and superiorly displaced third molar

Presentation Small KCOTs are asymptomatic and incidentally discovered during routine radiographic examinations. Larger KCOTs may cause swelling, pain, or become secondarily infected.

Differential Diagnosis

- Dentigerous cyst
- Ameloblastoma
- Ameloblastic fibroma
- Langerhans cell histiocytosis
- Giant cell tumor
- Aneurysmal bone cyst

Diagnosis and Evaluation

Physical Examination

- Majority of the lesions occur in the posterior mandible in the third molar region [21].
- Teeth may be displaced but root resorption is rare.
- Bony expansion and fluctuance, if present, is resorption or perforation of the cortex.

Imaging Evaluation

- Panoramic radiograph: well-defined radiolucency with smooth, well-corticated margins (Figs. 33.7 and 33.8). Twenty-five to forty percent of cases are associated with an unerupted tooth [2]. It may displace the inferior alveolar nerve inferiorly.

Pathology On gross examination, the cystic lumen may contain cheesy material or clear liquid. The lining is thin and fragile. Microscopically, the epithelial lining is composed of uniform layer of stratified squamous epithelium, 5–8 cell layers thick, without rete ridges. The luminal surface shows parakeratinized epithelium. There is a well-defined, palisaded basal layer of columnar or cuboidal cells [21].

Treatment Treatment of KCOT remains controversial, with recommendations including marsupialization, decompression,

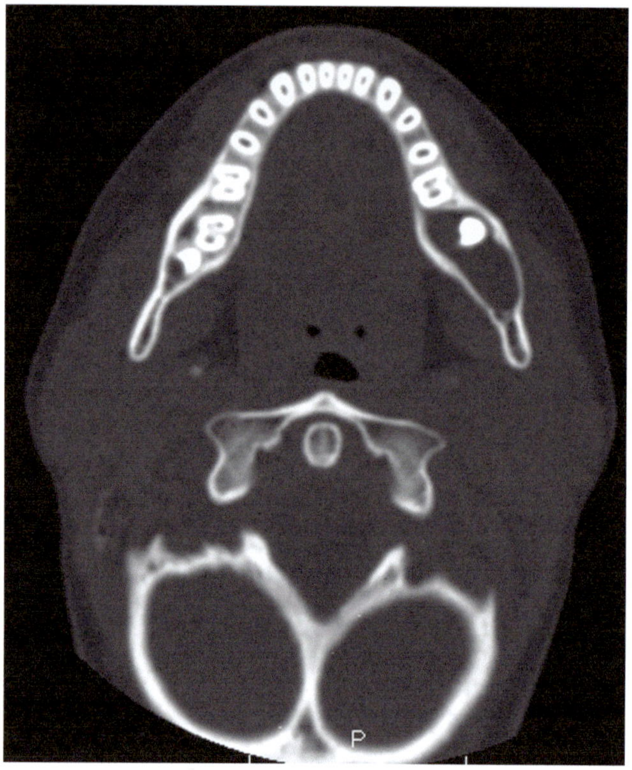

Fig. 33.8 Axial computed tomography (CT) scan of left mandible showing radiolucent lesion with intact cortex and minor buccal and lingual cortical expansion

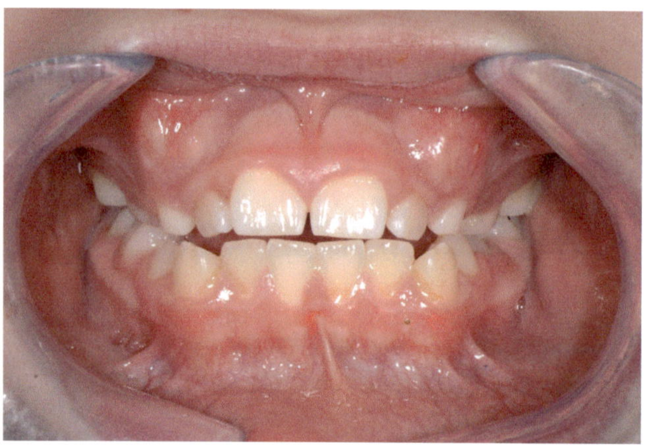

Fig. 33.9 Intraoral photograph showing expansion of maxillary alveolus and mandibular body

enucleation with or without curettage, peripheral ostectomy and/or cryotherapy, and resection.

- No consensus as to which is the most appropriate treatment. Although resection offers the highest cure rate and reduces recurrences, it is associated with the greatest morbidity. Enucleation with or without curettage, peripheral ostectomy, or cryotherapy preserves the jaw structure but has a higher recurrence rate.

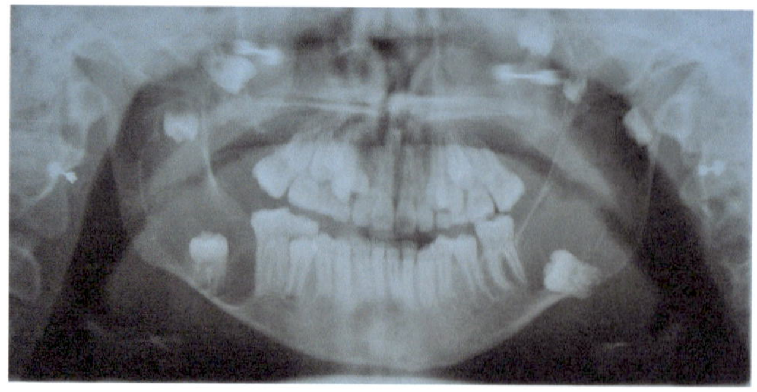

Fig. 33.10 Panoramic radiograph demonstrates bilateral mandibular radiolucent lesions extending from first molars filling entire rami bilaterally. The second molars are displaced to inferior border, and the developing, third molar tooth buds are displaced superiorly. There are also radiolucent lesions in the right and left maxilla with displacement of multiple teeth

- Recent studies have demonstrated that decompression of the lesion and placement of a stent with daily irrigation for 9 months, followed by cystectomy [13], results in dedifferentiation of the residual epithelium [22] and a lower recurrence rate.

Outcome The high recurrence rate for KCOT may result from incomplete removal or residual epithelial islands (daughter cysts).

- Acutely infected or multilocular KCOTs tend to have a higher recurrent rate because it may be more difficult to remove all the cystic components.
- Enucleation is associated with the highest recurrence rates, ranging from 17 to 56%, particularly when the KCOT is removed in fragments [23].
- Marker et al. found a lower recurrence rate (8.7%) in a series of patients who underwent decompression followed by cystectomy [24].

Relationships with Other Disease States and Syndromes

- Nevoid basal cell carcinoma syndrome (NBCCS): nevoid basal cell carcinoma syndrome, also known as Gorlin or Gorlin–Goltz syndrome [25], was first described by Gorlin and Goltz in 1960 as a triad of multiple basal cell carcinomas, odontogenic keratocysts, and bifid ribs.
- KCOT occurs in 74% of patients with NBCCS, with the first tumor occurring in 80% patients by the age of 20 years [26].
- Expanded spectrum also includes epidermal cysts, calficied falx cerebri, palmar/plantar pits, bifid ribs (splayed, fused, partially missing), and hypertelorbitism (Figs. 33.9 and 33.10). Less frequent clinical findings include spina bifida occulta of cervical or thoracic vertebrae, medulloblastomas, calficied ovarian fibromas, and mental retardation [26].

- An autosomal dominant condition with high penetrance and variable expressivity. Recently, this disorder has been associated with a mutation in the PTCH gene located on chromosome 9q22.3-q31 [26].

Tumors of Odontogenic Mesenchyme

Odontogenic Myxoma

Introduction The odontogenic myxoma is an uncommon benign tumor representing only 3–6% of all odontogenic tumors [27, 28].

Biology and Epidemiology It is an intraosseous neoplasm thought to arise from odontogenic ectomesenchyme. It behaves in a locally aggressive, infiltrating fashion. When a relatively greater amount of collagen is seen, the term myxofibroma is used.

- Commonly associated with an unerupted tooth or an area with a developmentally absent tooth [29].
- Found in young adults with an average age of 30 years. Kafee et al. reviewed 164 cases and found 75% occurred between second and fourth decades. In this study, 7% cases were found in the first decade of life.
- Female predilection of 1.5:1 ratio [30].

Presentation The mandible is more commonly involved. In Kafee's study, 109 (66%) cases were seen in the mandible and 55 (34%) in the maxilla.

- Small lesions are typically asymptomatic and incidentally found on radiographs.
- Larger lesions cause painless expansion of the bone resulting in facial deformity.

Differential Diagnosis

- Dental follicle
- Keratocyst odontogenic tumor
- Ameloblastoma
- Ameloblastic fibroma
- Odontogenic fibroma

Diagnosis and Evaluation

Physical Examination

- Seen in the molar and premolar region and commonly associated with an unerupted tooth. If it is in the maxilla, it tends to obliterate the maxillary sinus.
- Cortical expansion and perforation are commonly seen.
- Can cause displacement or, less frequently, resorption of teeth in the area of the tumor.
- Does not typically cause sensory changes.

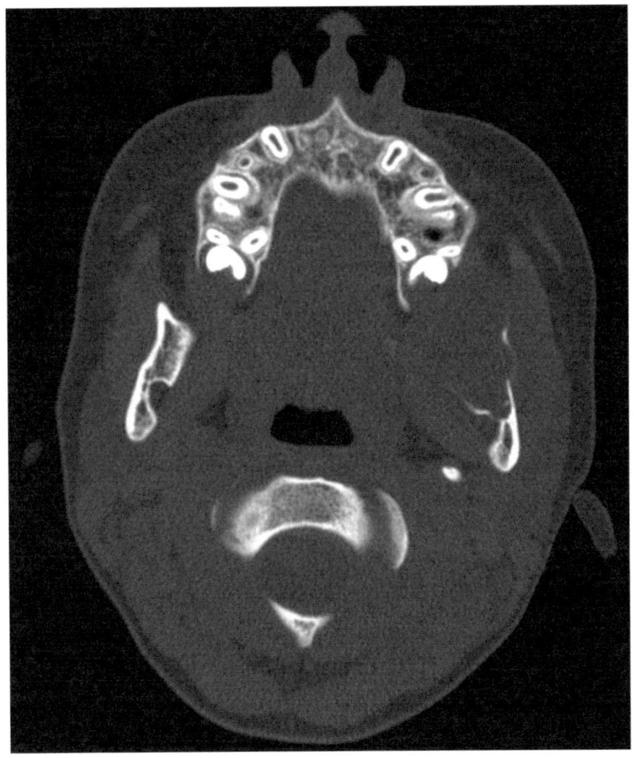

Fig. 33.11 Axial computed tomography (CT) scan of lesion in left mandibular ramus, with erosion of cortical bone and buccal and lingual expansion

Imaging

- Panoramic radiograph: findings are variable, from small unilocular to large multilocular radiolucencies (Fig. 33.11). Although most lesions are radiolucent, 12.5% are mixed, and 7% are radiopaque [30]. The margins are often irregular or scalloped. The thin trabeculae pattern has been described as "soap bubble," "honey comb," "tennis racket," "wispy," and/or "spider web" in appearance [2, 29]. These radiographic terms are not pathognomonic for the disease.

Pathology On gross examination, the tumor is unencapsulated, gray-white to tan-yellow in color. It is glistening, translucent, and homogenous on visual inspection. It is also rubbery, soft, and gelatinous in texture [2]. Margins of the tumor are ill-defined. On microscopic examination, stellate, spindle-shaped, and round cells in a loose myxoid stroma are seen with a few collagen fibrils [31, 32]. The myxoid matrix is rich in hyaluronic acid and chondroitin sulfate. Of note, mitosis is not a feature of myxoma.

Treatment Treatment is controversial [28].

- Surgical resection with 1 cm margins and one uninvolved anatomic barrier has been advocated because myxomas are not encapsulated and tend to infiltrate the surrounding tissues [13, 28, 33].

- In the pediatric population, there is reluctance to perform expertative surgery because of the resulting facial disfigurement and interference with facial growth [28, 33]. Wachter suggested a combination of enucleation along with peripheral ostectomy, removing a substantial circumferencial margin of bone, 0.5–1.0 mm, around the tumor [34]. Furthermore, a study by Rotenberg et al. discusses that conservative resection (narrow resection margins or one clear tissue plane) was an effective therapy for myxomas in pediatric patients with tumors in the maxilla [35].

Outcome The recurrence rate is approximately 25 %.
- If it recurs, it does so within the first two years after treatment [35].
- Its high recurrence rate is likely due to incomplete removal rather than the intrinsic biologic behavior of the neoplasm. It is the result of local invasion into cancellous bone beyond radiographically visible margins and absent encapsulation [36].

Cementoblastoma

Introduction Cementoblastoma is a rare neoplasm representing less than 1 % of all odontogenic tumors [2]. It occurs by connective tissue forming a cementum-like calcification, continuous to a tooth root [1].

Biology and Epidemiology Cementoblastoma is a benign ectomesenchymal odontogenic neoplasm that forms a mass of cementum or cementum-like tissue, continuous with the tooth root, usually a mandibular premolar or first molar.
- No gender predilection
- Age distribution: over a hundred cases have been reported, with an age range of 8–44 years, and a mean of 20 years [1]

Presentation The lesion is more common in the mandible than in the maxilla [1, 2]. There is commonly a painful swelling associated with this lesion.

Differential Diagnosis
- Calcifying odontogenic tumor
- Cementoblastoma
- Cementoossifying fibroma
- Odontoma
- Osteoblastoma

Diagnosis and Evaluation

Physical Examination
- Tender fullness at the buccal and/or lingual/palatal aspect of the alvelous.

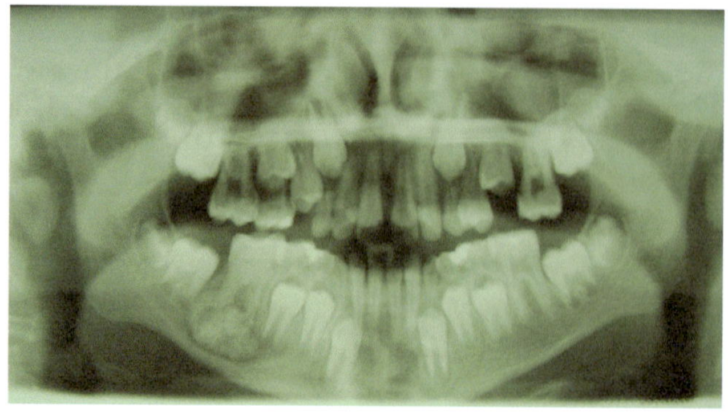

Fig. 33.12 Panoramic radiograph demonstrates a radiopaque mass encompassing and replacing the apical portion of the right first molar root. There is also a thin peripheral radiolucent zone

- Lesions range from 0.5 cm to 5.5 cm in diameter [13].
- Vitality of the affected tooth is intact.
- Paresthesia is rare [37].

Imaging Evaluation
- Panoramic radiograph: a well defined radiopaque or mixed radiolucent lesion (Fig. 33.12) surrounded by a thin radiolucent rim attached to the root of a tooth. It may be round or irregular in shape and often has a mottled texture [37]. There is often root resorption with loss of the root outline and obliteration of the periodontal ligament space.

Pathology On gross examination, there is a rounded or nodular mass attached to the tooth roots (Fig. 33.13). Microscopically, there are sheets of cementum-like calcified tissue, often being arranged in radiating columns [1]. The tumor mass blends with root of tooth, and there can be root resorption.

Treatment Treatment is the removal of the lesion and affected tooth or teeth followed by curettage or peripheral ostectomy [13].

Outcome The recurrence rate has been reported to be 37.1 % [37], and is likely due to incomplete removal.

Mixed Odontogenic Tumors

Ameloblastic Fibroma

Introduction Ameloblastic fibroma is a rare tumor, representing only 2 % of odontogenic tumors [38]. It is a mixed epithelial and mesenchymal odontogenic benign neoplasm, with no dental hard tissues present.

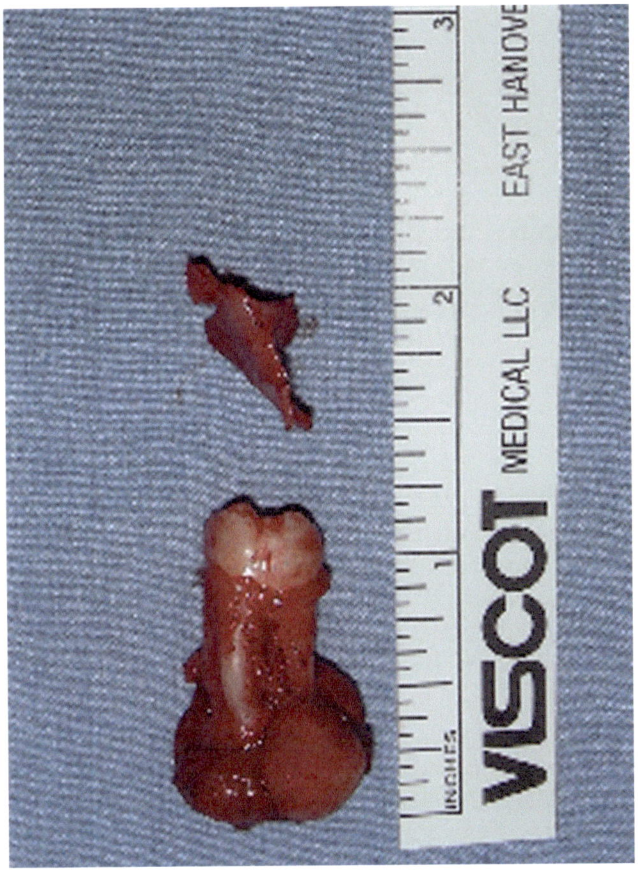

Fig. 33.13 Gross specimen showing rounded/nodular mass attached to tooth roots

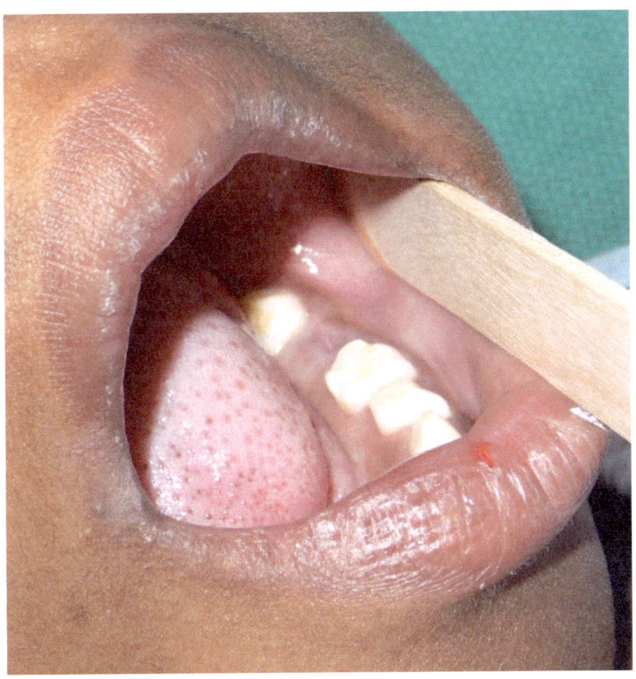

Fig. 33.14 Intraoral exam shows displaced left mandibular first molar with expansion of buccal plate of mandible

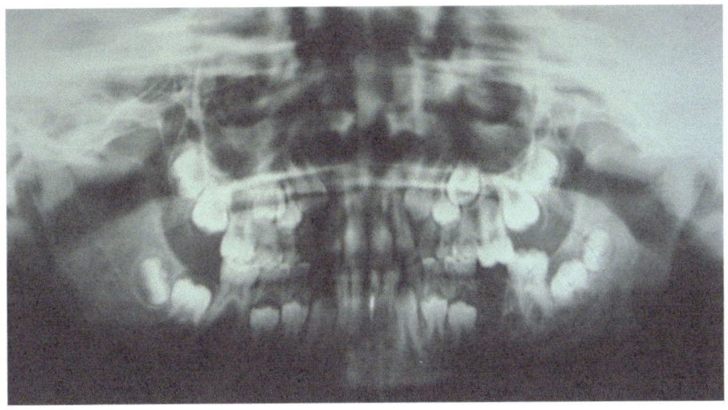

Fig. 33.15 Panoramic radiograph demonstrates left mandibular radiolucent lesion extending from sigmoid notch to the inferior border

Biology and Epidemiology Ameloblastic fibroma arises from epithelium of the enamel organ and odontogenic mesenchyme from the primitive dental pulp.

- Usually diagnosed in the first two decades of life [39]. The mean age is 16 years [39], although it has been reported in a 7-week-old infant as well [40].
- No gender predilection found.

Presentation Small tumors are asymptomatic while larger tumors are associated with painless swelling [1, 13].

Differential Diagnosis

- Dentigerous cyst
- Keratocystic odontogenic tumor
- Adenomatoid odontogenic tumor
- Ameloblastic fibroma
- Odontogenic myxoma
- Ameloblastoma
- Ossifying fibroma
- Giant cell lesion

Diagnosis and Evaluation

Physical Examination

- Nontender fullness in the affected area (Fig. 33.14).
- Posterior mandible is the most common site, with 70 % of lesions occurring in this area [2].
- Cortical expansion may cause tooth movement, but it will rarely cause root resorption [13].

Imaging Evaluation

- Panoramic radiograph: appears as a unilocular or multilocular radiolucent lesion with a well-demarcated border [1, 13] (Fig. 33.15). The size ranges from 1 cm to 8 cm [41]. In 75 % of the cases, this tumor is associated with an unerupted tooth similar to a dentigerous cyst [41].

Pathology On gross exam, the specimen is a solid, soft tissue mass with a smooth outer surface. Microscopically, there is cell-rich mesenchymal tissue (resembling primitive dental

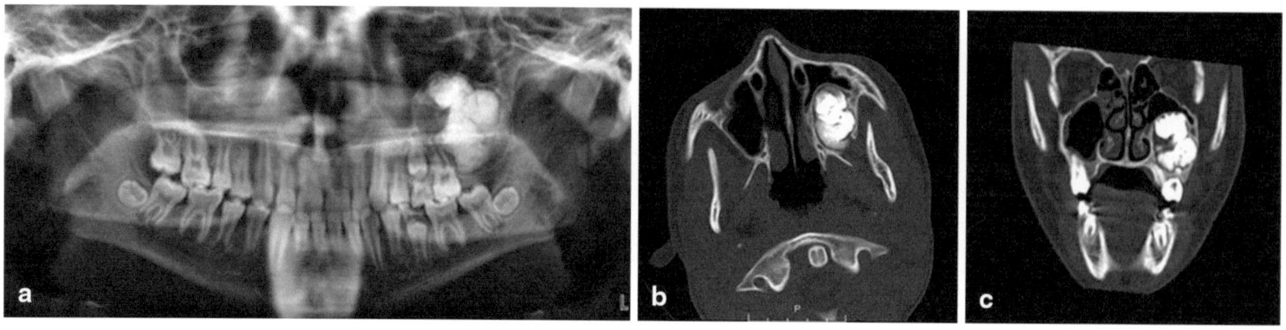

Fig. 33.16 Panoramic radiograph and computed tomography (CT) scan showing large mixed radiolucent/radiopaque lesion in left posterior maxilla (**a**, **b**, **c**). The lesion contains material of tooth density with a thin soft tissue rim

papilla) admixed with proliferating odontogenic epithelium. The epithelial pattern consists of long, narrow strands of odontogenic epithelium, two cuboidal or columnar cells in thickness. The mesenchymal portion consists of plump stellate and ovoid cells in loose matrix (resembling dental papilla), and not collagenized [1, 41].

Treatment Local excision or curettage has a substantial risk of recurrence and there is a chance for malignant transformation with inadequate treatment.

- Chen et al. [39] found a significantly lower rate of malignant transformation in younger patients (less than 22 years of age) with the five-year malignant transformation rate of 3.3 %. Therefore, it is reasonable to treat patients younger than 22 years by conservative approach [1, 6, 13, 41].
- For patients with a recurrent ameloblastic fibroma, patients older than 22 years, or when the tumor is massive in size, the treatment of choice is resection [39].

Outcome The overall recurrence rate is 33.3 % [39] with 90 % recurrences occurring in patients treated with enucleation and curettage. The longest recurrence interval was 96 months.

- High recurrence rate is likely due to regrowth of residual tumor.
- Rate of malignant transformation to fibroscarcoma is 11.4 %. Approximately 45 % of ameloblastic fibrosarcomas develop in the setting of recurrent ameloblastic fibroma [13].

Ameloblastic Fibro-odontoma/ Fibrodentinoma

Introduction The ameloblastic fibro-odontoma is less common than the ameloblastic fibroma, making up only 1–3 % of odontogenic tumors [41]. It is thought to represent an aberrant attempt at tooth formation occurring during the formation of enamel and dentin, and as such, is similar to the odontoma. If there is dentin material only, the lesion is referred to as ameloblastic fibrodentinoma.

Biology and Epidemiology This is an intraosseous lesion caused by a limited proliferation of both odontogenic epithelium and mesenchyme, producing some enamel, but mostly dentin. It is not invasive, reaches a maximum size, and then, ceases to grow.

- Etiology of these lesions is not known, but it has been postulated that it is related to trauma, infection, or genetic factors.
- Majority of these lesions (98 %) occur before the age of 20, with the average age being 9.
- Slight male predilection is found [1].

Presentation The lesion is usually asymptomatic and incidentally found when radiographs are taken particularly when there is a failure in tooth eruption. It presents as a painless, slow-growing, expansile lesion [1].

Differential Diagnosis

- Odontoma
- Ameloblastic fibro-odontoma
- Calcifying odontogenic cyst
- Cementoblastoma
- Fibrous dysplasia
- Osteoblastoma

Diagnosis and Evaluation:

Physical Examination

- Majority of these tumors (54 %) are found in the posterior mandible, with the second most common area in the posterior maxilla [2, 42].
- Most lesions are associated with unerupted teeth [1].

Imaging Evaluation

- Panoramic radiograph: unilocular radiolucency with variable amounts of calcified material similar to the radiodensity of a tooth [1] (Figs. 33.16a–c). There may also be root resorption of neighboring teeth.

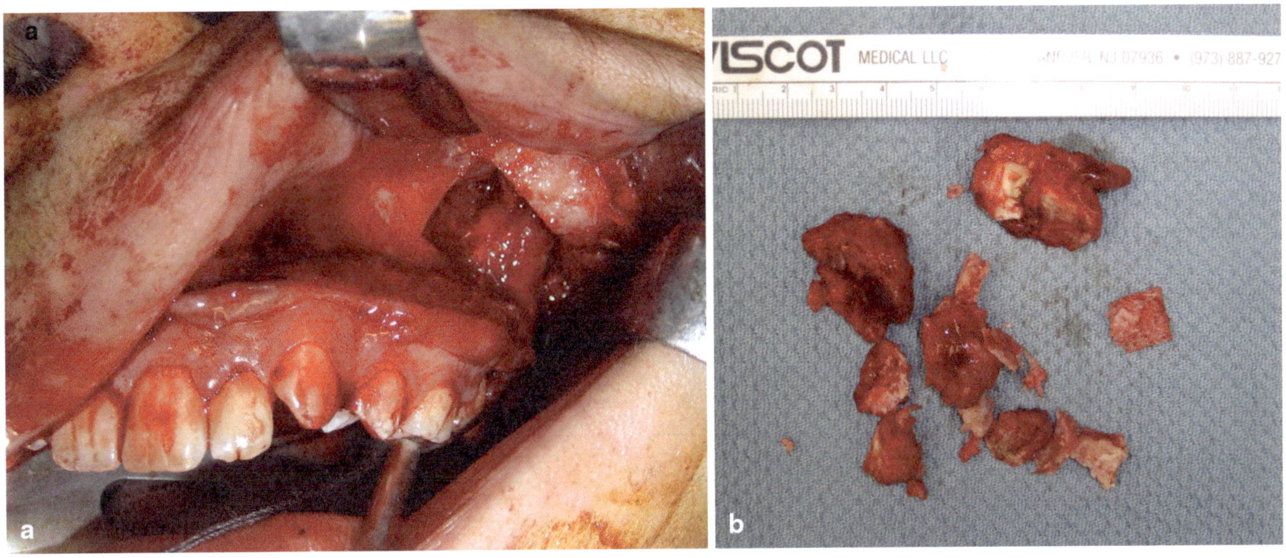

Fig. 33.17 a Intraoperative photograph showing hard-tissue lesion (20) and b specimen (21)

Pathology Microscopically, the tumor is well-circumscribed. Some regions of the tumor demonstrate the same composition of the tissue elements as in ameloblastic fibroma (cords and strands of odontogenic epithelium dispersed in a cell-rich mesenchymal tissue), but it is also admixed in areas in which odontogenic epithelium and the mesenchymal tissue form dental papillae and enamel organs [1, 2, 13] (Figs. 33.17a, b). The calcified component consists of foci of enamel matrix and dentin.

Treatment Treatment is enucleation and curettage [38].

- Intraoperatively, the lesion is well-circumscribed and easily separates from the surrounding bone.

Outcome The prognosis is excellent and recurrences are rare [1].

- After enucleation and curettage, there is spontaneous osteogenesis, filling in the defect, within 9–12 months in young patients [8].

Odontoma (Compound vs. Complex)

Introduction Odontoma is the most common odontogenic tumor of the jaws [1, 2, 8]. It is a mixed odontogenic tumor which is derived from a combination of epithelial and mesenchymal elements [1, 2, 6, 8]. There are two types of odontomas: compound and complex. The compound odontoma consists of multiple, small tooth-like structures, while the complex odontoma is a mass made up of enamel and dentin, without discernible tooth structures. A combination of two variants can also occur [1].

Biology and Epidemiology This lesion is a developmental anomaly rather than a true neoplasm. The odontoma can be associated with a calcifying odontogenic cyst (Chap. 32) [9].

- A slight prevalence difference exists between the compound, which occurs more often in the maxilla and anterior jaw, while the complex occurs more often in the mandible and posterior jaw.
- Most odontomas are diagnosed during the first two decades of life [1].
- No gender predilection found.

Presentation Odontomas are almost always asymptomatic, and discovered during routine dental radiographs for retained deciduous teeth and/or delayed eruption of permanent teeth. It is unlikely to cause facial swelling or pain.

Differential Diagnosis

- Fibro-odontoma
- Osteoma
- Gardner syndrome
- Odontoameloblastoma
- Calcifying odontogenic cyst with odontoma
- Calcifying epithelial odontogenic tumor (Pindborg tumor) with odontoma.

Diagnosis and Evaluation

Physical Examination:

- Diagnosed on radiographic examination
- If the lesion is large, the expansion of alveolar bone can be seen clinically

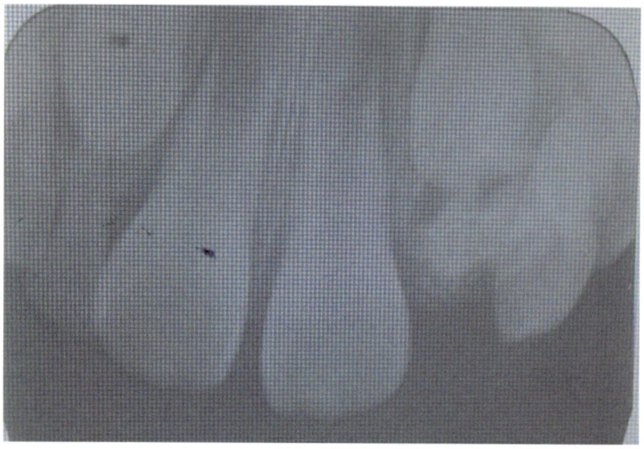

Fig. 33.18 Compound odontoma with multiple radiopaque structures preventing normal eruption of upper left lateral incisor

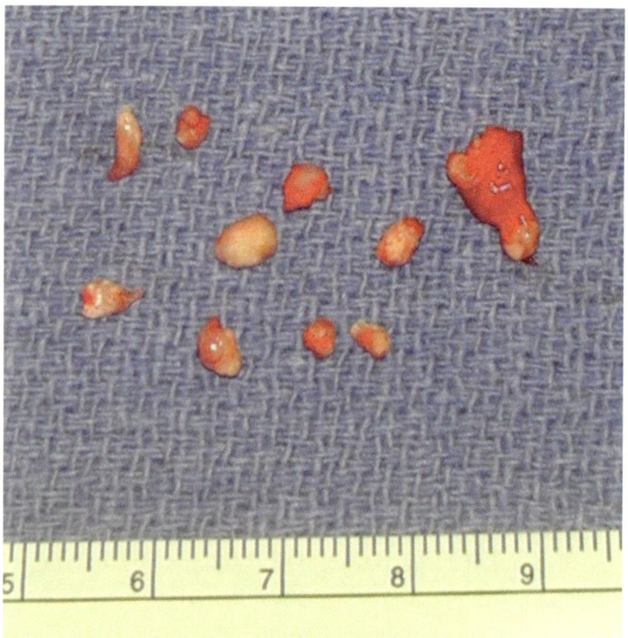

Fig. 33.19 Multiple tooth like structures with a dental sac typical of a compound odontoma

Imaging Evaluation Panoramic radiograph:

- Compound odontoma: radiopaque mass, with a collection of multiple tooth-like structures that can be of various sizes (Fig. 33.18).
- Complex odontoma: densely radiopaque calcified mass, without discernable tooth-like structures.

Pathology The histopathologic differentiation between compound and complex odontoma is not always possible and clinically insignificant since the treatment is the same for both types. Compound odontoma is usually found within a connective tissue capsule (Fig. 33.19).

Treatment

- Simple enucleation or curettage.
- Prognosis is good without recurrence.

References

1. Barnes L, Eveson J, Reichart P, Sidransky D. World health organization classification of tumours: pathology and genetics of the head and neck tumours. Lyon: IARC Press; 2005. pp 283–327.
2. Neville BW, Damm DD, Allen CM, Bouquot JE. Oral and maxillofacial pathology. 3rd ed. St. Louis: Saunders; 2009. pp 678–732.
3. Miloro M, Ghali GE, Larsen PE, Waite P. Peterson's oral and maxillofacial surgery. 2nd ed. Hamilton: BC Decker; 2004.pp 575–96.
4. Ord RA, Blanchaert RH Jr, Nikitakis NG, Sauk JJ. Ameloblastoma in children. J Oral Maxillofac Surg. 2002;60(7):762–70; discussion, 770–1.
5. Kessler HP. Intraosseous ameloblastoma. Oral Maxillofac Surg Clin North Am. 2004;16(3):309–22.
6. Kaban LB, Troulis MJ. Pediatric oral and maxillofacial surgery. Philadelphia: Saunders; 2004. pp 212–46.
7. Philipsen HP, Reichart PA. Unicystic ameloblastoma. A review of 193 cases from the literature. Oral Oncol. 1998;34(5):317–25.
8. Marx RE, Stern D. Oral and maxillofacial pathology: a rationale for diagnosis and treatment. Carol Stream: Quintessence Publishing Co; 2003. pp 637–85.
9. Becker R, Pertl A. [On the therapy of ameloblastoma]. Dtsch Zahn Mund Kieferheilkd Zentralbl Gesamte. 1967;49:423.
10. Fitzgerald GW, Frenkiel S, Black MJ, Rochon L, Baxter JD. Ameloblastoma of the jaws: a 12 year review of the McGill experience. J Otolaryngol. 1982;11(1):23–8.
11. Pullon PA, Shafer WG, Elzay RP, Kerr DA, Corio RL. Squamous odontogenic tumor. report of six cases of a previously undescribed lesion. Oral Surg Oral Med Oral Pathol. 1975;40(5):616–30.
12. Baden E, Doyle J, Mesa M, Fabie M, Lederman D, Eichen M. Squamous odontogenic tumor. report of three cases including the first extraosseous case. Oral Surg Oral Med Oral Pathol. 1993;75(6):733–8.
13. Fonseca R, Marciani R, Turvey T. Oral and maxillofacial surgery. 2nd ed. St. Louis: Saunders; 2009. pp 466–538.
14. Cillo JE Jr, Ellis E 3rd, Kessler HP. Pericoronal squamous odontogenic tumor associated with an impacted mandibular third molar: a case report. J Oral Maxillofac Surg. 2005;63(3):413–6.
15. Lin YL, White DK. Squamous odontogenic tumor. Oral Maxillofac Surg Clin North Am. 2004;16(3):355–7.
16. Philipsen HP, Srisuwan T, Reichart PA. Adenomatoid odontogenic tumor mimicking a periapical (radicular) cyst: a case report. Oral Surg Oral Med Oral Pathol Oral Radiol Endod. 2002;94(2):246–8.
17. Lee JK, Lee KB, Hwang BN. Adenomatoid odontogenic tumor: a case report. J Oral Maxillofac Surg. 2000;58(10):1161–4.
18. Philipsen HP, Reichart PA, Zhang KH, Nikai H, Yu QX. Adenomatoid odontogenic tumor: Biologic profile based on 499 cases. J Oral Pathol Med. 1991;20(4):149–58.
19. Madras J, Lapointe H. Keratocystic odontogenic tumour: reclassification of the odontogenic keratocyst from cyst to tumour. J Can Dent Assoc. 2008;74(2):165–165h.
20. Stoelinga PJ. Etiology and pathogenesis of keratocysts. Oral Maxillofac Surg Clin North Am. 2003;15(3):317–24.
21. Shear M. Odontogenic keratocysts: clinical features. Oral Maxillofac Surg Clin North Am. 2003;15(3):335–45.
22. August M, Faquin WC, Troulis MJ, Kaban LB. Dedifferentiation of odontogenic keratocyst epithelium after cyst decompression. J Oral Maxillofac Surg. 2003;61(6):678–83; discussion 683–4.

23. Forssell K, Forssell H, Kahnberg KE. Recurrence of keratocysts. A long-term follow-up study. Int J Oral Maxillofac Surg. 1988;17(1):25–8.
24. Marker P, Brondum N, Clausen PP, et al. Treatment of large odontogenic keratocysts by decompression and later cystectomy. a long-term follow-up and a histologic study of 23 cases. Oral Surg Oral Med Oral Pathol Oral Radiol Endod. 1996;82(2):122–31.
25. Gorlin RJ, Goltz RW. Multiple nevoid basal-cell epithelioma, jaw cysts and bifid rib: a syndrome. N Engl J Med. 1960;262:908–12.
26. Kimonis VE, Goldstein AM, Pastakia B, et al. Clinical manifestations in 105 persons with nevoid basal cell carcinoma syndrome. Am J Med Genet. 1997;69:299–308.
27. White SC, Pharoah MJ. Oral radiology: principles and interpretation. 6th ed. St Louis: CV Mosby; 2009. pp 366–404.
28. King TJ 3rd, Lewis J, Orvidas L, Kademani D. Pediatric maxillary odontogenic myxoma: a report of 2 cases and review of management. J Oral Maxillofac Surg. 2008 May;66(5):1057–62.
29. Brannon RB. Central odontogenic fibroma, myxoma (odontogenic myxoma, fibromyxoma), and central odontogenic granular cell tumor. Oral Maxillofac Surg Clin North Am. 2004;16(3):359–74.
30. Kaffe I, Naor H, Buchner A. Clinical and radiological features of odontogenic myxoma of the jaws. Dentomaxillofac Radiol. 1997;26(5):299–303.
31. Halfpenny W, Verey A, Bardsley V. Myxoma of the mandibular condyle. A case report and review of the literature. Oral Surg Oral Med Oral Pathol Oral Radiol Endod. 2000;90(3):348–53.
32. Lo Muzio L, Nocini P, Favia G, Procaccini M, Mignogna MD. Odontogenic myxoma of the jaws: a clinical, radiologic, immunohistochemical, and ultrastructural study. Oral Surg Oral Med Oral Pathol Oral Radiol Endod. 1996;82(4):426–33.
33. Fenton S, Slootweg PJ, Dunnebier EA, Mourits MP. Odontogenic myxoma in a 17-month-old child: a case report. J Oral Maxillofac Surg. 2003;61(6):734–6.
34. Wachter BG, Steinberg MJ, Darrow DH, McGinn JD, Park AH. Odontogenic myxoma of the maxilla: a report of two pediatric cases. Int J Pediatr Otorhinolaryngol. 2003;67(4):389–93.
35. Rotenberg BW, Daniel SJ, Nish IA, et al. Myxomatous lesions of the maxilla in children: a case series and review of management. Int J Pediatr Otorhinolaryngol. 2004;68:1251–6.
36. Pahl S, Henn W, Binger T, Stein U, Remberger K. Malignant odontogenic myxoma of the maxilla: case with cytogenetic confirmation. J Laryngol Otol. 2000;114(7):533–5.
37. Brannon RB, Fowler CB, Carpenter WM, Corio RL. Cementoblastoma: an innocuous neoplasm? A clinicopathologic study of 44 cases and review of the literature with special emphasis on recurrence. Oral Surg Oral Med Oral Pathol Oral Radiol Endod. 2002;93(3):311–20.
38. Cohen DM, Bhattacharyya I. Ameloblastic fibroma, ameloblastic fibro-odontoma, and odontoma. Oral Maxillofac Surg Clin North Am. 2004;16(3):375–84.
39. Chen Y, Wang JM, Li TJ. Ameloblastic fibroma: a review of published studies with special reference to its nature and biological behavior. Oral Oncol. 2007;43(10):960–9.
40. Mosby EL, Russell D, Noren S, Barker BF. Ameloblastic fibroma in a 7 week old infant, a case report and review of the literature. J Oral Maxillofac Surg. 1998;56:368–72.
41. Philipsen HP, Reichart PA, Praetorius F. Mixed odontogenic tumours and odontomas. considerations on interrelationship. review of the literature and presentation of 134 new cases of odontomas. Oral Oncol. 1997;33(2):86–99.
42. Miller AS, Lopez A-CF, Pullon PA, et al. Ameloblastic fibro-odontoma: report of seven cases. Oral Surg. 1976;41:354–65.

Parathyroid Tumors

34

Biren P. Modi and Stephen A. Huang

Introduction

Parathyroid tumors in children are exceedingly rare. In addition to sporadic parathyroid adenomas, many cases of parathyroid pathophysiology in young children are related to syndromic endocrinopathies, specifically multiple endocrine neoplasia syndromes 1 and 2a (MEN 1 and MEN 2a) or disorders of renal function [1]. Operative intervention for definitive therapy of parathyroid dysfunction in these instances may be indicated.

Parathyroid dysfunction typically presents in the form of hyperparathyroidism. However, even hyperparathyroidism is quite rare in children, and is never the result of a neoplasm (parathyroid adenocarcinoma or paraneoplastic syndrome) [2]. Hyperparathyroidism can be primary, as in the case of the MEN syndromes, or secondary or tertiary, as in the setting of renal dysfunction.

Key Points

- Parathyroid tumors in children are exceedingly rare.
- Parathyroid dysfunction typically presents in the form of hyperparathyroidism, and can be primary, secondary, or tertiary.
- In most cases of syndromic or disease-related hyperparathyroidism, subtotal parathyroidectomy with preservation of one-half of the most normal appearing gland is the surgical procedure of choice.

B. P. Modi (✉)
Department of Surgery, Boston Children's Hospital, Harvard Medical School, 300 Longwood Avenue, Fegan 3, Boston, MA 02115, USA
e-mail: Biren.Modi@childrens.harvard.edu

S. A. Huang
Department of Medicine, Boston Children's Hospital, Harvard Medical School, 300 Longwood Avenue, Fegan 3, Boston, MA 02115, USA

Biology and Epidemiology

The parathyroid glands derive from the third and fourth pharyngeal pouches in the 5th and 6th week of gestation. The derivatives of the third pouch descend with the thymic primordium and develop into the inferior parathyroid glands. The glands from the fourth pouch descend in the neck, finishing their descent cephalad to the inferior glands and developing into the superior parathyroids.

The chief cells of the parathyroid glands perform their function of calcium and phosphate homeostasis via their protein product, parathyroid hormone (PTH). This function is carried out through direct action on bone and kidneys as well as through vitamin D metabolism to regulate the intestinal absorption of calcium. Thus, hyperparathyroidism, the most common manifestation of parathyroid abnormalities, presents through hypercalcemia and its symptoms. Understanding of the feedback controls involved in the delicate balance of calcium homeostasis allows for proper interpretation of laboratory parameters to identify the cause of abnormal parathyroid function (Table 34.1).

Pathophysiology

- In general, hyperplasia of the parathyroid glands due to dysregulation of the normal calcium homeostatic feedback mechanisms results in the inappropriate production of parathyroid hormone despite elevated calcium levels.
- Alternatively, a single adenoma can become autonomous in its function.
- This results in increased conversion of 25-hydroxyvitamin D to 1, 25-dihydroxyvitamin D with increased intestinal calcium absorption, increased renal calcium excretion due to hypercalcemia resulting in the propensity for stone formation, and, most concerning, increased cortical bone resorption.
- Secondary hyperparathyroidism occurs due to an inciting stimulus. Most commonly, this is seen in vitamin

R. Rahbar et al. (eds.), *Pediatric Head and Neck Tumors*,
DOI 10.1007/978-1-4614-8755-5_34, © Springer Science+Business Media New York 2014

Table 34.1 Laboratory parameters in the various forms of hyperparathyroidism

Form	Serum calcium	Serum PTH	Notes
Primary	↑	↑ or normal	PTH normal in 15 %
Secondary	↓ or normal	↑	Assess for etiology
Tertiary	↑	↑	Clinical history gives diagnosis

↑ increased levels, ↓ decreased levels

D deficiency or in renal disease with urinary calcium losses and poor conversion of 25-hydroxyvitamin D to 1,25-dihydroxyvitamin D.

Molecular/Genetic Pathology

- The genetic defect in MEN1 is an autosomal dominant loss-of-function mutation in the *MEN1* gene, located on chromosome 11. This gene codes for menin, which is involved in the regulation of DNA replication and transcription [3, 4].
- The genetic defect in MEN2a is a gain-of-function mutation in the *RET* proto-oncogene, located on chromosome 10. Though hyperparathyroidism occurs in a minority of patients with MEN2a, it is more prevalent in patients with mutations in codon 634 of the *RET* proto-oncogene [3].
- The molecular pathways linking these genetic mutations to the development of hyperparathyroidism are incompletely understood.
- The genetic defect in familial hypocalciuric hypercalcemia (FHH) and neonatal severe hyperparathyroidism is in the calcium-sensing receptor gene (*CASR*) on chromosome 3 [4, 5].

Incidence and Prevalence

- Primary hyperparathyroidism is extremely rare in children, with an incidence of 2–5 per 100,000 [2, 6].
- MEN1 is the most common of the familial forms of primary hyperparathyroidism, accounting for 2–4 % of all cases of hyperparathyroidism, approximately 20 % of primary hyperparathyroidism, and 57 % of hyperplasia. MEN1 has a prevalence of 2–3 per 100,000 [3, 4, 6].
- Hyperparathyroidism occurs in approximately 20 % of patients with MEN2a. In contrast to MEN1, the other features of MEN2a, specifically medullary thyroid cancer (~90 %) and pheochromocytoma (50 %), have a higher penetrance than does hyperparathyroidism [3].

Age Distribution

- In adults, the peak incidence of hyperparathyroidism occurs in the seventh decade [5].
- Hyperparathyroidism in infancy is rare and can be associated with severe neonatal primary hyperparathyroidism, usually due to biallelic loss-of-function mutation(s) in the calcium sensing receptor gene [2, 4, 5].
- In MEN1, primary hyperparathyroidism is usually the first detected endocrinopathy, can often be diagnosed by age 20, and is present in 95 % of patients by age 40 [3].

Sex Predilection

- Primary hyperparathyroidism is found to be more common in females than males, with a ratio somewhere between 3:1 and 3:2 [2].
- MEN1 has equal incidence in males and females [3].

Geographic/Ethnic Distribution

- There is not a known specific ethnic or geographic distribution of parathyroid disease in children.

Risk Factors

- Primary hyperparathyroidism has been linked to childhood neck irradiation and to long-term lithium use [5].

Relationships to Other Disease States and Syndromes

- As mentioned above, parathyroid disease in children is related to several other disease states and syndromes. Specifically, MEN1 and MEN2a both result in hyperparathyroidism. In addition, renal failure can result in secondary hyperparathyroidism due to chronic calcium losses and poor vitamin D production. Tertiary hyperparathyroidism occurs when hyperparathyroidism becomes autonomous of the inciting stimulus in secondary hyperparathyroidism, such as when hyperparathyroidism persists after renal transplantation in cases of renal failure with secondary hyperparathyroidism [2, 3].
- Diagnosis of MEN1 requires a genetic confirmation, which is sometimes difficult due to variable genotype/phenotype correlation and a significant prevalence (10 %)

of de novo germline mutation [7]. Alternatively, a clinical diagnosis may be given if the patient has a tumor in two of the three classic organ systems (parathyroid, pancreas/duodenum, pituitary) or a family history of MEN1 and a tumor in one of the three organs [3].

- In cases of known or newly diagnosed MEN1, first-degree relatives and known gene carriers should be screened with annual serum calcium tests. The utility of concomitant PTH levels is not clear. A similar screening plan for MEN2a may be used, especially as less aggressive surgery for parathyroid disease at the time of childhood thyroidectomy for medullary thyroid cancer prevention is becoming more widespread [3].
- Specific features of hyperparathyroidism and the differential management of this entity in these related disease states and syndromes are discussed throughout this chapter.

Presentation

Symptoms

- A neck mass in the setting of parathyroid pathology is extremely rare, even in the case of parathyroid adenoma.
- Hypercalcemia due to overactive parathyroid function can result in weakness and fatigue, polyuria, nephrolithiasis, and pancreatitis. Neuropsychiatric manifestations, such as depression or difficulty with concentration, are also common [2, 3, 5]. Patients may complain of nausea, abdominal pain, and other nonspecific gastrointestinal symptoms.
- Increased catabolism of cortical bone can result in osteopenia or osteoporosis or, in extreme cases, pathologic fractures or osteitis fibrosa cystica.
- In severe and chronic cases of hyperparathyroidism, ectopic calcium deposition can result in organ damage, as is the case in nephrocalcinosis.

Patterns of Evolution

- In children, unless familial involvement is known, symptoms have often been present for several years prior to definitive diagnosis. As mentioned above, this can often result in end organ damage from prolonged hypercalcemia [6].
- A late finding resulting from the bony destruction that occurs with hyperparathyroidism is osteitis fibrosa cystica. This results in subperiosteal bony resorption, especially in the phalanges and skull. The latter can be demonstrated by the finding of a "salt-and-pepper" skull radiograph. This late development, thankfully, is rarely seen in modern settings.

Table 34.2 Differential diagnosis of hypercalcemia in children. (Adapted from Safford et al.[2] with permission from Elsevier)

Differential diagnosis of hypercalcemia in children
Disorders with elevated or inappropriate parathyroid hormone (PTH) levels
• Primary hyperparathyroidism
• Secondary hyperparathyroidism
• Tertiary hyperparathyroidism
• Ectopic PTH production
Hypervitaminosis D
Hypervitaminosis A
Sarcoid disease
Significant subcutaneous fat necrosis
Familial hypocalciuric hypercalcemia (FHH)
Idiopathic hypercalcemia of infancy
Thyrotoxicosis
Hypophosphatasia
Prolonged immobilization
Medication effects: e.g., thiazide diuretics, lithium

Differential Diagnosis

- The differential diagnosis of hypercalcemia is broad and can involve pathology related to multiple organ systems. A sample differential diagnosis is provided in Table 34.2, adapted from Safford et al. [2].

Diagnosis and Evaluation

Physical Examination

- As mentioned, a neck mass in the setting of parathyroid pathology is extremely rare, even in the case of parathyroid adenoma.
- Muscle weakness may be demonstrated in cases of symptomatic hypercalcemia.
- Neuropsychiatric evaluation may demonstrate signs of difficulty with concentration or evidence of depression.

Laboratory Data

- Table 34.1 depicts the typical laboratory findings in the various types of hyperparathyroidism. Clinical correlation with associated disease states will help to differentiate the various types of hyperparathyroidism. Because normal serum calcium concentrations are higher in children than in adults, age-appropriate normal ranges should be applied. Total serum calcium measurements should be corrected for serum albumin to rule out pseudohypercalcemia from hyperalbuminemia.

- Most children with primary hyperparathyroidism present with hypercalcemia and an overtly high serum PTH concentration. However, in a minority of patients, parathyroid levels may be within the normal range for serum levels. In concert with elevated serum calcium levels, however, this represents inappropriately high parathyroid hormone levels, and the absence or inadequacy of appropriate feedback regulation.
- Secondary and tertiary hyperparathyroidism are typically diagnosed by virtue of their clinical context.
- Urinary studies are helpful to distinguish primary hyperparathyroidism (which is characterized by hypercalciuria) from FHH (which usually displays a low urine calcium/creatinine ratio <0.01) [5]. This distinction is critical as parathyroidectomy is rarely indicated in FHH.
- Hypercalcemic children found to have low serum PTH concentrations should undergo testing for nonparathyroid causes, including measurement of vitamin D metabolites and parathyroid hormone-related protein (PTHrp).

Imaging Evaluation

- In the absence of family history of hypercalcemia or syndromic involvement, primary hyperparathyroidism in children is usually the result of a single adenoma. In this clinical setting, neck US may be helpful in identifying an isolated enlarged gland.
- Correlation of US findings with technetium-99 sestamibi radionuclide scan can help to verify the identification of a single adenomatous gland. In the identification of adult parathyroid gland disease, correlation between these two studies is highly sensitive and specific for single gland disease and has been used for directed parathyroid surgery.
- More recently, the use of 4D computed tomography (CT) of the neck has been reported to have improved sensitivity and specificity over both ultrasound and sestamibi [8].
- Since directed or mini parathyroidectomy is seldom used in children, and a full four-gland exploration is usually performed, localizing studies are often not necessary. In reoperative intervention, however, localizing imaging studies are essential, to allow for localization of active parathyroid tissue and the identification of potential supernumerary and/or ectopic glands [3].
- Other imaging modalities aimed at assessing for organ damage as a result of longstanding hypercalcemia may be useful. These include renal ultrasound when nephrolithiasis or nephrocalcinosis are a consideration and bone mineral density evaluation with a dual-energy X-ray absorptiometry (DEXA) scan [5].

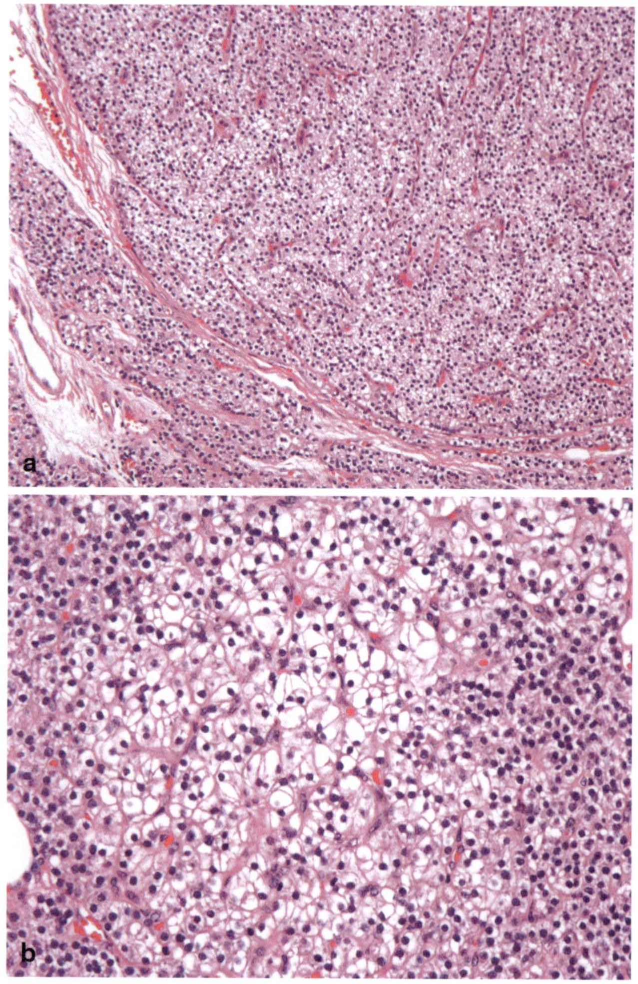

Fig. 34.1 Parathyroid hyperplasia. **a** Nodular hyperplasia of parathyroid gland showing a multinodular hypercellular parenchyma devoid of adipose tissue. **b** A mixture of chief and clear cells is present. Clear cells are clustered at the center

Pathology

- Histopathology of resected specimens in the setting of single gland disease reveals benign, chief cell adenoma.
- In the setting of hyperplasia, histology reveals hypercellularity of otherwise normal parathyroid tissue (Fig. 34.1). MEN1 patients have asymmetric nodular hyperplasia, with polyclonal hyperplasia resulting in multiple monoclonal nodules [3].
- Hyperplasia can often be asymmetric, affecting some glands more than others, making surgical decision making more difficult. This issue is discussed in more detail in the surgical section below.

Treatment

Goal

The goal of therapy for hyperparathyroidism in children is to normalize serum calcium in order to prevent or reverse end organ damage and manage symptoms. This includes reversal of bone resorption with rebuilding of osteopenic bone, normalization of renal calcium clearance to prevent nephrolithiasis, prevention and reversal of calcium deposition in tissue, and improvement of muscle weakness or associated neuropsychiatric disorders.

Surgical therapy is warranted in almost all pediatric cases of primary and tertiary hyperparathyroidism due to their relationship to syndromes and related diseases. In cases of secondary hyperparathyroidism, medical therapy is usually successful, along with eradication of the inciting factor. However, in any case with severe symptoms such as bone loss, pathologic fractures, or nephrocalcinosis, surgery is appropriate [2, 6].

Surgical Therapy

Choice of Operation In the case of de novo hyperparathyroidism without evidence of familial syndrome involvement, an adenoma is the likely culprit. Nonetheless, this can be a difficult assessment as younger patients are often the index case in the kindred [3]. Since involvement of the glands in the hyperplastic process can be asymmetric and metachronous, the appearance of the glands may support a diagnosis of adenoma when the eventual diagnosis will turn out to be hyperplasia. Certainly in secondary and tertiary hyperparathyroidism, all four glands are nearly universally involved to varying degrees.

Given the possibility of multiglandular hyperplasia, so called mini-parathyroidectomy or directed parathyroidectomy does not seem to be an appropriate surgical choice. The best option in young children is a full exploration of both sides of the neck to identify and visualize all four glands. If clear-cut single gland involvement is present, resection of the adenoma with marking of the remaining glands is a reasonable option.

In cases of hyperplasia, especially in MEN1 and neonatal severe hyperparathyroidism, any resection less than a subtotal (3½) parathyroidectomy has been shown to result in persistent or recurrent hyperparathyroidism with unacceptable rates [3, 4]. The decision between subtotal and total parathyroidectomy with autotransplantation is debatable, though most findings support the use of subtotal parathyroidectomy to avoid the development of hypoparathyroidism [4, 9].

As a result, the best surgical option is subtotal parathyroidectomy, with resection of the three most abnormal glands and removal of half of the fourth gland on its vascular pedicle, combined with cervical thymectomy to remove potential supernumerary parathyroid glands. In this setting, partial removal of the most normal gland should be conducted prior to removal of the other glands to ensure viability of the remnant [3]. In addition, the use of nonabsorbable suture or a hemoclip to mark the site of the remnant is useful for reoperations. If all four glands are markedly abnormal, or if there is vascular compromise, or at reoperation for persistent or recurrent disease, total parathyroidectomy with reimplantation into the muscle of the non-dominant forearm should be considered. This will place the patient at significant risk for prolonged or permanent postoperative hypoparathyroidism [3]. When available, cryopreservation of parathyroid tissue has been described [4].

In cases where all four glands cannot be localized, ectopic locations must be considered. These include the carotid sheath, retroesophageal space, perithyroid fatty tissue, and the thymus itself. Cervical thymectomy and routine exploration for ectopic glands should likely be performed with subtotal parathyroidectomy regardless of identification of all glands due to the greater than 15 % incidence of supernumerary parathyroid glands [3, 4]. If all glands cannot be identified, adding a thyroid lobectomy on the side of the "missing" gland is appropriate [2]. The utility of intraoperative parathyroid hormone measurement has not been clearly shown, though its utility in reoperative surgery may be more evident [4].

Classic teaching for MEN2a was to perform subtotal parathyroidectomy at the time of prophylactic thyroidectomy (usually around age 5 years). However, given the relatively low incidence of hyperparathyroidism in MEN2a (20 %), and the more mild nature of the hyperparathyroidism in these patients, a more thoughtful approach has been advocated. In general, the surgical approach should be to avoid hypoparathyroidism, especially given the need for prophylactic thyroidectomy and lymph node dissection. The operative intervention in these cases, even in the setting of eucalcemia, should therefore be removal of only enlarged glands at the time of thyroidectomy, with marking of the remaining glands [4]. If all glands appear involved, then subtotal parathyroidectomy should be performed [3]. Inadvertently injured or removed glands should be autotransplanted.

Timing Due to the significant risk for end-organ damage, including bone loss and nephrocalcinosis, primary and tertiary hyperparathyroidism in children is usually surgically treated at the time of diagnosis. In cases of secondary hyperparathyroidism, medical therapy aimed at mitigating the effects of the disease and at eradicating the underlying etiology is attempted. However, evidence of significant symptoms or organ damage should result in a low threshold for proceeding to operative intervention. In cases of MEN1, surgical therapy is performed at the time of diagnosis of hyperparathyroidism, using routine yearly surveillance of laboratory parameters as a monitoring method to determine onset of disease.

Complications Recurrence occurs in up to 30 % of patients during 10 years with MEN1 when treated with subtotal parathyroidectomy. Recurrence can be minimized with this operative strategy, however, as any resection less than a subtotal parathyroidectomy results in a much higher (> 50 %) recurrence rate [3, 9, 10]. If recurrence occurs, localizing studies preoperatively, including sestamibi, ultrasound, and perhaps 4D CT scan or selective venous sampling, are paramount to help guide surgical intervention. In most cases, the goal for surgery in the setting of recurrence is completion/total parathyroidectomy with reimplantation of a portion of the most normal appearing residual gland.

Technical complications, as with any central neck surgery, include inadvertent hypoparathyroidsm, especially in cases of total parathyroidectomy with reimplantation of a remnant, and recurrent laryngeal nerve injury. Recurrence, with the need for reoperative parathyroidectomy, places the nerve at increased risk. Using nonabsorbable suture or hemoclips to mark remaining gland(s) at the time of initial surgery can be quite helpful in this scenario.

Medical Therapy

Medical therapy in hyperparathyroidism in children is typically preserved for cases of secondary hyperparathyroidism. In this setting, medical therapy can consist of repletion of vitamin D in the case of vitamin D deficiency. In chronic kidney disease, the goal of medical therapy is to decrease parathyroid hormone levels to the normal range in order to optimize bone health and prevent ectopic calcification. Therapies used to achieve this include limitation of dietary phosphate intake, the use of phosphate binders, and the use of vitamin D and vitamin D analogs. The use of calcimimetics may also be of benefit. Indications for surgical intervention include evidence of end-organ damage, such as significant bone density compromise, or symptoms, such as significant persistent nephrolithiasis.

Short term medical therapy of primary hyperparathyroidism may be indicated to correct hypercalcemia prior to surgery. First-line therapy is hydration, with or without loop diuretics, to increase urinary calcium excretion. In addition, calcitonin may be used to inhibit osteoclastic bone resorption. Severe cases may warrant treatment with bisphosphonates or dialysis.

Outcomes

In cases of familial hyperparathyroidism, recurrence is quite high. As described above, less aggressive surgery in MEN1 has a recurrence rate over 50 % which can be brought down to 30 % over 10 years by using subtotal parathyroidectomy with cervical thymectomy as the procedure of choice. A conservative management strategy, however, can be used with good effect in MEN2a, by only resecting large glands at the time of prophylactic thyroidectomy. This results in a cure rate approaching 100 %, with a recurrence rate less than 5 % [3].

Follow-up

Frequency of Office Visits

In the early postoperative period, office visits, or at least phone consultation with assessment of lab results, should be relatively frequent. Patients in most cases are administered vitamin D (calcitriol) and calcium supplementation in the immediate postoperative period to control potential hypoparathyroidism and to prevent sudden deposition of cortical bone which can result in profound hypocalcemia (so-called hungry bone syndrome). After the stabilization or normalization of these issues, follow-up is dictated by lability of calcium levels and parathyroid function if this is still an issue. If normal parathyroid function and calcium levels are achieved, which should be in the majority of patients, then periodic checks of serum calcium level can help monitor for persistence or recurrence of hyperparathyroidism.

Frequency of Imaging

The use of imaging is limited to the localization of recurrent or ectopic hyperfunctioning glands in the case of recurrence of hyperparathyroidism. Additional studies, such as DEXA or renal ultrasound, are used as needed to monitor for bone and kidney health.

References

1. Lietman SA, Germain-Lee EL, Levine MA. Hypercalcemia in children and adolescents. Curr Opin Pediatr. 2010;22:508–15.
2. Safford SD, Skinner MA. Thyroid and parathyroid disease in children. Semin Pediatr Surg. 2006;15:85–91.
3. Akerstrom G, Stalberg P. Surgical management of MEN-1 and -2: state of the art. Surg Clin North Am. 2009;89:1047–68.
4. Stalberg P, Carling T. Familial parathyroid tumors: diagnosis and management. World J Surg. 2009;33:2234–43.

5. Marcocci C, Cetani F. Clinical practice. Primary hyperparathyroidism. N Engl J Med. 2011;365:2389–97.
6. Kollars J, Zarroug AE, Heerden J van, et al. Primary hyperparathyroidism in pediatric patients. Pediatrics. 2005;115:974–80.
7. Thakker RV, Newey PJ, Walls GV, et al. Clinical practice guidelines for multiple endocrine neoplasia type 1 (MEN1). J Clin Endocrinol Metab. 2012;97(9):2990–3011.
8. Rodgers SE, Hunter GJ, Hamberg LM, et al. Improved preoperative planning for directed parathyroidectomy with 4-dimensional computed tomography. Surgery. 2006;140:932–40; discussion 40–1.
9. Elaraj DM, Skarulis MC, Libutti SK, et al. Results of initial operation for hyperparathyroidism in patients with multiple endocrine neoplasia type 1. Surgery. 2003;134:858–64.
10. Hellman P, Skogseid B, Oberg K, Juhlin C, Akerstrom G, Rastad J. Primary and reoperative parathyroid operations in hyperparathyroidism of multiple endocrine neoplasia type 1. Surgery. 1998;124:993–9.

35 Pilomatrixoma

Christian J. Vercler and John G. Meara

Introduction

In 1880, Malherbe and Chenantais [1] used the term *calcifying epithelioma* to describe a benign subcutaneous tumor thought to be of sebaceous origin. Forbis and Helwig [2] suggested the term *pilomatrixoma* in 1961 to more accurately refer to this benign neoplasm originating from hair follicle matrix cells. This tumor is common in children and is often misdiagnosed as other skin conditions. It most commonly presents in the head and neck and is more common in girls. Surgical excision is the treatment of choice and the recurrence rate is low [3, 4].

Biology and Epidemiology

After epidermoid cysts, pilomatrixoma is the second most common superficial lesion in children [5]. Sixty percent of pilomatrixomas present in the first two decades of life [6]. They are more common in girls, with a male-to-female ratio of 1:1.5 to 1.75 [4, 7].

These lesions are almost always solitary, but reports of multiple or recurring tumors have been associated with Gardner syndrome [8], myotonic dystrophy [9], or Turner syndrome [10]. Mutations that activate the β-catenin gene have been described with the locus mapped to the CTNNB1 gene on 3p22-p21.3 [11, 12].

While there have been reports of aggressive behavior of these lesions in children [13, 14], pilomatrix carcinoma has never been reported in the pediatric population. Malignant behavior in pilomatrixoma is rare, but has been observed and has been described as behaving like basal cell carcinoma [15].

Presentation

Pilomatrixomas most commonly occur in the head and neck, with the cheek and preauricular area being the most frequent site of occurrence (Table 35.1). The typical presentation is a slow-growing, well-circumscribed, firm, nontender, subcutaneous nodule. They never arise in glabrous skin, which is consistent with the understanding of the hair cell as of the origin of the tumor.

Differential Diagnosis

Although this tumor is commonly seen in children, accurate preoperative diagnosis is made in only 28.9–46% of cases [4, 16–19]. Differential diagnosis includes dermoid cyst, branchial cyst, sebaceous cyst, preauricular cyst, ossifying hematoma, chondroma, foreign body reaction, giant cell tumor, osteoma cutis, fibroxanthoma, and lymphadenopathy (see Table 35.2).

Diagnosis and Evaluation

Physical Examination

Pilomatrixoma often presents as a hard, subcutaneous, slow-growing mass that may be tender, although usually not. The tumor is fixed to the skin but mobile over deeper underlying structures. They most often have a discoloration, with blue being the most common color [4], but this can be obscured by telangiectasia, hyperkeratosis, hemosiderin deposition, and erosion. The "tent sign" described by Graham and Mer-

J. G. Meara (✉)
Department of Plastic and Oral Surgery, Boston Children's Hospital, Harvard Medical School, Boston, MA, USA
e-mail: john.meara@childrens.harvard.edu

C. J. Vercler
Section of Plastic Surgery, University of Michigan, Ann Arbor, MI, USA

R. Rahbar et al. (eds.), *Pediatric Head and Neck Tumors*,
DOI 10.1007/978-1-4614-8755-5_35, © Springer Science+Business Media New York 2014

Table 35.1 Locations of presenting lesions (reprinted from Pirouzmanesh et al. [4], with permission)

Location	No. of cases
Head	
Cheek	175 (50.6 %)
Periauricular region	65 (18.8 %)
Orbital region	19 (5.5 %)
Forehead	15 (4.3 %)
Eyelid	13 (3.8 %)
Scalp	11 (3.2 %)
Temporal region	9 (2.6 %)
Ear	7 (2.0 %)
Submental/submandibular region	5 (1.4 %)
Occipital region	5 (1.4 %)
Lips	3 (0.9 %)
Neck	61 (17.6 %)
Trunk	50 (14.4 %)
Back	25 (7.2 %)
Shoulder	15 (4.3 %)
Chest	9 (2.6 %)
Axillary region	1 (0.3 %)
Upper extremities	53 (15.3 %)
Lower Extremities	7 (2.0 %)

Table 35.2 Preoperative diagnoses (reprinted from Pirouzmanesh et al. [4], with permission)

Preoperative diagnosis	No. of cases
Pilomatrixoma	100 (28.9 %)
Unidentified mass	98 (28.3 %)
Epidermoid cyst	41 (11.8 %)
Sebaceous cyst	30 (8.7 %)
Dermoid cyst	24 (6.9 %)
Nonspecific cyst	21 (6.1 %)
Foreign body	5 (1.4 %)
Calcified hematoma	3 (0.9 %)
Vascular malformation	3 (0.9 %)
Subcutaneous abscess	2 (0.6 %)
Dermoid tumor	2 (0.6 %)
Lobule hemangioma	2 (0.6 %)
Fusiform incision	1 (0.3 %)
Lipoma	1 (0.3 %)
Ankyloglossia	1 (0.3 %)
Atypical tuberculosis	1 (0.3 %)
Inflammatory lymph node	1 (0.3 %)
Thyroglossal duct cyst	1 (0.3 %)
Posttransplantation lymphoproliferative disorder	1 (0.3 %)

win in 1978 [20] is the demonstration of the pilomatrixoma's multifaceted, often calcified nature by stretching the skin tightly over the tumor.

Laboratory Data

Currently there is no laboratory test for pilomatrixoma, nor does this neoplasm cause any systemic physiologic changes that can be detected via laboratory testing. While fine-needle aspiration of these lesions is sometimes performed, the results can often be misleading [21–23]. Definitive diagnosis is most frequently made upon excisional biopsy.

In cases of patients who present with multiple pilomatrixomas, genetic screening may be warranted, as there have been cases where these lesions present as an early marker of myotonic dystrophy and adenomatous polyposis coli [24–26].

Imaging Evaluation

There is no specific imaging modality that provides a definitive diagnosis of pilomatrixoma; generally, imaging is not necessary. CT scan shows well-circumscribed masses in the subcutaneous tissue that may or may not have calcification. MRI reveals a nonenhancing, low to intermediate signal abnormality [7]. Ultrasound may be helpful in detecting the presence of calcifications and determining the position of the lesion with relation to deeper structures. This is particularly useful for tumors that may be large or in the parotid region [27]. Compared to CT and MRI, ultrasound is a less expensive noninvasive modality that does not require sedation or anesthesia, making it an attractive initial choice for evaluation in children.

Pathology

Histology provides the definitive diagnosis in all cases. The tumor is in the deep subepidermal layer. Classic findings include a mass of cells in a circular configuration with enucleated "shadow cells" or "ghost cells" in the center and basophilic nucleated cells in the periphery. These cells are the immature basaloid cells' attempt to manufacture hair. Hair shafts are absent in these lesions, as the basaloid cells fail to differentiate into follicles. These cells invoke a foreign body reaction and giant cell formation. Calcifications are typically present [7, 28, 29] and most commonly noted as stippled areas of cytoplasm [19]. The overlying epidermis is generally not involved, but is separated by a fibrous component (pseudocapsule) that gives the impression on physical exam of adherence to the skin (see Fig. 35.1 and Table 35.3).

In a review of 336 cases[4], the presence of giant cells was the most common finding (50.6 %). Inflammation was present in 40.8 %. Blue cells were present in 31.5 %. Calcification was found in 19.1 % and ossification in 2.6 %. Pigmentation was noted in only 2.6 % of cases.

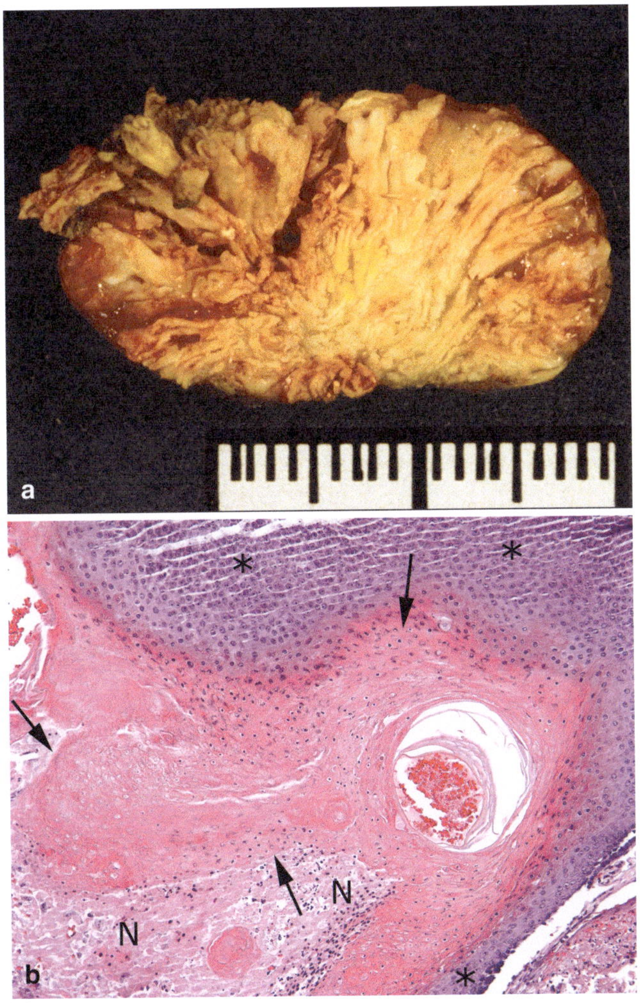

Fig. 35.1 **a** Macroscopy of pilomatrixoma. Well-circumscribed, solid tumor with a granular, soft, gritty, and grayish-yellow cut surface. **b** Light microscopy of pilomatrixoma: a hair follicle-like structure with an external layer of basaloid cells*, an internal coat of squamous cell "ghosts" (coagulative necrosis, between *arrows*) and a central area with cellular and keratinaceous debris as well as inflammation (*N*)

Table 35.3 Histopathological features (reprinted from Pirouzmanesh et al. [4], with permission)

Histopathological features	No. of cases
Giant cell	175 (50.6 %)
Inflammation	141 (40.8 %)
Blue cells	109 (31.5 %)
Calcification	66 (19.1 %)
Ossification	9 (2.6 %)
Pigmentation	9 (2.6 %)

Despite a high mitotic activity, these tumors are benign. More aggressive types of pilomatrixoma with potential for malignant degeneration are rare and will present with infiltration of surrounding structures [30–32].

Treatment

Medical

No medical therapy currently exists to treat this tumor.

Surgical

Excision of these lesions is the treatment of choice, with exceedingly low recurrence rates, even with close margins [2, 4]. As these tumors primarily occur on the face, the excision should be planned to leave the smallest possible scar keeping in mind the principles of placing elective incisions on this aesthetically important area. Excessive margins are unwarranted. As there is no histological adherence to the epidermis, technically these can be excised without taking the overlying skin. Practically, however, excising a small ellipse of overlying skin at the most superficial extent of the tumor can facilitate removal.

Adjuvant Treatment

There is no adjuvant treatment for pilomatrixoma.

Outcome

Recurrence occurs in 1.5–6 % of cases, and in the largest series reviewed the average time to recurrence was 1.6 years [4]. Given the benign, slow growth of these tumors, this course is logically consistent with an incomplete initial excision. An excellent clinical outcome is assured with complete excision of the lesion.

References

1. Malherbe A, Chenantais J. Note sur l'épithélioma calcifidés glandes sébacées. Prog Med. 1880;8:826–37.
2. Forbis R, Helwig EB. Pilomatrixoma (calcifying epithelioma). Arch Dermatol. 1961;83:606–17.
3. Julian CG, Bowers PW. A clinical review of 209 pilomatricomas. J Am Acad Dermatol. 1998;39:191–5.
4. Pirouzmanesh A, Reinisch JF, Gonzalez-Gomez I, Smith EM, Meara JG. Pilamatrixoma: a review of 346 cases. Plast Reconstr Surg. 2003;112:1784–9.
5. Knight PJ, Reiner CB. Superficial lumps in children: what, when, and why? Pediatrics. 1983;72:147–53.
6. Moehlenbeck FW. Pilomatrixoma (calcifying epithelioma): a statistical study. Arch Dermatol. 1973;108:606–18.
7. Agarwal RP, Handler SD, Matthews MR, Carpentieri D. Pilomatrixoma of the head and neck in children. Otolaryngol Head Neck Surg. 2001;125:510–5.

8. Cooper PH, Fechner RE. Pilomatricoma-like changes in the epidermal cysts of Gardner's syndrome. J Am Acad Dermatol. 1983;8:639–44.
9. Harper PS. Calcifying epithelioma of Malherbe: association with myotonic muscular dystrophy. Arch Dermatol. 1972;106:41–4.
10. Noguchi H, Kayashimi K, Nishimaya S, et al. Two cases of pilomatrixoma in Turner's syndrome. Dermatology. 1999;4:338–40.
11. Chan EF, Gat U, McNiff JM, Fuchs E. A common human skin tumour is caused by activating mutation in beta-catenin. Nat Genet. 1999;21:410–3.
12. Chan EF. Pilomatricomas contain activating mutation in β-catenin. J Am Acad Dermatol. 2000;43:701–2.
13. Marrogi A, Wick M, Dehner L. Pilomatrical neoplasms in children and young adults. Am J Dermatopathol. 1992;14:87–94.
14. Nield D, Saad M, Ali M. Aggressive pilomatrixoma in a child: a case report. Br J Plast Surg. 1986;39:139–41.
15. Black SJ, Marble BF, Vuitch F. Multiple giant pilomatrix carcinomas of the head and neck. Otolaryngol Head Neck Surg. 1993;109:543–7.
16. Jacobsen AS, Bowen J, Bruce J, Gough DCS. The calcifying epithelioma of Malherbe in children: a 15-year experience. Pediatr Surg Int. 1995;10:44–5.
17. Wells NJ, Blair GK, Magee JF, Whiteman DM. Pilomatrixoma: a common, benign childhood skin tumor. Can J Surg. 1994;37:483–6.
18. Colver GB, Buxton PK. Pilomatrixoma an elusive diagnosis. Int J Dermatol. 1988;27:177–8.
19. Kumaran N, Azmy A, Carachi R, Rainie PAM, Macfarlane JH, Howatson AG. Pilomatrixoma—accuracy of clinical diagnosis. J Pediatr Surg. 2006;41:1755–8.
20. Graham JL, Merwin CF. The tent sign of pilomatricoma. Cutis. 1978;22(5):577–80.
21. Bansal C, Handa U, Mohan H. Fine needle aspiration cytology of pilomatrixoma. J Cytol. 2011;28:1–6.
22. Sanyal S, Monickam A, Komala G, Verma SK. Fine needle aspiration cytology of pilomatrixoma. J Cytol. 2004;21:109–10.
23. Ma KF, Tsui MS, Chan SK. Fine-needle aspiration diagnosis of pilomatrixoma: a monomorphic population of basaloid cells with squamous differentiation not to be mistaken for carcinoma. Acta Cytol. 1991;35:570–4.
24. Geh JLC, Moss ALH. Multiple pilomatrixomata and myotonic dystrophy: a familial association. Br J Plast Surg. 1999;52:143–5.
25. Sherrod QJ, Chiu MW, Gutierrez MA. Multiple pilomatricomas: cutaneous marker for myotonic dystrophy. Dermatol Online J. 2008;14:22.
26. Trufant J, Kurz W, Frankel A, Muthusamy V, McKinnon W, Greenblatt M, Lazar A, Cook D, Bosenberg M. Familial multiple pilomatrixomas as a presentation of adenomatous polyposis coli. J Cutan Pathol. 2012;39:440–3.
27. Brander MD, Bunkis J. Pilomatrixoma presenting as a parotid mass. Plast Reconstr Surg. 1986;78:518–21.
28. Duflo S, Nicollas R, Roman S, Roman M, Triglia JM. Pilomatrixoma of the head and neck in children: a study of 38 cases and a review of the literature. Arch Otolaryngol Head Neck Surg. 1998;124:1239–42.
29. Demircan M, Balik E. Pilomatricoma in children: a prospective study. Pediatr Dermatolog. 1997;14:430–2.
30. Lopansi S, Mihm MC Jr. Pilomatrix carcinoma or calcifying epitheliocarcinoma of Malherbe: a case report and review of literature. Cancer. 1980;45:2368–73.
31. Inglefield CJ, Muir IF, Gray ES. Aggressive pilomatricoma in childhood. Ann Plast Surg. 1994;33:656–8.
32. Sasaki CT, Yue A, Enriques R. Giant calcifying epithelioma. Arch Otolaryngol. 1976;102:753–5.

Pituitary Region Tumors

36

Edward R. Smith

Introduction

There are numerous lesions which can present in the region of the pituitary gland in children. This chapter will focus on primary lesions of the pituitary gland including pituitary adenomas, Rathke's cleft cysts (RCC) and pars intermedia cysts. (Craniopharyngioma is covered in another chapter and pituitary carcinoma is extraordinarily rare in children.) Hormonally active adenomas can have effects far greater than might be expected from their size alone, while the developmental Rathke's and pars intermedia cysts often can be managed expectantly.

Key Points

- Pituitary tumors are rare in children, with the most common entity being a prolactinoma.
- Symptomatic lesions commonly present with hormonal dysfunction (growth arrest, pubertal delay), visual complaints (bitemporal hemianopsia, double vision from cavernous sinus injury), or headache.
- While asymptomatic lesions can often be managed with observation, with the exception of prolactinoma, most symptomatic pituitary region lesions are treated surgically.

Biology and Epidemiology

The etiology of pituitary adenomas remains uncertain, with most cases being apparently spontaneous. Adenomas are neoplastic lesions that can grow over time and are usually characterized by the cell of origin and capacity for hormone production [1–14].

RCCs are generally considered to be developmental lesions derived from embryonic remnants of Rathke's pouch, an invagination of the upper part of the roof of the nasopharynx. They are lined with squamous epithelium (which can secrete mucous) and can enlarge with mucous, serous, or—rarely—blood products (Fig. 36.1) [5].

Pars intermedia cysts are embryonic fluid-filled cavities between the adenohypophysis and neurohypophysis. They differ from RCC in not being derived from Rathke's pouch, not being lined with epithelium, and generally not enlarging over time [5, 6].

Pathophysiology

- All lesions of this region can cause symptoms by local mass effect, compressing the optic apparatus (classically causing a bitemporal hemianopsia), the hypothalamus (causing obesity), the third ventricle (causing hydrocephalus), or the cavernous sinus (causing injury to the cranial nerves with visual or pain complaints).
- Adenomas can cause symptoms by overexpression of specific hormones or—in larger lesions—impairment of glandular function by mass effect (commonly manifested as growth arrest or impaired sexual maturation).
- Rarely, pituitary lesions can present with apoplexy, although this is far less common in children than in adults.

Molecular/Genetic Pathology

Associations with multiple endocrine neoplasia type I (MEN-1), GSPT1, p53, and p16 have all been implicated in the development of adenomas, although the high rate of reported tumor incidence (0.3 %) suggests that a large number of factors may be involved in tumorigenesis [2, 7].

E. R. Smith (✉)
Department of Neurosurgery, Boston Children's Hospital, Harvard Medical School, Boston, MA, USA
e-mail: Edward.smith@childrens.harvard.edu

R. Rahbar et al. (eds.), *Pediatric Head and Neck Tumors*,
DOI 10.1007/978-1-4614-8755-5_36, © Springer Science+Business Media New York 2014

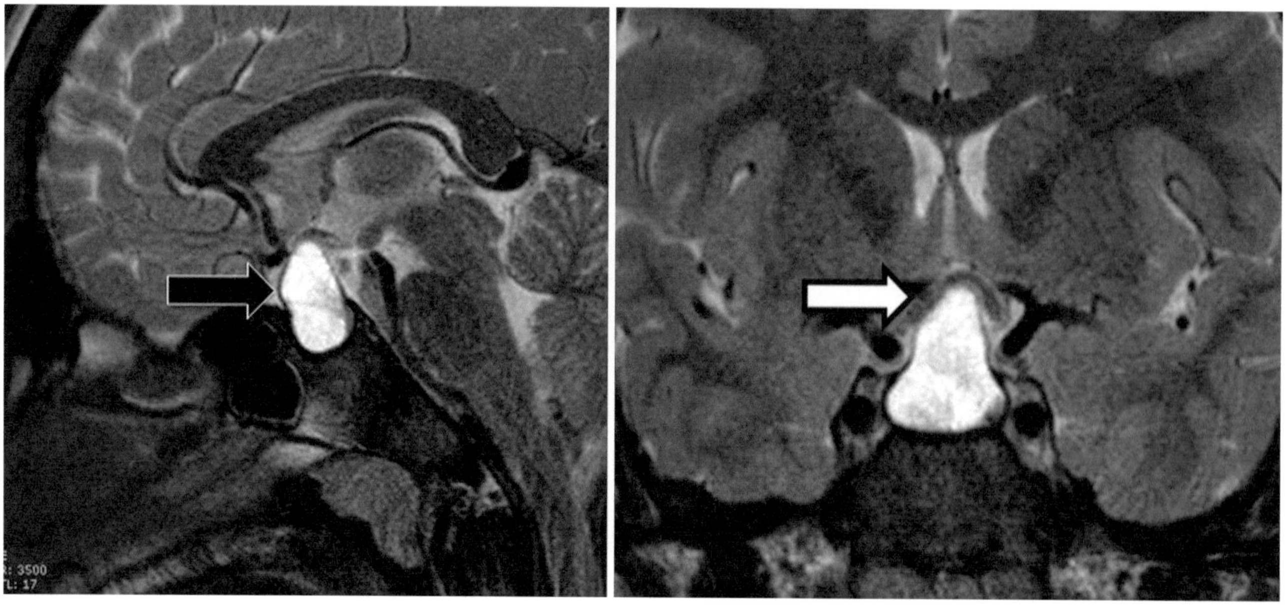

Fig. 36.1 Magnetic resonance imaging (MRI) appearance of Rathke's cleft cyst (RCC), with sagittal (**a**) and coronal (**b**) T2-weighted images. Note lesion rising out of sella (*black arrow*) and compressing optic chiasm (*white arrow*)

Incidence and Prevalence

Pituitary adenomas are <5 % of pediatric brain tumors [1, 4].

Up to 10 % of all individuals will have occult pituitary lesions [8, 9].

Secretory adenomas that produce growth hormone (GH) and adrenocorticotropic hormone (ACTH) are most common in preadolescent children, while prolactin-secreting adenomas are most common in older children (and are also the most common overall, at nearly 50 %, of all adenomas in children).

Gonadotropin- and thyrotropin-secreting tumors are extremely rare at <1 % [1, 10].

RCCs are found in up to 25 % of all adults, implying a similar number in children [6].

Age Distribution

GH-producing adenomas are most common in infants, while all other adenomas tend to present across all ages, with some reports suggesting an increased detection (up to 66 % of all adenomas) during teen years [4].

ACTH-secreting tumors are most commonly seen in young children and prolactinomas are the most common tumors in teens [3, 4].

Sex Predilection

- Females more commonly present with adenomas (3:1) than males in the pediatric population, except for ACTH-secreting tumors, which are found predominantly in males (2:1) [10, 11].

Geographic Distribution

- None

Risk Factors—Environmental, Life Style

- None

Relationships to Other Disease States, Syndromes

MEN-1 has been associated with adenomas, although it remains extremely rare in children.

RCCs are often found in association with adenomas, although some have suggested that this is a "bystander" effect, in which a symptomatic adenoma is what prompts imaging, and then an incidental finding of a RCC is noted (given the high incidence in the general population of RCC at about 25 %, see above).

Presentation

In general, lesions of this region are either found incidentally or present in one of three ways. These include:

- Visual loss (usually bitemporal hemianopsia from chiasmal compression)
- Endocrine or hypothalamic dysfunction (from tumoral hormone production or injury to the hypothalamus)
- Symptoms of mass effect in the sellar region (headache, hydrocephalus, and dysfunction of the cranial nerves in the cavernous sinus leading to double vision or facial pain)

Differential Diagnosis

The differential diagnosis of lesions in the pituitary region in children include:

- Adenoma
- RCC
- Pars intermedia cyst
- Craniopharyngioma
- Germinoma/nongerminomatous germ cell tumors
- Optic pathway tumor
- Lipoma
- Dermoid/epidermoid
- Arachnoid cyst/encephalocoele
- Lymphocytic hypophysitis/infection (tuberculosis)
- Aneurysm

Diagnosis and Evaluation

Physical Examination and History

Symptoms

Hormonal symptoms often include growth arrest (especially in younger children, and especially with Cushing's disease—oversecretion of ACTH), pubertal delay (including amenorrhea and menstrual irregularity which can be due to either primary hypogonadism or secondary to hyperprolactinemia), and galactorrhea (prolactinoma). Cushing's disease can result in obesity, hirsutism, fatigue, and acne.

Headache is variable in patients, but an association with RCC has been reported.

Visual loss is often a bitemporal hemianopsia, although acute, severe loss of all vision can occur in the extremely rare entity of apoplexy [12].

Diabetes insipidus (DI) is extremely rare (except in the setting of nongerminomatous germ cell tumors.)

- *Prolactinoma*—pubertal delay, menstrual irregularities, galactorrhea, gynecomastia
- *ACTH-secreting (Cushing's disease)*—obesity, growth delay, menstrual irregularities, acne, hypertension (and rare psychiatric issues)
- *GH-secreting*—acromegaly, hypertension, gigantism (may be tall if prior to bone plate fusion, otherwise may have acromegalic facies and stature)

Patterns of Evolution

- Nearly all symptoms are subacute to chronic, presenting over a period of months to years.
- Apoplexy, however, can present over minutes to hours with extreme headache, vision loss, extraocular motor palsies and—in some cases—unconsciousness. However, apoplexy is vanishingly rare in children [12].

Evaluation at Presentation

- Visual fields and a dilated fundoscopic examination can be useful to assess for compression of the optic chiasm.
- Imaging and laboratory studies (see below).
- Consider referral to endocrinology.

Laboratory Data

- Endocrine panel—serum prolactin (PRL), cortisol, ACTH, insulin-like growth factor-1 (IGF-1), lutenizing hormone (LH), follicle stimulating hormone (FSH), thyroid stimulating hormone (TSH), free T4, GH, glucose, sodium, alpha-feto protein (AFP), and quantitative human chorionic gonadotrophin (hCG). Urine 24 h cortisol levels should be evaluated as well.
- In rare cases, inferior petrosal sinus sampling with transvenous catheterization can be useful to attempt to identify and localize ACTH-secreting tumors. However, this is a difficult technique and generally should be reserved for select cases.
- Decadron can be used to perform high- and low-dose cortisol suppression testing to distinguish between central (Cushing's disease) and peripheral (ectopic) sources of elevated cortisol. The administration of low-dose decadron will *not* suppress adenoma-related hypercortisolemia, but high doses *will* suppress pituitary-related hypercortisolemia (but will *not* suppress ectopic (nonpituitary) cortisol sources).
- Glucose testing can be done to detect the presence of a GH secreting tumor. Oral glucose is administered and serum GH levels checked 1–2 h afterwards. In healthy individuals, there is a normal suppression of GH levels to less than 5 ng/ml. In children with GH-secreting tumors, the levels will remain above 5 ng/ml and may actually increase to > 10 ng/ml.

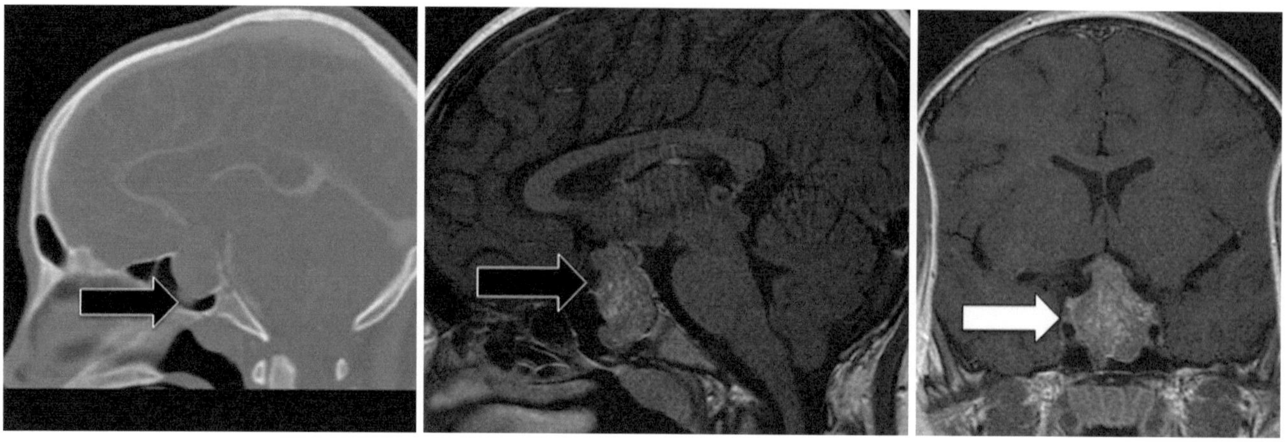

Fig. 36.2 Radiographic appearance of pituitary macroadenoma. **a** Sagittal CT demonstrates erosion of bone at base of lesion into the sphenoid sinus (*black arrow*). **b** Same lesion seen on sagittal T1-weighted MRI with gadolinium; note patchy enhancement of lesion (*black arrow*). **c** On coronal image, note involvement of tumor into cavernous sinus and around carotid artery (*white arrow*)

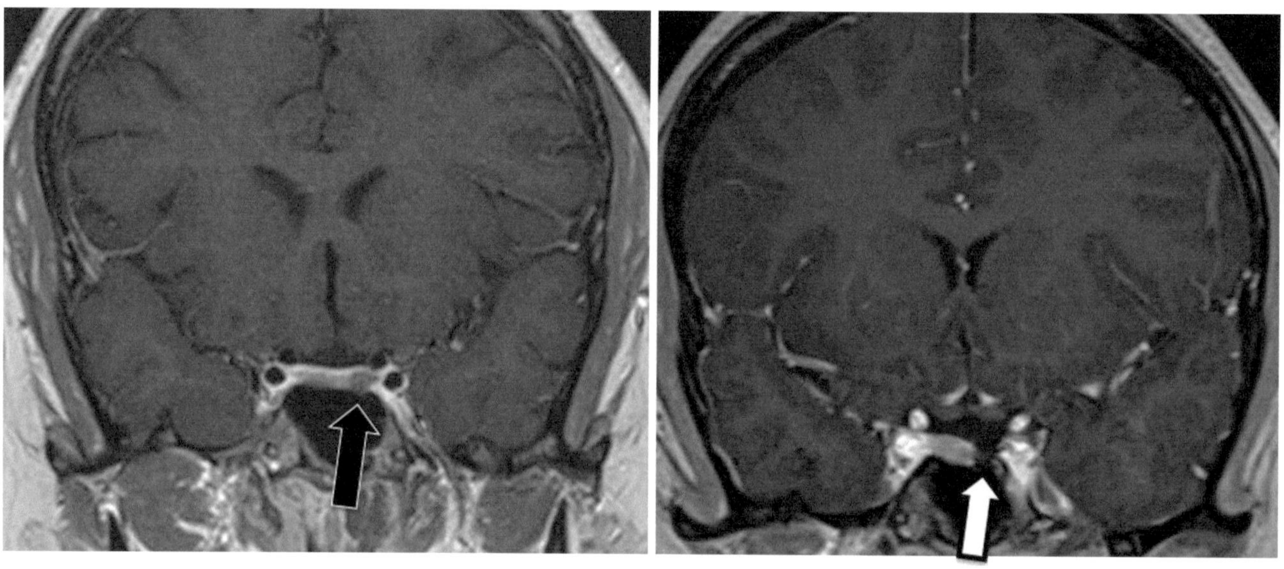

Fig. 36.3 Pituitary microadenoma (ACTH-producing). **a** Preoperative coronal T1-weighted MRI with gadolinium reveals nonenhancing left-sided pituitary lesion (*black arrow*). **b** Postoperative image shows resection cavity (*white arrow*)

Imaging Evaluation

- MRI of the brain with and without gadolinium, with thin cuts through the sella turcica in the coronal and sagittal planes. Macroadenomas (>1 cm), prolactinomas, and GH-secreting tumors are often well-visualized, while ACTH-secreting tumors are far more difficult to find (being nonvisualized in up to 50 % of cases) (Figs. 36.2 and 36.3) [11, 13].
- If the question of craniopharyngioma is raised, computerized tomography (CT) can be useful to identify the presence of calcium (often found with craniopharyngiomas in children). CT can also be useful for surgical planning, particularly if a transsphenoidal approach is being considered.
- Careful attention to surrounding structures, such as pneumatization of the sphenoid sinus, size and anatomy of the carotid arteries/cavernous sinus, and relationship to the optic nerves should be addressed.

Pathology

Adenomas are benign lesions, with almost no cases of carcinoma reported in children. Diagnosis is made based on immunohistochemistry identifying specific hormonal

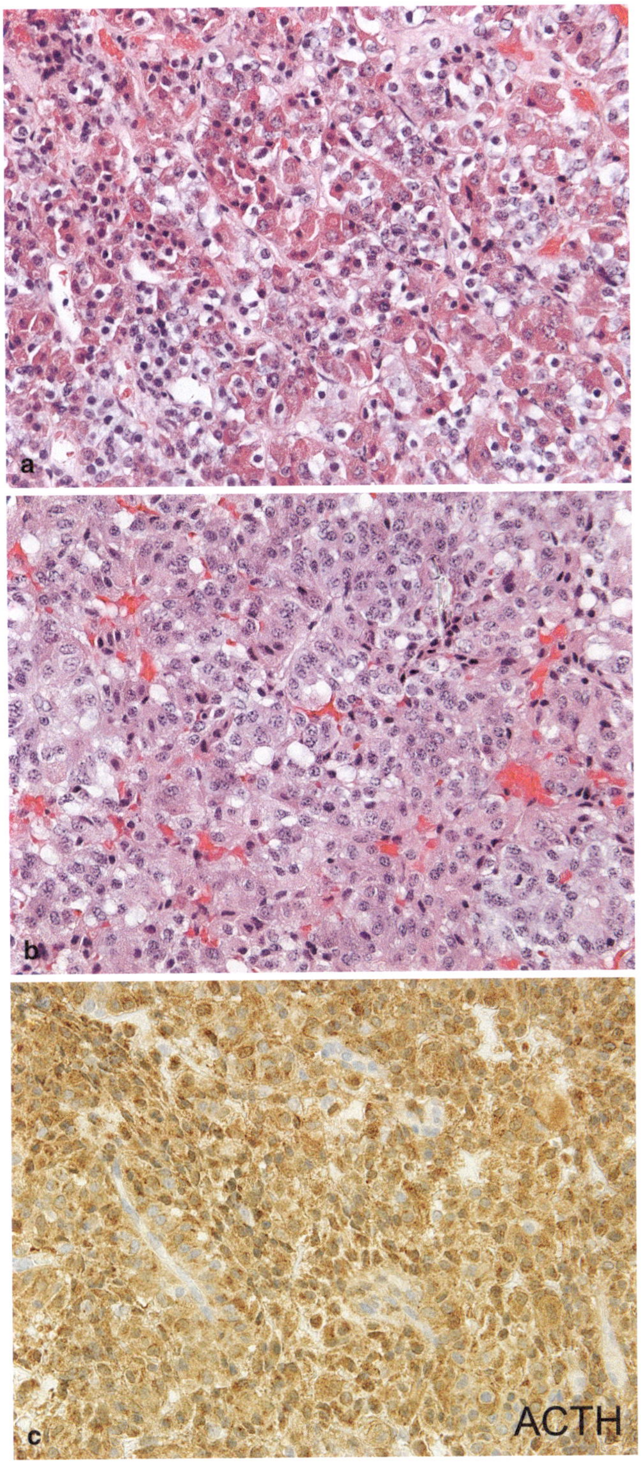

Fig. 36.4 Pituitary adenoma. **a** Normal anterior pituitary gland composed of a mixture of acidophilic, basophilic, and chromophobe cells. **b** Classical basophil adenoma of Cushing's disease composed of uniform basophilic cells. There is no significant pleomorphism or mitoses. **c** Tumor cells have diffuse cytoplasmic immunoreactivity for ACTH

species. Of interest, some studies have suggested that up to 29 % of pediatric pituitary adenomas may be plurihormonal (Fig. 36.4) [3, 4].

RCC are epithelial-lined lesions of presumed embryonic origin, as contrasted to pars intermedia cysts, which occupy the same location between the anterior and posterior gland, but lack an epithelial lining [6].

Treatment

Goal To prevent mass effect on neural structures (especially the optic apparatus) and to obviate hormonal symptoms (if present). In rare cases of RCC, treatment may be predicated on reduction in headache symptoms. It is important to note that many pituitary lesions do not require any treatment.

The majority of lesions will be managed either with observation or with surgical resection. However, an important exception is the prolactinoma, for which the first line of therapy is usually medical management.

In the surgical management of RCC, it is often possible to alleviate the symptoms by partial excision and marsupialization of the base of the cyst into the sphenoid sinus, without needing to perform a total resection (which can increase the risk of glandular injury) [14, 15].

Medical therapy

In the case of the symptomatic prolactinoma (or lesions with serum PRL levels greater than 200 ng/ml), the primary treatment is medical. Typically, a dopamine agonist, such as bromocriptine (or an analog), is used. Effectiveness is measured by following serum PRL levels and with serial imaging. Typically, medical therapy is indefinite in length, but effective in up to 90 % of cases. Surgical therapy is limited to nonresponders or individuals unable to tolerate side effects of medical therapy. It is worth noting that medical treatment of macroadenomas with skull base erosion can result in problematic cerebrospinal fluid (CSF) leaks, as the tumor regresses and exposes defects in the bone.

Medical therapy may also be indicated for GH-secreting tumors that do not respond to surgical resection. Somatostatin analogs are commonly used for these tumors.

Surgical Therapy

Timing If a child presents with symptoms of increased intracranial pressure (ICP) or acute visual loss in the rare case of apoplexy, then urgent operation may be necessary. However, this is the exception rather than the norm, and most pituitary cases can be scheduled electively.

For nearly all pituitary lesions, transsphenoidal surgery is used for resection of the lesion. Surgery is the first-line therapy for ACTH and GH-secreting tumors, for RCCs with

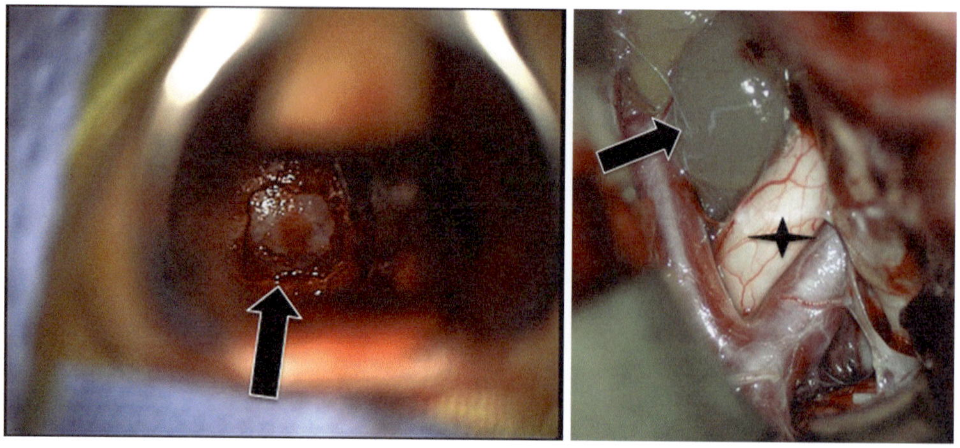

Fig. 36.5 Operative images of pituitary lesions. **a** Typical transphenoidal view of exposed sella turcica with dural window (*black arrow*, dura not opened). **b** View of large RCC from right pterional craniotomy approach, showing lesion pushing through front of optic chiasm (*black arrow*) and displacing optic nerve (*black star*, internal carotid artery just below)

symptomatic mass effect, and for refractory prolactinomas. While surgery has historically been microscope-based, recent advances in endoscopy have improved the efficacy and safety of transsphenoidal surgery in this population. However, in young children—particularly those in whom the sphenoid sinus is not yet pneumatized—transsphenoidal surgery may not be feasible and a craniotomy may be required for symptomatic adenomas. (Fig. 36.5)

Complications

- CSF leaks
- Injury to the carotid arteries
- Injury to the pituitary gland (including transient or permanent DI, panhypopituitarism)
- Infection
- Cranial nerve injury

It is critical to remember that patients with pituitary lesions may be deficient in their ability to mount a stress response to surgery and, as such, supplemental corticosteroids should be considered in all pituitary tumor cases.

Radiation Therapy

Radiation therapy is of markedly limited use in pituitary tumors, being restricted to refractory GH-secreting tumors (which have failed surgical and medical therapy), ACTH-secreting tumors, and almost no prolactinomas. There is no role for radiation in the treatment of RCC or pars intermedia cysts.

Outcomes

Outcomes for patients vary based on the type of lesions that they harbor.

- Prolactinomas are successfully treated in up to 90% of patients with medical therapy [1]. Success is measured by decrease in serum levels of hormone, radiographic evidence of tumor reduction, and symptomatic relief. Duration of therapy and cessation of treatment remain controversial. For patients who fail medical therapy, surgery can offer cure rates of up to 70%. However, larger tumors are harder to treat and in all cases, recurrence rates can be as high as one-third [10].
- Surgical management is the first choice for ACTH-secreting tumors and cures Cushing's disease in up to 76% of children in whom tumors are identified at operation [16]. This number increases to 90% when additional medical or radiation therapy is employed [13, 16]. However, recurrence can occur in up to 40% of cases and can be delayed by years. Recurrent cases can be very refractory to treatment and this type of tumor thus merits particular attention for aggressive treatment and careful long-term follow-up.
- GH-secreting tumors can be cured surgically, but have very poor success rates, with some groups reporting rates of less than 15% long-term control [17]. The option of medical treatment with somatostatin exists, with up to 50% success rates, but the drug is expensive and difficult to administer.
- RCCs have symptomatic improvement (in vision, endocrine issues, or headache) in about two-thirds of patients when carefully selected preoperatively [14, 15]. Recurrence rates in many series are high, sometimes approaching 50%.

Follow-up

- Postoperative care will frequently consist of an office visit approximately 1 month postoperatively, then annually thereafter. Radiation therapy also involves annual posttreatment visits.
- It is often useful to have coordination of follow-up with endocrinology and—in symptomatic patients—ophthalmology.
- An MRI/MRA at 6–12 weeks postoperatively may be helpful as a baseline study, to then be compared to subsequent annual MRI. Imaging is commonly performed annually for 5 years, if feasible.

- Serial laboratory studies (if in the setting of a hormonally active tumor) may be useful.

References

1. Haddad SF, VanGilder JC, Menezes AH. Pediatric pituitary tumors. Neurosurgery. 1991;29:509–14.
2. Jagannathan J, Kanter AS, Sheehan JP, Jane JA Jr, Laws ER Jr. Benign brain tumors: sellar/parasellar tumors. Neurol Clin. 2007;25:1231–49, xi.
3. Mindermann T, Wilson CB. Pituitary adenomas in childhood and adolescence. J Pediatr Endocrinol Metab. 1995;8:79–83.
4. Mindermann T, Wilson CB. Pediatric pituitary adenomas. Neurosurgery. 1995;36:259–68 (discussion 69).
5. Fager CA, Carter H. Intrasellar epithelial cysts. J Neurosurg. 1966;24:77–81.
6. Voelker JL, Campbell RL, Muller J. Clinical, radiographic, and pathological features of symptomatic Rathke's cleft cysts. J Neurosurg. 1991;74:535–44.
7. Levy A, Hall L, Yeudall WA, Lightman SL. p53 gene mutations in pituitary adenomas: rare events. Clin Endocrinol (Oxf). 1994;41:809–14.
8. Hall WA, Luciano MG, Doppman JL, Patronas NJ, Oldfield EH. Pituitary magnetic resonance imaging in normal human volunteers: occult adenomas in the general population. Ann Intern Med. 1994;120:817–20.
9. Vernooij MW, Ikram MA, Tanghe HL, et al. Incidental findings on brain MRI in the general population. N Engl J Med. 2007;357:1821–8.
10. Kane LA, Leinung MC, Scheithauer BW, et al. Pituitary adenomas in childhood and adolescence. J Clin Endocrinol Metab. 1994;79:1135–40.
11. Partington MD, Davis DH, Laws ER Jr, Scheithauer BW. Pituitary adenomas in childhood and adolescence. Results of transsphenoidal surgery. J Neurosurg. 1994;80:209–16.
12. Sugita S, Hirohata M, Tokutomi T, Yamashita M, Shigemori M. A case of pituitary apoplexy in a child. Surg Neurol. 1995;43:154–7.
13. Magiakou MA, Mastorakos G, Oldfield EH, et al. Cushing's syndrome in children and adolescents. Presentation, diagnosis, and therapy. N Engl J Med. 1994;331:629–36.
14. Cavallo LM, Prevedello D, Esposito F, et al. The role of the endoscope in the transsphenoidal management of cystic lesions of the sellar region. Neurosurg Rev. 2008;31:55–64 (discussion 64).
15. Frank G, Sciarretta V, Mazzatenta D, Farneti G, Modugno GC, Pasquini E. Transsphenoidal endoscopic approach in the treatment of Rathke's cleft cyst. Neurosurgery. 2005;56:124–8 (discussion 9).
16. Kanter AS, Diallo AO, Jane JA Jr, et al. Single-center experience with pediatric Cushing's disease. J Neurosurg. 2005;103:413–20.
17. Dyer EH, Civit T, Visot A, Delalande O, Derome P. Transsphenoidal surgery for pituitary adenomas in children. Neurosurgery. 1994;34:207–12 (discussion 12).

Retinoblastoma

37

Carlos Rodriguez-Galindo, Darren B. Orbach and Deborah Vanderveen

Introduction

Retinoblastoma is the most frequent neoplasm of the eye in childhood, and the third most common intraocular malignancy in all ages, following malignant melanoma and metastatic carcinoma, representing 2.5–4 % of all pediatric cancers. The average age-adjusted incidence rate of retinoblastoma in the United States and Europe is 2–5 per million children (approximately one in 14,000–18,000 live births) [1, 2]. Retinoblastoma is a cancer of the very young; two-thirds are diagnosed before 2 years of age, and 95 % before 5 years [1]. For these reasons, therapeutic approaches need to consider not only the cure of the disease, but also the need to preserve vision with minimal long-term side effects.

Retinoblastoma presents in two distinct clinical forms: (1) A bilateral or multifocal, heritable form (25 % of all cases), characterized by the presence of germ line mutations of the *RB1* gene. Multifocal retinoblastoma may be inherited from an affected survivor (25 %) or be the result of a new germ line mutation (75 %); and (2) a unilateral or unifocal form (75 % of all cases), 90 % of which are nonhereditary. About 10 % of germ line cases are unilateral; in the absence of a positive family history, however, it is not possible without genetic screening to determine which unilateral cases are capable of being transmitted to the next generation.

Key Points

- Retinoblastoma is the most common cancer of the eye in children, accounting for 3 % of all childhood malignancies.
- Retinoblastoma affects very young children: two-thirds of the cases are diagnosed before 2 years of age, and more than 90 % before 5 years.
- Two clinical forms are identified: (1) Unilateral retinoblastoma, which accounts for approximately 75 % of the cases, and (2) bilateral retinoblastoma, which accounts for 25 % of the cases. Patients with bilateral disease carry a germ line mutation of the *RB1* gene; this mutation is inherited from an affected parent in 25 % of the cases, and results from a de novo mutation in utero in 75 % of the cases.
- Treatment of retinoblastoma is risk-adapted. Factors to be considered in the treatment decisions include intraocular and extraocular stage, laterality, and potential for vision.
- Ocular salvage treatments include systemic or intra-arterial chemotherapy, aggressive focal treatments (photocoagulation, thermotherapy, cryotherapy, and brachytherapy) and external-beam radiation therapy.
- Children with bilateral disease are at very high risk of developing second malignancies and therefore need to be followed closely. Radiation therapy is avoided whenever possible in this group of children.

Biology and Epidemiology

The incidence of retinoblastoma is not distributed equally around the world. It appears to be higher (6–10 cases per million children) in Africa, India, and among children of native American descent in the North American continent. The increased incidence in those groups occurs primarily in unilateral cases. Whether these geographical variations are due to ethnic or socio-economic factors is not well known. However, the fact that even in industrialized countries an

C. Rodriguez-Galindo (✉)
Department of Pediatric Oncology, Dana-Farber/Boston Children's Hospital Cancer and Blood Disorders Center, Harvard Medical School, Boston, MA, USA
e-mail: carlos_rodriguez-galindo@dfci.harvard.edu

D. B. Orbach
Interventional & Neurointerventional Radiology, Department of Radiology, Boston Children's Hospital, Harvard Medical School, Boston, MA, USA

D. Vanderveen
Boston Children's Hospital, Harvard Medical School, Boston, MA 02215, USA

R. Rahbar et al. (eds.), *Pediatric Head and Neck Tumors*,
DOI 10.1007/978-1-4614-8755-5_37, © Springer Science+Business Media New York 2014

increased incidence of retinoblastoma is associated with poverty and low levels of maternal education, suggests a role for the environment [3].

In recent years, studies have suggested a role for human papilloma viruses (HPV) in the pathogenesis of retinoblastoma. The viral oncoprotein E7 of high-risk HPV types has been shown to bind to and inactivate the *RB1* gene product (pRB). Therefore, it is plausible that HPV infection could be functionally equivalent to the biallelic loss of *RB1*. High-risk HPV sequences have been detected in 28–36% of tumors [4].

Biology

In 1971, based on the mathematical analysis of the age at presentation of bilateral (hereditary) and unilateral (mostly nonhereditary) cases of retinoblastoma, Knudson proposed the "two-hit hypothesis," in which two mutational events in a developing retinal cell lead to the development of retinoblastoma [5]. This hypothesis was subsequently extended to suggest that the two events could be mutations of both alleles of the *RB1* gene. *RB1,* located in chromosome 13q14, was identified and cloned in 1986 [6, 7]. Its product, pRb, is a key substrate for G1 cyclin-cdk complexes, which phosphorylate target gene products required for the transition of the cell through the G1 phase of the cell cycle. The active pRb functions as a tumor suppressor and stands as the major gatekeeper to control this critical point in growth regulation. The lack of pRb or its inactivation will remove the pRb constraint on cell cycle control, with the consequence of deregulated cell proliferation. Bi-allelic loss of *RB1* function is required for tumor development; this loss is germ line and somatic for patients with bilateral disease, and somatic in a single cell in patients with unilateral disease. However, additional events may be required for tumor progression. Approximately two-thirds of tumors have *MDM4/MDM2* amplification leading to inactivation of the *p53* pathway [8]. Other genes and pathways are probably also involved; studies using comparative genomic hybridization have consistently shown chromosomal gains and amplifications at 6p and 1q, and losses at 16q1. Finally, a very small proportion of tumors appear to develop in the context of normal *RB1;* amplification of *N-MYC* has been described in those cases [9].

Prevention, Early Detection, and Genetic Counseling

The successful management of retinoblastoma depends on the ability to detect the disease while it is still intraocular; disease stage correlates with delay in diagnosis [10]. In developing countries, late referrals are strongly associated with orbital and metastatic disease [11]. It is for this reason

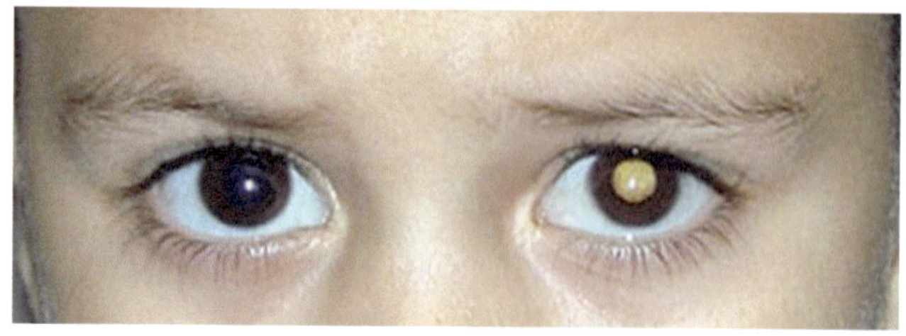

Fig. 37.1 3-year-old boy presenting with left leukocoria

that eye assessment should be performed in all newborns and at all subsequent health supervision visits by the primary care provider. Mass screening is also being considered, especially where the tumor is common, such as areas of South America and Asia. Retinoblastoma is a unique neoplasm, in that the genetic form imparts a predisposition to developing tumor in an autosomal dominant fashion with almost complete penetrance (85–95%) [12]. The majority of such children acquire the first mutation as a new germ line mutation, with only 15–25% having a positive family history. Genetic counseling is of the utmost importance to assist parents in understanding the genetic consequences of each form of retinoblastoma and to estimate the risk in relatives. Regardless of the clinical presentation, it is recommended that all patients undergo genetic testing. With the refinement in methods of mutational analysis over the last decade, detection rates have increased to greater than 90% at present [13].

Clinical Manifestations, Patient Evaluation, and Staging

Retinoblastoma is by definition a tumor of the young child, and the age at presentation correlates with laterality. Patients with bilateral retinoblastoma tend to present at a younger age (usually before 1 year of age) than patients with unilateral disease (often in the second or third year of life) [12, 14]. In more than half of the cases, the presenting sign is leukocoria, which is occasionally first noticed after a flash photograph (Fig. 37.1). Strabismus is the second most common presenting sign, and usually correlates with macular involvement. Very advanced intraocular tumors may become painful as a result in secondary glaucoma. Differential diagnosis must be made from other childhood diseases that can present with leukocoria, such as persistent hyperplastic primary vitreous, retrolental fibrodysplasia, Coat's disease, congenital cataracts, toxicariasis, and toxoplasmosis.

A small proportion of patients with bilateral disease (5–6%) carry a deletion involving the 13q14 locus, which is large enough to be detected by karyotype analysis. In those cases, retinoblastoma is part of a more complex syndrome resulting from the loss of additional genetic material.

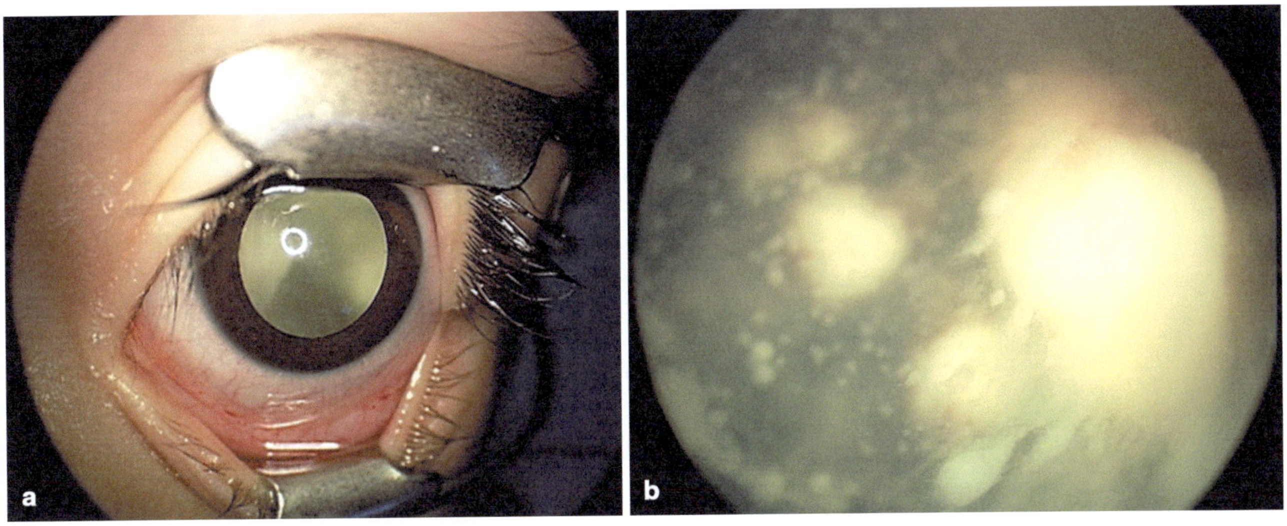

Fig. 37.2 Examination under anesthesia for retinoblastoma. Maximally dilated pupil shows a mass in the posterior chamber (**a**), closer examination reveals a large endophytic mass with massive vitreous seeding (**b**)

Patients with the "13q- syndrome" are characterized by typical facial dysmorphic features, subtle skeletal abnormalities, and different degrees of mental retardation and motor impairment [15]. Dysmorphic features more consistently found include thick anteverted ear lobes, high and broad forehead, prominent philtrum, and short nose. A proportion of patients also have overlapping fingers and toes, microcephaly, and delayed skeletal maturation.

Trilateral retinoblastoma refers to the association of bilateral retinoblastoma with an asynchronous intracranial tumor, which occurs in less than 10% of bilateral cases [16]. Tumors comprising trilateral retinoblastoma are primitive neuroectodermal tumors (PNETs) exhibiting varying degrees of neuronal or photoreceptor differentiation, suggesting an origin from the germinal layer of primitive cells. The majority of these tumors are pineal region PNETs (pineoblastomas), but in 20–25% of the cases, the tumors are suprasellar or parasellar. The median age at diagnosis of trilateral retinoblastoma is 23–48 months and the interval between the diagnosis of bilateral retinoblastoma and the diagnosis of the brain tumor is usually more than 20 months [17]. Approximately 5% of patients with bilateral disease develop pineal cysts; these appear to be a forme fruste of trilateral retinoblastoma [18].

The diagnosis of intraocular retinoblastoma is usually made without pathologic confirmation. An examination under anesthesia with a maximally dilated pupil and scleral indentation is required to examine the entire retina (Fig. 37.2). Endophytic tumors are those that grow inward to the vitreous cavity. Because of its friability, endophytic retinoblastoma may seed the vitreous cavity. Exophytic retinoblastoma grows into the subretinal space, thus causing progressive retinal detachment and subretinal seeding. A very detailed documentation of the number, location, and size of tumors, the presence of retinal detachment and subretinal fluid, and the presence of vitreous and subretinal seeds must be performed. Wide-angle real-time retinal imaging systems such as RetCam® provide a 130° field of view and digital recording, facilitating diagnosis and monitoring.

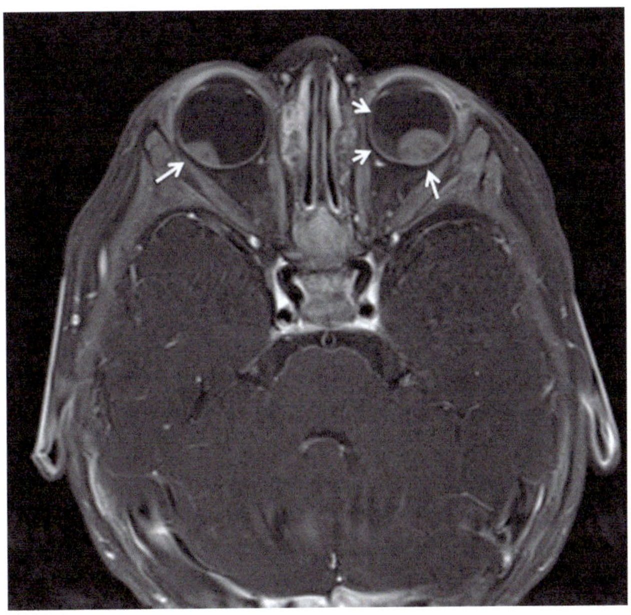

Fig. 37.3 Axial T1 MRI image showing bilateral intraocular masses in an 8-month-old infant with retinoblastoma (*arrows*)

Additional imaging studies that aid in the diagnosis include bi-dimensional ultrasound, computerized tomography (CT) and magnetic resonance imaging (MRI). These imaging studies are particularly important to evaluate extraocular extension and to differentiate retinoblastoma from other causes of leukocoria (Fig. 37.3). Evaluation for the presence of metastatic disease also needs to be considered in a sub-

Table 37.1 R-E grouping for suitability for treatment of retinoblastoma by radiation therapy

Group I. very favorable		
	Ia	Solitary tumor smaller than 4 dd at or behind the equator
	Ib	Multiple tumors, none larger than 4 dd, all at or behind equator
Group II. favorable		
	IIa	Solitary tumor 4–10 dd
	IIb	Multiple tumors 4–10 dd
Group III. doubtful		
	IIIa	Any lesion anterior to equator
	IIIb	Solitary tumor larger than 10 dd behind equator
Group IV. unfavorable		
	IVa	Multiple tumors, some larger than 10 dd
	IVb	Any lesion extending anteriorly to the ora serrata
Group V. very unfavorable		
	Va	Massive tumors involving more than half the retina
	Vb	Vitreous seeding

dd disk diameter (1.5 mm)

group of patients. Metastatic disease occurs in approximately 10–15% of patients, and it usually occurs in association with distinct intraocular histological features, such as deep choroidal and scleral invasion, or with involvement of the iris or ciliary body and optic nerve beyond the lamina cribrosa. In these cases, additional staging procedures, including bone scintigraphy, bone marrow aspirates and biopsies, and lumbar puncture, must be performed.

The Reese-Ellsworth (R-E) grouping system has been generally accepted as the standard for intraocular disease. This grouping system was initially designed to predict the outcome after external beam radiation therapy. It divides eyes into five groups on the basis of the size, location, and number of lesions, and on the presence of vitreous seeding (Table 37.1) [19]. However, developments in the conservative management of intraocular retinoblastoma have made the R-E grouping system less predictable of eye salvage, and less helpful in guiding treatment. A new staging system (International Classification of Retinoblastoma) has been developed, with the goal of providing a simpler, more user-friendly classification more applicable to current therapies. This new system is based on extent of tumor seeding within the vitreous cavity and subretinal space, rather than on tumor size and location, and seems to be a better predictor of treatment success (Fig. 37.4 and Table 37.2) [20].

For patients undergoing enucleation, pathologic staging that incorporates other features known to influence the modality of treatment and the prognosis, such as choroidal and scleral involvement, optic nerve extension and presence of metastatic disease are used. A newly proposed staging system developed by an international consortium of ophthalmologists and pediatric oncologists incorporates the most important elements of the older systems (Table 37.3) [21]. Growth and invasion occur as a sequence of events, and extraretinal extension occurs only once the tumor has reached large intraocular dimensions. As part of this process, retinoblastoma extends into the ocular coats (choroids and sclera), the optic nerve, and the anterior segment. Extraocular disease is the next step in this progression; locoregional dissemination occurs by direct extension through the sclera into the orbital contents and preauricular lymph nodes, and extraorbital disease manifests as intracranial dissemination and hematogenous metastases.

Pathology and Pathways of Spread

Macroscopically, retinoblastoma is soft and friable, and it tends to outgrow its blood supply, with resulting necrosis and calcification. Because of its friability, dissemination within the vitreous and retina in the form of small, white nodules (seeds) is common (Fig. 37.2b) [22]. Microscopically, the appearance of retinoblastoma depends on the degree of differentiation. Undifferentiated retinoblastoma is composed of small, round, densely packed cells with hypochromatic nuclei and scant cytoplasm. Several degrees of photoreceptor differentiation have been described and are characterized by distinctive arrangements of tumor cells. The Homer-Wright rosettes are composed of irregular circlets of tumor cells arranged around a tangle of fibrils with no lumen or internal limiting membrane. They are infrequently seen in retinoblastoma and are most often seen in other neuroblastic tumors such as neuroblastoma and medulloblastoma. The Flexner-Wintersteiner rosettes, on the other hand, are specific for retinoblastoma. These structures consist of a cluster of low columnar cells arranged around a central lumen that is bounded by an eosinophilic membrane analogous to the external membrane of the normal retina. These rosettes are seen in 70% of tumors. The fleurettes are less often seen. In this case, the cells exhibit even more ultrastructural characteristics of photoreceptor differentiation. They are composed of larger cells with abundant eosinophilic cytoplasm arranged in a distinctive fleur-de-lis pattern. Especially well-differentiated tumors composed almost entirely of fleurettes have been called retinomas or retinocytomas. Ultrastructurally, retinoblastoma cells also demonstrate photoreceptor differentiation with the presence of the 9-0 microtubule doublet pattern, abundant cytoplasmic microtubules, synaptic ribbons, and neurosecretory granules. The typical macroscopic and microscopic characteristics of retinoblastoma are depicted in Fig. 37.5.

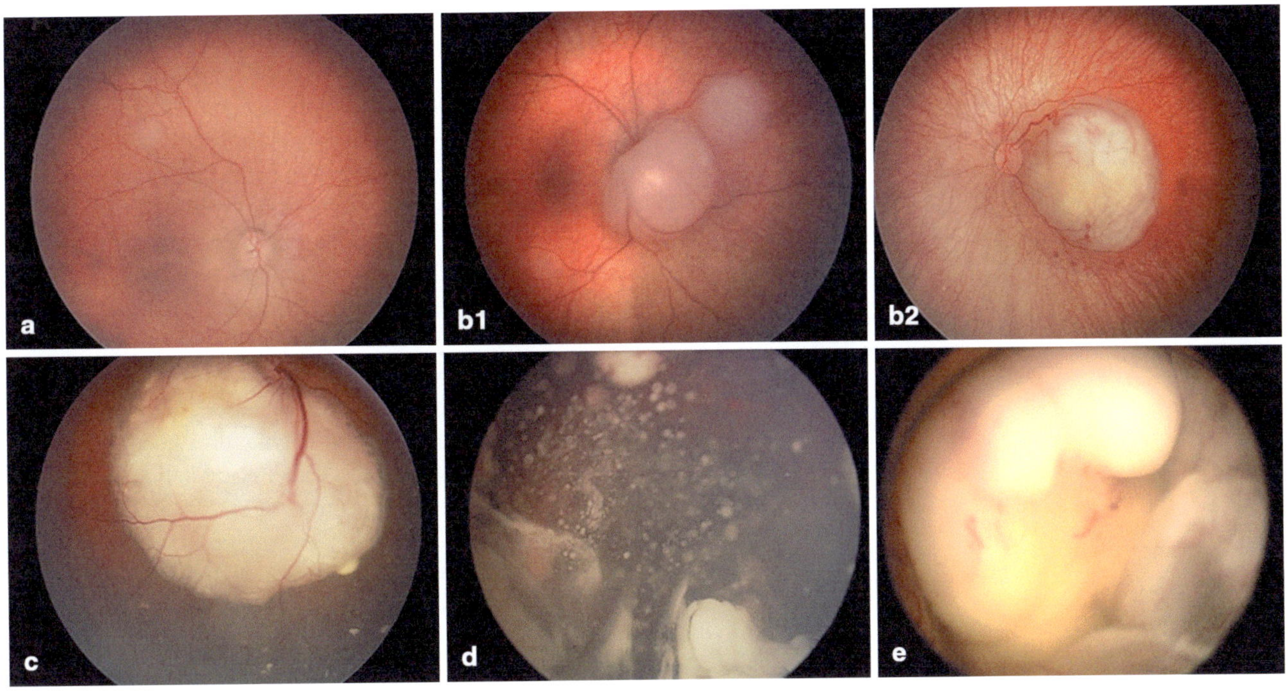

Fig. 37.4 International Classification for Intraocular Retinoblastoma. **a** Small tumor confined to the retina and distant from the foveola and the optic nerve (Group A). **b1** Two small tumors confined to the retina but adjacent to the optic nerve (Group B). **b2** Tumor with small amount of subretinal fluid and no subretinal seeding (Group B). **c** Exophytic retinoblastoma with subretinal fluid and seeding (Group C). **d** Endophytic retinoblastoma with massive vitreous seeding (Group D). **e** Large retinoblastoma filling more than two-thirds of the globe (Group E)

Table 37.2 International Classification for Intraocular Retinoblastoma

Group A
Small tumors away from foveola and disc
Tumors ≤ 3 mm in greatest dimension confined to the retina, and
Located at least 3 mm from the foveola and 1.5 mm from the optic disc
Group B
All remaining tumors confined to the retina
All other tumors confined to the retina not in Group A
Subretinal fluid (without subretinal seeding) ≤ 3 mm from the base of the tumor
Group C
Local subretinal fluid or seeding
Local subretinal fluid alone > 3 to ≤ 6 mm from the tumor
Vitreous seeding or subretinal seeding ≤ 3 mm from the tumor
Group D
Diffuse subretinal fluid or seeding
Subretinal fluid alone > 6 mm from the tumor
Vitreous seeding or subretinal seeding > 3 mm from tumor
Group E
Presence of any or more of these poor prognosis features
More than 2/3 globe filled with tumor
Tumor in anterior segment
Tumor in or on the ciliary body
Iris neovascularization
Neovascular glaucoma
Opaque media from hemorrhage
Tumor necrosis with aseptic orbital cellulitis
Phthisis bulbi

Table 37.3 International retinoblastoma staging system

Stage 0	Patients treated conservatively
Stage I	Eye enucleated, completely resected histologically
Stage II	Eye enucleated, microscopic residual tumor
Stage III	Regional extension
	a. Overt orbital disease
	b. Preauricular or cervical lymph node extension
Stage IV	Metastatic disease
	a. *Hematogenous metastasis* (without central nervous system (CNS) involvement)
	1. Single lesion
	2. Multiple lesions
	b. *CNS extension* (with or without any other site of regional or metastatic disease)
	1. Prechiasmatic lesion
	2. CNS mass
	3. Leptomeningeal and cerebral spinal fluid (CSF) disease

Principles of Treatment

Treatment of retinoblastoma aims to save life and preserve vision, and thus needs to be individualized. Factors that need to be considered include unilaterality or bilaterality of the disease, potential for preserving vision, intraocular and extraocular staging [23].

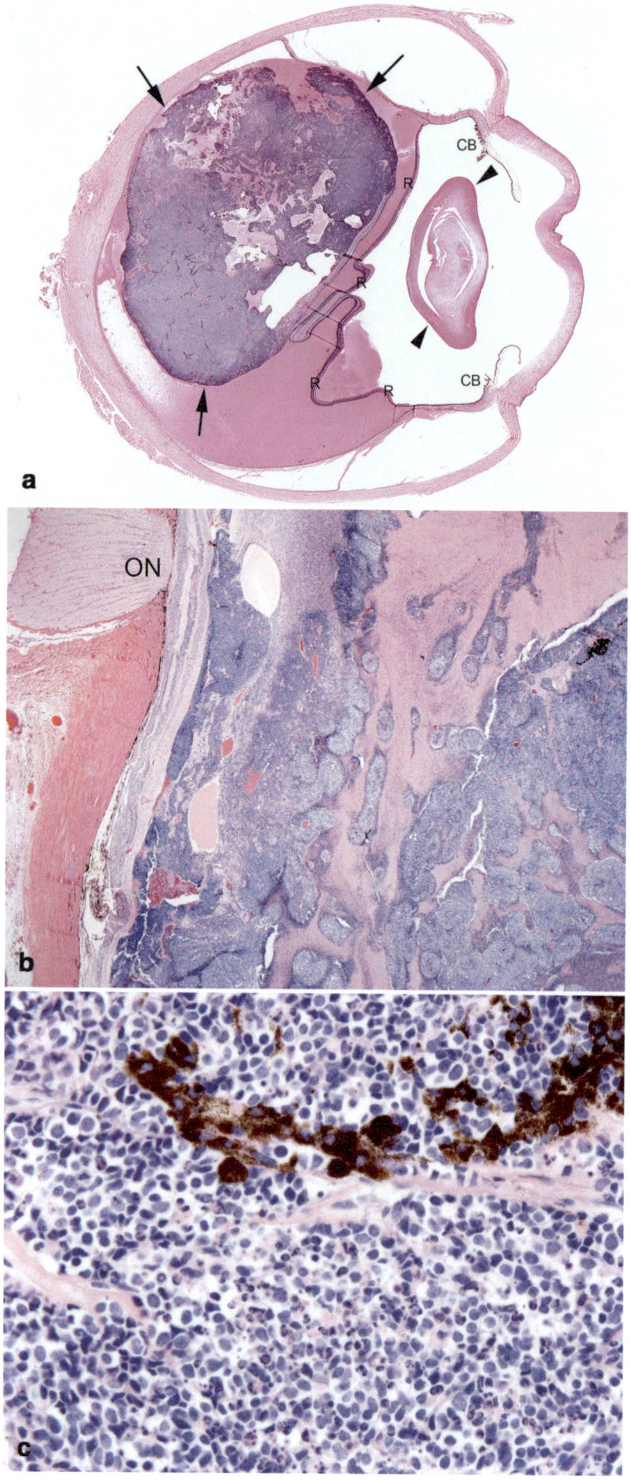

Fig. 37.5 Retinoblastoma. **a** Cut section of an enucleated eye with posteriorly located retinoblastoma (*between arrows*) detaching the retina (*R*). The lens is indicated by *arrowheads* and the ciliary bodies as *CB*. **b** Poorly differentiated retinoblastoma with areas of geographic necrosis. Optic nerve (*ON*). **c** Retinoblastoma composed of densely cellular small round cells with numerous apoptotic bodies. A cluster of dark-staining, melanin-laden cells are also observed

Surgery

Enucleation is indicated for large tumors filling the vitreous for which there is little or no likelihood of restoring vision, and in cases of tumor present in the anterior chamber or in the presence of neovascular glaucoma. Enucleation should be performed by an experienced ophthalmologist; the eye must be removed intact, without seeding the malignancy into the orbit and avoiding globe perforation [24]. For optimal staging, a long section (10–15 mm) of the optic nerve needs to be removed with the globe. An orbital implant is usually fitted during the same procedure, and the extraocular muscles are attached to it. A ceramic prosthetic eye is later fitted in the orbital socket. Orbital exenteration is very seldom indicated. For patients presenting with orbital disease, a judicious use of chemotherapy, surgery (enucleation), and radiation therapy will result in good tumor control, avoiding the need for orbital exenteration.

Focal Therapies

Focal treatments are used for small tumors (less than 3–6 mm), usually in patients with bilateral disease, and in combination with chemotherapy. *Photocoagulation* with Argon laser is used for the treatment of tumors situated at or posterior to the equator of the eye, and for the treatment of retinal neovascularization due to radiation therapy [25]. This technique is limited to tumors measuring no greater than 4.5 mm in base, and no greater than 2.5 mm in thickness. The treatment is directed to coagulate all blood supply to the tumor. *Cryotherapy* is used for the treatment of small equatorial and peripheral lesions, measuring no more than 3.5 mm in base and no more than 2 mm thickness [26]. One or two monthly sessions of triple freeze and thaw are performed, and tumor control rates are usually excellent. Finally, an important focal method is *transpupillary thermotherapy,* which applies focused heat at subphotocoagulation levels, usually with diode laser [27]. In thermotherapy, the goal is to deliver a temperature of 42–60 °C for 5–20 min to the tumor, sparing retinal vessels from photocoagulation. The use of focal treatments is especially important in conjunction with chemotherapy, and both treatment modalities appear to have a synergistic effect. In general, local control rates of 70–80 % can be achieved. Complications of focal treatments include transient serous retinal detachment, retinal traction and tears, and localized fibrosis.

Chemotherapy

Chemotherapy is indicated in patients with extraocular disease, in the subgroup of patients with intraocular disease with high-risk histological features, and in patients with bilateral disease in conjunction with aggressive focal therapies. Agents effective in the treatment of retinoblastoma include platinum compounds, etoposide, cyclophosphamide, doxorubicin, vincristine, and ifosfamide [23].

Radiotherapy

The goal of radiation therapy is to minimize integral dose to the patient to avoid the risk of complications: late normal tissue damage and second malignancies. The incidence of second malignancies in this patient population is very high even if radiation is not used. Radiation therapy can be delivered in form of brachytherapy or external beam radiation. Brachytherapy is used for the control of small tumors, usually in conjunction with other therapies; implants of radioactive material are placed in the form of episcleral plaques for a period of time to deliver high doses of radiation well focused to the tumor, sparing the normal structures. The majority of implants today use iodine-125 (^{125}I). Many other agents can be used such as gold, cobalt, palladium, ruthenium, and others [28–31]. External beam technique is used for treatment of the entire eye globe for ocular salvage, or for the management of extraocular disease to the orbit, CNS, or metastatic sites. Photons are commonly used; however, the use of proton therapy has significant advantages for patients with bilateral disease in terms of potentially lower risk of second malignancies [32].

Treatment of Intraocular Retinoblastoma

Unilateral Retinoblastoma

In the absence of extraocular disease, enucleation alone is curative for 85–90 % of children with unilateral retinoblastoma. The outcome for patients with unilateral disease that has been enucleated is excellent, with good functional results and minimal long-term effects [33]. In view of the apparent success in treating bilateral intraocular disease with chemoreduction, a conservative approach with chemotherapy and focal measures, is being increasingly used. With the use of intra-arterial chemotherapy, ocular salvage rates above 70–80 % can be achieved [34]. For patients undergoing enucleation, adjuvant treatment is indicated in those cases with scleral invasion and in patients with positive tumor at the transection line of the optic nerve. Adjuvant treatment for the remaining patients with intraocular disease is debatable. In the absence of randomized studies, available information would suggest that the use of adjuvant chemotherapy is beneficial for the selected group of patients with higher risk of extraocular dissemination (patients with concurrent retrolaminar and choroidal involvement, and possibly patients with massive choroidal involvement). Adjuvant chemotherapy is not indicated for patients with prelaminar involvement or isolated focal choroidal involvement [23]. Different chemotherapy regimens have been proposed. Six-month treatment with VDC (vincristine, cyclophosphamide, and doxorubicin), VCE (vincristine, carboplatin, and etoposide), or a hybrid with alternating courses of both regimens appear to be effective. Radiation therapy is only indicated when there is transscleral disease or involvement of the cut end of the optic nerve.

Bilateral Retinoblastoma

In the past, the treatment for patients with bilateral retinoblastoma has been enucleation of those eyes with advanced intraocular disease and no visual potential, and the use of external beam radiation therapy for the remaining eyes. However, there are several complications associated with radiation therapy. Irradiation of the orbit during a period of rapid growth results in a major decrease in orbital volume, resulting in midfacial deformities. More importantly, however, is the greatly increased risk for the development of a sarcoma within the radiation therapy field, compared to the underlying increased risk of secondary neoplasms in these predisposed individuals. This risk may be age-related and decreases as irradiation is delayed [35]. These concerns have resulted in the development of more conservative approaches. The treatment of patients with bilateral retinoblastoma now incorporates up-front chemotherapy, which is intended to achieve maximum chemoreduction of the intraocular tumor burden early in the treatment, followed by aggressive focal therapies. Chemoreduction coupled with intensive use of sequential focal therapies has resulted in an increase in the eye salvage rates and in a decrease (and delay) in the use of radiation therapy. Different chemotherapy combinations are used, although the best results are achieved with a combination of vincristine, carboplatin, and etoposide. For patients with early intraocular stages (R-E Groups I–III, International Group B), a less intensive regimen with vincristine and carboplatin alone appears to be effective [23]. Salvage rates for Group A and B eyes approache 100 % using these techniques. For patients with advanced intraocular tumors (Groups C and D), ocular salvage rates are not better than 50–70 %, and external beam radiation therapy is usually required [36]. However, the use of radiation therapy is usually delayed for several months, which allows for better orbital growth and a decrease in the risk of second malignancies.

Table 37.4 Recommended approach to the treatment of intraocular retinoblastoma

R-E group	ABC group	Treatment			
		Focal Tx	Intra-arterial chemotherapy	Systemic chemotherapy	Radiation
I–II	A	+	If PD	If PD	If PD
I–III	B	+	MEL 3–5 mg x 3–6 courses	VCR 0.05 mg/kg d 1 CBP 18.6 mg/kg d 1 X 2–6 courses	If PD
IV–V	C–D[a]	+	MEL 3–5 mg x 3–6 courses consider addition of second agent (TOP, CBP)	VCR 0.05 mg/kg d 1 CBP 14 mg/kg d 1, 2 ETO 6 mg/kg d 1, 2 X 6 courses	If PD consider early EBRT if massive vitreous seeding at completion of chemotherapy
V b	E	Enucleation			

PD progressive disease, *MEL* melphalan, *TOP* topotecan, *CBP* carboplatin, *VCR* vincristine, *ETO* etoposide, *EBRT* external beam radiation therapy

[a] Consider upfront enucleation if unilateral

Intravitreal and Intra-arterial Chemotherapy for Intraocular Retinoblastoma

Japanese investigators have pioneered the administration of intravitreal and intra-arterial melphalan for patients with advanced or recurrent intraocular retinoblastoma [37]. Clinical responses in patients with progressive retinoblastoma were obtained using intravitreal melphalan followed by hyperthermia [37]. Kaneko et al. initially reported the feasibility of injecting melphalan into the ipsilateral carotid artery, with documented efficacy [37]. The technique was later perfected by Mohri using a balloon catheter that allowed for selective injection into the ophthalmic artery [38]. More recently, Abramson et al. reported a variation of this technique that includes a direct cannulation of the ophthalmic artery using a microcatheter [39]. Using this approach, high ocular salvage rates can be achieved after the administration of 3–5 mg of intra-arterial melphalan, although other agents such as topotecan and carboplatin are also used [34, 39, 40]. The use of this new treatment modality is being progressively incorporated into the frontline of ocular salvage for intraocular retinoblastoma. Direct administration of melphalan into the vitreous is also a promising approach for cases with vitreous disease [41].

The approach to the ocular salvage management for intraocular retinoblastoma is summarized in Table 37.4.

Treatment of Extraocular Retinoblastoma

Extraocular dissemination of retinoblastoma bears a close relationship with the socio-economic conditions that result in delayed diagnosis and treatment. In Europe and the United States, fewer than 5 % of patients present with extraocular disease, in contrast to up to 40–80 % in less developed countries [42, 43]. Three patterns of extraocular disease have been recognized: (1) Locoregional dissemination, including orbital disease, tumor extending to the cut end of the optic nerve, and lymphatic spread to the preauricular lymph nodes; (2) CNS dissemination; and (3) metastatic retinoblastoma.

Orbital and Locoregional Retinoblastoma

Orbital retinoblastoma occurs as a result of progression of the tumor through the emissary vessels and sclera. For this reason, scleral disease is considered to be extraocular and should be treated as such. Orbital retinoblastoma is isolated in 60–70 % of cases; lymphatic, hematogenous, and CNS metastases occur in the remaining patients [44]. Treatment should include systemic chemotherapy and radiation therapy; with this approach, 60–85 % of patients can be cured. Since most recurrences occur in the CNS, regimens using drugs with well-documented CNS penetration are recommended. Different chemotherapy regimens have proven to be effective, including vincristine, cyclophosphamide, and doxorubicin, platinum- and epipodophyllotoxin-based regimens, or a combination of both [23]. For patients with macroscopic orbital disease, it is recommended that surgery is delayed until response to chemotherapy has been obtained (usually two or three courses of treatment). Enucleation should then be performed, and an additional four to six courses of chemotherapy administered. Local control should then be consolidated with orbital irradiation (40–45 Gy). Using this approach, orbital exenteration is not indicated [45]. Similar management should be followed for patients with scleral disease, including radiation therapy, although good outcomes without irradiation have also been reported [42]. Patients with isolated involvement of the optic nerve at the transection level should also receive similar systemic treatment, and irradiation should include the entire orbit (36 Gy) with 9–10 Gy boost to the chiasm (total 45–46 Gy). The preauricular and cervical lymph nodes should be explored carefully, since 20 % of patients with orbital retinoblastoma have lymphatic metastases [44]. Lymphatic dissemination does not carry a worse prognosis, provided that the involved lymph nodes are also irradiated.

Central Nervous System Disease

Intracranial dissemination occurs by direct extension through the optic nerve, and its prognosis is dismal [42, 45]. Treatment for these patients should include platinum-based intensive systemic chemotherapy and CNS directed therapy. Although intrathecal chemotherapy has been traditionally used, there is no preclinical or clinical evidence to support its use. Although the use of irradiation in these patients is controversial, responses have been observed with craniospinal irradiation, using 23.4–36 Gy to the entire craniospinal axis, and a boost to achieve up to 45 Gy to sites of measurable disease. Therapeutic intensification with high-dose, marrow-ablative chemotherapy and autologous hematopoietic progenitor cell rescue has been explored but its role is not yet clear [46, 47]. Despite the intensity of the treatment and the documented responses of the intracranial disease patients succumb to their disease, and survivors are anecdotal. These patients should be evaluated on protocols if possible.

(Extracranial) Metastatic Retinoblastoma

Hematogenous metastases may develop in the bones, bone marrow, and, less frequently, in the liver. Although long-term survivors have been reported with conventional chemotherapy, these cures should be considered anecdotal. In recent years, however, small series of patients have shown that metastatic retinoblastoma can be cured using high-dose, marrow-ablative chemotherapy and autologous hematopoietic progenitor cell rescue. The approach is similar to metastatic neuroblastoma; patients receive short and intensive induction regimens usually containing alkylating agents, anthracyclines, etoposide, and platinum compounds and are then consolidated with marrow-ablative chemotherapy and autologous hematopoietic cell rescue. Using this approach, the outcome appears to be excellent [47]. An interesting observation is that patients with distant (outside orbit and skull) bone metastases that show good response to induction chemotherapy may not require radiation therapy when treated with marrow-ablative chemotherapy.

Long-Term Effects of Retinoblastoma and Its Treatment

The cumulative incidence of second cancers in patients with germ line mutations of the *RB1* gene is greatly increased with the use and dose of radiation therapy, and this incidence is reported to increase steadily with age, to up to 40–60 % at 40–50 years of age, although a more recent study estimates a considerably lower risk [48, 49]. Patients with nonhereditary retinoblastoma are not inherently at an increased risk. Almost any neoplasm has been described in survivors of retinoblastoma and 60–70 % of the tumors occur in the head and neck areas [48, 49]. The most common second tumor is osteogenic sarcoma, arising both inside and outside the irradiation field, which accounts for approximately one-third of all cases of second cancers. Soft tissue sarcomas and melanomas are second in frequency, accounting for 20–25 % of cases. In recent years, it has become apparent that patients with hereditary retinoblastoma are also at risk of developing epithelial cancers late in adulthood [50]. Of those, lung cancer appears to be the most common.

Because their orbital growth is still in progress, children treated for retinoblastoma are at risk of functionally and cosmetically significant bony orbital abnormalities. These sequelae become evident by early adolescence, when orbital growth is largely complete, and results in the "hour-glass facial deformity." Both enucleation, which causes orbital contraction, and radiotherapy, which induces arrest of bone growth, adversely affect orbital growth. In children treated for bilateral retinoblastoma, the impact of enucleation in orbital development is not different from that of irradiation. However, final orbital volumes after enucleation correlate with the size of the prosthetic implant.

References

1. Young JL, Smith MA, Roffers SD, Liff JM, Bunin GR. Retinoblastoma. Bethesda: SEER; 1999. p. 73–8. (Monograph)
2. Parkin DM, Stiller CA, Draper GJ, Bieber CA. The international incidence of childhood cancer. Int J Cancer. 1988;42:511–20.
3. Bunin GR, Meadows AT, Emanuel BS, Buckley JD, Woods WG, Hammond GD. Pre- and postconception factors associated with sporadic heritable and nonheritable retinoblastoma. Cancer Res. 1989;49:5730–5.
4. Orjuela M, Ponce Castaneda V, Ridaura C, et al. Presence of human papilloma virus in tumor tissue from children with retinoblastoma: an alternative mechanism for tumor development. Clin Cancer Res. 2000;6(10):4010–6.
5. Knudson AG. Mutation and childhood cancer: a probabilistic model for the incidence of retinoblastoma. Proc Natl Acad Sci USA. 1971;68:820–3.
6. Lee WH, Bookstein R, Hong F, Young LJ, Shew JY, Lee EY. Human retinoblastoma susceptibility gene: cloning, identification, and sequence. Science. 1987;235(4794):1394–9.
7. Friend SH, Bernards R, Rogelj S, et al. A human DNA segment with properties of the gene that predisposes to retinoblastoma and osteosarcoma. Nature. 1986;323(6089):643–6.
8. Laurie NA, Donovan SL, Shih CS, et al. Inactivation of the p53 pathway in retinoblastoma. Nature. 2006;444(7115):61–6.
9. Rushlow DE, Mol BM, Kennett JY, et al. Characterisation of retinoblastomas without RB1 mutations: genomic, gene expression, and clinical studies. Lancet Oncology. 2013;14:327–34.
10. Goddard AG, Kingston JE, Hungerford JL. Delay in diagnosis of retinoblastoma: risk factors and treatment outcome. Br J Ophthalmol. 1999;83:1320–3.

11. Chantada GL, Qaddoumi I, Canturk S, et al. Strategies to manage retinoblastoma in developing countries. Pediatr Blood Cancer. 2011;56:341–8.
12. Draper GJ, Sanders BM, Brownhill PA, Hawkins MM. Patterns of risk of hereditary retinoblastoma and applications to genetic counselling. Br J Cancer. 1992;66(1):211–9.
13. Richter S, Vandezande K, Chen N, et al. Sensitive and efficient detection of RB1 gene mutations enhances care for families with retinoblastoma. Am J Hum Genet. 2003;72(2):253–69.
14. Abramson DH, Frank CM, Susman M, Whalen MP, Dunkel IJ, Boyd NW. Presenting signs of retinoblastoma. J Pediatr. 1998;132:505–8.
15. Baud O, Cormier-Daire V, Lyonnet S, Desjardins L, Turleau C, Doz F. Dysmorphic phenotype and neurological impairment in 22 retinoblastoma patients with constitutional cytogenetic 13q deletion. Clin Genet. 1999;55:478–82.
16. Holladay DA, Holladay A, Montebello JF, Redmond KP. Clinical presentation, treatment, and outcome of trilateral retinoblastoma. Cancer. 1991;67:710–5.
17. Kivel T. Trilateral retinoblastoma: a meta-analysis of hereditary retinoblastoma associated with primary ectopic intracranial retinoblastoma. J Clin Oncol. 1999;17(6):1829–37.
18. Beck-Popovic M, Balmer A, Maeder P, Braganca T, Munier FL. Benign pineal cysts in children with bilateral retinoblastoma: a new variant of trilateral retinoblastoma? Pediatr Blood Cancer. 2006;46:755–61.
19. Reese AB, Ellsworth RM. The evaluation and current concept of retinoblastoma therapy. Trans Am Acad Ophthalmol Otolaryngol. 1963;67:164–72.
20. Shields CL, Mashayekhi A, Au AK, et al. The international classification of retinoblastoma predicts chemoreduction success. Ophthalmology. 2006;113(12):2276–80.
21. Chantada G, Doz F, Antonelli CBG, et al. A proposal for an international retinoblastoma staging system. Pediatr Blood Cancer. 2006;47(6):801–5.
22. Sang DN, Albert DM. Retinoblastoma: clinical and histopathologic features. Hum Pathol. 1982;13(2):133–47.
23. Rodriguez-Galindo C, Chantada GL, Haik B, Wilson MW. Retinoblastoma: current treatment and future perspectives. Curr Treat Options Neurol. 2007;9(4):294–307.
24. Shields CL, Shields JA. Recent developments in the management of retinoblastoma. J Pediatr Ophthalmol Strabismus. 1999;36(1):8–18.
25. Shields JA, Shields CL, DePotter P. Photocoagulation of retinoblastoma. Int Ophthalmol Clin. 1993;33:95–9.
26. Shields JA, Parsons H, Shields CL, Giblin ME. The role of cryotherapy in the management of retinoblastoma. Am J Ophthalmol. 1989;108(3):260–4.
27. Shields CL, Santos MCM, Diniz W, et al. Thermotherapy for retinoblastoma. Arch Ophthalmol. 1999;117(7):885–93.
28. Fass D, McCormick B, Abramson D, Ellsworth R. Cobalt60 plaques in recurrent retinoblastoma. Int J Radiat Oncol Biol Phys. 1991;21:625–7.
29. Freire JE, De Potter P, Brady LW, Longton WA. Brachytherapy in primary ocular tumors. Semin Surg Oncol. 1997;13:167–76.
30. Al-Haj AN, Lobriguito AM, Lagarde CS. Radiation dose profile in 125I brachytherapy: an 8-year review. Radiat Prot Dosimetry. 2004;111:115–9.
31. Abouzeid H, Moeckli R, Gaillard MC, et al. (106)Ruthenium brachytherapy for retinoblastoma. Int J Radiat Oncol Biol Phys. 2008;71:821–8.
32. Reisner ML, Viegas CM, Grazziotin RZ, et al. Retinoblastoma–comparative analysis of external radiotherapy techniques, including an IMRT technique. Int J Radiat Oncol Biol Phys. 2007;67:933–41.
33. Ross G, Lipper EG, Abramson D, Preiser L. The development of young children with retinoblastoma. Arch Pediatr Adolesc Med. 2001;155(1):80–3.
34. Gobin YP, Dunkel IJ, Marr BP, Brodie SE, Abramson DH. Intra-arterial chemotherapy for the management of retinoblastoma: four-year experience. Arch Ophthalmol. 2011;129:732–7.
35. Abramson DH, Frank CM. Second nonocular tumors in survivors of bilateral retinoblastoma. A possible age effect on radiation-related risk. Ophthalmology. 1998;105:573–80.
36. Shields CL, Honavar SG, Meadows AT, et al. Chemoreduction plus focal therapy for retinoblastoma: factors predictive of need for treatment with external beam radiotherapy or enucleation. Am J Ophthalmo. 2002;133:657–64.
37. Kaneko A, Suzuki S. Eye-preservation treatment of retinoblastoma with vitreous seeding. Jpn J Clin Oncol. 2003;33:601–7.
38. Mohri M. The technique of selective ophthalmic arterial infusion for conservative treatment of recurrent intraocular retinoblastoma. Keio Igaku. 1993;70:679–87.
39. Abramson DH, Dunkel IJ, Brodie SE, Kim JW, Gobin YP. A phase I/II study of direct intraarterial (ophthalmic artery) chemotherapy with melphalan for intraocular retinoblastoma: initial results. Ophthalmology. 2008;115:1398–404.
40. Abramson DH, Dunkel IJ, Brodie SE, Marr B, Gobin YP. Bilateral superselective ophthalmic artery chemotherapy for bilateral retinoblastoma: tandem therapy. Arch Ophthalmol. 2010;128:370–2.
41. Munier FL, Gaillard M-C, Balmer A, et al. Intravitreal chemotherapy for vitreous disease in retinoblastoma revisited: from prohibition to conditional indications. Br J Ophthalmol. 2012;96:1078–83.
42. Antonelli CBG, Steinhorst F, Ribeiro KCB, et al. Extraocular retinoblastoma: a 13-year experience. Cancer. 2003;98:1292–8.
43. Menon BS, Reddy SC, Maziah W, Ham A, Rosline H. Extraocular retinoblastoma. Med Pediatr Oncol. 2000;35:75–6.
44. Doz F, Khelfaoui F, Mosseri V, et al. The role of chemotherapy in orbital involvement of retinoblastoma. Cancer. 1994;74(2):722–32.
45. Chantada G, Fandiño A, Casak S, Manzitti J, Raslawski E, Schvartzman E. Treatment of overt extraocular retinoblastoma. Med Pediatr Oncol. 2003;40:158–61.
46. Namouni F, Doz F, Tanguy ML, et al. High-dose chemotherapy with carboplatin, etoposide and cyclophosphamide followed by a haematopoietic stem cell rescue in patients with high-risk retinoblastoma: a SFOP and SFGM study. Eur J Cancer. 1997;33(14):2368–75.
47. Dunkel IJ, Khakoo Y, Kernan NA, et al. Intensive multimodality therapy for patients with stage 4a metastatic retinoblastoma. Pediatr Blood Cancer. 2010;55:55–9.
48. Kleinerman RA, Tucker MA, Tarone RE, et al. Risk of new cancers after radiotherapy in long-term survivors of retinoblastoma: an extended follow-up. J Clin Oncol. 2005;23:2272–9.
49. Kleinerman RA, Tucker MA, Abramson DH, Seddon JM, Tarone RE, Fraumeni JF. Risk of soft tissue sarcomas by individual subtype in survivors of hereditary retinoblastoma. J Natl Cancer Inst. 2007;99:24–31.
50. Fletcher O, Easton D, Anderson K, Gilham C, Jay M, Peto J. Lifetime risks of common cancers among retinoblastoma survivors. J Natl Cancer Inst. 2004;96(5):357–63.

Rhabdomyoma

38

Karen Watters and Reza Rahbar

Introduction and Classification

Rhabdomyomas are rare benign tumors arising from striated muscle. They are divided topographically into cardiac and extracardiac. Cardiac rhabdomyomas, the most common type, are believed to be hamartomas and represent 90% of cardiac tumors of infancy. Extracardiac rhabdomyomas, which are neoplastic, are further classified into three subtypes—adult, fetal, and genital type, based on their distinct clinical and histological presentations (Table 38.1). The head and neck region is the principle site of involvement in 95% of cases of extracardiac rhabdomyomas [1]. They are extremely rare tumors accounting for less than 2% of all neoplasms showing striated muscle differentiation—their malignant counterpart, rhabdomyosarcomas, are far more common, representing 98% of all skeletal muscle tumors. Rhabdomyoma and rhabdomyosarcoma are considered independent entities [2].

Etiology

No racial or geographic predilection for rhabdomyoma has been identified to date. Unlike the cardiac type, which is typically seen in patients with tuberous sclerosis, extracardiac rhabdomyomas have no association with tuberous sclerosis. Due to the rarity of rhabdomyomas, an incidence cannot be estimated.

K. Watters (✉)
Boston Children's Hospital, Harvard Medical School, 300 Longwood Avenue, LO-367, Boston, MA 02115, USA
e-mail: karen.watters@childrens.harvard.edu

R. Rahbar
Department of Otolaryngology, Boston Children's Hospital; Harvard Medical School, 300 Longwood Ave, LO-367, Boston, MA 02115, USA

Clinical Presentation

Fetal rhabdomyomas: These are the least common of all rhabdomyoma types. Since their first description by Dehner in 1972, case reports and small series have attempted to characterize them [3]. It is hypothesized that fetal rhabdomyomas may in fact arise from fetal rests. They are seen primarily in the head and neck region of male infants usually less than 3 years of age, and typically present as a solitary mass, with symptoms related to their specific site—they may present with hoarseness, dysphasia, dysphagia, or respiratory distress [4–6].

Two variants, *classic* and *intermediate*, have been described:

- The *classic or myxoid* subtype is the most common and usually presents in the head and neck region as a well-demarcated subcutaneous mass, particularly affecting the preauricular and postauricular regions. It has been described only in infants during the first year of life.
- The *intermediate or cellular* form occurs more often in soft tissue and mucosal sites of the head and neck region, typically the tongue, nasopharynx, larynx, orbit, and neck. It has been described in case reports in the infratemporal fossa and cricopharyngeus [7, 8].

Adult rhabdomyomas These are thought to arise from the branchial musculature of third and fourth branchial arches. They occur most often in the upper aerodigestive tract and neck musculature of male adults over the age of 40. The most common sites include the mucosa of the larynx, oropharynx, floor of the mouth, and lip. They usually present as slow-growing masses with symptoms often related to aerodigestive tract obstruction, dyspnoea, hoarseness, dysphagia, and new-onset sleep apnea. They are usually solitary but there have been reports of multifocality [9, 10].

R. Rahbar et al. (eds.), *Pediatric Head and Neck Tumors*,
DOI 10.1007/978-1-4614-8755-5_38, © Springer Science+Business Media New York 2014

Table 38.1 Classification of rhabdomyoma

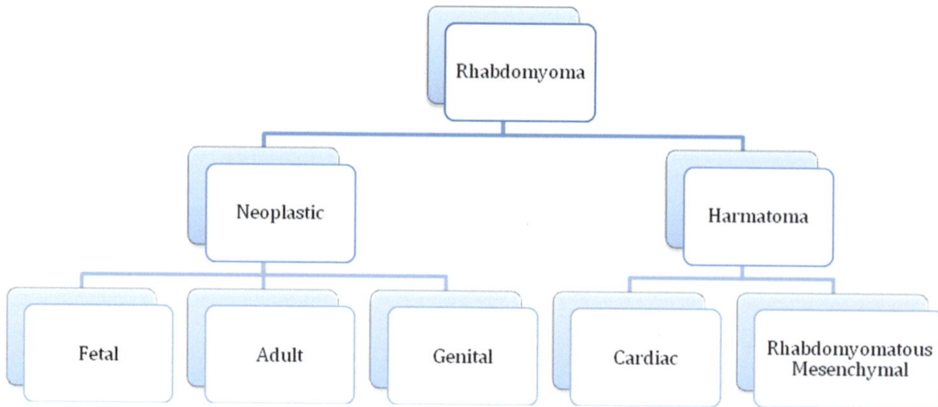

Histology

Macroscopically, rhabdomyomas are well circumscribed and encapsulated, of soft consistency, tan to grayish in color, and homogenous and mucoid when cut. Fetal and adult rhabdomyomas can be differentiated by histologic criteria and immunohistochemistry (Fig. 38.1).

Fetal rhabdomyoma

- The *classic* immature form, is identified by the presence of a mixture of bland primitive spindle cells with elongated muscle cells containing indistinct cytoplasm and muscle fibers. These spindle cells are haphazardly arranged in a fibromyxoid stroma and resemble myoblasts at 6–10 weeks of embryonic development. Myoblasts may be seen at different stages of differentiation.
- The *intermediate* form shows a greater degree and a greater number of cells with skeletal muscle differentiation, "rhabdomyoblastic maturation". Overlapping features can also be seen between the two forms. Immunohistochemically fetal rhabdomyoma typically expresses desmin, muscle specific actin and myoglobin. Primitive mesenchymal cells unpredictably express S-100 protein, glial fibrillary acidic protein, smooth muscle actin, and vimentin.

Adult rhabdomyoma This is characterized by the presence of sheets of well-differentiated large cells that resemble striated muscle cells. The cells are deeply eosinophilic polygonal cells, with small peripherally placed nuclei and occasional intracellular vacuoles. Cross-striations are a hallmark of identification and minimal or no mitotic activity is present. Muscle specific actin, desmin, and myoglobin are expressed to a higher degree than fetal rhabdomyomas, but vimentin is not expressed in the adult form.

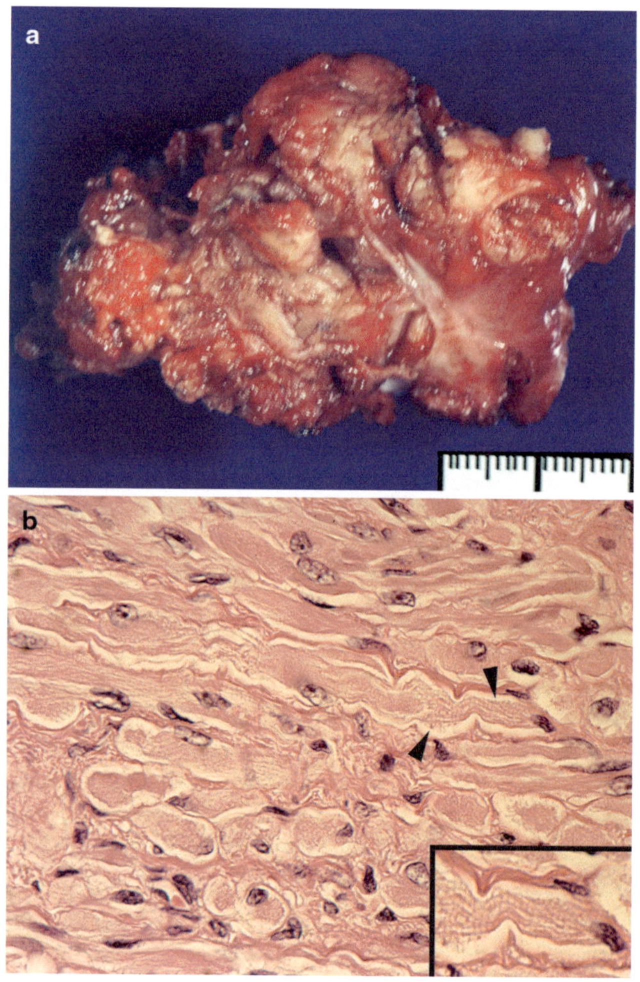

Fig. 38.1 Rhabdomyoma of neck. **a** Cut surface of lobulated soft tissue mass with a meaty appearance and a *red* and *white-gray* color. The mass had a soft rubbery consistency and absence of necrosis. **b** Tumor cells have the appearance of well-differentiated rhabdomyoblasts, some with visible striations (seen between *arrowheads* and in inset)

Table 38.2 Histological characteristics of tumors in the differential diagnosis

Tumor	Histology	Immunohistochemistry
Rhabdomyoma		
Fetal	Primitive spindle cells, myoblasts, no mitotic figures	Express muscle specific actin, desmin, and myoglobin. Weak S-100, vimentin expression
Adult	Well-differentiated skeletal muscle cells, cross striations	Strong actin, desmin and myoglobin expression. Do not express vimentin
Rhabdomyosarcoma	Cellular pleomorphism, nuclear atypia, mitotic figures, necrosis, invasion	
Granular cell tumor	Smaller cells	Strong staining for S-100
Hibernoma	Mixture of granulated and smaller vacuolated cells, lipocytes (resembles fetal fat)	May express S-100, Do not express muscle immunostains

Differential Diagnosis

The diagnosis of fetal rhabdomyoma is complicated due to the paucity of cases and the similarities between *rhabdomyosarcoma*. Distinction from the spindle cell variant of embryonal rhabdomyosarcoma can be notoriously difficult. Unlike fetal rhabdomyomas, which are well circumscribed and do not invade and destroy adjacent soft tissue, rhabdomyosarcomas, have infiltrative margins and invade normal tissues. Histologically, rhabdomyosarcomas can be differentiated by the presence of cellular atypia, increased mitotic activity, lack of differentiation, and similarity to other sarcomas. Foci of necrosis and hemorrhage are often also present in rhabdomyosarcoma.

Other tumors in the differential diagnosis include benign hamartomatous lesions, such as neuromuscular hamartomas and rhabdomyomatous mesenchymal hamartomas of the skin, teratoma, vascular malformation, neurofibroma, schwannoma, granular cell tumor, hibernoma, paraganglioma, and malignant tumors with skeletal muscle differentiation. Immunohistochemical stains including S-100, desmin, and myoglobulin may also be helpful in making exclusive diagnosis (Table 38.2). For example, granular cell tumors express S-100 protein but skeletal muscle markers usually are absent.

Evaluation

Clinical diagnosis of fetal rhabdomyoma can be challenging due to the absence of distinctive clinical characteristics.

Biopsy Diagnosis is made histologically via trucut biopsy (under radiographic guidance), open biopsy or excision biopsy of the lesion. Fine needle aspiration may also be a helpful tool in the work-up of rhabdomyomas. Cytological features suggestive of rhabdomyomas include cohesive clusters of spindle cells and rhabdomyoblasts with abundant eosinophilic granular cytoplasm, often peripherally located nuclei, cross-striations, elongated intracytoplasmic inclusions, and absence of mitotic figures. It is important to differentiate findings from a rhabdomyosarcoma, which will typically show pleomorphic nuclei and cellular atypical. There have been number of reports of solitary rhabdomyomas, which were correctly diagnosed with fine needle aspiration cytology preoperatively [11, 12].

Radiology The radiographic appearances of extracardiac rhabdomyomas have not been well defined. Although, imaging alone may not clearly differentiate rhabdomyomas from other benign neoplasms, the submucosal location of rhabdomyomas and the absence of invasion into surrounding tissues may help to distinguish them from malignant lesions. Both computed tomography (CT) and magnetic resonance imaging (MRI) are helpful in determining tumor characteristics, including the size, extent of local involvement, necrosis, nature of the tumor, including its occasional multilobar feature, and multifocality. Imaging is recommended prior to biopsy or excision. Fetal ultrasound and MRI can identify rhabdomyoma in utero at approximately 12–16 weeks gestation.

CT Imaging Rhabdomyoma appears as a well-defined, often multilobed, mass with the same density as surrounding muscle on unenhanced CT. With administration of contrast media, the tumor shows mild homogeneous enhancement with regular margins (Fig. 38.2).

MRI Imaging On T1-weighted images rhabdomyoma appears the same density as surrounding muscle. Intensity is heightened on T2-weighted images. Enhancement with gadolinium demonstrates a mild diffusely homogenous mass with regular margins.

Management

Complete excision of a rhabdomyoma with negative margins is usually curative. No cases of aggressive local tumor growth or metastasis have been documented. In cases where

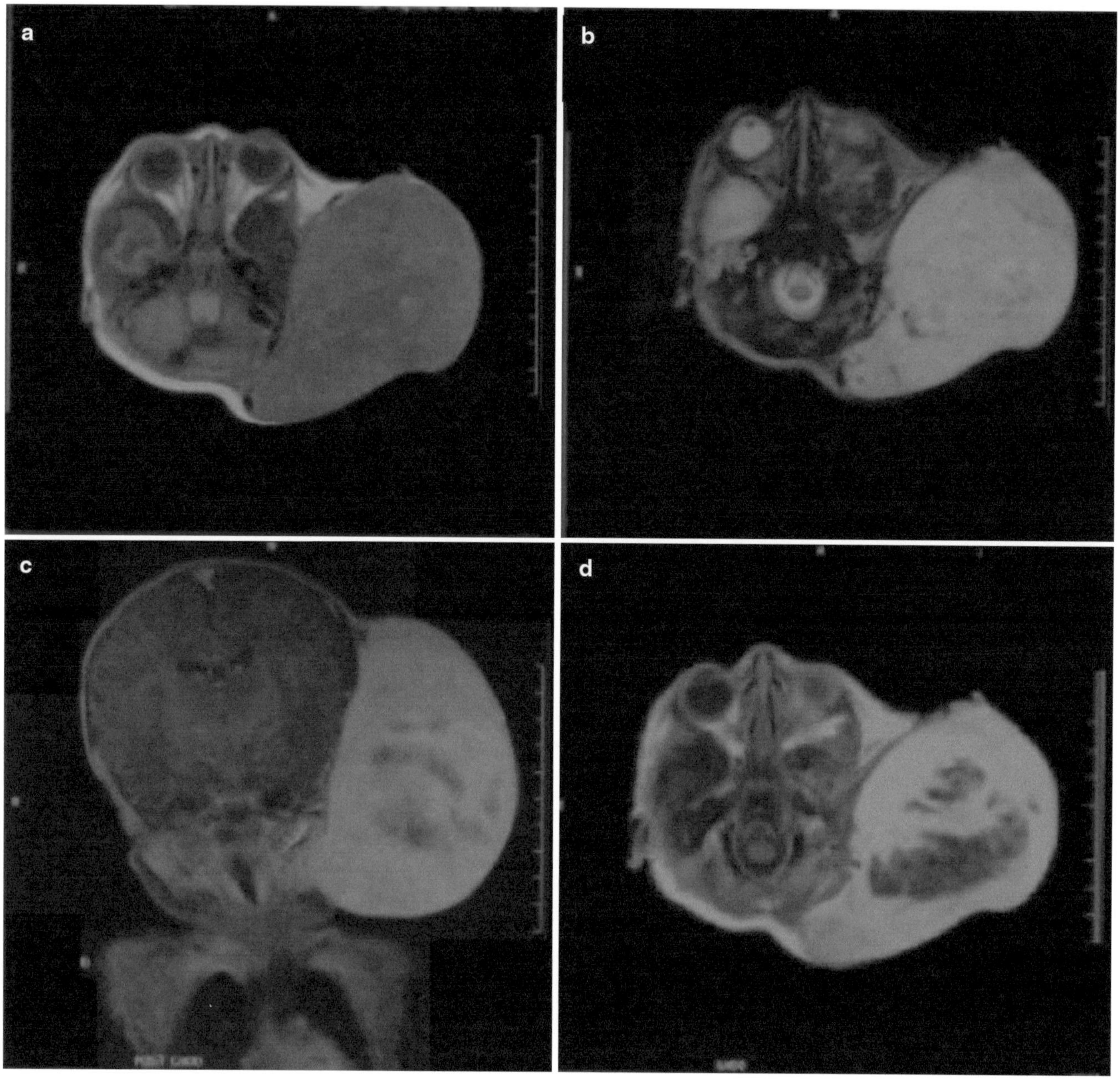

Fig. 38.2 An axial CT scan showing a left cervical fetal rhabdomyoma in a male newborn infant. T1 weighted-images (**a**), the tumor is diffusely homogenous to muscle with regular margins; T2 weighted-images (**b**), the intensity of the tumor is increased. Coronal (**c**) and axial (**d**) CT images with gadolinium (**c**) show hyperintensity of the tumor to surrounding muscle with areas of central necrosis

the tumor is extensive, craniofacial resection may be necessary with reconstruction (Figs. 38.3 and 38.4). Rare local tumor recurrences have been reported, possibly attributed to incomplete excision [13]. A complete workup to exclude rhabdomyosarcoma is essential in all cases of recurrence. Recurrence is treated with further excision. Malignant transformation of rhabdomyomas is very rare although it has been reported [2]. Chemotherapy and radiotherapy do not have a role to play.

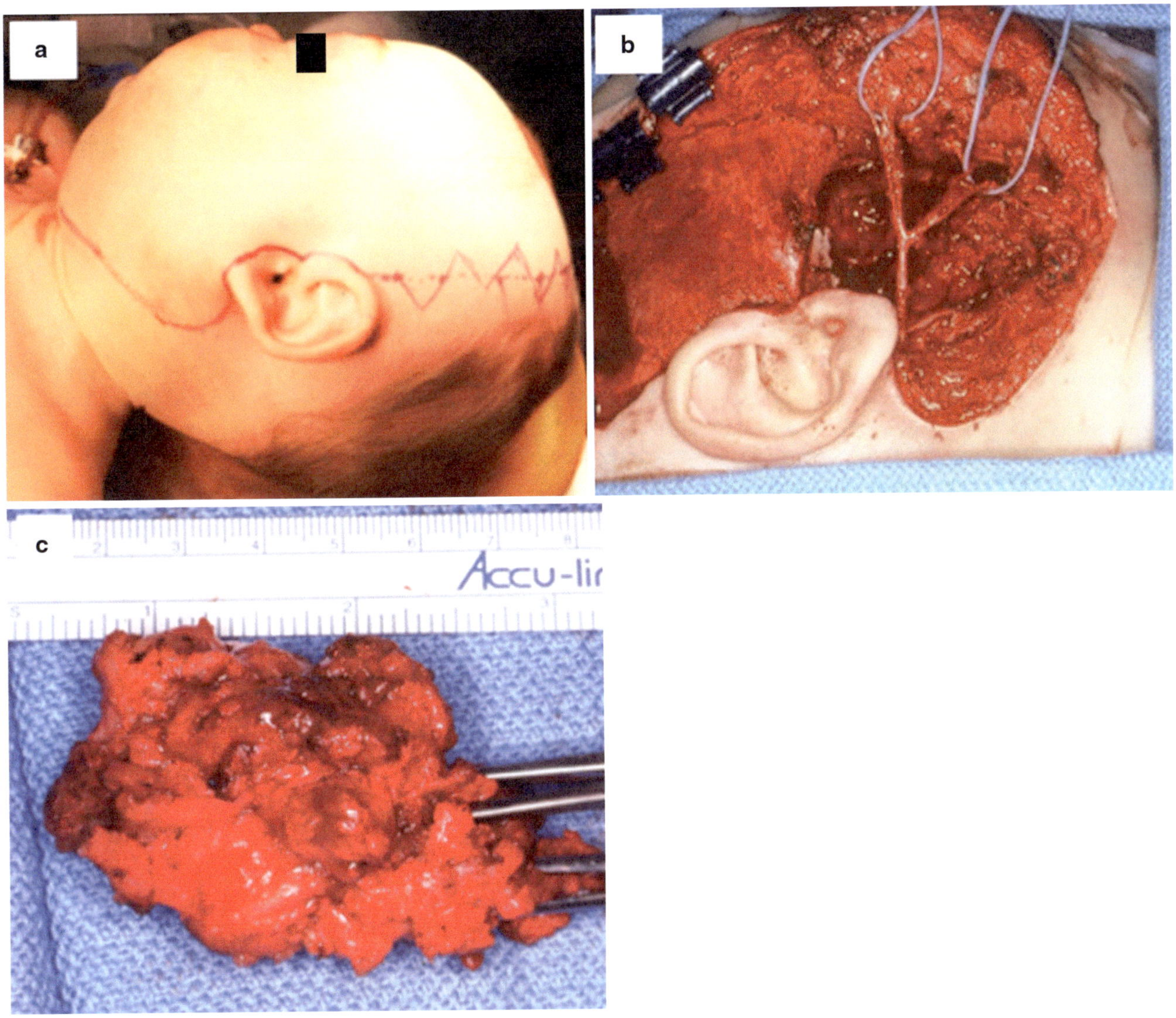

Fig. 38.3 A newborn male infant with a fetal rhabdomyoma involving the left parotid gland and extending into the left mandible and maxillary bone. A left modified Blair parotidectomy incision was used to approach the tumor (**a**). The left facial nerve was dissected and preserved (**b**). The resected tumor was deep to the facial nerve, measuring approximately 7 × 6 cm in size (**c**).

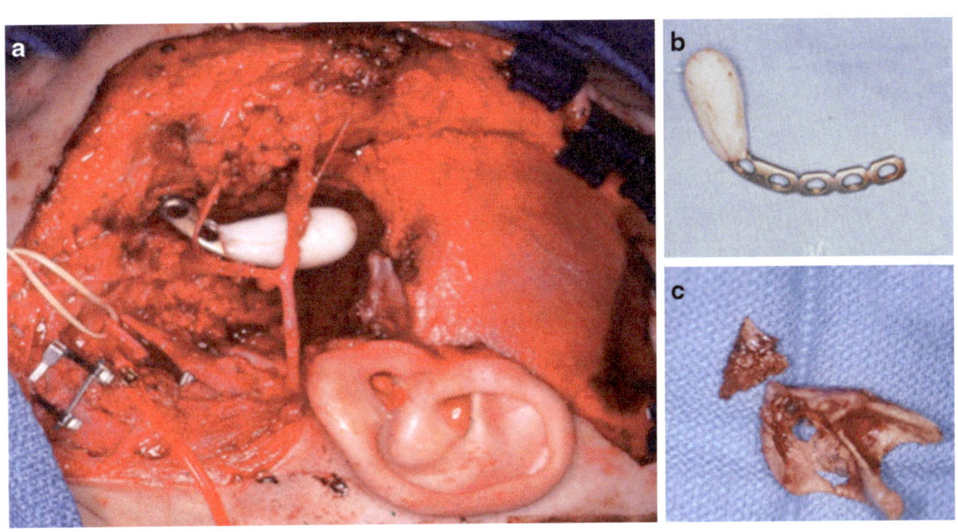

Fig. 38.4 Intra-operative images of the patient in Fig. 38.2. A titanium prosthesis was used to reconstruct the mandible. The prosthesis is seen in situ deep to main trunk and upper branches of the facial nerve (**a**). The titanium prosthesis (**b**). The resected sphenoid bone (**c**).

References

1. Helliwell TR, Sissons MC, Stoney PJ, Ashworth MT. Immunochemistry and electron microscopy of head and neck rhabdomyoma. J Clin Pathol. 1988;41(10):1058–63.
2. Kodet R, Fajstavr J, Kabelka Z, Koutecky J, Eckschlager T, Newton WA Jr. Is fetal cellular rhabdomyoma an entity or a differentiated rhabdomyosarcoma? A study of patients with rhabdomyoma of the tongue and sarcoma of the tongue enrolled in the intergroup rhabdomyosarcoma studies I, II, and III. Cancer. 1991;67(11):2907–13.
3. Dehner LP, Enzinger FM, Font RI. Fetal rhabdomyoma: an analysis of nine cases. Cancer. 1972;30:160–6.
4. Carron JD, Darrow DH, Karakla DW. Fetal rhabdomyoma of the posterior cervical triangle. Int J Pediatr Otorhinolaryngol. 2001;61(1):77–81.
5. Cacciari A, Predieri B, Mordenti M, Ceccarelli PL, Maiorana A, Cerofolini E, Bernasconi S. Rhabdomyoma of a rare type in a child: case report and literature review. Eur J Pediatr Surg. 2001;11(1):66–8.
6. Pichi B, Manciocco V, Marchesi P, Pellini R, Ruscito P, Vidiri A, Covello R, Spriano G. Rhabdomyoma of the parapharyngeal space presenting with dysphagia. Dysphagia. 2008;23(2):202–4.
7. Leboulanger N, Picard A, Roger G, Garabedian EN. Fetal rhabdomyoma of the infratemporal fossa in children. Eur Ann Otorhinolaryngol Head Neck Dis. 2010;127(1):30–2.
8. Pownell PH, Brown OE, Argyle JC, Manning SC. Rhabdomyoma of the cricopharyngeus in an infant. Int J Pediatr Otorhinolaryngol. 1990;20(2):149–58. Review.
9. Koutsimpelas D, Weber A, Lippert BM, Mann WJ. Multifocal adult rhabdomyoma of the head and neck: a case report and literature review. Auris Nasus Larynx. 2008;35(2):313–7.
10. Liess BD, Zitsch RP 3rd, Lane R, Bickel JT. Multifocal adult rhabdomyoma: a case report and literature review. Am J Otolaryngol. 2005;26(3):214–7. Review.
11. Wan WK, Sng TY, Goh HK, Hwang SG. Foetal rhabdomyoma with fine-needle aspirate cytology correlation. Singapore Med J. 2009;50(4):e138–40.
12. Eigenbrodt ML, Cunningham LF. Fine needle aspiration cytology of a rhabdomyoma of the pharynx. Acta Cytol. 1986;30(5):528–32.
13. Valdez TA, Desai U, Volk MS. Recurrent fetal rhabdomyoma of the head and neck. Int J Pediatr Otorhinolaryngol. 2006;70(6):1115–8.

Salivary Gland Tumors

39

Paul Lennon and Michael J. Cunningham

Introduction

Malignant neoplasms of the salivary glands are rare in the pediatric population. The vast majority of those that do occur arise in the parotid gland. An asymptomatic firm mass in the preauricular region is the most common presentation. Surgical resection is the principal treatment. Adjuvant radiation therapy or chemotherapy may be indicated depending on clinical presentation and tumor type. Prognosis is chiefly determined by histopathologic findings.

Pathophysiology

Salivary gland tumors have been described as 'the orphans of oncologic research' [1]. Little is known about their genesis or the factors that promote them. Some benign tumors, such as pleomorphic adenoma (PA) can undergo malignant transformation, while some malignant tumors, such as adenoid cystic carcinomas (AdCCs) are notorious for their indolent course. There is a wide range of morphological diversity between different tumor types and sometimes within an individual tumor mass. These features have resulted in an unclear concept of salivary gland tumorgenesis [1].

Two major hypotheses attempt to explain the wide variety of histopathology demonstrated by salivary gland neoplasms. The bicellular theory suggests that basal cells found in the excretory and intercalated ducts act as stem cells for the eventual differentiated cells of the salivary gland unit [2]. According to this theory, intercalated duct stem cells are the origin of adenomatoid tumors including PA, Warthin's tumor, oncocytoma, acinic cell carcinomas (ACC), and AdCC, whereas the excretory duct stem cells give rise to epidermoid tumors, such as squamous cell carcinoma and mucopeidermoid carcinoma.

The multicellular theory, in contrast, matches each tumor type with a particular cell of origin within the salivary gland unit. For example, the striated duct cells give rise to oncocytic tumors, acinar cells give rise to ACC, excretory duct cells give rise to squamous cell carcinoma and mucoepidermoid carcinoma, and the intercalated duct cells and myopeithelial cells give rise to pleomorphic tumors.The bicellular hypothesis has been challenged by studies demonstrating all glandular cell types, including acinar cells, to be capable of rapidly entering the cell cycle and therefore be possible targets for neoplastic transformation [3].

Molecular or Genetic Pathology

The goal of the molecular biological studies of salivary gland tumors is to define objective markers that may aid in the evaluation, diagnosis, and biological assessment of patients so afflicted [4]. A wide variety of oncogenes whose function becomes enhanced in carcinogenesis are implicated in salivary gland tumorgenesis [5].

The C-erbB-2/HER-2/neu gene, a member of the EGFR signal transduction family known for its role in breast cancer, has been identified in salivary gland adenocarinoma and mucoepidermoid carcinoma with over expression of HER-2 linked to adverse clinicopathological features [5]. The KIT protein, a proto-oncogene, has been shown to appear in certain tumor types, such as AdCC, lymphoepithelioma-like carcinoma, and myoepithelial carcinoma. An inhibitor of the KIT protein has been used with some success in treating AdCC [6].

Other oncogenes and their associated salivary gland malignancies include Maml2 (mucoepidermoid carcinoma), H-ras (mucoepidermoid carcinoma and adenocarcinoma), WNT1 (epithelial-myoepithelial carcinoma), and the Sox4 (AdCC) [7]. The role of tumor suppressor genes, whose

P. Lennon (✉)
Department of Otolaryngology and Communication Enhancement, Boston Children's Hospital, Harvard Medical School, Boston, MA, USA
e-mail: paullennon81@gmail.com

M. J. Cunningham
Department of Otolaryngology and Communication Enhancement, Boston Children's Hospital, Harvard Medical School, Boston, MA, USA

R. Rahbar et al. (eds.), *Pediatric Head and Neck Tumors*,
DOI 10.1007/978-1-4614-8755-5_39, © Springer Science+Business Media New York 2014

function is lost in carcinogenesis, is comparatively less clear. Results, thus far assessing TP53 located on the short arm of chromosome 17 have been quite variable [8].

Incidence and Prevalence

The epidemiology of salivary gland tumors in adults and particularly in children is not well documented [9]. The global annual incidence for all salivary gland tumors, both benign and malignant, varies from 0.4 to 13.5 cases per 100,000, whereas the frequency of malignant salivary neoplasms ranges from 0.4 to 2.6 cases per 100,000 [9, 10]. Malignancies of the salivary glands in children and adolescents are exceedingly rare with an estimate annual incidence of 0.08 per 100,000 [11]. An Armed Forces Institute of Pathology database review of almost 10,000 salivary gland lesions revealed only 35 salivary gland epithelial carcinomas in children under 14 years of age [12].

The majority of information available on salivary gland neoplasms consists of retrospective studies at tertiary care oncological institutions [13–33]. These longitudinal studies span durations of up to 58 years. The total number of pediatric epithelial carcinomas compiled in such studies varies from 3 to 46, corresponding to an average of only one pediatric patient diagnosed every 2 years even at major institutions (Table 39.1). When vascular anomalies are excluded, up to 50% of major salivary gland tumors in the pediatric age group are malignant, more than twice the proportion reported in the adult population [17, 23]. This relative percentage of malignancy is even higher with respect to minor salivary gland tumors.

Table 39.1 Composite of pediatric salivary gland malignancy publications

Primary author (year of publication)	Study duration (years)	Pediatric malignancies (number)
Castro 1972	34	19
Dahlqvist 1982	22	9
Byers 1884	37	26
Baker 1985	25	13
Shikhani 1988	30	3
Lack 1988	58	15
Fonseca 1991	30	7
Callender 1992	43	21
Otago 1994	26	11
Rogers 1994	19	8
Kessler 1994	9	8
Bull 1999	18	5
Orvidas 2000	21	19
Ribeiro Khe 2002	44	27
Yu 2002	25	46
Ethunandan 2003	26	3
De cruz Peres 2004	34	26
Verdine 2006	20	18
Guzzo 2006	30	15
Rahbar 2006	10	7
Ellies 2006	34	9
Castro 1972	34	19

Anatomical Distribution

The most common anatomical site for salivary gland tumors in the pediatric population is the parotid gland [24]. Analysis of the 20 pediatric retrospective studies [13–33] previously mentioned reveals 82% of the composite 315 tumors to have arisen within the parotid gland; the submandibular gland accounted for approximately 7%, and the sublingual gland for less than 1%. The minor salivary glands accounted for the remaining 11%. These respective incidences are similar to those reported in adults. Rarely the accessory parotid tissue can be the site of origin of a pediatric salivary gland malignancy [34].

Tumor Classification

The histopathology of salivary gland malignancies in the pediatric population is similar to that in adults. The World Health Organization (WHO) has categorized 14 benign and 24 malignant salivary gland neoplasms [4] (Table 39.2). The relative frequency of occurrence of the various histological types does, however, vary. Mucoepidermoid carcinoma is by far the most common in children, accounting for 61% of the total number of tumors in the twenty retrospective studies [13–33]. Acinic cell (11%) and adenocarcinoma (10%) account for a relatively large number, whereas adenoid cystic (9%), carcinoma ex PA (1%), and squamous cell carcinomas (0%) are comparatively rare (Fig. 39.1). Sarcomas, particularly rhabdomyosarcoma, and lymphomas can also arise within the salivary glands in children [35].

Age and Sex Distribution

Although salivary gland tumors have been reported in children of all ages, the vast majority occur in older children and adolescents. Recognizing the upper age limit varying from 14 to 20 years, composite analysis of retrospective studies identifies a median age of 12 years (28, 31, and 47). One epidemiology study similarly documented an average age of 13.4 years [36]. Benign salivary gland neoplasms present at the slightly older average age of 15 years [17]. Although isolated studies have suggested a strong female predominance (35), composite retrospective article review [13–33] suggests a near equal distribution between the sexes with a 53%

Table 39.2 WHO classifications of salivary gland tumors. (Reprinted with permission from [4])

Malignant epithelial tumors	
Acinic cell carcinoma (ACC)	8550/3
Mucoepidermoid carcinoma	8430/3
Adenoid cystic carcinoma (AdCC)	8200/3
Polymorphous low-grade adenocarcinoma	8525/3
Epithelial-myoepithelial carcinoma	8562/3
Clear cell carcinoma, not otherwise specified	8310/3
Basal cell adenocarcinoma	8147/3
Sebaceous carcinoma	8410/3
Sebaceous lymphadenocarcinoma	8410/3
Cystadenocarcinoma	8440/3
Low-grade cribriform cystadenocarcinoma	
Mucinous adenocarcinoma	8480/3
Oncocytic carcinoma	8290/3
Salivary duct carcinoma	8500/3
Adenocarcinoma, not otherwise specified	8140/3
Myoepithelial carcinoma	8982/3
Carcinoma ex pleomorphic adenoma	8941/3
Carcinosarcoma	8980/3
Metastasizing pleomorphic adenoma	8940/1
Squamous cell carcinoma	8070/3
Small cell carcinoma	8041/3
Large cell carcinoma	8012/3
Lymphoepithelial carcinoma	8082/3
Sialoblastoma	8974/1
Benign epithelial tumors	
Pleomorphic adenoma	8940/0
Myoepithelioma	8982/0
Basal cell adenoma	8147/0
Warthin tumor	8561/0
Oncocytoma	8290/0
Canalicular adenoma	8149/0
Sebaceous adenoma	8410/0
Lymphadenoma	
Sebaceous	8410/0
Nonsebaceous	8410/0
Ductal papillomas	
Inverted ductal papilloma	8503/0
Intraductal papilloma	8503/0
Sialadenoma papilliferum	8406/0
Cystadenoma	8440/0
Soft tissue tumors	
Hemangioma	9120/0
Hematolymphoid tumors	
Hodgkin lymphoma	
Diffuse large B-cell lymphoma	9680/3
Extranodal marginal zone B-cell lymphoma	9699/3
Secondary tumors	

Behavior is coded /0 for benign tumors, /3 for malignant tumors, and /1 for borderline or uncertain behavior

Morphology code of the international classification of diseases for oncology (ICD-O) {821} and the systematized nomenclature of medicine (http://snomed.org)

prevalence of salivary gland malignancies in females and a 47 % prevalence in males.

Geographic Distribution

There is surprisingly little international variation in the incidence of salivary gland cancers [10]. Of the 20 studies listed in (Table 39.1), 11 separate countries are represented, with little variation in individual tumor prevalence.

Risk Factors

One of the few well established risk factors for salivary gland cancer is exposure to radiation [10]. The evidence in this respect comes principally from research into the atomic bomb survivors of Hiroshima and Nagasaki, study of whom shows an increased relative risk for benign and malignant salivary gland neoplasms of 3.5 and 11 %, respectively [37]. A strong dose response relationship exists for mucoepidermoid carcinomas [38], and the latent period in salivary tissues was found to be 20 years or more. Data from other studies has also indicated a causative relationship with prior radiation therapy, again with a disproportionately greater representation of mucoepidermoid carcinomas within irradiated patient groups [39].

Second malignant neoplasms in children have emerged as one of the most troublesome complications in pediatric oncology [40]. Over the past few decades, a number of studies have demonstrated a relationship between previously treated childhood cancer, particularly leukemia and lymphoma, and salivary gland cancer [16, 40, 41]. The median latent time between the primary and secondary malignancies was seven years in one study [16], and this was shown by meta-analysis to be significantly shorter in patients treated with both chemotherapy and radiotherapy than radiotherapy alone [42]. It is unclear whether this is a result solely of the cytotoxic treatments or combined to a greater or lesser extent with genetic factors [16].

There is a strong association between Epstein Barr virus (EBV) and lymphoepithelial carcinomas of the salivary glands [43]. No association between salivary gland malignancies and other viruses, such as the human immunodeficiency virus (HIV), polyoma virus and papilloma virus has been convincingly demonstrated [4, 10].

Presentation

The most common presentation of a salivary gland neoplasm is a firm mass in the lateral cervicofacial or submandibular region. A firm salivary gland mass in a child is uncommon,

Fig. 39.1 Frequency distribution of malignant salivary gland tumor types in the pediatric population

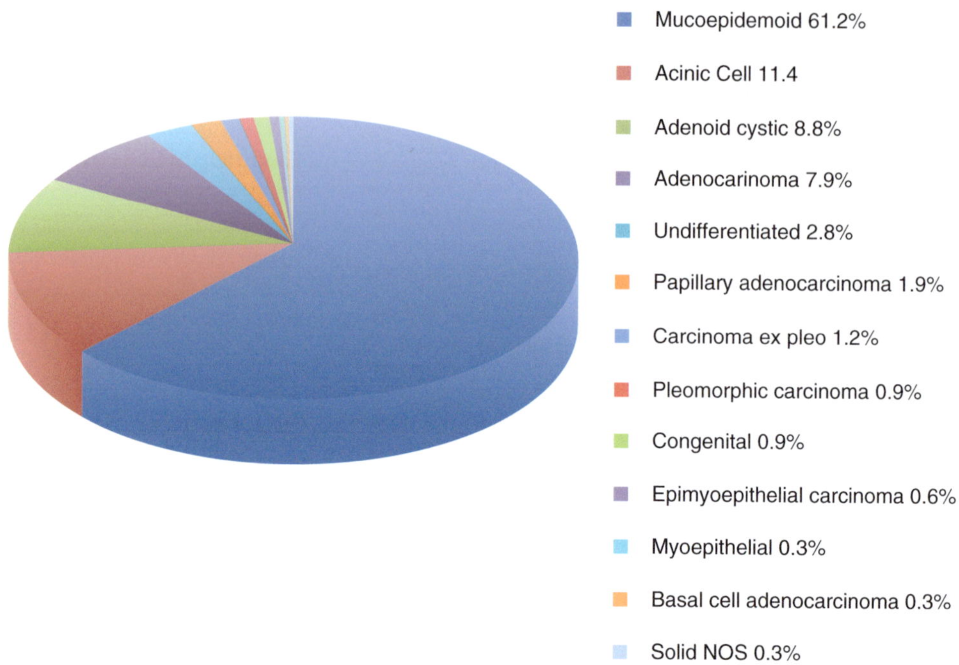

and the fact that over 50% of these tumors are malignant dictates a thorough diagnostic evaluation by the head and neck surgeon [44]. Unfortunately, the duration from mass documentation until definitive diagnosis varies greatly, ranging in one study from 2 to 156 months [20]. An average time prior to presentation of 8–12 months is often quoted [17, 18, 25]. Parotid gland tumors are usually asymptomatic; rarely adenoid cystic and acinar cell carcinomas may be painful [15, 30]. The incidence of facial nerve paresis on presentation approximates 4% [16, 19, 21, 22, 26, 30, 33]. Associated regional lymphatic metastases are documented at presentation in 3.5% children [16, 17, 24, 28]. Intraoral masses in the vicinity of the tonsil or the soft palate can be an uncommon presentation of deep lobe tumors of the parotid. In one review, 1.7% of patients with parotid tumors were found to present in such a fashion [45].

The usual presentation of submandibular gland tumors is a painless swelling below the mandible. The differential diagnosis includes the much more frequent entities of sialoadenitis of this gland or submandibular region lymphadenopathy. Sublingual gland tumors typically manifest as a palpable fullness in the floor of the mouth. Bimanual palpation of submandibular and sublingual masses may reveal fixation to surrounding structures. Although typically asymptomatic, pain may occur with progressive glandular enlargement. Advanced tumors may involve neural structures including the marginal mandibular branch of the facial nerve, the lingual nerve and the hypoglossal nerve [46] with resultant cranial nerve palsies.

Tumors of the minor salivary glands can be more difficult to diagnose because of their site-dependent presentation. For example, a minor salivary gland malignancy of the hard palate can mimic a bone lesion [47], whereas one of laryngeal origin may produce airway obstruction, dysphagia, or hoarseness. Friability may be an indication of malignancy [17]. The oral cavity accounts for over 50% of minor salivary gland malignancies in the pediatric population [48]. A painless mass on the palate or floor of mouth is the most common presentation.

Diagnosis and Evaluation

Imaging Evaluation

High-resolution ultrasound is an imaging modality of potential applicability for the evaluation of a parotid or submandibular region mass in a child. Ultrasound can be particularly helpful in distinguishing solid from cystic masses. Doppler ultrasound can evaluate the vascularity of the lesion. Ultrasound has the additional advantages of being noninvasive, not involving radiation, and typically being able to be performed with or without the need for sedation [49]. Any solid mass of the parotid or submandibular region, particularly one without associated inflammatory manifestations, should signal the need for more detailed imaging via computed tomography (CT) or magnetic resonance imaging (MRI) [23]. The age of the child with respect to the need for sedation or general anesthesia may dictate which procedure is initially performed.

Even younger children may tolerate the performance of a relatively short duration CT without sedation. CT is useful in evaluating lymph node metastasis (LNM) and is particularly beneficial if there is a concern of osseous involvement or tumor invasion of neural foramina [50]. Glandular signal intensity and enhancement pattern can, however, parallel that of adjacent musculature on CT. This is particularly true in children, because of the relative lack of fat in the parotid space, soft tissue differentiation in this region may be obscured [41].

MRI, on the other hand, clearly demarcates tumor from glandular tissue in multiplanar fashion. MRI also has the advantage of being free of radiation. T1-weighted images of normal parotid have an image signal intermediate between fat and muscle, whereas submandibular tissue is closer to muscle in intensity [51]. Parotid tumors are well visualized on T1-weighted MR images because of the hyperintense background of the gland. The T1-weighted image gives an excellent assessment of the margin of the tumor, its deep extent, and its pattern of infiltration [52]. Coupled with fat-saturation, contrast enhanced T1-weighted imaging can be used to assess for perineural spread [53]. MR features strongly suggestive of parotid malignancy are poorly defined margins with infiltration into the parapharyngeal space and surrounding musculature [54]. The conventional wisdom is that a hyperintense mass on T2-weighted images is benign and a mass of low to intermediate signal intensity is malignant [52]. A number of studies have, however, shown this not to be a reliable discriminative factor [54]. Innovative techniques, such as diffusion weighted MRI and intravoxel incoherent motion MRI [55] have shown some early promise in distinguishing benign from malignant tumors.

Fine Needle Aspiration or Biopsy

Fine needle aspiration (FNA) cytology in adults is a diagnostic tool that has a reliable sensitivity and specificity for the assessment of salivary gland pathology [56]. Although, its use in children has some advocates [57], the role of FNA is controversial because of the limited established specificity in pediatric salivary gland tumors [58] and because of the need for sedation or even general anesthesia for its performance in younger children [22]. Retrospective study review reveals FNA to be rarely undertaken and the accuracy to be as low as 33 % when it was performed [16].

Incisional biopsy is a consideration in masses involving the tail of the parotid region, and is particularly indicated in clinically unresectable lesions for which a diagnostic biopsy alone is required. Under most circumstances, total excision of the submandibular gland or superficial parotidectomy are the preferred techniques, providing both an excisional biopsy specimen and potential definitive therapy [59]. The marginal mandibular and facial nerves, respectively, need be identified and preserved during these procedures.

Staging

There is no specific staging system for pediatric salivary gland tumors. For parotid, submandibular, and sublingual neoplasms, the adult tumor node metastases (TNM) clinicopathologic staging system unified between the American Joint Committee on Cancer (AJCC) and the International Union Against Cancer (UICC) is often applied (Table 39.3; [60]). For minor salivary gland malignancies, the staging system for squamous cell carcinomas, depending on tumor site (oral cavity/oropharynx/nasal cavity/nasopharynx) is alternatively used. Children are often diagnosed at an earlier stage than adults [11].

Grade

Owing to the wide range of neoplasms and the diversity of their biological behavior, there is no single grading system for salivary gland cancers. Certain cancers are acknowledged as low grade (for example some adenocarcinomas, basal cell adenocarcinoma, and acinic cell adenocarcinoma) and others as high grade (for example some adenocarcinomas, squamous cell carcinoma, and undifferentiated carcinoma) [60]. Alternatively, salivary gland malignancies have been stratified into low-risk and high-risk tumors, low-risk tumors being those that do not require treatment beyond excision, whereas high-risk being those that do (Table 39.4) [61]. The caveat is that high grade versions of 'intrinsically' low grade tumors exist as do low grade versions of typically high grade tumors [61].

For some of the more common adult salivary gland malignancies, specific grading systems have been utilized. For example, three grades of AdCC have been described based on their growth pattern. The tubular and cribriform patterns are considered low grade, with increasing solid components contributing to higher grade, grade 3 being almost entirely solid [60, 61]. This system is controversial as some authors grade any tumor over 30 % solid as high grade [62], while others deem that up to 50 % of the tumor can be solid and still be termed intermediate [63].

A number of quantitative point scoring grading schemes also exist for mucoepidermoid carcinoma [64]. These assess characteristics, such as intracystic component, presence of neural invasion or necrosis, mitotic rate, and cellular anaplasia to stratify tumors into low, intermediate, or high grade [60]. Most mucoepidemoid carcinomas in children have been found to be low grade, with relative frequencies of low (76 %), intermediate (14 %), and high (10 %) grade (Table 39.5).

Cellular differentiation has also been used to grade salivary gland malignancies into well, moderately, poorly, undifferentiated, or anaplastic categories. Using this system, a

Table 39.3 AJCC staging of salivary gland malignancies

T	*Primary tumor*		
TX:	Primary tumor cannot be evaluated		
T0:	No evidence of a tumor		
T1:	Tumor 2 cm or less at its greatest dimension, without extraparenchymal extension		
T2:	Tumor more than 2 cm but less than 4 cm, without extraparenchymal extension		
T3:	Tumor larger than 4 cm, and or tumor with extraparenchymal extension		
T4a:	The tumor invades the skin, jawbone, ear canal, and/or facial nerve		
T4b:	The tumor invades the skull base and/or the pterygoid plate. And/or encases the carotid arteries		
Note	Extraparenchymal extension is clinical or macroscopic evidence of invsion of soft tissue or nerve, except those listed in 4a or 4b. Microscopic evisence alone does not constitute extraparenchymal extension for classification purposes		
N	*Nodal status*		
NX:	Regional lymph nodes cannot be evaluated		
N0:	No regional lymph node metastasis (LNM)		
N1:	Metastasis in a single ipsilateral node, 3 cm or less in greatest dimension		
N2:	Metastasis in a single ipsilateral node, more than 3 cm but not more than 6 cm in greatest dimension, or in multiple ipsilateral lymph nodes, none more than 6 cm in greatest dimension; or in bilateral or contralateral lymph nodes, none more than 6 cm in greatest dimension		
	N2a: Metastasis in a single ipsilateral node, more than 3 cm but not more than 6 cm in greatest dimension		
	N2b: Metastasis in multiple ipsilateral lymph nodes, none more than 6 cm in greatest dimension		
	N2c: Metastasis in bilateral or contralateral lymph nodes, none more than 6 cm in greatest dimension		
N3:	Metastasis in lymph node more than 6 cm in greatest dimension		
M	*Distant metastases*		
Mx	Distant metastases cannot be assessed		
M0	No distant metastases		
M1	Distant metastases		
	Stage grouping		
I	T1	N0	M0
II	T2	N0	M0
III	T3	N0	M0
	T1 T2 T3	N1	M0
IVA	T4A, T4B	N0 N1	M0
	T1 T2 T3 T4A	N2	M0
IVB	T4B	Any N	M0
	Any T	N3	M0
IVC	Any T	Any N	M1

significantly higher percentage of tumors in children (88 %) are reported to be well differentiated or moderately differentiated in comparisom to adults (49 %) [11].

Table 39.4 Risk stratification of WHO recognized salivary gland malignancies. (Reprinted from Seethala [61] with permission from Springer Science+Business Media.)

Low risk	High risk
Acinic cell carcinoma (ACC)	Sebaceous carcinoma/ Lymphadenocarcinoma
Low grade MEC[a]	High grade MEC[a]
Epitheial-myoepithelial carcinoma	Adenoid cystic carcinoma[b](AdCC)
Polymorphous low grade adenocarcinoma	Mucinous adenocarcinoma
Clear cell carcinoma	Squamous cell carcinoma
Basal cell adenocarcinoma	Small cell carcinoma
Low grade salivary duct or cribiform adenocarcinoma	Large cell carcinoma
Myoepithelial carcinoma	Lymphoepithelial carcinoma
Oncocytic carcinoma	Metastasizing pleomorphic adenoma (PA)
Carcinoma ex pleo (low grade/intracapsular)	Carcinoma ex pleo (high grade/widely invasive)
Sialoblatoma	Carcinosarcoma
Adenocarcinoma NOS low grade[a]	Adenocarcinoma NOS low grade[a]
Cystadenocarcinoma low grade	Cystadenocarcinoma low grade

[a] Intermediate grade variants of these tumors are controversial in the assignment of risk. For MEC this may depend on the grading scheme used. For adenocarcinoma NOS there is little data, but what is present suggests that intermediate grade should be placed in the high-risk group

[b] AdCC are all considered high risk in terms of local recurrence, but only solid AdCC is considered high risk for metastases

Table 39.5 Grading of mucoepidemoid carcinoma. (Reprinted from Auclair et al. [81] with permission of John Wiley & Sons, Inc.)

Author/year	Low grade	Intermediate	High
Dahlqvist 1982	5	0	0
Byers 1884	9	4	2
Baker 1985	3	0	0
Lack 1988	6	0	0
Fonseca 1991	5	0	0
Otago 1994	6	0	0
Rogers 1994	2	3	1
Kessler 1994	8	0	0
Bull 1999	1	0	0
Orvidas 2000	7	1	0
Ribeiro Khe 2002	6	6	5
Ethunandan 2003	3	0	0
De cruz Peres 2004	18	2	1
Verdine 2006	11	3	2
Guzzo 2006	9	1	2
Rahbar 2006	7	0	0
Ellies 2006	3	0	1
Total	109	20	14
Percentage (%)	76	14	10

Treatment

Children and adolescents with salivary gland neoplasms should be referred to specialized centers where they can be treated by a multidisciplinary team incorporating pediatric oncologists, radiation oncologists, and head and neck surgeons in order to optimize their management [29].

Surgery

The treatment of choice of most salivary gland neoplasms is complete removal with adequate margins [14]. For submandibular tumors, complete excision of the gland is recommended [59]. In the case of parotid tumors, depending on the lesion, superficial or total parotidectomy is indicated. Parotidectomy is considered a safer and more definitive procedure than tumor enucleation as the latter results in higher rates of recurrence and facial nerve dysfunction. Superficial parotidectomy is the treatment of choice when the tumor is lateral to the facial nerve and subsequent histology reveals a low-grade malignancy. Total parotidectomy is recommended when there is deep lobe involvement, suspected or confirmed high-grade tumors, or tumors with aggressive malignant potential, such as those with facial nerve involvement, multiple intraparotid masses, or cervical metastasis [14, 59]. Definitive surgery allows for very good local control rates approximating 97% in some series [16, 42].

Resection of the facial nerve is controversial. Factors that historically have influenced facial nerve resection include a tumor completely encapsulating the nerve, large tumors (>3 cm), and undifferentiated tumors [18, 31]. Resection is currently recommended only when there is gross anatomic or histopathologic evidence of neural invasion at the time of the surgery [59]. When there is no direct involvement, sparing the facial nerve does not appear to worsen the prognosis [65]. When resection of the nerve is necessary, immediate reanimation by means of primary anastomosis or free nerve graft is advocated [66]. Timely management in this respect is critical for achieving optimal facial function results.

The role of neck dissection in salivary gland cancer in children is also debatable. The overall incidence of LN metastases at presentation for primary parotid carcinomas in all age groups ranges between 18 and 28% [67, 68]. In the adult literature, recommendations range from routine elective neck dissection in all patients with primary carcinoma of the parotid gland [67] to neck dissection under specific circumstances including patients with tumors larger than 3 cm, high-grade tumors, facial paralysis, extra-glandular extension, and perilymphatic invasion [69]. Others argue in support of a supra-omohyoid neck dissection in patients with high-grade tumors for staging purposes, reserving an elective full neck dissection for patients with undifferentiated and squamous cell carcinomas [70]. In children, simultaneous neck dissection at the time of primary tumor excision is typically recommended only when cervical nodal metastases are clinically detected [15, 20, 23, 26]. Some advocate concurrent neck dissection when there is clinical evidence of high TNM stage or known high histological grade [14]. The clinical picture in children is further complicated by the fact that the presence of lymph node hyperplasia is common, particularly in younger children [59]. Under such circumstances, nodal biopsy is indicated, and a formal modified neck dissection undertaken if there is intraoperative frozen section confirmation of nodal metastases [26, 30, 69].

Permanent facial nerve paresis or paralysis after surgery for benign parotid tumors in adults ranges from 3 to 5% [71, 72], while transient facial nerve dysfunction ranges from 46 to 65% [71, 72]. These figures are notably higher when tumor enucleation rather than formal parotidectomy is undertaken [73]. In children, rates of facial nerve palsy following parotidectomy range from 5 to 33% [11, 15, 18, 21, 30]. This risk of facial weakness may be greater in children compared with adults, with one study reporting 10 of 21 cases had one or more branches of the facial nerve sectioned intraoperatively [26]. This risk is also higher in infants than older children [21]. Preoperative planning for facial nerve grafting should be considered if facial nerve resection is required [14]. As would be expected, complete parotidectomy has higher rates of transient facial nerve dysfunction and secondary Frey syndrome than superficial parotidectomy [74].

Frey's Syndrome, also known as gustatory sweating, is characterized by hyperhidrosis and flushing of the lateral cervicofacial skin following parotid surgery. These symptoms are due to abnormal skin innervation by auriculotemporal nerve parasympathetic fibers that communicate with the sympathetic nervous system. Subjective symptoms may be mentioned by 5–50% of patients, but formal evaluation via the starch iodine test can reveal the presence of this syndrome in the majority of postparotidectomy patients [75]. In children, reports of Frey's syndrome ranges from 0 to 47% [15, 18, 21, 22, 76]. Children are typically managed expectantly [76]. In adults botulinum toxin type A injection is the treatment of choice [75].

Additional potential postoperative complications include hypertrophic scars and keloid formation, which may need to be treated with intralesional steroids [18], and sialocele development, which may result from either parotid or submandibular gland resection [18].

Radiotherapy

There are well-documented studies that demonstrate the efficacy of postoperative radiation therapy in improving local and regional control of salivary gland malignancies in patients of all ages [77]. The principal indications for radiotherapy include high-grade malignancies, such as AdCC, squamous cell carcinoma, carcinoma ex pleomorphic and undifferentiated carcinomas, gross or histopathologic evidence of perineural invasion or soft tissue extension, multiple level cervical metastases, and incomplete primary lesion resection [14, 15, 26]. Children receive adjuvant radiation therapy less frequently than adults due to the higher risk of postradiotherapy complications (51 %vs 27 %) [11, 29]. Of particular significance in the pediatric population are facial growth retardation [78] and secondary malignant neoplasms [16, 40–42]. To minimize these potential risks, careful treatment planning with conformal techniques, such as intensity-modulated radiation therapy or proton beam therapy should be used in children whenever possible [79].

Chemotherapy

The role of chemotherapy in the management of salivary gland cancers remains poorly defined. Chemotherapy is generally reserved for patients with progressive local or metastatic disease that is not amenable to surgical or radiation therapy [14]. There is a scarcity of high quality data regarding the role of chemotherapy in the palliative management of salivary gland cancers in adults, and far less when it comes to children. While response rates of up to 50 % have been reported with some chemotherapeutic protocols, the duration of response is typically short, ranging from 6 to 12 months. High-grade mucoepidermoid carcinoma has demonstrated some chemotherapeutic sensitivity, but there is no clear evidence that such treatment improves survival [80]. The main goals of such therapy are palliative for prevention of symptoms secondary to rapid disease progression.

Prognosis and Outcomes

Tumor recurrence has been reported in 7–20 % of patients [15, 81]. Local and regional recurrence is more likely to occur in patients with positive margins, regardless of tumor grade. The 5 year overall survival (OS) for children with malignancies of the major salivary glands approximates 95 %, in comparison to a contrasting figure of 59 % for adults [11]. Data also suggests a more favorable prognosis for pediatric minor salivary gland malignancies compared to adults [48]. These survival figures reflect the fact that the majority of tumors presenting in younger patients are low-grade lesions with an inherent better prognosis [82, 83]. Data suggests that childhood malignancies of the same stage and grade have similar outcomes to their adult counterparts [15, 20, 21].

In a large single institution series in which 16 children were reported deceased at study cut-off, 13 were reported to have cancer related mortality, 4 had distant spread at diagnosis, and 2 were reported to have developed terminal second malignancies (acute lymphoblastic leukemia and osteosarcoma) [11]. Factors associated with a poor outcome in all age groups include male sex, high-grade tumors, large size (>2.5 cm), perineural invasion, LNM, soft tissue extension, macroscopic residual disease, and pathologic diagnoses other than mucoepidermoid or acinar cell carcinoma [11, 31, 77]. When different grades are examined in patients of all ages, the published 5 year survival rates range from 92 to 100 % in cases involving low-grade tumors, 62–92 % in those involving intermediate-grade tumors, and 0–43 % in those involving high-grade tumors [15, 70, 82, 83]. Children with salivary gland malignancies, regardless of histopathologic type, have a 3.2 % risk of the development of a second cancer during the following 20 years [84].

Follow-up

The follow-up of children with salivary gland malignancies will depend on the specific tumor histopathology, grade, stage and modality of treatment. Various protocols have been suggested, such as quarterly to semiannual checks for 5 years, and annual assessments thereafter for children with mucoepidermoid carcinoma [85]. There is a general consensus that long-term follow-up is necessary given the unpredictable nature of these neoplasms, as well as the risk of secondary malignancies. Some advocate follow-up over a minimum of 20 years [86].

Mucoepidermoid Carcinoma

Mucoepidermoid carcinoma (MEC) is the most common primary salivary gland malignancy in both adults and children [11]. MEC accounts for approximately 30 % of the total epithelial carcinomas in patients of all age and up to 60 % of pediatric salivary gland malignancies [12]. Macroscopically, MEC tumors are firm, smooth, often cystic, masses, of tan, white or pink color, with well-defined borders, or infiltrative edges [4]. Microscopically, they are composed of epidermoid cells, mucous secreting cells, and intermediate cells sharing both epidermoid and secretory features. Clear cells are also common. The proportion of different cell types and their architectural configuration, including cyst formation, varies in and between tumors (Fig. 39.2).

Several grading systems have been proposed without universal acceptance; these include the Armed Forces Institute of Pathology (AFIP) grading system (Table 39.6), the modified Healey system [87], and the Brandwein system [64]. Although, none of these systems has been shown to be ideal, there is evidence to suggest that the consistent use of a grad-

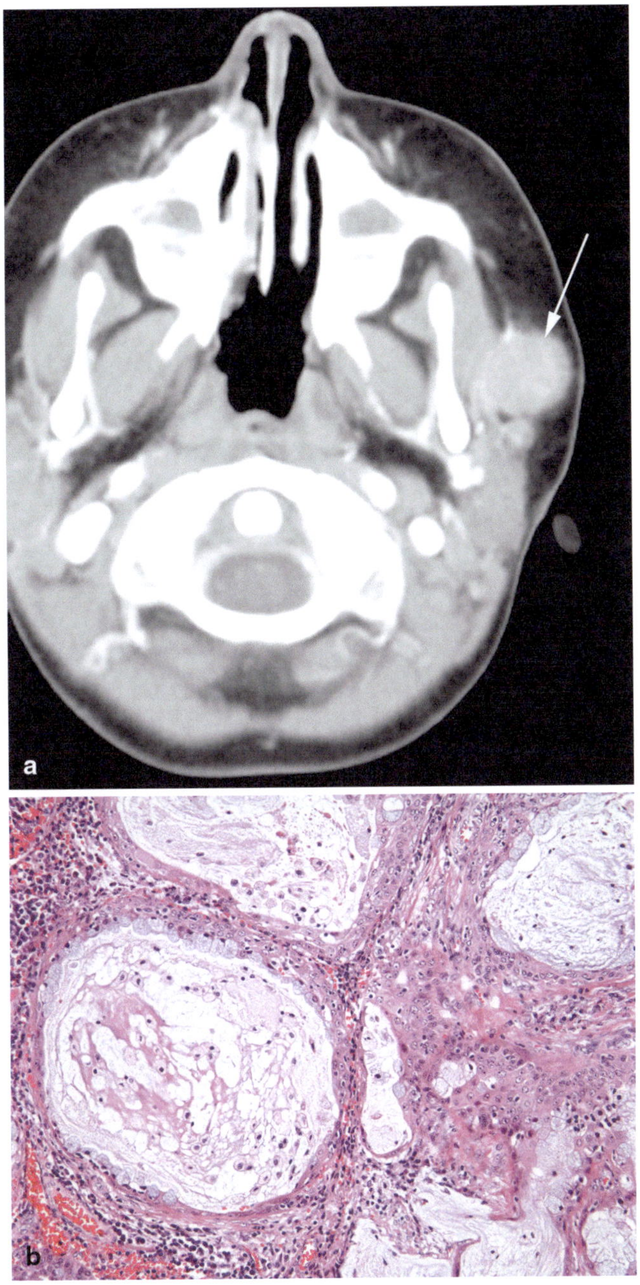

Fig. 39.2 Mucoepidermoid carcinoma. **a** Computer tomography (CT) showing a moderately well-defined mass within the parotid mass (*arrow*). **b.** Microscopically, the tumor reveals mucous-filled cysts with intervening squamoid tumor cells

ing scheme shows greater reproducibility than an alternative intuitive approach [61]. With regard to low-grade mucoepidermoid carcinoma, in less than 5 % of the cases is lymphatic metastatic spread observed, while in cases of high grade mucoepidermoid, LN metastases occur in up to 80 % [88].Low-grade MEC is generally treatable by primary tumor surgical resection alone, while high-grade MEC requires ipsilateral neck dissection and adjuvant radiation therapy [89]. The reported overall 5 year survival for MEC ranges from 92 to

Table 39.6 AFIP grading system for mucoepidermoid carcinomas

Histological features	*Point value*
Cystic component < 20 %	2
Neural invasion	2
Necrosis	3
4 or more mitosis/10 hpf	3
Anaplasia	4
Tumor grade	*Point score*
Low	0–4
Intermediate	5–6
High	7 or more

100 % for low grade tumors, 62–92 % for intermediate grade tumors, and 0–43 % for high-grade tumors [61].

Acinic Cell Carcinoma

ACCs make up approximately 10 % of all malignant salivary gland tumors, accounting for 9–17 % of parotid, 1–4 % of submandibular, and 1–3 % of minor salivary gland malignancies [90–92]. A similar percentage of ACC involvement is reported in children [19, 26]. This salivary gland malignancy is more common in women, with up to a 2:1 female to male predominance in adult series.

ACC classically presents as a slow growing mass. Pain may also be a feature in up to a third of patients although, unlike other salivary gland malignancies, pain does necessarily indicate a poor prognosis [93]. The overwhelming majority of ACC (88 %) present locally [94]. Facial nerve palsy may occur in up to 10 % of patients [95]. If metastases are present, the cervical chain is the most common site, followed by the lungs and bone [93]. Macroscopically most ACC are well-circumscribed, solitary nodules but some are ill defined. The cut surface appears lobular and tan to red in color. They vary from firm to soft, and solid to cystic [4]. Histologically four architectural patterns have been described including solid, microcystic, papillary-cystic, and follicular. Classifying ACC according to these subtypes is difficult because different patterns may occur in a single lesion [96].

Owing to the indolent nature of these tumors, they were initially classified as benign, with the term acinic cell "tumor" rather than "carcinoma" being used in some early classification systems. The recognition of recurrence and metastases led to the more appropriate categorization as a true carcinoma [97]. Typically thought of as a tumor with low malignant potential, many studies suggest an unusually high rate of LNM and recurrence in comparison to other low-risk tumors [61]. Grading systems have been proposed, in which features such as tumor infiltration, medullary architecture, tubular morphology, desmoplasia, atypia, increased mitotic activity, and prominence of undifferentiated cells are employed to define high-grade tumors with a poor prognosis [98]. However, these grading systems are not widely used as the histological features of these tumors often do not correlate with the clinical course [99]. Currently, there is no consensus on the grading of ACC [100]. Staging is often a better predictor of prognosis in ACC, with large size, involvement of the deep lobe of the parotid gland, local invasion, metastases on presentation, and incomplete resection predictive of recurrence and a poor outcome [4, 100]. Rates of local control according to stage (I, II, and III) have been found to be 85, 63 and 43 %, respectively [101]. A number of studies have also shown a link between prognosis and growth fraction assessed by the MiB1 monoclonal antibody, with high indices of the antibody indicative of a poor outcome [99].

As with other salivary gland tumors, surgical excision with negative margins is the principal treatment. Elective neck dissection has not been shown to provide any survival benefit [102]. Ipsilateral neck dissection is indicated if there are clinically positive cervical chain lymph nodes, and radiotherapy is recommended in recurrent tumors, equivocal or positive margins, when there is evidence of tumor spillage, nodal metastases, extraglandular extension, or with large tumors greater than 4 cm [94].

In adults, ACC is biologically less aggressive than AdCC or intermediate and high-grade mucoepidermoid carcinoma. Such appears to be true of ACC in children as well [33]. For the most part (82 %), first recurrences and metastases occur within 5 years of initial therapy [93], however, similar to AdCC, delayed development of local recurrence may be seen [30], In all ages, ACCs have the longest tumor-free interval and best prognosis with a 10-year relative survival of 85–88 % [92].

Adenoid Cystic Carcinoma

AdCC accounts for 20–30 % of all malignant salivary gland tumors in adults. Although a large number of studies describe mucoepidermoid carcinoma to be the most frequent subtype [103, 104], many series, particularly those from northern Europe, report a predominance of AdCC or nearly equal frequencies of adenoid cystic and mucoepidermoid carcinomas [90, 92, 105]. Composite analysis of the a large number of pediatric retrospective studies reveals 8.8 % of the malignant salivary gland tumors in children to be AdCC [13–15, 18–20, 25, 26, 28–30, 32, 33]. Unlike mucoepidermoid and ACCs, the majority of AdCCs in adults arise in the minor salivary gland (36 %) or the submandibular and sublingual glands (27 %) [106, 107]. AdCCs are also found in greater numbers in the paranasal sinuses, lacrimal glands and trachea than other salivary gland tumors. In children, almost all reported AdCCs have occurred in the parotid gland (Table 39.7), with a few case reports of childhood AdCC arising in the lacrimal glands [108], larynx and minor salivary glands [109].

Table 39.7 Anatomic distribution of AdCCs in children

Paper/year	Ref	Parotid	Submand/ sublingual	Minor	Other	Total
Baker 85	30	5	0	0	0	5
Ribeiro 02	20	2	1	0	0	3
Yu 02	19	2	0	1	0	3
Ellies 06	13	3	0	0	0	3
Guzzo 06	15	1	0	0	0	1
Ogato 94	25	1	0	0	0	1
Total		14	1	1	0	16
Percentage (%)		88	6	6	0	100

Table 39.8 Comparison of common pattern grading schemes in AdCC. (Reprinted from Seethala 2009 [61] with permission from Springer Science+Business Media)

Grade	Perzin 1978 [113]; Szanto 1984 [62]	Grade	Spiro 1992 [63]
1	Predominantly tubular, no solid component	1	Mostly tubular or cribriform (no stipulation on solid component)
2	Predominantly cribriform, solid component <30 %		
3	Solid component >30 %	2	50 % solid
		3	Mostly solid

Like other salivary neoplasms, AdCC presents as a slow growing mass, but because of its proclivity for perineural invasion, symptoms of pain and numbness are frequent [106]. Pain was a noted symptom at presentation in almost 50 % of adults [110] and 40 % of children [30]. This correlates strongly with rates of perineural invasion, which have been reported from 43 to 51 % [111]. Large tumors (T3 and T4) have been shown to have a much higher incidence of perineural invasion (60 %) than smaller (T1 and T2) tumors (23.5 %). A variety of other presenting complaints can be associated with AdCC including ulceration, nasal obstruction, hoarseness, and dysphagia because of the varied location of such tumors [110]. Up to 10 % of patients may present with distant metastases, predominantly in the lungs [106].

The gross appearance of AdCC is typically a firm, light tan, well defined but nonencapsulated mass that invariably infiltrates surrounding normal tissues [4]. Despite the name, these are solid tumors that rarely display obvious cystic spaces on the cut surface. Microscopically they have been described as biphasic, composed of ducts and basal or myoepithelial cells with small basaloid cells surrounding cystic spaces [30]. Such cells are arranged into three prognostically significant patterns: cribriform, tubular, and solid. The cribriform type is most common and classically contains multiple cylindric cyst-like spaces resembling 'Swiss cheese'. The grading systems used for AdCC are summarized in Table 39.8. Any solid component imparts a poor prognosis, and the current WHO classification system refers to tumors by predominant pattern rather than actually assigning a numeric grade [61]. Other prognostic factors include age over 45 years, rapid progression of disease prior to presentation, presence of numbness (paresthesia) on presentation, tumor size, lymph node involvement, distant metastases, solid histological type, and presence of residual tumor [112].

In adults, multimodality therapy, specifically surgery followed by radiation, is considered the standard of care for AdCC. Postoperative radiotherapy has been shown to improve the 5 year local recurrence rate and disease-free survival compared to surgery alone [107]. As with all malignancies of the head and neck, the benefits of radiotherapy must be weighed against the potential long-term side effects. The clinical course of this tumor overall is characteristically slow but relentless growth. Five year survival is favorable at roughly 75–80 %, but 15 year survival is poor at about 35 % [63, 111]. In the largest series of pediatric AdCC, only one of five patients was alive with no evidence of disease 7 years after initial treatment; the other four patients, followed on a longer term basis, had died of disease 11–28 years following presentation [30]. Lifelong follow-up of AdCC patients is clearly required.

Sialoblastoma

Sialoblastoma is an extremely rare tumor with less than 50 cases reported in the literature [114]. Sialoblastoma was not recognized as a distinct entity in early classifications of salivary gland malignancies. Initially considered to be a benign salivary gland tumor [115], reports of aggressive lesions with rapid growth, recurrence, metastases [116] and tumor-related mortality [116, 117] led to sialoblastoma being eventually categorized as a malignancy [4, 103].

This neoplasm is often described as congenital because sialoblastomas are usually diagnosed on antenatal ultrasound scans [118], at birth, or shortly thereafter [118]. There are, however, reported sialoblastoma diagnoses as late as 5 years of age [119]. Approximately 75 % of sialoblastomas arise from the parotid gland [4, 120], with the remainder of primarily submandilular gland origin [121]. There are case reports of sialoblastomas arising in ectopic salivary gland tissue [122] and in minor salivary glands [123]. The male to female ratio is 2:1 [4]. The majority of patients present with an asymptomatic mass in the parotid or submandibular region, but massive tumors with skin necrosis [124] and facial nerve palsy are described [125]. Radiographically, these tumors appear as expansile lobulated masses. MRI shows an isointense tumor on T1-weighted images, and a hyperintense tumor on T2-weighted images with heterogeneous contrast enhancement [124]. Incisional biopsy of massive lesions is necessary to rule out other malignancies such as rhabdomyosarcoma [4].

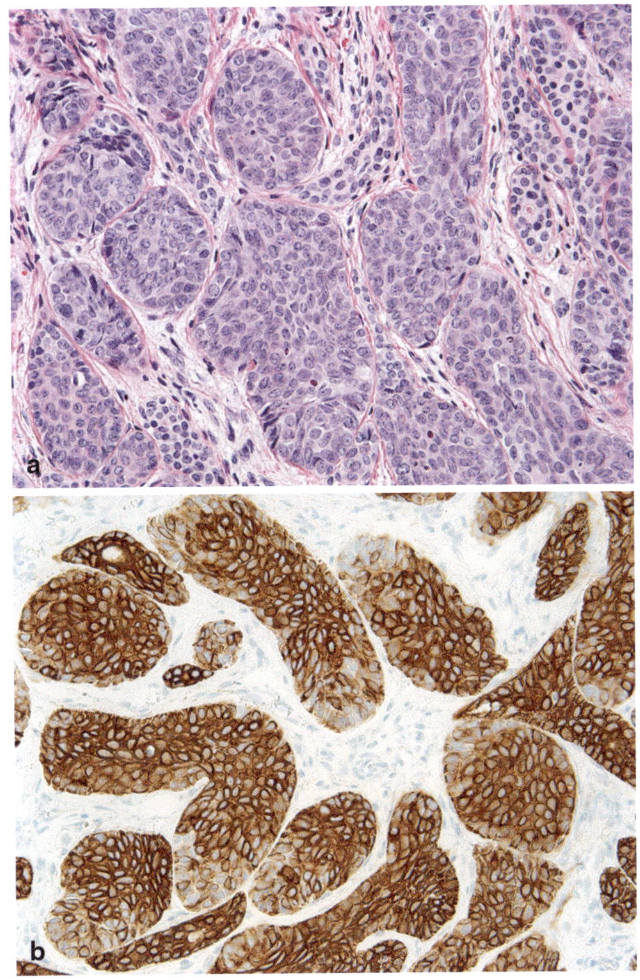

Fig. 39.3 Silaoblastoma. **a** The tumor is composed of well circumscribed nests surrounded by a well-developed basal lamina. Mitoses are frequently present. **b** Tumor cells are strongly immunoreactive for low molecular weight cytokeratins (CK19 immunostain)

Although, there is histologic variability, characteristically sialoblastomas are composed of numerous small, individual, and solid hypercellular islands of primitive basaloid epithelial cells with scant cytoplasm, round to oval nuclei, single or few nucleoli, and a relatively fine chromatin pattern, separated by fibrous or fibromyxomatous stroma [4, 114] (Fig. 39.3). Based on histological features, such as mitotic figures, necrosis, and anaplasia, histological prognostic factors have been proposed with characterization of favorable and unfavorable tumors [116]. The accuracy of such categorization is arguably questionable as some tumors with initially favorable features have been shown to recur with increasingly unfavorable characteristics on subsequent histopathologic examination [126]. Sialoblastomas express S-100 and vimentin, smooth muscle actin, and p63 diffusely. Cytokeratin classically accentuates the ductal structures [126].

Surgical excision with tumor-free margins is the desired therapy. Massive tumors, however, are often unresectable and require some form of adjuvant therapy. Although, external beam radiotherapy is controversial in this age group, treatment with brachytherapy has been reported with successful outcome [127]. In patients with extensive or metastatic disease, chemotherapy has been used with some success [120, 122]. In some cases, chemotherapy may induce tumor reduction, thereby facilitating subsequent surgical resection [120]. Local recurrence is a common (38 %) feature of sialoblastoma [120]. Local recurrences, along with distant metastases, have been successfully treated with further surgical excision [116], chemotherapy [118], radiotherapy or a combination of treatment modalities [116, 122]. As a result, the overall prognosis is relatively quite good [4, 120]. Two of the reported deaths in the literature occurred in neonates prior to any diagnosis or treatment and were judged to be due to unrelated causes [116, 128]. The third mortality involved a patient who initially presented with a parotid mass at 1 year of age but with delayed diagnosis until age 4; this patient had extensive surgery but recurred within 15 months and subsequently failed chemotherapy and further surgery [117].

Pleomorphic Adenoma

PA are rare in children and adolescents, accounting for approximately 2 % of all salivary gland tumors [18, 129], in contrast to their commonality (65 % of all salivary neoplasms) in adults [130]. Composite analysis of a number of studies reveals the majority (62 %; range 56–77 %) to occur in the parotid gland, with the submandibular gland (26 %; range 11–40 %) and the minor salivary glands (12 %; range 0–21 %) being comparatively less frequents sites of origin [12, 19, 25, 26, 28, 29, 129]. Similar to adults, a female predominance has been documented with an approximate 1.4:1 female to male ratio [129]. The typical presentation is a slow growing mass with an average duration of symptoms prior to presentation of approximately 12 months [18, 129]. Pain is a rare symptom and, when present, often implies tumor necrosis [131]. Rarely facial nerve paresis has been reported secondary to PA [132]; in such situations malignancy should be suspected.

On gross inspection, PAs are well circumscribed and lobulated with a smooth surface (Fig. 39.4). The appearance of the cut surface may reflect the tumor's cellular composition. Predominantly, epithelial or myoepithelial tumors may appear white and solid, whereas a bluish or semitransparent tumor is indicative chondroid tissue, and a soft mucoid tumor appearance corresponds with myxoid predominance. The microscopic characteristics vary from lesion to lesion, and also within different parts of the tumor [133]. Classic histologic features include epithelial or myoepithelial cells in a myxochondroid matrix [134]. The relative amounts of cellular and stromal tissue have no bearing on the aggressiveness of the tumor [133].The optimal treatment of PA is

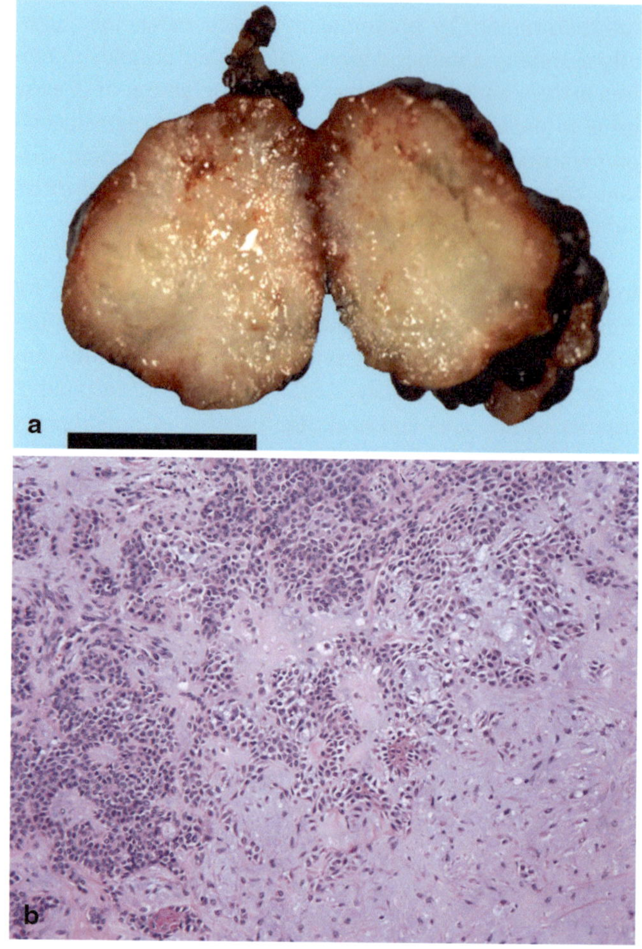

Fig. 39.4 Pleomorphic adenoma (PA). **a** Gross specimen showing a well-circumscribed mass with a *glistening*, *white-gray* cut surface imparting a chondroid appearance. **b** Microscopically, there is variation in the cellularity of the tumor. Chondroid matrix is prominent on the *right lower* corner of the photograph while on the *left upper* corner the tumor is more cellular primarily composed of epithelial elements

wide surgical excision with negative margins. The preferred treatment for parotid lesions is superficial parotidectomy or total parotidectomy depending on lesion location [129]. This approach yields local control rates in excess of 95 % [135]. In contrast, the risk of PA recurrence following lesion enucleation reportedly approaches 43 % [136]. Postoperative radiotherapy is controversial. Some authors do advocate its use in cases of tumor spillage or residual tumors in order to decrease the morbidity from recurrence [137]. Such use must be weighed against the potential complications of radiotherapy, particularly in the pediatric age group [138].

Although PA is a benign neoplasm, there is potential for malignant transformation. The average incidence of carcinoma ex PA has been estimated to be 6.2 % [139]. The risk of malignant degeneration in an untreated patient appears to be related, in part, to the duration of the lesion, increasing from about 1.5 % in the first 5 years to 9.5 % for adenomas present longer than 15 years [140]. Carcinomas ex PA are extremely rare in children, with only four cases total in the composite review of retrospective series [20, 25, 32]. Long life expectancy, combined with documented recurrences of up to 30 years after initial resection, increases the recurrence risk in children, with resultant long-term follow-up mandatory [134].

References

1. Levin RJ, Bradley MK. Neuroectodermal antigens persist in benign and malignant salivary gland tumor cultures. Arch Otolaryngol Head Neck Surg. 1996;122:551–7 (discussion 577–8).
2. Eversole LR. Histogenic classification of salivary tumors. Arch Pathol. 1971;92:433–43.
3. Dardick I, Burford-Mason AP. Current status of histogenetic and morphogenetic concepts of salivary gland tumorigenesis. Crit Rev Oral Biol Med. 1993;4:639–77.
4. Barnes L, Eveson JW, Reichart P, Sidransky D. Tumours of the salivary glands. World Health Organization Classification of Tumours, Pathology and Genetics of Head and Neck Tumours. Lyon: IARC Press; 2005. p. 209–81.
5. Gibbons MD, Manne U, Carroll WR, Peters GE, Weiss HL, Grizzle WE. Molecular differences in mucoepidermoid carcinoma and adenoid cystic carcinoma of the major salivary glands. Laryngoscope. 2001;111:1373–8.
6. Alcedo JC, Fabrega JM, Arosemena JR, Urrutia A. Imatinib mesylate as treatment for adenoid cystic carcinoma of the salivary glands: report of two successfully treated cases. Head Neck. 2004;26:829–31.
7. Frierson HF Jr, El-Naggar AK, Welsh JB, et al. Large scale molecular analysis identifies genes with altered expression in salivary adenoid cystic carcinoma. Am J Pathol. 2002;161:1315–23.
8. Kiyoshima T, Shima K, Kobayashi I, et al. Expression of p53 tumor suppressor gene in adenoid cystic and mucoepidermoid carcinomas of the salivary glands. Oral Oncol. 2001;37:315–22.
9. Pinkston JA, Cole P. Incidence rates of salivary gland tumors: results from a population-based study. Otolaryngol Head Neck Surg. 1999;120:834–40.
10. Sun EC, Curtis R, Melbye M, Goedert JJ. Salivary gland cancer in the United States. Cancer Epidemiol Biomarkers Prev. 1999;8:1095–100.
11. Sultan I, Rodriguez-Galindo C, Al-Sharabati S, Guzzo M, Casanova M, Ferrari A. Salivary gland carcinomas in children and adolescents: a population-based study, with comparison to adult cases. Head Neck. 2011;33:1476–81.
12. Krolls SO, Trodahl JN, Boyers RC. Salivary gland lesions in children. A survey of 430 cases. Cancer. 1972;30:459–69.
13. Ellies M, Schaffranietz F, Arglebe C, Laskawi R. Tumors of the salivary glands in childhood and adolescence. J Oral Maxillofac Surg. 2006;64:1049–58.
14. Rahbar R, Grimmer JF, Vargas SO, et al. Mucoepidermoid carcinoma of the parotid gland in children: a 10-year experience. Arch Otolaryngol Head Neck Surg. 2006;132:375–80.
15. Guzzo M, Ferrari A, Marcon I, et al. Salivary gland neoplasms in children: the experience of the Istituto Nazionale Tumori of Milan. Pediatr Blood Cancer. 2006;47:806–10.
16. Vedrine PO, Coffinet L, Temam S, et al. Mucoepidermoid carcinoma of salivary glands in the pediatric age group: 18 clinical cases, including 11 s malignant neoplasms. Head Neck. 2006;28:827–33.
17. da Cruz PDE, Pires FR, Alves FA, Almeida OP, Kowalski LP. Salivary gland tumors in children and adolescents: a clinicopathologic and immunohistochemical study of fifty-three cases. Int J Pediatr Otorhinolaryngol. 2004;68:895–902.
18. Ethunandan M, Ethunandan A, Macpherson D, Conroy B, Pratt C. Parotid neoplasms in children: experience of diagnosis and management in a district general hospital. Int J Oral Maxillofac Surg. 2003;32:373–7.
19. Yu GY, Li ZL, Ma DQ, Zhang Y. Diagnosis and treatment of epithelial salivary gland tumours in children and adolescents. Br J Oral Maxillofac Surg. 2002;40:389–92.
20. Ribeiro Kde C, Kowalski LP, Saba LM, de Camargo B. Epithelial salivary glands neoplasms in children and adolescents: a forty-four-year experience. Med Pediatr Oncol. 2002;39:594–600.
21. Orvidas LJ, Kasperbauer JL, Lewis JE, Olsen KD, Lesnick TG. Pediatric parotid masses. Arch Otolaryngol Head Neck Surg. 2000;126:177–84.
22. Bull PD. Salivary gland neoplasia in childhood. Int J Pediatr Otorhinolaryngol. 1999;49 Suppl 1:S235–8.
23. Kessler A, Handler SD. Salivary gland neoplasms in children: a 10-year survey at the children's hospital of Philadelphia. Int J Pediatr Otorhinolaryngol. 1994;29:195–202.
24. Rogers DA, Rao BN, Bowman L, et al. Primary malignancy of the salivary gland in children. J Pediatr Surg. 1994;29:44–7.
25. Ogata H, Ebihara S, Mukai K. Salivary gland neoplasms in children. Jpn J Clin Oncol. 1994;24:88–93.
26. Callender DL, Frankenthaler RA, Luna MA, Lee SS, Goepfert H. Salivary gland neoplasms in children. Arch Otolaryngol Head Neck Surg. 1992;118:472–6.
27. Fonseca I, Martins AG, Soares J. Epithelial salivary gland tumors of children and adolescents in southern Portugal. A clinicopathologic study of twenty-four cases. Oral Surg Oral Med Oral Pathol. 1991;72:696–701.
28. Lack EE, Upton MP. Histopathologic review of salivary gland tumors in childhood. Arch Otolaryngol Head Neck Surg. 1988;114:898–906.
29. Shikhani AH, Johns ME. Tumors of the major salivary glands in children. Head Neck Surg. 1988;10:257–63.
30. Baker SR, Malone B. Salivary gland malignancies in children. Cancer. 1985;55:1730–6.
31. Byers RM, Piorkowski R, Luna MA. Malignant parotid tumors in patients under 20 years of age. Arch Otolaryngol. 1984;110:232–5.
32. Dahlqvist A, Ostberg Y. Malignant salivary gland tumours in children. Acta Otolaryngol. 1982;94:175–9.
33. Castro EB, Huvos AG, Strong EW, Foote FW Jr. Tumors of the major salivary glands in children. Cancer. 1972;29:312–7.
34. Leuin SC, Cunningham MJ, Curtin H, Faquin WC. Childhood acinic cell carcinoma of the accessory parotid gland: a rare combination. Int J Pediatr Otorhinolaryngol Extra. 2007;2:1–5.
35. Walterhouse DO, Pappo AS, Baker KS, et al. Rhabdomyosarcoma of the parotid region occurring in childhood and adolescence. A report from the Intergroup Rhabdomyosarcoma Study Group. Cancer. 2001;92:3135–46.
36. Shapiro NL, Bhattacharyya N. Clinical characteristics and survival for major salivary gland malignancies in children. Otolaryngol Head Neck Surg. 2006;134:631–4.
37. Takeichi N, Hirose F, Yamamoto H, Ezaki H, Fujikura T. Salivary gland tumors in atomic bomb survivors, Hiroshima, Japan. II. Pathologic study and supplementary epidemiologic observations. Cancer. 1983;52:377–85.
38. Saku T, Hayashi Y, Takahara O, et al. Salivary gland tumors among atomic bomb survivors, 1950–1987. Cancer. 1997;79:1465–75.
39. Spitz MR, Tilley BC, Batsakis JG, Gibeau JM, Newell GR. Risk factors for major salivary gland carcinoma. A case-comparison study. Cancer. 1984;54:1854–9.
40. Loy TS, McLaughlin R, Odom LF, Dehner LP. Mucoepidermoid carcinoma of the parotid as a second malignant neoplasm in children. Cancer. 1989;64:2174–7.

41. Kaste SC, Hedlund G, Pratt CB. Malignant parotid tumors in patients previously treated for childhood cancer: clinical and imaging findings in eight cases. AJR Am J Roentgenol. 1994;162:655–9.
42. Verma J, Teh BS, Paulino AC. Characteristics and outcome of radiation and chemotherapy-related mucoepidermoid carcinoma of the salivary glands. Pediatr Blood Cancer. 2011;57:1137–41.
43. Tsai CC, Chen CL, Hsu HC. Expression of Epstein-Barr virus in carcinomas of major salivary glands: a strong association with lymphoepithelioma-like carcinoma. Hum Pathol. 1996;27:258–62.
44. Schuller DE, McCabe BF. The firm salivary mass in children. Laryngoscope. 1977;87:1891–8.
45. Byrne MN, Spector JG. Parotid masses: evaluation, analysis, and current management. Laryngoscope. 1988;98:99–105.
46. Tincani AJ, Del Negro A, Araujo PP, et al. Management of salivary gland adenoid cystic carcinoma: institutional experience of a case series. Sao Paulo Med J. 2006;124:26–30.
47. Moraes P, Pereira C, Almeida O, Perez D, Correa ME, Alves F. Paediatric intraoral mucoepidermoid carcinoma mimicking a bone lesion. Int J Paediatr Dent. 2007;17:151–4.
48. Galer C, Santillan AA, Chelius D, et al. Minor salivary gland malignancies in the pediatric population. Head Neck. 2012;34(11):1648–51.
49. Oldham KT, Aiken JA. Pediatric head and neck. In: Mulholland MW, Lillemoe KD, Doherty GM, Maier RV, Simeone DM, Upchurch GR, editors. Greenfield's surgery: scientific principles & practice. 5th ed. Philadelphia: Lippincott Williams & Wilkins; 2010.
50. Yuh WT, Sato Y, Loes DJ, et al. Magnetic resonance imaging and computed tomography in pediatric head and neck masses. Ann Otol Rhinol Laryngol. 1991;100:54–62.
51. Kaneda T, Minami M, Ozawa K, et al. MR of the submandibular gland: normal and pathologic states. AJNR Am J Neuroradiol. 1996;17:1575–81.
52. Yousem DM, Kraut MA, Chalian AA. Major salivary gland imaging. Radiology. 2000;216:19–29.
53. Parker GD, Harnsberger HR. Clinical-radiologic issues in perineural tumor spread of malignant diseases of the extracranial head and neck. Radiographics. 1991;11:383–99.
54. Freling NJ, Molenaar WM, Vermey A, et al. Malignant parotid tumors: clinical use of MR imaging and histologic correlation. Radiology. 1992;185:691–6.
55. Sumi M, Van Cauteren M, Sumi T, Obara M, Ichikawa Y, Nakamura T. Salivary gland tumors: use of intravoxel incoherent motion MR imaging for assessment of diffusion and perfusion for the differentiation of benign from malignant tumors. Radiology. 2012;263(3):770–7.
56. Colella G, Cannavale R, Flamminio F, Foschini MP. Fine-needle aspiration cytology of salivary gland lesions: a systematic review. J Oral Maxillofac Surg. 2010;68:2146–53.
57. Liu ES, Bernstein JM, Sculerati N, Wu HC. Fine needle aspiration biopsy of pediatric head and neck masses. Int J Pediatr Otorhinolaryngol. 2001;60:135–40.
58. Cho HW, Kim J, Choi J, et al. Sonographically guided fine-needle aspiration biopsy of major salivary gland masses: a review of 245 cases. AJR Am J Roentgenol. 2011;196:1160–3.
59. Cunningham MJ. Salivary gland surgery. In: Bluestone CD, editor. Surgical Atlas of Pediatric Otolaryngology. 1st ed. Hamilton: BC Decker Inc; 2002. p. 515–38.
60. Zarbo RJ. Salivary gland neoplasia: a review for the practicing pathologist. Mod Pathol. 2002;15:298–323.
61. Seethala RR. An update on grading of salivary gland carcinomas. Head Neck Pathol. 2009;3:69–77.
62. Szanto PA, Luna MA, Tortoledo ME, White RA. Histologic grading of adenoid cystic carcinoma of the salivary glands. Cancer. 1984;54:1062–9.
63. Spiro RH, Huvos AG. Stage means more than grade in adenoid cystic carcinoma. Am J Surg. 1992;164:623–8.
64. Brandwein MS, Ferlito A, Bradley PJ, Hille JJ, Rinaldo A. Diagnosis and classification of salivary neoplasms: pathologic challenges and relevance to clinical outcomes. Acta Otolaryngol. 2002;122:758–64.
65. Longo F, Manola M, Villano S, et al. Treatment of the facial nerve and the neck in malignant parotid gland tumors. Tumori. 2003;89:257–9.
66. Revenaugh PC, Knott PD, Scharpf J, Fritz MA. Simultaneous anterolateral thigh flap and temporalis tendon transfer to optimize facial form and function after radical parotidectomy. Arch Facial Plast Surg. 2012;14:104–9.
67. Zbaren P, Schupbach J, Nuyens M, Stauffer E. Elective neck dissection versus observation in primary parotid carcinoma. Otolaryngol Head Neck Surg. 2005;132:387–91.
68. Rodriguez-Cuevas S, Labastida S, Baena L, Gallegos F. Risk of nodal metastases from malignant salivary gland tumors related to tumor size and grade of malignancy. Eur Arch Otorhinolaryngol. 1995;252:139–42.
69. Medina JE. Neck dissection in the treatment of cancer of major salivary glands. Otolaryngol Clin North Am. 1998;31:815–22.
70. Spiro RH, Armstrong J, Harrison L, Geller NL, Lin SY, Strong EW. Carcinoma of major salivary glands. Recent trends. Arch Otolaryngol Head Neck Surg. 1989;115:316–21.
71. Mehle ME, Kraus DH, Wood BG, et al. Facial nerve morbidity following parotid surgery for benign disease: the Cleveland Clinic Foundation experience. Laryngoscope. 1993;103:386–8.
72. Laccourreye H, Laccourreye O, Cauchois R, Jouffre V, Menard M, Brasnu D. Total conservative parotidectomy for primary benign pleomorphic adenoma of the parotid gland: a 25-year experience with 229 patients. Laryngoscope. 1994;104:1487–94.
73. Donovan DT, Conley JJ. Capsular significance in parotid tumor surgery: reality and myths of lateral lobectomy. Laryngoscope. 1984;94:324–9.
74. Witt RL. The significance of the margin in parotid surgery for pleomorphic adenoma. Laryngoscope. 2002;112:2141–54.
75. Kyrmizakis DE, Pangalos A, Papadakis CE, Logothetis J, Maroudias NJ, Helidonis ES. The use of botulinum toxin type A in the treatment of Frey and crocodile tears syndromes. J Oral Maxillofac Surg. 2004;62:840–4.
76. Xie CM, Kubba H. Parotidectomy in children: indications and complications. J Laryngol Otol. 2010;124:1289–93.
77. Weber RS, Byers RM, Petit B, Wolf P, Ang K, Luna M. Submandibular gland tumors. Adverse histologic factors and therapeutic implications. Arch Otolaryngol Head Neck Surg. 1990;116:1055–60.
78. Denys D, Kaste SC, Kun LE, Chaudhary MA, Bowman LC, Robbins KT. The effects of radiation on craniofacial skeletal growth: a quantitative study. Int J Pediatr Otorhinolaryngol. 1998;45:7–13.
79. Schoenfeld JD, Sher DJ, Norris CM Jr, et al. Salivary gland tumors treated with adjuvant intensity-modulated radiotherapy with or without concurrent chemotherapy. Int J Radiat Oncol Biol Phys. 2012;82:308–14.
80. Airoldi M, Brando V, Giordano C, Gabriele P, Bussi M, Cortesina G. Chemotherapy for recurrent salivary gland malignancies: experience of the ENT Department of Turin University. ORL J Otorhinolaryngol Relat Spec. 1994;56:105–11.
81. Auclair PL, Goode RK, Ellis GL. Mucoepidermoid carcinoma of 2 salivary glands. Evaluation and application of grading criteria in 143 cases. Cancer. 1992;69:2021–30.
82. Clode AL, Fonseca I, Santos JR, Soares J. Mucoepidermoid carcinoma of the salivary glands: a reappraisal of the influence of tumor differentiation on prognosis. J Surg Oncol. 1991;46:100–6.
83. Nascimento AG, Amaral LP, Prado LA, Kligerman J, Silveira TR. Mucoepidermoid carcinoma of salivary glands: a clinicopathologic study of 46 cases. Head Neck Surg. 1986;8:409–17.

84. Neglia JP, Friedman DL, Yasui Y, et al. Second malignant neoplasms in five-year survivors of childhood cancer: childhood cancer survivor study. J Natl Cancer Inst. 2001;93:618–29.
85. April MM, Brodsky LS, Cunningham MJ, Harari PM, Harrison L, Poje CP. Mucoepidermoid carcinoma in a 10-year-old girl. Head Neck. 1997;19:431–5.
86. Batsakis JG. Staging of salivary gland neoplasms: role of histopathologic and molecular factors. Am J Surg. 1994;168:386–90.
87. Batsakis JG, Luna MA. Histopathologic grading of salivary gland neoplasms: I. Mucoepidermoid carcinomas. Ann Otol Rhinol Laryngol. 1990;99:835–8.
88. Moll R, Ramaswamy A. The pathology of lymphogenic metastatic spread. In: Werner JA, Davis RK, editors. Metastases in head and neck cancer. Berlin: Springer; 2005. p. 75.
89. Aro K, Leivo I, Makitie AA. Management and outcome of patients with mucoepidermoid carcinoma of major salivary gland origin: a single institution's 30-year experience. Laryngoscope. 2008;118:258–62.
90. Bjorndal K, Krogdahl A, Therkildsen MH, et al. Salivary gland carcinoma in Denmark 1990–2005: a national study of incidence, site and histology. Results of the Danish Head and Neck Cancer Group (DAHANCA). Oral Oncol. 2011;47:677–82.
91. Eveson JW, Cawson RA. Salivary gland tumours. A review of 2410 cases with particular reference to histological types, site, age and sex distribution. J Pathol. 1985;146:51–8.
92. Wahlberg P, Anderson H, Biorklund A, Moller T, Perfekt R. Carcinoma of the parotid and submandibular glands—a study of survival in 2465 patients. Oral Oncol. 2002;38:706–13.
93. Ellis GL, Corio RL. Acinic cell adenocarcinoma. A clinicopathologic analysis of 294 cases. Cancer. 1983;52:542–9.
94. Hoffman HT, Karnell LH, Robinson RA, Pinkston JA. Menck HR. National cancer data base report on cancer of the head and neck: acinic cell carcinoma. Head Neck. 1999;21:297–309.
95. Laskawi R, Rodel R, Zirk A, Arglebe C. Retrospective analysis of 35 patients with acinic cell carcinoma of the parotid gland. J Oral Maxillofac Surg. 1998;56:440–3.
96. Schwarz S, Zenk J, Muller M, et al. The many faces of acinic cell carcinomas of the salivary glands: a study of 40 cases relating histological and immunohistological subtypes to clinical parameters and prognosis. Histopathology. 2012;61(3):395–408.
97. Guimaraes DS, Amaral AP, Prado LF, Nascimento AG. Acinic cell carcinoma of salivary glands: 16 cases with clinicopathologic correlation. J Oral Pathol Med. 1989;18:396–9.
98. Batsakis JG, Luna MA, el-Naggar AK. Histopathologic grading of salivary gland neoplasms: II. Acinic cell carcinomas. Ann Otol Rhinol Laryngol. 1990;99:929–33.
99. Suzzi MV, Alessi A, Bertarelli C, et al. Prognostic relevance of cell proliferation in major salivary gland carcinomas. Acta Otorhinolaryngol Ital. 2005;25:161–8.
100. Timon CI, Dardick I. The importance of dedifferentiation in recurrent acinic cell carcinoma. J Laryngol Otol. 2001;115:639–44.
101. Spiro RH, Huvos AG, Strong EW. Acinic cell carcinoma of salivary origin. A clinicopathologic study of 67 cases. Cancer. 1978;41:924–35.
102. Zbaren P, Schupbach J, Nuyens M, Stauffer E, Greiner R, Hausler R. Carcinoma of the parotid gland. Am J Surg. 2003;186:57–62.
103. Ellis GL, Auclair PL. Tumors of the salivary glands. AFIP Atlas of Tumor Pathology. 4th ed. Silver Spring MD: ARP Press; 2008. p. 225–30.
104. Etit D, Ekinci N, Tan A, Altinel D, Dag F. An analysis of salivary gland neoplasms: A 12-year, single-institution experience in Turkey. Ear Nose Throat J. 2012;91:125–9.
105. Onyango JF, Awange DO, Muthamia JM, Muga BI. Salivary gland tumours in Kenya. East Afr Med J. 1992;69:525–30.
106. Sur RK, Donde B, Levin V, et al. Adenoid cystic carcinoma of the salivary glands: a review of 10 years. Laryngoscope. 1997;107:1276–80.
107. Shen C, Xu T, Huang C, Hu C, He S. Treatment outcomes and prognostic features in adenoid cystic carcinoma originated from the head and neck. Oral Oncol. 2012;48:445–9.
108. Thavaraj V, Sridhar MR, Sethi A, Arya LS. Adenoid cystic carcinoma of the lacrimal gland. Indian J Pediatr. 2003;70:751–3.
109. Ustundag E, Iseri M, Aydin O, Dal H, Almac A, Paksoy N. Adenoid cystic carcinoma of the tongue. J Laryngol Otol. 2000;114:477–80.
110. Nascimento AG, Amaral AL, Prado LA, Kligerman J, Silveira TR. Adenoid cystic carcinoma of salivary glands. A study of 61 cases with clinicopathologic correlation. Cancer. 1986;57:312–9.
111. Fordice J, Kershaw C, El-Naggar A, Goepfert H. Adenoid cystic carcinoma of the head and neck: predictors of morbidity and mortality. Arch Otolaryngol Head Neck Surg. 1999;125:149–52.
112. da Cruz PDE, de Abreu AF, Nobuko Nishimoto I, de Almeida OP, Kowalski LP. Prognostic factors in head and neck adenoid cystic carcinoma. Oral Oncol. 2006;42:139–46.
113. Perzin KH, Gullane P, Clairmont AC. Adenoid cystic carcinomas arising in salivary glands: a correlation of histologic features and clinical course. Cancer. 1978;42:265–82.
114. Ellis GL. What's new in the AFIP fascicle on salivary gland tumors: a few highlights from the 4th Series Atlas. Head Neck Pathol. 2009;3:225–30.
115. Ellis GL, Auclair PL. Tumors of the salivary glands. Atlas of Tumor Pathology. 3rd ed. Washington DC: Armed Forces Instiute of Pathology; 1996. p. 132–42.
116. Williams SB, Ellis GL, Warnock GR. Sialoblastoma: a clinicopathologic and immunohistochemical study of 7 cases. Ann Diagn Pathol. 2006;10:320–6.
117. Tatlidede S, Karsidag S, Ugurlu K, Sadikoglu B, Tanik C, Bas L. Sialoblastoma: a congenital epithelial tumor of the salivary gland. J Pediatr Surg. 2006;41:1322–5.
118. Siddiqi SH, Solomon MP, Haller JO. Sialoblastoma and hepatoblastoma in a neonate. Pediatr Radiol. 2000;30:349–51.
119. Alvarez-Mendoza A, Calderon-Elvir C, Carrasco-Daza D. Diagnostic and therapeutic approach to sialoblastoma: report of a case. J Pediatr Surg. 1999;34:1875–7.
120. Prigent M, Teissier N, Peuchmaur M, et al. Sialoblastoma of salivary glands in children: chemotherapy should be discussed as an alternative to mutilating surgery. Int J Pediatr Otorhinolaryngol. 2010;74:942–5.
121. Vidyadhar M, Amanda C, Thuan Q, Prabhakaran K. Sialoblastoma. J Pediatr Surg. 2008;43:e11–3.
122. Shet T, Ramadwar M, Sharma S, Laskar S, Arora B, Kurkure P. An eyelid sialoblastoma-like tumor with a sarcomatoid myoepithelial component. Pediatr Dev Pathol. 2007;10:309–14.
123. Saffari Y, Blei F, Warren SM, Milla S, Greco MA. Congenital minor salivary gland sialoblastoma: a case report and review of the literature. Fetal Pediatr Pathol. 2011;30:32–9.
124. Yekeler E, Dursun M, Gun F, et al. Sialoblastoma: MRI findings. Pediatr Radiol. 2004;34:1005–7.
125. Simpson PR, Rutledge JC, Schaefer SD, Anderson RC. Congenital hybrid basal cell adenoma—adenoid cystic carcinoma of the salivary gland. Pediatr Pathol. 1986;6:199–208.
126. Brandwein M, Al-Naeif NS, Manwani D, et al. Sialoblastoma: clinicopathological/immunohistochemical study. Am J Surg Pathol. 1999;23:342–8.
127. Shan XF, Cai ZG, Zhang JG, Zhang J, Gao Y, Yu GY. Management of sialoblastoma with surgery and brachytherapy. Pediatr Blood Cancer. 2010;55:1427–30.

128. Stones DK, Jansen JC, Griessel D. Sialoblastoma and hepatoblastoma in a newborn infant. Pediatr Blood Cancer. 2009;52:883–5.
129. Fu H, Wang J, Wang L, Zhang Z, He Y. Pleomorphic adenoma of the salivary glands in children and adolescents. J Pediatr Surg. 2012;47:715–9.
130. Mendenhall WM, Mendenhall CM, Werning JW, Malyapa RS, Mendenhall NP. Salivary gland pleomorphic adenoma. Am J Clin Oncol. 2008;31:95–9.
131. Chen YK, Lin CC, Lai S, et al. Pleomorphic adenoma with extensive necrosis: report of two cases. Oral Dis. 2004;10:54–9.
132. Jecker P, Hartwein J. Facial paralysis in benign parotid tumor: case report and review of the literature. Laryngorhinootologie. 1993;72:204–6.
133. Michaels L, Hellquist HB. Ear, nose and throat histopathology. 2nd ed. New York:Springer; 2001.
134. Rodriguez KH, Vargas S, Robson C, et al. Pleomorphic adenoma of the parotid gland in children. Int J Pediatr Otorhinolaryngol. 2007;71:1717–23.
135. Leverstein H, van der Wal JE, Tiwari RM, van der Waal I, Snow GB. Surgical management of 246 previously untreated pleomorphic adenomas of the parotid gland. Br J Surg. 1997;84:399–403.
136. Krolls SO, Boyers RC. Mixed tumors of salivary glands. Long-term follow-up. Cancer. 1972;30:276–81.
137. Barton J, Slevin NJ, Gleave EN. Radiotherapy for pleomorphic adenoma of the parotid gland. Int J Radiat Oncol Biol Phys. 1992;22:925–8.
138. Wang CC. Unnecessary morbidity following irradiation of lateralized head and neck carcinoma. Int J Radiat Oncol Biol Phys. 1992;22:1155–6.
139. Gnepp DR. Malignant mixed tumors of the salivary glands: a review. Pathol Annu. 1993;28 Pt 1:279–328.
140. Seifert G. Histopathology of malignant salivary gland tumours. Eur J Cancer B Oral Oncol. 1992;28B(1):49–56.

Sarcoma: Bony Lesion

40

Lillian M. Guenther and Katherine A. Janeway

Osteosarcoma of the Head and Neck in Children

Introduction and Epidemiology

Osteosarcoma is the most common malignant bone tumor in children. With an annual incidence of approximately 400/year in the United States, osteosarcoma represents 56 % of all malignant pediatric bone tumors [18]. Osteosarcoma occurs most often in the metaphysis of the distal femur, proximal tibia, and the humerus in children, and, less often, in the pelvis. The peak incidence is in the second decade of life, correlating with the adolescent growth spurt. In many data sets, there is a slight increased incidence in boys [18].

The literature on head and neck osteosarcoma (HNOS), in adults and children, is confined largely to case reports and case series due to its low frequency. Approximately 8 % of all osteosarcomas occur in the head and neck, and most of these are gnathic [9]. In pediatric patients the proportion of osteosarcoma occurring in the head and neck is even less. In a St. Jude Children's Research Hospital cohort of 812 pediatric bone tumors, only 18, or 4.8 %, were HNOS [9]. Unlike osteosarcoma of the appendicular skeleton, which occurs typically in the second decade of life, HNOS seems to present approximately a decade later, pushing most of the HNOS diagnoses into the adult age range [13] (Fig. 40.1).

Clinical Presentation

When all HNOS, pediatric and adult, are considered together, tumors occur most commonly in the mandible (45–49 %) with the maxilla closely following as the second most common site (47–40 %) [17, 23]. In one of the only reports on pediatric HNOS, of 18 individuals the maxilla and mandible were equally involved (44.5 % each) and other sites were involved 11 % of the time [9]. The majority of patients with HNOS present with a mass lesion or swelling which can be accompanied by pain [12, 15]. Trismus is rarely described as an isolated symptom in HNOS, likely because it is almost always accompanied by pain. It is also important to recognize that symptoms of gnathic osteosarcoma may mimic dental infection. In fact, in one study, 44 % of individuals with these tumors presented to their dentist first for presumed tooth etiology [15]. Other rarer signs and symptoms of HNOS can include cranial nerve palsies, proptosis, or increased intracranial pressure [31].

Etiology and Biology

Like with all osteosarcomas, the etiology for most primary osteosarcoma of the head and neck is unknown. The most significant risk factor for HNOS in children is hereditary retinoblastoma. Other risk factors include prior radiation therapy, and additional cancer predisposition syndromes. Li–Fraumeni and Rothmund–Thomson syndromes predispose individuals to osteosarcoma in general but not specifically HNOS. Paget's Disease of bone also results in predisposition to osteosarcoma; however, because it causes osteosarcoma in older individuals, Paget's disease will not be discussed here.

Li–Fraumeni syndrome is an autosomal dominant familial condition involving germline mutations of the *TP53* gene that manifests with a very high incidence of malignancies, including osteosarcoma. A study of a large database of *TP53* mutation carriers published in 2003 demonstrated that 13.4 % of these individuals with tumors had osteosarcoma [32]. However, the literature does not suggest that anatomic distribution of osteosarcoma in Li–Fraumeni syndrome differs from sporadic osteosarcoma.

K. A. Janeway (✉)
Department of Pediatric Oncology, Boston Children's Hospital, Harvard Medical School, Boston, MA 02115, USA
e-mail: Katherine_Janeway@dfci.harvard.edu

L. M. Guenther
Department of Medicine, Boston Children's Hospital, Harvard Medical School, Boston, MA 02115,USA

R. Rahbar et al. (eds.), *Pediatric Head and Neck Tumors*,
DOI 10.1007/978-1-4614-8755-5_40, © Springer Science+Business Media New York 2014

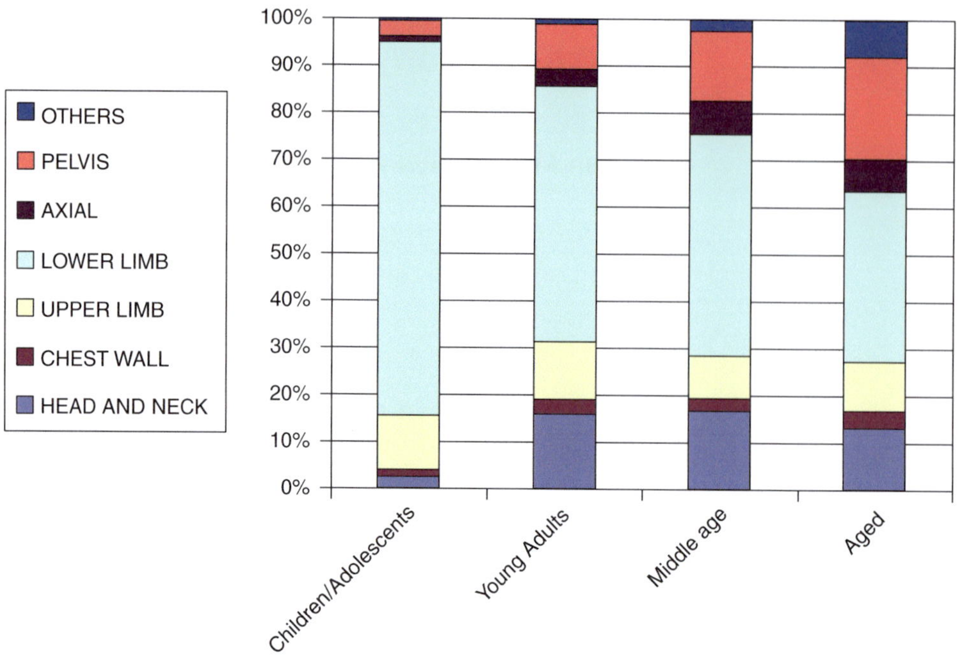

Fig. 40.1 Frequency of primary sites of osteosarcoma according to age. (Data obtained from SEER 17 database) [30]

Rothmund–Thomson syndrome is an autosomal recessive disorder associated with poikiloderma and other skin abnormalities, as well as bone developmental defects. An increased likelihood of osteosarcoma was first shown in 1990. There are no reported cases of Rothmund–Thomson-syndrome-associated HNOS; rather, these are appendicular skeleton tumors [24].

Hereditary retinoblastoma is caused by a heterozygous germline mutation in the *RB1* gene, on the long arm of chromosome 13 [1]. In children who suffer from hereditary retinoblastoma, about 50 % of secondary tumors (after occurrence of retinoblastoma) are osteosarcomas [20]. Originally, the increased risk of osteosarcoma in hereditary retinoblastoma was thought to be strictly secondary to DNA damage inflicted by radiation therapy delivered to the orbit to treat retinoblastoma. However, it is now known that the genetic defect in hereditary retinoblastoma contributes to increased osteosarcoma incidence independent of radiation therapy as demonstrated by an increased prevalence of osteosarcoma in patients with hereditary retinoblastoma at sites distant from radiation fields, such as the extremities. Radiation exposure does further increase HNOS risk in hereditary retinoblastoma. Children who have been irradiated for hereditary retinoblastoma therapy are 2,000 times more likely to get osteosarcoma of the skull than the average person, while they are 500 times more likely to develop osteosarcoma of the extremities [26]. Among children and adults with HNOS, a history of hereditary retinoblastoma is common. Four percent of 173 children and adults with HNOS [23] and 33 % of a group of 18 children with HNOS had a history of hereditary osteosarcoma [9]. While retinoblastoma is almost always diagnosed before the age of five, secondary osteosarcoma may not be diagnosed until adulthood.

Secondary osteosarcoma due to radiation from other pediatric tumors of the head and neck, such as leukemia, brain tumors, and other soft tissue tumors, such as rhabdomyosarcoma, does occur in very small numbers, and the latency period is often a decade or more [34]. It is notable that throughout the literature HNOS secondary to radiation is statistically linked to decreased survival compared to other non-radiation-associated primary HNOS, suggesting that this is a more aggressive tumor type [17, 15].

Diagnosis and Staging

Complete assessment of a newly identified head and neck bone tumor with imaging is required prior to biopsy in order to allow for appropriate planning of the best biopsy approach. Plain films are a good initial imaging modality to help identify the bone or region of interest for further evaluation and to define the extent of periosteal new bone formation or osteolysis present, but plain films are of limited utility because superimposed bony structures in the head and neck region permit only crude visualization of mass lesions. On cross-section imaging, osteosarcomas typically appear as a tumor arising from bone, causing cortical destruction and resulting in a soft tissue mass containing calcification. Computerized tomography (CT) shows more details of bony involvement and invasion into surrounding structures, and 3D modeling from CT can be helpful for presurgical mapping of the tumor (Fig. 40.2). Magnetic resonance imaging (MRI) provides the

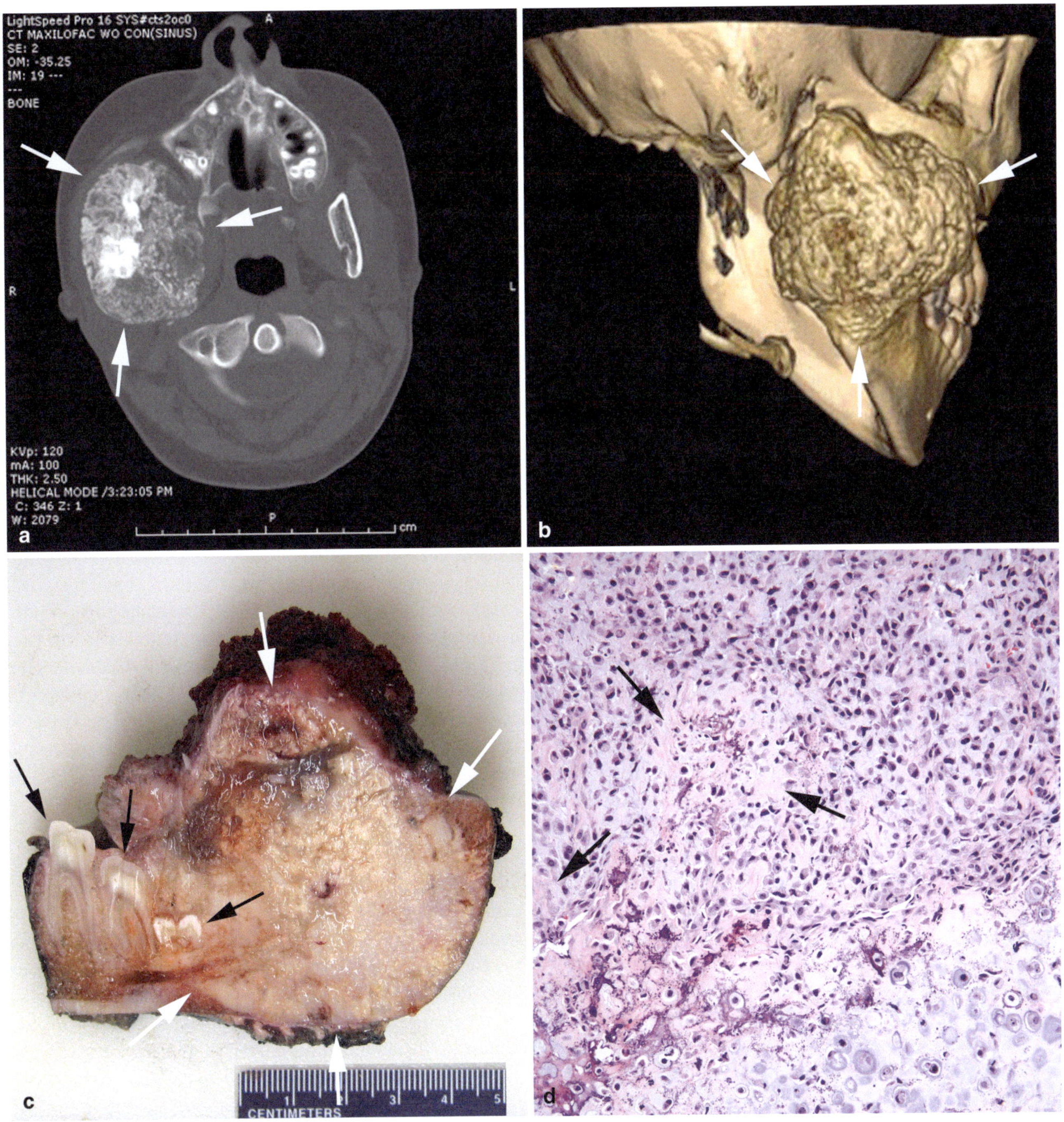

Fig. 40.2 Chondroblastic osteosarcoma of the mandible. **a** Bone-destructive, irregularly spherical mass centered in the right posterior mandible (between *arrows*). The mass reveals prominent spotty calcifications. **b** Three-dimensional reconstruction of the posterior mandibular mass (between *arrows*). **c** Cut section of the resected specimen showing the firm, destructive mass (between *white arrows*) with white-gray color, granular calcifications and areas of necrosis and hemorrhage. Cut section of the molars is indicated by *black arrows*. **d** Cellular tumor composed of large atypical cells with focal osteoid formation (*arrows*). Chondroid matrix is seen on the *right lower corner* of the photograph

most details of soft tissue involvement [9]. Up to 15–20% of patients with osteosarcoma have metastatic spread at the time of diagnosis; sites of distant metastases in osteosarcoma are, most commonly, the lungs followed by bones. Chest CT and bone scan are performed as part of staging work up to look for distant metastases [42].

Definitive diagnosis of HNOS requires a tissue biopsy. Surgical open biopsy is the traditional approach for obtaining a tissue biopsy. More recently, interventional radiology-guided, percutaneous, core needle biopsy has become a common approach, especially at tertiary care centers with interventional radiology specialists and large volumes of

Table 40.1 Differential diagnosis of HNOS

Other malignant primary bone tumors
Ewing sarcoma
Chondrosarcoma
Fibrosarcoma
Other malignancies presenting as bone tumor(s)
Lymphoma
Neuroblastoma
Metastatic rhabdomyosarcoma
Metastatic melanoma
Langerhans cell histiocytosis
Benign bone tumors
Aneurysmal bone cyst
Osteoblastoma
Osteoid osteoma
Giant cell tumor
Unicameral bone cyst
Hemangioma
Infectious/inflammatory
Osteomyelitis
Chronic recurrent multifocal osteomyelitis

pediatric solid tumor patients. The diagnostic yield of a core needle biopsy is operator dependent and ranges between 78 and 94% [4, 22, 41]. More recent studies that benefit from updated technology and user familiarity with the technique demonstrate diagnostic percentages on the higher end of this range. Regardless of the biopsy approach, it is important to sample the soft tissue component of the mass if possible, as this usually provides the greatest diagnostic yield. Surgical biopsy is most often incisional rather than excisional given that neo-adjuvant chemotherapy is often given prior to surgical resection. Osteosarcoma has been reported to recur into the tract left by the biopsy apparatus, so it is essential for the physician performing the biopsy, either percutaneously or surgically, to choose an entry point that will be removed en bloc with the tumor when it is surgically excised [8].

Differential diagnosis of HNOS includes other malignant primary bone tumors, other malignancies involving bone, benign bone tumors, and infectious and inflammatory conditions (Table 40.1). On pathologic examination osteosarcoma is a malignant tumor composed of pleomorphic cells associated with osteoid matrix production. Based on the degree of atypia, differentiation, and necrosis, the tumors can be classified as low, intermediate, or high grade. In children, low-grade tumors are very uncommon. In the head and neck, osteosarcomas are usually rich in chondroid matrix (Fig. 40.2).

Natural History

One interesting difference between HNOS and osteosarcoma of the long bones is the difference in propensity for metastases, both at time of diagnosis and following initial surgical and/or medical therapy for the primary tumor. The available case series on these tumors, in both adults and children, suggest that metastasis at time of diagnosis is very rare in primary HNOS, as opposed to in osteosarcoma in general, where 25% of initial diagnoses are made in the presence of distant metastases. In the St. Jude pediatric cohort, none of the 18 patients with HNOS had distant metastases at time of diagnosis [9]. A small case series of five pediatric patients of St. Louis, published in 1973 concluded that none of their cases had metastasized at time of diagnosis [10]. At M.D. Anderson, too, in a cohort of 12 patients between the ages of 12 and 21 years that were retrospectively examined none had evidence of distant metastases at time of diagnosis [21].

Management

In non-head and neck osteosarcoma the standard treatment approach is a combination of systemic chemotherapy and local control, most often accomplished by complete surgical resection with wide margins. The current and historical data show that with surgery alone, more than 80% of non-head and neck osteosarcoma will recur with distant metastases because of micro-metastatic disease [26]. Chemotherapy when added to surgical resection has been proven to improve overall survival [25]. However, in HNOS some controversy exists regarding whether to administer chemotherapy due to lack of data concerning the utility of chemotherapy in this disease.

Chemotherapy

Standard of care for chemotherapy treatment of osteosarcoma in sites other than the head and neck is four cycles of treatment with doxorubicin, cisplatin, and high-dose methotrexate and two cycles of treatment with doxorubicin and high-dose methotrexate (Fig. 40.3). This regimen is typically abbreviated as MAP. Some institutions, particularly in Europe, add ifosfamide to MAP and, in doing so, decrease the cumulative dose of doxorubicin given [3, 27]. Typically two cycles of MAP therapy are given prior to surgery in order to facilitate early initiation of chemotherapy and surgical planning, but upfront resection followed by chemotherapy is also an acceptable approach. Because of the differences in the natural history of HNOS compared to all other osteosarcomas, the role of chemotherapy is less certain.

As discussed above, HNOS differs in that it metastasizes infrequently. Retrospective studies to evaluate whether the use of chemotherapy impacts survival in HNOS are difficult to interpret due to the inevitable issue of confounding factors. In one study from Memorial Sloan–Kettering Cancer Center that included adults and children who were treated with radical surgery following neo-adjuvant chemotherapy, chemotherapy did not significantly improve event-free survival. However, only patients who were determined to

Week	1	2	3	4	5	6	7	8	9	10	11	12	13	14	15	16	17	18	19	20	21	22	23	24	25	26	27	28	29
Chemo	A			M	M	A			M	M	Surgery	A			M	M	A			M	M	A		M	M	A		M	M
	P					P						P					P												

A = Doxorubicin 75 mg/m² continuous infusion over 48 hours

P = Cisplatin 60 mg/m²/day x 2 days

M = Methotrexate 12 gm/m² x 1 dose, maximum dose 20 gm

Fig. 40.3 MAP chemotherapy regimen for the treatment of osteosarcoma

have high-grade tumors, unresectable tumors, or predisposing factors to HNOS such as retinoblastoma were offered chemotherapy in this study [33]. In patients who have positive surgical margins following resection or an unresectable HNOS, retrospective studies suggest that patients receiving chemotherapy have a better outcome; however, the study populations are small [31].

Two meta-analyses of combined adult and pediatric data published in 1997 assessed the role of chemotherapy in HNOS. These studies oppose one another. In the first, only adjuvant chemotherapy was addressed, and the authors concluded that there was no significant difference in 5-year survival between the groups that received chemotherapy (50 %) versus surgery alone; however, the study did not address the question of surgical margins or resectability of the tumors—both important prognostic factors [23]. In the second study, the authors concluded that the addition of chemotherapy led to significantly prolonged survival and better outcomes in general for patients with HNOS, both for individuals who had complete surgical removal and who had incomplete resections. They recommended the same protocol for HNOS as for non-head and neck osteosarcoma [38].

In pediatrics, the practice is generally to offer chemotherapy for HNOS patients, and children with HNOS have been permitted to enroll on Children's Oncology Group studies of chemotherapeutic regimens in osteosarcoma [14, 27]. In order to determine the impact of chemotherapy in HNOS in children, randomized control trials would be needed but patient numbers are too small to permit studies of this type.

Local Control: Surgery

Because osteosarcoma is relatively resistant to radiotherapy, definitive local control of HNOS, like any osteosarcoma, requires complete surgical resection with negative surgical margins. In non-head and neck osteosarcomas, surgical resectability is an important prognostic factor. For this reason osteosarcoma of the pelvis has a significantly worse outcome than osteosarcoma involving other sites [19]. Similarly, retrospective studies have shown that complete surgical resection of HNOS with negative margins is the most significant prognostic factor influencing overall survival [17, 33, 42]. This includes a retrospective study in a pediatric cohort, where a Kaplan–Meier survival analysis of HNOS patients showed a 75 % 5-year survival of individuals who underwent complete resection as compared to a 35 % 5-year survival of those who underwent incomplete resection or biopsy, regardless of adjuvant therapy [9]. The surgical management of HNOS is complicated by anatomical challenges of resection of the gnathic, neck, and skull bones. Mandibular tumors have the highest rates of negative margins because of ease of surgical access, and therefore have the best outcome, followed by maxillary lesions and skull tumors, which are the most difficult to resect. Therefore, the goal should always be complete removal with negative margins, which, unfortunately, is not always achievable in the head and neck region.

The extent of surgical margin required in osteosarcoma in order to be considered adequate to decrease the risk of local recurrence is a topic of great debate. Marginal and intralesional margins are associated with a poor outcome and an increased risk of local recurrence [5]. In general, orthopedic surgeons treating osteosarcoma of the limb aim for margins of 2–5 mm for soft tissue and 2–3 cm for bone marrow. The pathological/surgical staging system utilized in osteosarcoma is the Enneking staging system (Table 40.2) [11]. Most osteosarcomas in children are high grade (G2) and extracompartmental, meaning that the tumor has broken through the cortex of the bone. Consequently, most osteosarcomas in children are Enneking stage IIB or III.

Local Control: Radiation

In the head and neck region, radiotherapy has not been well studied, particularly in pediatrics, where the number of patients in published retrospective studies who have received radiation is too small to come to definitive conclusions about its effects [9, 12]. The Smeele 1997 retrospective study of chemotherapy regimens in HNOS reported that 34 % of the patients included in the study had received radiation, either in combination with chemotherapy and/or surgery, or as a single modality. In their analysis, they found that radiation therapy was insignificant as a modifier of disease outcome [38]. However, radiation may play a key role, especially in patients with positive surgical margins, as demonstrated in a retrospective 2009 study from M.D. Anderson where 5-year local control of tumors in patients with incomplete surgical resection or positive margins who received radiation therapy was 80 % as opposed to 31 % with surgery alone [17]. Therefore,

Table 40.2 Enneking staging system for osteosarcoma [11]

Stage	Grade	Site	Metastasis
IA	G1	T1	M0
IB	G1	T2	M0
IIA	G2	T1	M0
IIB	G2	T2	M0
III	G1,2	T1,2	M1

G1 Low grade, characterized by few mitoses and a relatively well-differentiated appearance
G2 High grade characterized by higher mitotic rate and a less differentiated appearance
T1 Tumor is intracompartmental or confined to the anatomic compartment of origin
T2 Tumor is extracompartmental or extends beyond the anatomic compartment of origin
M0 No distant metastases present
M1 Distant metastases present

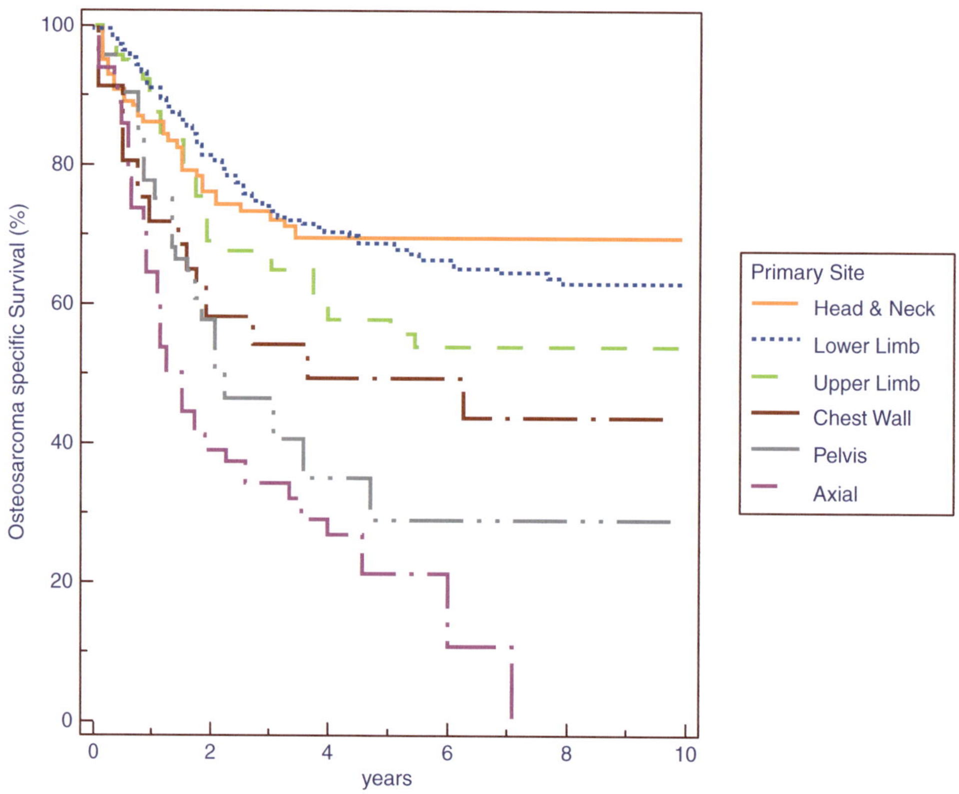

Fig. 40.4 Osteosarcoma-specific survival by site. (SEER 9 database, 1996–2005) [30]

the generally accepted role of radiation therapy in osteosarcoma is for treatment of positive surgical margins where re-resection to achieve negative margins is not feasible.

Outcome

Five-year overall survival in osteosarcoma ranges from 65 to 70%. Five-year overall survival in HNOS is slightly higher, ranging from 60 to 75% in individuals who underwent complete surgical resection [9, 39] (Fig. 40.4). There is evidence to support the fact that gnathic osteosarcomas have significantly higher 5-year survival rates than extra-gnathic HNOS [23].

Recurrences of non-head and neck osteosarcomas are almost always distant, usually affecting lung or bone, with <5% recurring locally. HNOS tumors, instead, usually recur locally; while only 7–17% have distant metastatic recurrence [42]. In one study of all pediatric patients, 32% had local recurrence following surgical intervention, with no differences in the recurrence rate between gnathic and skull lesions [12]. This is similar in more aggressive, radiation-related HNOS, where in one study of these individuals, 86% of the study population that recurred did so locally, instead of with distant metastases [31]. When HNOS does metastasize, it behaves like other osteosarcomas, occurring most commonly in the lung [15]. Also, it is important to point out that local recurrence is not a positive outcome, given that these tumors are oftentimes unresectable and lead to a large local tumor burden with eventual development of significant morbidity and mortality.

Ewing Sarcoma of the Head and Neck in Children

Introduction and Epidemiology

Ewing sarcoma is the second most common primary bone malignancy in children with approximately 200 cases occurring in children each year in the United States. As with osteosarcoma, incidence peaks in adolescence coincident with the peak in growth velocity. For girls peak incidence occurs at age 10–14 and in boys peak incidence occurs at age 15–19 years. One particularly interesting demographic feature of Ewing sarcoma is that the disease is extremely rare in people of African or Asian descent [29].

Only 4–9% of Ewing sarcomas occur in the head and neck making this a rare entity [2, 37]. As with HNOS, published data regarding Ewing sarcoma of the head and neck are limited to case reports and case series. The most comprehensive manuscript, reporting on patients enrolled on four intergroup Ewing's Sarcoma Studies, describes 29 patients with head and neck Ewing sarcoma [37].

Clinical Presentation

As with Ewing sarcoma in other sites, Ewing sarcoma of the head and neck most often present as a painful mass lesion. The most common sites in the head and neck for Ewing sarcoma are the skull bones, mandible, and maxilla. Ewing sarcoma has also been reported to occur in the orbit, nasal cavity, and cervical vertebrae. Clinical presentation of Ewing sarcoma in these less common sites includes proptosis, occulomotor dysfunction, and symptoms of cord compression [2, 37]. Rare head and neck locations described in case reports include the larynx, sinuses, and thyroid [6, 7, 45].

Up to 15–20% of patients with Ewing sarcoma have metastatic disease at the time of diagnosis; in those cases the most common sites of metastasis are lung, bone, and bone marrow. Patients with metastatic disease often have multiple sites involved. Loco-regional lymph nodes are rarely involved with metastatic disease at the time of diagnosis [28, 35]. Although data are limited, it appears as though a similar proportion of patients with head and neck Ewing sarcoma present with metastatic disease [2].

Etiology and Biology

As with most pediatric malignancies, the cause of Ewing Sarcoma is not known. Ninty-five percent of Ewing sarcomas have a translocation involving the *EWSR1* gene. In most cases the translocation partner is *FLI1*, an E-twenty-six (ETS) family transcription factor [36]. How this translocation leads to transformation is not known and this is an active area of ongoing research. Unlike osteosarcoma, Ewing sarcoma does not frequently occur in the setting of a cancer predisposition syndrome and it is not a common second malignancy following radiation therapy [40]. While Ewing sarcoma is classified as a primary bone tumor, the cell of origin is not known and 25% of tumors arise in extra-skeletal locations. Most of the rare head and neck locations for Ewing sarcoma are extra-skeletal.

Diagnosis and Staging

While radiographic features of Ewing sarcoma differ from those in osteosarcoma, it is not possible to distinguish these two primary bone tumors on the basis of imaging alone. As with osteosarcoma, tissue biopsy is required for definitive diagnosis. The best imaging modality for evaluation of the primary tumor for the purposes of planning for biopsy and ultimate surgical resection is MRI. CT scan can be helpful in bone tumors in some cases. A complete staging evaluation in Ewing sarcoma consists of, at a minimum, a CT scan of the chest and a bone scan. Ewing sarcoma is positive on fluorodeoxyglucose positron emission tomography (FDG-PET), and this diagnostic modality is often performed in addition to bone scan. Bilateral bone marrow aspirates and biopsies are routinely performed for staging in pediatric patients.

Differential diagnosis of Ewing sarcoma of the head and neck includes those considerations listed for osteosarcoma (Table 40.1). When head and neck Ewing sarcoma occurs in rare extra-skeletal locations, the differential diagnosis is broader and includes soft tissue sarcomas such as rhabdomyosarcoma and other soft tissue sarcomas as well as malignant tumors occurring in the location from which the Ewing sarcoma is arising, such as nasopharyngeal carcinoma.

Considerations in the approach to biopsy of Ewing sarcoma are essentially the same as those in the approach to biopsy in osteosarcoma (see previous discussion). Acceptable methods of obtaining a tissue biopsy are open surgical incisional biopsy and interventional radiology-guided, core needle biopsy. Regardless of approach, biopsy should be performed at a center with experience in the diagnosis and treatment of pediatric sarcomas of the head and neck. With rare exceptions, upfront resection or excisional biopsy should not be performed for Ewing sarcoma. This is particularly true for Ewing sarcoma of the head and neck in which radiation therapy rather than surgery is often used for definitive local control (see local control: surgery and radiation below).

On histologic examination, Ewing sarcoma is a small, round, blue cell tumor (Fig. 40.5). Immunohistochemistry for CD99 can aid in the diagnosis as Ewing sarcoma has a membranous staining pattern for CD99. Fluorescence in situ hybridization (FISH) for a translocation involving *EWSR1*

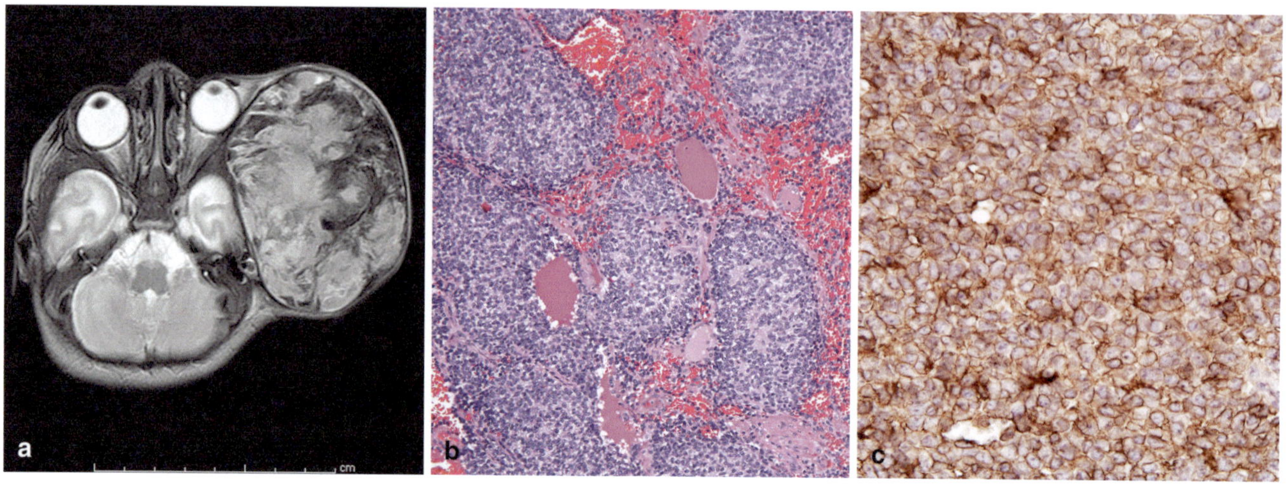

Fig. 40.5 Ewing sarcoma/malignant primitive neuroectodermal tumor. **a** Large heterogeneous destructive mass involving the skull. **b** Islands of undifferentiated small, round cells with focally poorly formed rosettes. **c** Diffuse, strong membranous immunoreactivity for CD99 in tumor cells

can also be informative as 95 % of Ewing sarcomas contain translocations involving *EWSR1* [36].

Management

Because the natural history of head and neck Ewing sarcoma appears to be similar to that of non-head and neck Ewing sarcoma, the approach to treatment for head and neck Ewing sarcoma is the same as the approach to treatment of non-head and neck Ewing sarcoma. The standard approach to management of Ewing sarcoma is a multi-modality approach with chemotherapy administration and local control accomplished by either surgery or radiation therapy.

Chemotherapy

Prior to uniform use of modern multi-modality therapy for Ewing sarcoma overall survival was less than 45 % [18]. With modern multi-modality therapy including chemotherapy overall survival is now 80 % in those with localized disease [44]. Over the past 30 years, chemotherapy regimens have been studied in large prospective phase III trials. The current approach to standard of care is based on the results of these trials. The best reported outcomes in Ewing sarcoma are from chemotherapy regimens including five drugs: vincristine, doxorubicin, cyclophosphamide, ifosfamide, and etoposide with chemotherapy cycles administered in an interval-compressed manner of every 2 weeks [16, 44] (Fig. 40.6).

Local Control: Surgery and Radiation

In stark contrast to osteosarcoma, both radiation therapy and surgical resection with negative margins are effective methods of local control in Ewing sarcoma. Whether surgical resection with negative margins results in a decreased risk of local recurrence when compared to radiation therapy is a subject of considerable debate. As randomized controlled trials to answer this question are not feasible, data are limited to retrospective studies, which are subject to confounding by additional prognostic variables such as tumor size, tumor site, and the presence of metastatic disease. Retrospective studies, including a recently presented large study of patients treated on prospective Children's Oncology Group trials, suggest that there is a slightly increased risk of local recurrence when local control is performed with radiation alone as compared to surgery or surgery plus radiation therapy [35, 43]. However, because local recurrence is a rare event, this slight increased risk of local recurrence does not appear to translate into an increased risk of disease-related death [43]. Consequently, selection of the optimal approach to local control for patients with Ewing sarcoma is an individualized decision in which disease control, acute complications, late-effects, functional compromise, and cosmesis resulting from surgery and radiation are considered in a multi-disciplinary discussion. Patients being treated in centers without experience in local control for Ewing sarcoma should consider referral to a center with this expertise for consultation regarding the optimal approach to local control. In head and neck Ewing sarcoma, because of the challenges in achieving complete surgical resection with negative margins without significant functional compromise and impact on cosmesis, radiation therapy is the most common approach utilized for local control [2, 37].

When performed, local control surgery should occur after induction chemotherapy as Ewing sarcoma primary tumors often undergo considerable shrinkage in response to chemotherapy making surgical resection easier. In order for surgery alone to constitute adequate local control, resection margins must be free of involvement by tumor. As with osteosarcoma, the extent of normal tissue margin needed to reduce the

Induction (Before local control):

Week	1	3	5	7	9	11	13
Vincristine	*		*		*		Local Control[1]
Doxorubicin	*		*		*		
Cyclophosphamide	*		*		*		
Ifosfamide		*		*		*	
Etoposide		*		*		*	
Filgrastim	*	*	*	*	*	*	

Consolidation (After or during local control):

Week[2]	13	15	17	19	21	23	25	27
Vincristine	*		*		*		*	
Doxorubicin[3]	*		*					
Cyclophosphamide	*		*		*		*	
Ifosfamide		*		*		*		*
Etoposide		*		*		*		*
Filgrastim	*	*	*	*	*	*	*	*

[1] Local control is achieved with surgery, radiation or, on occasion, both.

[2] Chemotherapy continues during radiation therapy (if given).

[3] Two of the vincristine, doxorubicin and cyclophosphamide cycles include only vincristine and cyclophosphamide without doxorubicin. When chemotherapy is continued during radiation therapy doxorubicin is not administered concurrently with radiation and is held for several weeks following completion of radiation therapy to prevent radiation recall.

Fig. 40.6 Standard of care chemotherapy regimen for the treatment of Ewing sarcoma used in North America

risk of local recurrence is not known. The dose of radiation therapy utilized in treatment of Ewing sarcoma varies depending on the clinical scenario. For definitive local control of gross disease doses of 55.8 Gy are utilized.

Outcome

Overall survival at 5 years in localized Ewing sarcoma following treatment with modern multi-modality therapy is 80% [16, 44]. Outcomes are much worse in patients with metastatic Ewing sarcoma where overall survival at 5 years is approximately 30–40% [35]. In addition to metastatic disease, prognostic factors in Ewing sarcoma are age, size, and anatomic site with older patients and those with larger tumors having worse outcomes. Head and neck appears to be a good prognostic variable. Case series consistently demonstrate a better outcome for head and neck Ewing sarcoma when compared to other sites with the exception of cervical Ewing sarcoma which appears to have a similar outcome to non-head and neck sites [2, 37]. However, these case series include patients who did not receive modern therapy. Whether the improved outcomes in non-head and neck Ewing sarcoma with modern therapy have eliminated this difference in outcomes between non-head and neck and head and neck sites is not know.

References

1. Albright JT, Topham AK, Reilly JS. Pediatric head and neck malignancies: US incidence and trends over 2 decades. Arch Otolaryngol Head Neck Surg. 2002;128:655–9.
2. Allam A, El-Husseiny G, Khafaga Y, et al. Ewing's sarcoma of the head and neck: a retrospective analysis of 24 cases. Sarcoma. 1999;3:11–5.
3. Anninga JK, Gelderblom H, Fiocco M, et al. Chemotherapeutic adjuvant treatment for osteosarcoma: where do we stand? Eur J Cancer. 2011;47:2431–45.
4. Ayala AG, Zornosa J. Primary bone tumors: percutaneous needle biopsy. Radiologic-pathologic study of 222 biopsies. Radiology. 1983;149:675–9.
5. Bacci G, Longhi A, Versari M, et al. Prognostic factors for osteosarcoma of the extremity treated with neoadjuvant chemotherapy: 15-year experience in 789 patients treated at a single institution. Cancer. 2006;106:1154–61.

6. Chirila M, Muresan M, Ciuleanu E, et al. Extraosseous Ewing sarcoma and peripheral primitive neuroectodermal tumor of the thyroid gland: Case report and review. Ear Nose Throat J. 2013;92:E3–6.
7. Coskun BU, Cinar U, Savk H, et al. Isolated maxillary sinus Ewing's sarcoma. Rhinology. 2005;43:225–8.
8. Davies NM, Livesley PJ, Cannon SR. Recurrence of an osteosarcoma in a needle biopsy track. J Bone Joint Surg Br. 1993;75:977–8.
9. Daw NC, Mahmoud HH, Meyer WH, et al. Bone sarcomas of the head and neck in children: the St Jude Children's Research Hospital experience. Cancer. 2000;88:2172–80.
10. Dehner LP. Tumors of the mandible and maxilla in children. I. Clinicopathologic study of 46 histologically benign lesions. Cancer. 1973;31:364–84.
11. Enneking WF, Spanier SS, Goodman MA. A system for the surgical staging of musculoskeletal sarcoma. Clin Orthop Relat Res. 1980;106–20.
12. Gadwal SR, Gannon FH, Fanburg-Smith JC, et al. Primary osteosarcoma of the head and neck in pediatric patients: a clinicopathologic study of 22 cases with a review of the literature. Cancer. 2001;91:598–605.
13. Garrington GE, Scofield HH, Cornyn J, et al. Osteosarcoma of the jaws. Analysis of 56 cases. Cancer. 1967;20:377–91.
14. Goorin AM, Schwartzentruber DJ, Devidas M, et al. Presurgical chemotherapy compared with immediate surgery and adjuvant chemotherapy for nonmetastatic osteosarcoma: Pediatric Oncology Group Study POG-8651. J Clin Oncol. 2003;21:1574–80.
15. Granowski-LeCornu M, Chuang SK, Kaban LB, et al. Osteosarcoma of the jaws: factors influencing prognosis. J Oral Maxillofac Surg. 2011;69:2368–75.
16. Grier HE, Krailo MD, Tarbell NJ, et al. Addition of ifosfamide and etoposide to standard chemotherapy for Ewing's sarcoma and primitive neuroectodermal tumor of bone. N Engl J Med. 2003;348:694–701.
17. Guadagnolo BA, Zagars GK, Raymond AK, et al. Osteosarcoma of the jaw/craniofacial region: outcomes after multimodality treatment. Cancer. 2009;115:3262–70.
18. Gurney JG SA BM Malignant bone tumors. In: Ries LAG SM, Gurney JG, editors. Cancer incidence and survival among children and adolescents: United States SEER Program 1975–1995, NIH Pub; 1999
19. Isakoff MS, Barkauskas DA, Ebb D, et al. Poor survival for osteosarcoma of the pelvis: a report from the Children's Oncology Group. Clin Orthop Relat Res. 2012;470:2007–13.
20. Hansen MF, Koufos A, Gallie BL, et al. Osteosarcoma and retinoblastoma: a shared chromosomal mechanism revealing recessive predisposition. Proc Natl Acad Sci USA. 1985;82:6216–20.
21. Huh WW, Holsinger FC, Levy A, et al. Osteosarcoma of the jaw in children and young adults. Head Neck. 2012;34:981–4.
22. Jelinek JS, Murphey MD, Welker JA, et al. Diagnosis of primary bone tumors with image-guided percutaneous biopsy: experience with 110 tumors. Radiology. 2002;223:731–7.
23. Kassir RR, Rassekh CH, Kinsella JB, et al. Osteosarcoma of the head and neck: meta-analysis of nonrandomized studies. Laryngoscope. 1997;107:56–61.
24. Leonard A, Craft AW, Moss C, et al. Osteogenic sarcoma in the Rothmund–Thomson syndrome. Med Pediatr Oncol. 1996;26:249–53.
25. Link MP, Goorin AM, Miser AW, et al. The effect of adjuvant chemotherapy on relapse-free survival in patients with osteosarcoma of the extremity. N Engl J Med. 1986;314:1600–6.
26. Link MP, Gebhardt MC, Meyers PA. Osteosarcoma in principles and practice of pediatric oncology. In: Pizzo PA, Poplack DG, editors. Priciples and Practice of Pediatric Oncology. 5th edn. Philadelphia: Lippincott Williams & Wilkins; 2006. pp 1074–115.
27. Meyers PA, Schwartz CL, Krailo MD, et al. Osteosarcoma: the addition of muramyl tripeptide to chemotherapy improves overall survival—a report from the Children's Oncology Group. J Clin Oncol. 2008;26:633–8.
28. Miser JS, Goldsby RE, Chen Z, et al. Treatment of metastatic Ewing sarcoma/primitive neuroectodermal tumor of bone: evaluation of increasing the dose intensity of chemotherapy—a report from the Children's Oncology Group. Pediatr Blood Cancer. 2007;49:894–900.
29. National Cancer Institute. Cancer epidemiology in older adolescents and young adults 15–29 years of age, including SEER incidence and survival: 1975–2000. Bethesda: National Cancer Institute, NIH; 2006.
30. National Cancer Institute. Surveillance Epidemilogy and End Results. SEER*Stat Database. http://www.seer.cancer.gov.
31. Oda D, Bavisotto LM, Schmidt RA, et al. Head and neck osteosarcoma at the University of Washington. Head Neck. 1997;19:513–23.
32. Olivier M, Goldgar DE, Sodha N, et al. Li–Fraumeni and related syndromes: correlation between tumor type, family structure, and TP53 genotype. Cancer Res. 2003;63:6643–50.
33. Patel SG, Meyers P, Huvos AG, et al. Improved outcomes in patients with osteogenic sarcoma of the head and neck. Cancer. 2002;95:1495–503.
34. Patel AJ, Rao VY, Fox BD, et al. Radiation-induced osteosarcomas of the calvarium and skull base. Cancer. 2011;117:2120–6.
35. Rodriguez-Galindo C, Liu T, Krasin MJ, et al. Analysis of prognostic factors in ewing sarcoma family of tumors: review of St. Jude Children's Research Hospital studies. Cancer. 2007;110:375–84.
36. Sankar S, Lessnick SL. Promiscuous partnerships in Ewing's sarcoma. Cancer Genet. 2011;204:351–65.
37. Siegal GP, Oliver WR, Reinus WR, et al. Primary Ewing's sarcoma involving the bones of the head and neck. Cancer. 1987;60:2829–40.
38. Smeele LE, Kostense PJ, van der Waal I, et al. Effect of chemotherapy on survival of craniofacial osteosarcoma: a systematic review of 201 patients. J Clin Oncol. 1997;15:363–7.
39. Smith RB, Apostolakis LW, Karnell LH, et al. National Cancer Data Base report on osteosarcoma of the head and neck. Cancer. 2003;98:1670–80.
40. Spunt SL, Rodriguez-Galindo C, Fuller CE, et al. Ewing sarcoma-family tumors that arise after treatment of primary childhood cancer. Cancer. 2006;107:201–6.
41. Stoker DJ, Cobb JP, Pringle JA. Needle biopsy of musculoskeletal lesions. A review of 208 procedures. J.Bone Joint Surg Br. 1991;73:498–500.
42. Sturgis EM, Potter BO. Sarcomas of the head and neck region. Curr Opin Oncol. 2003;15:239–52.
43. DuBois SG, Krailo M, Gebhardt M, Donaldson S, Marcus KJ, Dormans J, Shamberger RC, Sailer S, Nicholas R, Healey J, Tarbell N, Devidas M, Meyer J, Granowetter L, Womer RB, Bernstein M, Marina N, Grier HE. Local and distant failure according to mode of local control in patients with localized Ewing sarcoma of bone: a report from the Children's Oncology Group. Connective Tissue Oncology Society Annual Meeting; 2012..
44. Womer RB, West DC, Krailo MD, et al. Randomized controlled trial of interval-compressed chemotherapy for the treatment of localized Ewing sarcoma: a report from the Children's Oncology Group. J Clin Oncol. 2012;30:4148–54.
45. Yang YS, Hong KH. Extraskeletal Ewing's sarcoma of the larynx. J Laryngol Otol. 2004;118:62–4.

Sarcoma: Non-Rhabdomyosarcoma Soft Tissue Sarcomas

41

Allison O'Neill and Carlos Rodriguez-Galindo

Introduction

Sarcomas are malignant tumors of mesenchymal origin. Roughly 1,500 children are diagnosed with bone or soft tissue sarcoma each year [1, 2]. The most common sarcoma involving the head and neck is rhadomyosarcoma (RMS) which accounts for an estimated 50 % of cases [3, 4]. Only 5 % of the remaining 50 % is comprised of non-RMS tumors arising from either bone or soft tissue [5]. Although the Intergroup Rhabdomyosarcoma Study (IRS) protocols have established a multidisciplinary approach to the treatment of pediatric RMS, there is very little published data agreeing on the approach for non-RMS tumors. The small subset of non-RMS tumors affecting the head and neck are the focus of this chapter.

Key Points

- Head and neck non-RMS tumors are extremely rare.
- Successful treatment hinges on full surgical resection and radiation therapy.
- The role of adjuvant chemotherapy and radiotherapy is continually debated.

A. O'Neill (✉)
Department of Pediatric Oncology, Harvard Medical School, Dana-Farber/Boston Children's Hospital Cancer and Blood Disorders Center, Boston, MA, USA
e-mail: allison_oneill@dfci.harvard.edu

C. Rodriguez-Galindo
Department of Pediatric Oncology, Harvard Medical School, Dana-Farber/Boston Children's Hospital Cancer and Blood Disorders Center, Boston, MA, USA
e-mail: carlos_rodriguez-galindo@dfci.harvard.edu

R. Rahbar et al. (eds.), *Pediatric Head and Neck Tumors*,
DOI 10.1007/978-1-4614-8755-5_41, © Springer Science+Business Media New York 2014

Biology and Epidemiology

The biology for non-RMS tumors of the head and neck varies depending on histologic diagnosis. Given the rarity of non-RMS head and neck tumors, data regarding the epidemiology is scarce.

Pathophysiology

- Non-RMS tumors of the head and neck can arise from a variety of structures including bone, primitive neuroectodermal tissue, fat, and connective tissue. As with most tumors of pediatric origin, the actual etiology of many of these tumors is unknown.
- The one known risk factor associated with head and neck sarcoma in pediatric patients is prior receipt of radiation therapy for a history of malignancy. The most common tumor to arise in the radiation field is osteosarcoma, however, a range of tumors has been reported [6, 7].

Histopathology

The histopathology for non-RMS tumors arising from the head and neck varies substantially depending on the diagnosis.

- A retrospective review by Nasri et al. describing the experience with non-RMS head and neck sarcomas at UCLA, found that of the 229 head and neck sarcoma cases from 1955 to 1988, 65 cases (29 %) were in the pediatric age group and 33 were non-RMS [4]. The diagnoses reported included: fibrosarcoma, synovial sarcoma, osteosarcoma, dermatofibrosarcoma protuberans (DFSP), malignant fibrous histiocytoma (MFH), chondrosarcoma, angiosarcoma, leiomyosarcoma, liposarcoma, and unclassified sarcomas.
- Smith et al. described this category to include (infantile) fibrosarcoma, DFSP, epitheliod sarcoma, synovial sarcoma, MFH, hemangiopericytoma, chondrosarcoma,

osteosarcoma, leiomyosarcoma, liposarcoma, and soft-tissue clear-cell sarcoma [5].

- Horowitz et al. reported that non-RMS tumors of all sites accounted for only 1.4% of childhood neoplasms at St. Jude Children's Research Hospital between 1962 and 1983 [8].
- An even larger retrospective review over 45 years of 55 pediatric tumor cases involving the nasal cavity and paranasal sinuses by Holsinger et al., demonstrated the majority of these tumors to be non-sarcomatous in etiology [9].

Molecular/Genetic Pathology:

Given the wide range of possible diagnoses affecting this region, the diagnosis must first be gleaned based on histology and tissue origin, with molecular/genetic testing tailored to the diagnosis of highest probability. Listed below are chromosomal translocations commonly linked to a subset of tumors:

Fibrosarcoma (infantile): t(12;15)(p13;q25) leading to the fusion of ETV6-NTRK3 [10]

DFSP: t(17;22)(q22;q13) leading to the fusion of the COL1A1 and PDGFB genes [11]

Synovial sarcoma: t(X;18)(p11.2;q11.2) leading to SS18-SSX1 or SS18-SSX2 fusions [12]

Ewing sarcoma: t(11;22)(q24;q12) leading to the EWS-FL1 fusion [13].

Fluorescent in situ hybridization (FISH) and reverse transcriptase-polymerase chain reaction (RT-PCR) can be helpful in assessing for the characteristic translocations described above, especially when cytogenetic studies are not possible.

Incidence and Prevalence

- As noted earlier, there are roughly 1,500 children diagnosed with bone or soft tissue sarcoma each year in the USA. The proportion of these patients with non-RMS tumors involving the head and neck is remarkably small. There is no reproducible incidence and prevalence data available.

Relationships to Other Disease States, Syndromes

- Although head and neck sarcomas have been reported in association with pre-existing conditions, numbers reported are too small to draw concrete associations [14].
- Survivors of retinoblastoma carrying a germline *RB1* mutation (long arm of chromosome 13), have been described to be at higher risk of secondary osteosarcoma and other soft tissue sarcomas in the radiation field [15]. This risk is up to 500 times higher than unaffected individuals.

Presentation

Symptoms are dependent upon the tumor's location at diagnosis. Head and neck non-RMS are not routinely divided into orbital, parameningeal, and nonorbital nonparameningeal, distinctions reserved for RMS tumors. This may be because non-RMS tumors can arise from multiple structures, including a range of soft tissues and bone [16]. Non-RMS tumors typically present as a firm, non-mobile mass. One can postulate, based on location, that non-RMS tumors can likewise be associated with cranial nerve deficits, changes in hearing or voice, proptosis, otalgia, nasal discharge, airway obstruction, or bony deformity.

Patterns of Evolution

- Patterns of metastatic spread are dependent on the histologic classification of the tumor. Sarcomas in general have the propensity to spread to the lungs, bone, and bone marrow. Lung metastases are often asymptomatic unless large or progressive, whereas bone metastases typically cause pain at the site of the lesion. Bone marrow disease may lead to diminished peripheral blood counts.

Evaluation at Presentation

Physical Examination

- Thorough history and physical examination of the head and neck region are recommended to determine the location and size of the mass, as well as the presence or absence of abnormal lymphadenopathy. Cranial nerves should be assessed. Flexible nasal endoscopy and laryngoscopy should be routinely performed. Referral to an ophthalmologist, audiologist, and ear, nose, and throat (ENT) surgeon are imperative.

Initial Imaging

Given the wide range of tumors on the differential diagnosis (see further) and the possibility for benign lesions, imaging studies should be selected carefully. Imaging must assess the origin and local extent of the primary tumor, its size in centimeters, extension beyond the skull base, meningeal involvement, and invasion into adjacent structures.

- Ultrasound can be used as a first-pass imaging technique to evaluate extracranial head and neck masses in children. Technical developments in high-resolution gray-scale ultrasound have improved the ability of this modality to

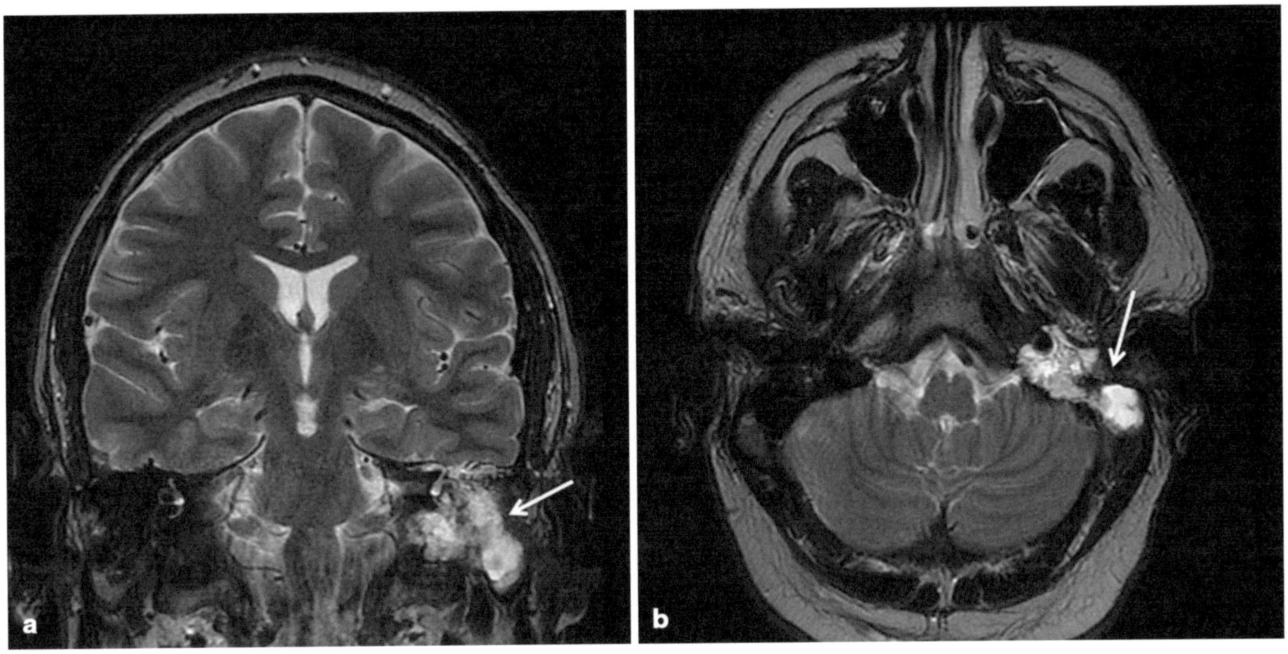

Fig. 41.1 Coronal (**a**) and Axial (**b**) T2 images showing a large angiosarcoma in the left temporal fossa (*arrows*) in a 16-year-old adolescent male

characterize the internal architecture of lesions. Doppler ultrasound can be particularly useful in assessing for vascular malformations [17].

- Tumors of the head and neck are best depicted with magnetic resonance imaging (MRI) due to superior soft-tissue contrast, excellent spatial resolution, multiplanar imaging, and absence of ionizing radiation associated with MRI (Fig. 41.1). With these benefits, come the downside of a 30–45 min examination requiring anesthesia for younger children [17].
- Routine spin-echo (SE) T1- and T2 weighted sequences before and after intravenous contrast administration are routine. Diffusion-weighted imaging plays a substantial role in characterizing head and neck masses. A recent study found a significant difference in apparent diffusion coefficient (ADC) values for malignant versus benign lesions with a 94 % sensitivity and 91 % specificity in distinguishing between the two [18].
- CT can more readily identify lesions arising from the bone, and can detect bony erosion.
- The role of positron emission tomography (PET) and PET-CT in childhood malignancies is continually being defined (see further, staging); it may have a distinct role in soft tissue sarcomas [19].

Biopsy

- Tissue sampling can occur either via open or needle biopsy. If possible, an open biopsy under anesthesia is preferred. Closed techniques such as fine needle aspiration and tru-cut biopsy are reserved for inaccessible lesions. They obtain smaller volumes of tissue, and thus increase sampling error and inconclusive findings and often preclude molecular studies [20]. Endoscopic techniques play an important role in exploring and biopsying sinonasal and nasopharyngeal tumors. A frozen section should be obtained at the time of open biopsy to ensure that the specimen is adequate.
- Lymph nodes have not been shown to be routinely involved in head and neck non-RMS. Should images or clinical exam yield concern, the patient should undergo concurrent lymph node dissection. Sarcomas with the propensity to spread to lymph nodes include synovial sarcoma, angiosarcoma, epitheliod sarcoma, and clear cell sarcoma, among others.
- Pathology of head and neck sarcomas is extremely varied as this entity encompasses a large group of mesenchymal tumors of different cell origin. The most common non-RMS tumors are represented in Figs. 41.2, 41.3, 41.4 and 41.5.

Differential Diagnosis

The differential diagnosis of head and neck non-RMS includes both benign and malignant conditions (Table 41.1).

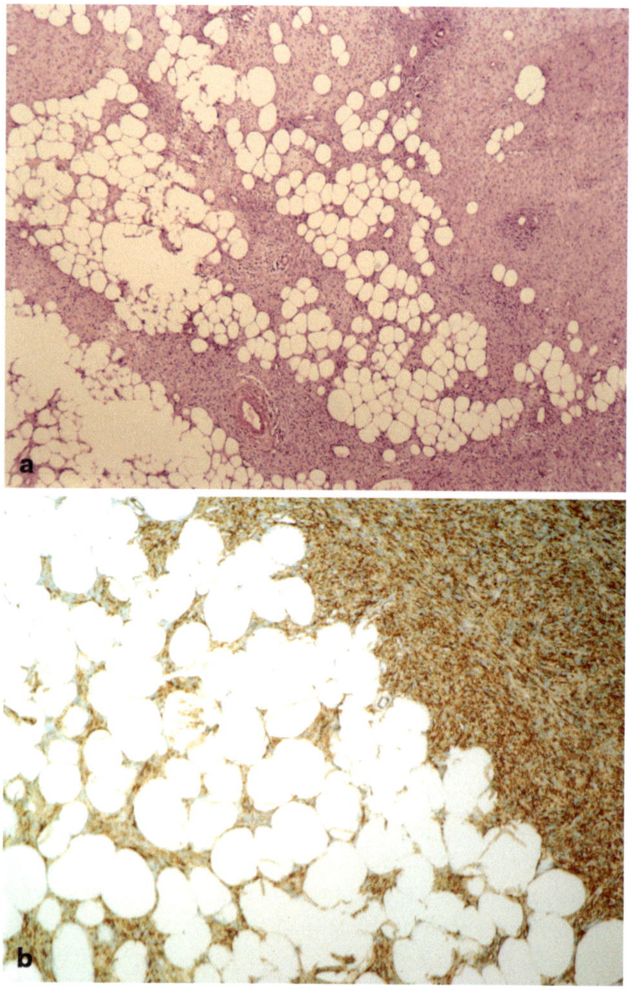

Fig. 41.2 Pathology of soft tissue sarcomas: dermatofibrosarcoma protuberans. **a** Poorly circumscribed proliferation of spindled cells infiltrating subcutaneous tissue. The tumor profusely infiltrates lobules of adipose tissue. **b** Immunohistochemically, tumor cells are diffusely and strongly reactive for CD34

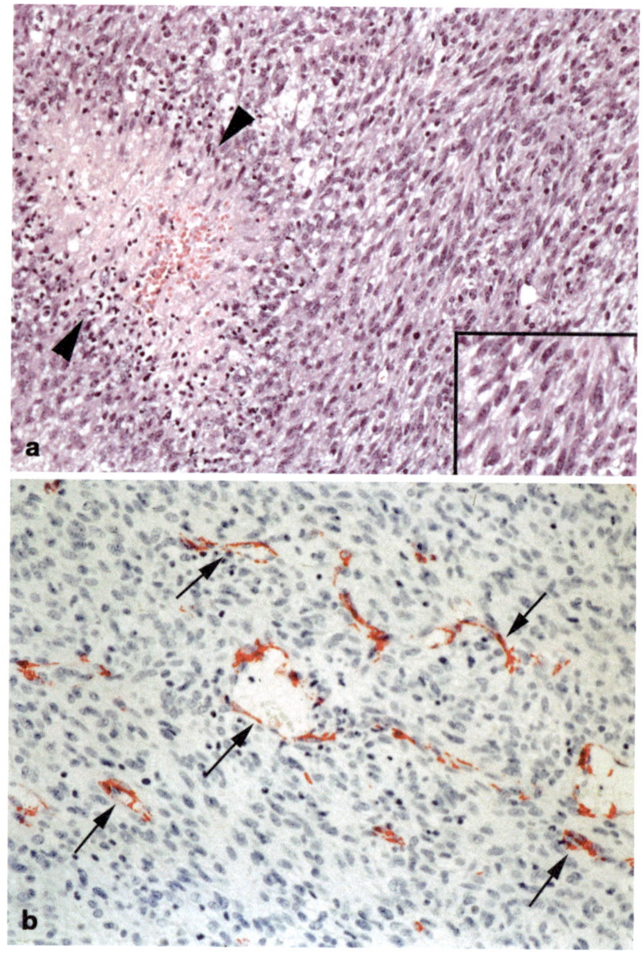

Fig. 41.3 Pathology of soft tissue sarcomas: infantile fibrosarcoma. **a** Cellular spindled cell tumor with numerous mitoses, apoptoses, and areas of necrosis (between *arrows heads*). **b** The tumor often exhibits numerous branching vessels imparting a hemangiopericytoma pattern (*arrows*). Endothelial cells are highlighted with CD31 antibody

Additional Workup/Staging

Laboratory Data

- Complete blood count with differential, liver function tests, electrolytes.
- Lumbar puncture should be performed if there is concern for bony erosion or leptomeningeal enhancement on CT or MRI.
- Bilateral bone marrow aspirates and biopsies (for sarcomas known to metastasize to the intramedullary space).

Imaging Evaluation

- In addition to imaging of the primary site of disease, diagnostic biopsy, and nodal assessment (as stated earlier), a metastatic work-up should be performed as follows:
  - CT scan of the chest: recommended to assess for pulmonary nodules. This modality is limited in many disease types by its inability to distinguish benign from malignant lesions [21].
  - Positron emission tomography: distant metastases and lymph node metastases have been reported to be superiorly detected by PET/CT over conventional imaging studies [19, 22]. The use of PET in pediatric patients with head and neck non-RMS is not yet routine, but will likely approach the standard of care.

Treatment

Treatment for non-RMS tumors is not as well defined as that for RMS. Regardless, treatment approach should be coordinated by a multidisciplinary pediatric oncology team comprised of medical and radiation oncologists, head and neck

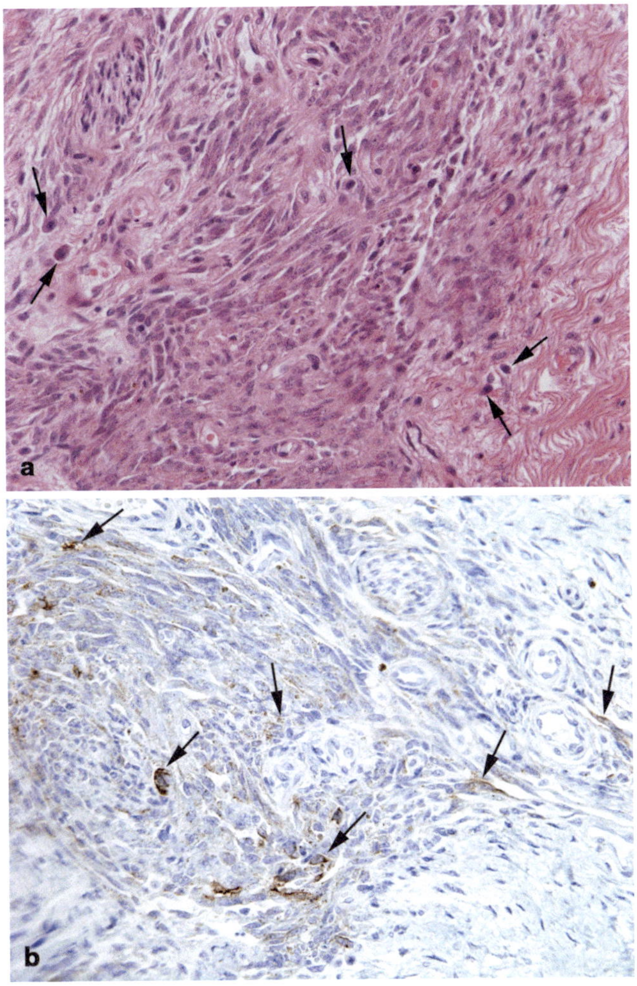

Fig. 41.4 Pathology of soft tissue sarcomas: synovial sarcoma. **a** Fascicles of spindled cells with variable mitotic rate and interspersed mast cells (*arrows*). **b** Tumor cells are focally immunoreactive for epithelial membrane antigen (*arrows*)

surgeons, plastic surgeons and neurosurgeons, in addition to a nutritionist, psychologist, and physiotherapist.

Surgery

A common approach to therapy is aggressive resection following biopsy [23]. The extent of surgical resection in RMS is clearly prognostic as shown by the IRS [24]. The extent of surgical resection and residual disease is likewise reported to be prognostic in non-RMS tumors [4, 8, 25, 26]. Nasri et al. demonstrated that tumors of the oral cavity, pharynx, and skin extent the best prognosis, likely due to their ease of surgical resection [4]. Although complete surgical resection with negative margins offers the best chance of survival, location often precludes clear margins and more aggressive surgical resection can lead to unacceptable morbidity.

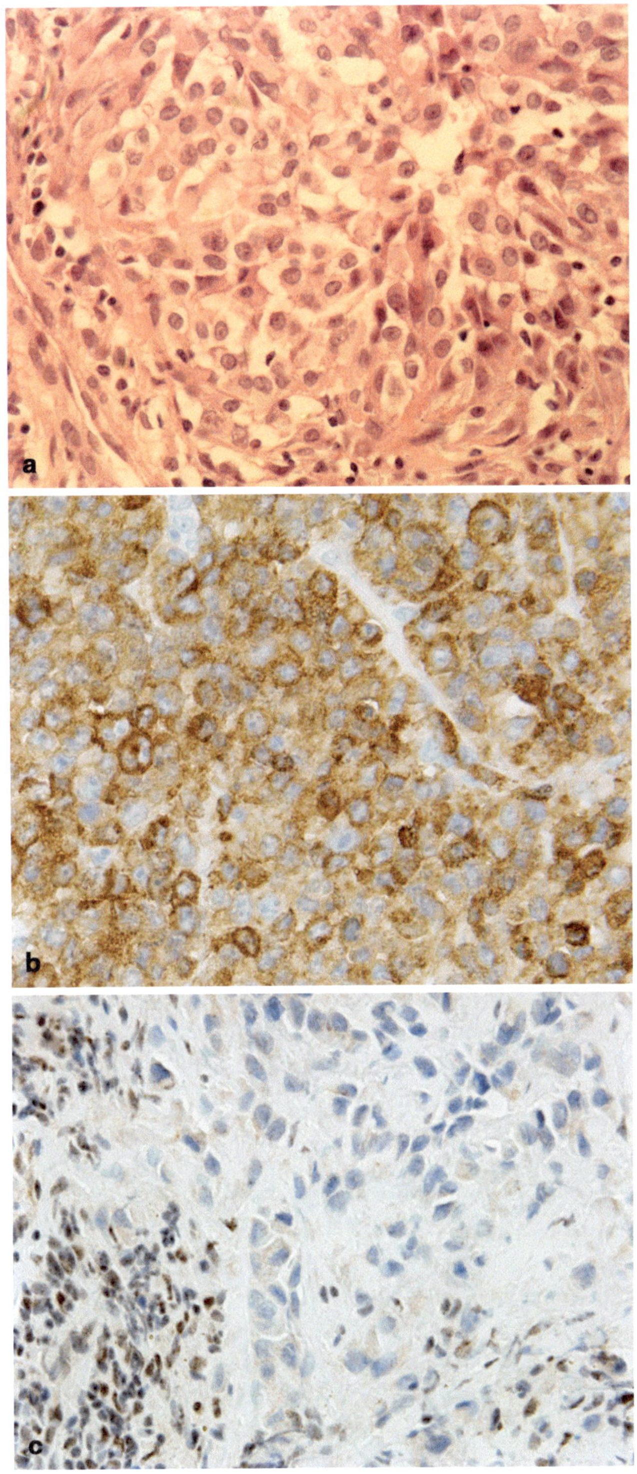

Fig. 41.5 Pathology of soft tissue sarcomas: epithelioid sarcoma. **a** Nests of medium to large size epithelioid cells with abundant eosinophilic cytoplasm, round to ovoid nuclei with open chromatin, and single distinct nucleoli. **b** Tumor cells show diffuse cytoplasmic staining for Cam5.2 cytokeratin by immunohistochemistry. **c** Characteristic nuclear INI-1 loss is observed in tumor cells. In contrast, the lymphocytes seen on the *lower left corner* of the photograph show retention of nuclear INI-1

Table 41.1 Differential diagnosis for non-RMS

Oncologic	Benign
1. Neuroblastoma	Hemangioma/Lymphangioma
2. Melanoma	Ossifying fibroma
3. Langerhans cell histiocytosis	Schwannoma
4. Nasopharyngeal carcinoma	Vascular malformation
5. Basal cell carcinoma	Benign fibrous histiocytoma
6. Lymphoma	Giant cell granuloma
7. Esthesioneuroblastoma	Neurofibroma
	Osteochondroma

Table 41.2 Disease grouping dependent upon extent of surgical resection

Group I	Localized disease, completely resected
	Confined to muscle/organ of origin
	Contiguous involvement-infiltration outside the muscle or organ of origin, as through fascial planes
Group II	Total gross resection with evidence of regional spread
	Microscopic residual disease
	Regional disease with involved nodes, completely resected with no microscopic residual
	Regional disease with involved nodes, grossly resected, but with evidence of microscopic residual and/or histologic involvement of the most distal regional node (from the primary site) in the dissection
Group III	Incomplete resection with gross residual disease
	After biopsy only
	After gross major resection of the primary
Group IV	Distant metastatic disease present at onset
	Lung, liver, bones, bone marrow, brain, distant muscle/nodes
	The presence of positive cytology in CSF, pleural or abdominal fluid, as well as implants on pleural or peritoneal surfaces

Given the role of surgery, non-RMS tumors are grouped similarly to the IRS RMS schematic, reflecting the extent of surgical resection. (Table 41.2).

Grading and Staging

Tumors are graded per the following schematic:

Grade I

- Myxoid and well-differentiated liposarcoma
- Deep-seated dermatofibrosarcoma protuberans
- Well-differentiated or infantile (≤4 years old) fibrosarcoma
- Well-differentiated or infantile (≤4 years old) hemangiopericytoma
- Well-differentiated malignant peripheral nerve sheath tumor
- Extraskeletal myxoid chondrosarcoma
- Angiomatoid malignant fibrous histiocytoma

Grade II

- Sarcomas not specifically included in Grade I or III and in which: less than 15% of the surface area shows necrosis, and/or the mitotic count is less than or equal to 5 mitotic figures per 10 high-power fields (hpf) using a 40x objective.
- As secondary criteria, nuclear atypia is not prominent and the tumor is not markedly cellular.

Grade III

- Pleomorphic or round cell liposarcoma
- Mesenchymal chondrosarcoma
- Extraskeletal osteosarcoma
- Malignant triton tumor
- Alveolar soft part sarcoma
- Angiosarcoma
- Synovial sarcoma
- Malignant peripheral nerve sheath tumor
- Malignant fibrous histiocytoma
- Sarcomas not specifically included in Grade I or II and in which: greater than 15% of the surface area shows necrosis, and/or the mitotic count is greater than 5 mitotic figures per 10 high-power fields (hpf) using a 40x objective.
- Marked atypia or cellularity are less predictive but may assist in placing tumors in this category.

Staging

Staging	Primary tumor	Regional LNs	Distant metastases	Histologic grade
I	Any	N0	M0	G1,G2
II	T1a, T1b, T2a	N0	M0	G3
III	T2b	N0	M0	G3
IV	Any	N1	Any	Any
	Any	Any	M1	Any

Primary Tumor

- T1a—Tumor less than or equal to 5 cm in maximal diameter, superficial
- T1b—Tumor less than or equal to 5 cm in maximal diameter, deep
- T2a—Tumor > 5 cm in maximal diameter, superficial
- T2b—Tumor > 5 cm in maximal diameter, deep

Note: Superficial tumors are located exclusively above the superficial fascia without invasion of the fascia; deep tumors are located either exclusively beneath the superficial fascia or superficial to the fascia with invasion of or through the fascia. The majority of head and neck tumors are classified as deep tumors.

Regional Lymph Nodes

- N0—No regional lymph node metastases
- N1—Regional lymph node metastases

Distant Metastases

- M0—No distant metastases
- M1—Distant metastases

Histologic Grade

- G1—Well differentiated
- G2—Moderately differentiated
- G3—Poorly differentiated

Chemotherapy and Radiotherapy

The role of chemotherapy and radiotherapy is unclear; many studies have shown both to be of little benefit in non-RMS tumors [4, 23]. Lyos et al. showed that inclusion of adjuvant radiotherapy and chemotherapy for high-grade lesions with residual disease following surgical resection resulted in a 75% 5-year survival [23]. Data from adult studies has shown the importance of postoperative RT for head and neck tumors with residual disease [27]. Doses above 4,500 cGy are usually required [4, 28].

In general, the following guidelines should be considered in the management of head and neck sarcomas:

- Upfront surgery should always be considered.
- Patients with small (≤5 cm) tumors, completely resected, can be followed without additional therapy. For patients with microscopic residual, adjuvant radiation is indicated (5,580 cGy).
- Patients with resected large (>5 cm) tumors should be considered for adjuvant radiation therapy (5,580 cGy) and chemotherapy (six cycles of ifosfamide and doxorubicin) due to the risks of local and systemic recurrence.
- Patients with unresectable disease should receive neoadjuvant chemotherapy, followed by surgery and radiation therapy. The concurrent administration of chemotherapy and radiation therapy prior to surgery may facilitate resection. This is the approach currently followed by the major cooperative groups in North America and Europe. According to this approach, patients receive two cycles of ifosfamide and doxorubicin, followed by concurrent chemoradiation with ifosfamide and 4,500 cGy to the primary tumor. Resection of the primary tumor is then performed with the goal of negative microscopic margins. For patients with complete resection, no additional radiation therapy is recommended. Patients with residual tumor receive a radiotherapy boost to the primary site (1,980 cGy for gross residual, 1,080 cGy for microscopic residual). For patients responding to preoperative chemotherapy, adjuvant treatment is recommended.

There are a few entities that require individualized treatment, with less aggressive approaches:

1. *Infantile fibrosarcomas* and commonly *infantile hemangiopericytomas* are treated very differently from the remainder of non-RMS tumors; their clinical behavior is more favorable despite their aggressive clinical presentation. A conservative approach with neoadjuvant chemotherapy (vincristine, dactinomycin—VA or VA with cyclophosphamide—VAC) and conservative surgery is favored; radical resection and radiation therapy should be avoided [29].
2. *Desmoid fibromatosis* has the potential to be either locally aggressive and destructive or to stabilize without intervention; both subtypes lack metastatic potential. Extra-abdominal head and neck desmoids correlate with a more indolent course and better prognosis [30]. The two growth patterns can be differentiated by means of observation or conservative therapies to allow determination of tumor behavior. Patients with progressive tumors can undergo upfront resection or trial of low-dose neoadjuvant chemotherapy to induce disease response or stabilization; the most commonly used regimen is the combination of methotrexate and vinblastine [31]. Neoadjuvant or adjuvant radiotherapy has also been utilized

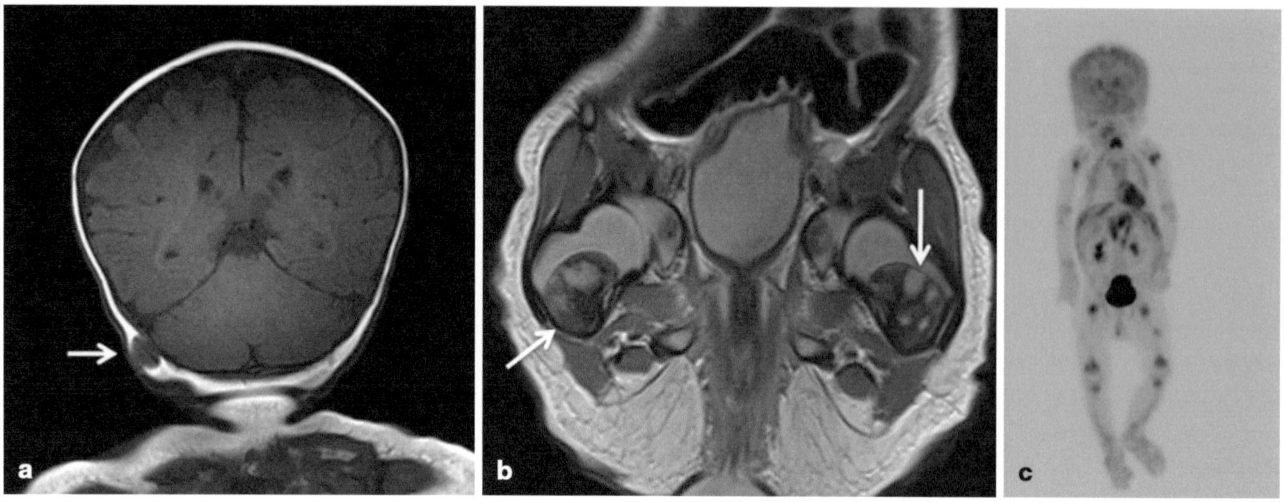

Fig. 41.6 Infantile myofibromatosis in a 2-month-old infant who presented with a right neck mass (**a**, *arrow*). Additional evaluation showed multiple bone and soft tissue myofibromas (involvement of both femoral heads, **b**, *arrows*), which were fludeoxyglucose (FDG) avid on PET scan (**c**)

but is typically deferred in pediatric patients due to effects on growth and concern for secondary malignancy [32]. Completeness of initial resection has been shown to be the main factor impacting event-free survival (EFS) [33]. Local failure rates are reported anywhere from 10 to 77% [32, 34–37].

3. *Infantile myofibroma and myofibromatosis* can involve the head and neck one-third of the time, as part of either a solitary or multicentric presentation—the latter being divided into soft tissue or visceral involvement (Fig. 41.6) [38]. Multicentric myofibromatosis with visceral involvement is associated with high morbidity and mortality despite chemotherapy; however the other forms have an excellent prognosis with surgery alone or observation [39]. Lesions limited to the skin have a high likelihood of spontaneous remission [40]. Rarely, chemotherapy (methotrexate/vinblastine extrapolated from desmoid therapy) is required for rapid growth or for lesions that might cause local damage upon growth (i.e., orbital). Recent evidence suggests that infantile hemangiopericytoma, myofibroma, and myofibromatosis are different stages of maturation of a single entity [41].

Complications to Radiation Therapy

Facial growth, neuroendocrine dysfunction, visual/orbital problems, dental abnormalities, asymmetry of the tissues at the primary tumor site, hypothyroidism, secondary malignancy, and intellectual and academic delays are all found to be associated with the receipt of head and neck radiotherapy [42].

Prognosis

- There is little information in the literature regarding overall prognosis in children with non-RMS of the head and neck. A 5-year survival rate of 50–60% has been reported.
- The influence of tumor grade on prognosis is well described in the adult literature; in the pediatric literature, Sollacio et al. reported tumor grade to influence local and distant failure as well as overall prognosis [43].
- Patients with metastatic disease fare very poorly with less than 20% surviving at 5 years.

Follow-Up

Frequency of Office Visits

- Imaging studies should be performed no sooner than 6 weeks post treatment to avoid confusion between residual disease and post-treatment changes. Enhancement of the tumor bed that remains stable for at least 3 months after treatment is suspicious for residual tumor.
- After completion of therapy, office visits with laboratory work (CBC, chemistry) should be performed q3 months × 1 year, q6 months for the second year, and annually starting at 3 years.

Frequency of Imaging

- At each of the above mentioned clinical visits, chest x-ray (CXR) should be performed along with imaging of the primary site of disease (preferably with MRI).

References

1. Gurney JG, Swensen AR, Bulterys M. Malignant bone tumors SEER data pediatrics. National Cancer Institute; 1975–1995. pp. 99–110.
2. Gurney JG, Young JL Jr, Roffers SD, Smith MA, Bunin GR. Soft tissue sarcomas SEER data pediatrics. National Cancer Institute; 1975–1995. pp. 111–124.
3. Pappo AS, Shapiro DN, Crist WM, Maurer HM. Biology and therapy of pediatric rhabdomyosarcoma. J Clin Oncol. 1995;13:2123–39.
4. Nasri S, Mark RJ, Sercarz JA, Tran LM, Sadeghi S. Pediatric sarcomas of the head and neck other than rhabdomyosarcoma. Am J Otolaryngol. 1995;16:165–71.
5. Smith R, Robinson RA. Head and neck malignancies, pediatric otolaryngology head and neck surgery. St. Louis:Mosby; 1998.
6. Koshy M, Paulino AC, Mai WY, Teh BS. Radiation-induced osteosarcomas in the pediatric population. Int J Radiat Oncol Biol Phys. 2005;63:1169–74.
7. Raney RB, Asmar L, Vassilopoulou-Sellin R, et al. Late complications of therapy in 213 children with localized, nonorbital soft-tissue sarcoma of the head and neck: a descriptive report from the Intergroup Rhabdomyosarcoma Studies (IRS)-II and—III. IRS Group of the Children's Cancer Group and the Pediatric Oncology Group. Med Pediatr Oncol. 1999;33:362–71.
8. Horowitz ME, Pratt CB, Webber BL, et al. Therapy for childhood soft-tissue sarcomas other than rhabdomyosarcoma: a review of 62 cases treated at a single institution. J Clin Oncol. 1986;4:559–64.
9. Holsinger FC, Hafemeister AC, Hicks MJ, Sulek M, Huh WW, Friedman EM. Differential diagnosis of pediatric tumors of the nasal cavity and paranasal sinuses: a 45-year multi-institutional review. Ear Nose Throat J. 2010;89:534–40.
10. Gadd S, Beezhold P, Jennings L, et al. Mediators of receptor tyrosine kinase activation in infantile fibrosarcoma: a children's oncology group study. J Pathol. 2012;228:119–30.
11. Salgado R, Llombart B, M Pujol R, et al. Molecular diagnosis of dermatofibrosarcoma protuberans: a comparison between reverse transcriptase-polymerase chain reaction and fluorescence in situ hybridization methodologies. Genes Chromosomes Cancer. 2011;50:510–7.
12. Przybyl J, Sciot R, Rutkowski P, et al. Recurrent and novel SS18-SSX fusion transcripts in synovial sarcoma: description of three new cases. Tumour Biol. 2012;33(6):2245–53.
13. Sankar S, Lessnick SL. Promiscuous partnerships in Ewing's sarcoma. Cancer Genet. 2011;204:351–65.
14. Hayani A, Mahoney DH Jr, Hawkins HK, Steuber CP, Hurwitz R, Fernbach DJ. Soft-tissue sarcomas other than rhabdomyosarcoma in children. Med Pediatr Oncol. 1992;20:114–8.
15. Goorin AM, Abelson HT. Frei E 3rd. Osteosarcoma: fifteen years later. N Engl J Med. 1985;313:1637–43.
16. Turner JH, Richmon JD. Head and neck rhabdomyosarcoma: a critical analysis of population-based incidence and survival data. Otolaryngol Head Neck Surg. 2011;145:967–73.
17. Lloyd C, McHugh K. The role of radiology in head and neck tumours in children. Cancer Imaging. 2010;10:49–61.
18. Abdel Razek AA, Gaballa G, Elhawarey G, Megahed AS, Hafez M, Nada N. Characterization of pediatric head and neck masses with diffusion-weighted MR imaging. Eur Radiol. 2009;19:201–8.
19. Jadvar H, Connolly LP, Fahey FH, Shulkin BL. PET and PET/CT in pediatric oncology. Semin Nucl Med. 2007;37:316–31.
20. Bisogno G, De Rossi C, Gamboa Y, et al. Improved survival for children with parameningeal rhabdomyosarcoma: results from the AIEOP soft tissue sarcoma committee. Pediatr Blood Cancer. 2008;50:1154–8.
21. Van Rijn RR, Wilde JC, Bras J, Oldenburger F, McHugh KM, Merks JH. Imaging findings in noncraniofacial childhood rhabdomyosarcoma. Pediatr Radiol. 2008;38:617–34.
22. Volker T, Denecke T, Steffen I, et al. Positron emission tomography for staging of pediatric sarcoma patients: results of a prospective multicenter trial. J Clin Oncol. 2007;25:5435–41.
23. Lyos AT, Goepfert H, Luna MA, Jaffe N, Malpica A. Soft tissue sarcoma of the head and neck in children and adolescents. Cancer. 1996;77:193–200.
24. Daya H, Chan HS, Sirkin W, Forte V. Pediatric rhabdomyosarcoma of the head and neck: is there a place for surgical management? Arch Otolaryngol Head Neck Surg. 2000;126:468–72.
25. Fontanesi J, Pratt C, Kun L, et al. Local-regional non-rhabdomyosarcomatous soft tissue sarcomas of the head and neck. Int J Radiat Oncol Biol Phys. 1990;19:995–9.
26. Brizel DM, Weinstein H, Hunt M, Tarbell NJ. Failure patterns and survival in pediatric soft tissue sarcoma. Int J Radiat Oncol Biol Phys. 1988;15:37–41.
27. Tran LM, Mark R, Meier R, Calcaterra TC, Parker RG. Sarcomas of the head and neck. Prognostic factors and treatment strategies. Cancer. 1992;70:169–77.
28. Kinsella TJ, Miser JS, Triche TJ, Horvath K, Glatstein E. Treatment of high-risk sarcomas in children and young adults: analysis of local control using intensive combined modality therapy. NCI Monogr. 1988;6:291–6.
29. Orbach D, Rey A, Cecchetto G, et al. Infantile fibrosarcoma: management based on the European experience. J Clin Oncol. 2010;28:318–23.
30. Salas S, Dufresne A, Bui B, et al. Prognostic factors influencing progression-free survival determined from a series of sporadic desmoid tumors: a wait-and-see policy according to tumor presentation. J Clin Oncol. 2011;29:3553–8.
31. Skapek SX, Ferguson WS, Granowetter L, et al. Vinblastine and methotrexate for desmoid fibromatosis in children: results of a Pediatric Oncology Group Phase II Trial. J Clin Oncol. 2007;25:501–6.
32. Francis WP, Zippel D, Mack LA, et al. Desmoids: a revelation in biology and treatment. Ann Surg Oncol. 2009;16:1650–4.
33. Meazza C, Bisogno G, Gronchi A, et al. Aggressive fibromatosis in children and adolescents: the Italian experience. Cancer. 2010;116:233–40.
34. Karakousis CP, Mayordomo J, Zografos GC, Driscoll DL. Desmoid tumors of the trunk and extremity. Cancer. 1993;72:1637–41.
35. Miralbell R, Suit HD, Mankin HJ, Zuckerberg LR, Stracher MA, Rosenberg AE. Fibromatoses: from postsurgical surveillance to combined surgery and radiation therapy. Int J Radiat Oncol Biol Phys. 1990;18:535–40.
36. Pritchard DJ, Nascimento AG, Petersen IA. Local control of extra-abdominal desmoid tumors. J Bone Joint Surg Am. 1996;78:848–54.
37. Rock MG, Pritchard DJ, Reiman HM, Soule EH, Brewster RC. Extra-abdominal desmoid tumors. J Bone Joint Surg Am. 1984;66:1369–74.
38. Behar PM, Albritton FD, Muller S, Todd NW. Multicentric infantile myofibromatosis. Int J Pediatr Otorhinolaryngol. 1998;45:249–54.
39. Wiswell TE, Davis J, Cunningham BE, Solenberger R, Thomas PJ. Infantile myofibromatosis: the most common fibrous tumor of infancy. J Pediatr Surg. 1988;23:315–8.
40. Gopal M, Chahal G, Al-Rifai Z, Eradi B, Ninan G, Nour S. Infantile myofibromatosis. Pediatr Surg Int. 2008;24:287–91.
41. Mentzel T, Calonje E, Nascimento AG, Fletcher CD. Infantile hemangiopericytoma versus infantile myofibromatosis. Study of a series suggesting a continuous spectrum of infantile myofibroblastic lesions. Am J Surg Pathol. 1994;9:922–30.
42. Fromm M, Littman P, Raney RB, et al. Late effects after treatment of twenty children with soft tissue sarcomas of the head and neck. Experience at a single institution with a review of the literature. Cancer. 1986;57:2070–6.
43. Sollaccio RJ, Conrad C, Mendenhall NP, Mareus RR, Million RR, Springfield DS, Enneking WF. Soft tissue sarcoma in children: analysis of prognostic factors. J Radiation Oncol Biol Phy. 1986;12:133 (abstract 82).

Sarcoma: Rhabdomyosarcoma

42

Allison O'Neill, Karen Watters, Reza Rahbar
and Carlos Rodriguez-Galindo

Introduction

Rhabdomyosarcoma (RMS) is a morphologically and clinically heterogeneous group of malignant tumors that resemble developing skeletal muscle. Head and neck RMS comprise nearly one-third of all pediatric RMS cases [1]. This group is subdivided into three types: orbital, parameningeal, and non-orbital non-parameningeal. While tumors of the head and neck are generally considered to have a favorable prognosis, those in the parameningeal region typically have a more adverse outcome. Treatment is stratified based on location, histology, and surgical resectability, and includes a combination of multi-agent chemotherapy and local control.

Key Points

- Head and neck RMS are classified as orbital, parameningeal, and non-orbital non-parameningeal. Parameningeal sites portend a poor prognosis, while orbital tumors have an excellent prognosis.
- Treatment consists of systemic chemotherapy with local control: surgery, radiotherapy, or both. Orbital and parameningeal tumors are less amenable to a surgical approach.
- Approximately 70% of patients with localized RMS are cured; however their outcome continues to be dependent on a number of prognostic factors including tumor size, location, histology, staging, and patient age [2].

Biology and Epidemiology

Rhabdomyosarcomas are malignant tumors that are derived from undifferentiated skeletal muscle and are histologically classified based on their resemblance to normal fetal muscle prior to innervation [3]. They are categorized into embryonal (60%) or alveolar (20%) subtypes with the remainder falling into a pleomorphic or undifferentiated category [4, 5]. Embryonal RMS occurs at sites throughout the body with the head and neck region being the most common representing 29% of cases. Orbital tumors comprise an additional 11% of embryonal RMS. Alveolar tumors tend to more frequently involve the extremities, however nearly 22% of cases involve the head and neck [6].

Pathophysiology

- RMS tumors express markers of developing skeletal muscle and are thought to arise from myogenic cells. As with most tumors of pediatric origin, the actual etiology is unknown.

Histopathology

RMS is one of the small, round blue cell tumors of childhood. The cells of an RMS, or "myoblasts," can have variable differentiation along the myogenesis pathway. Discernible muscle cross-striations may be visible under light mi-

A. O'Neill (✉)
Department of Pediatric Oncology, Harvard Medical School, Dana-Farber/Boston Children's Hospital Cancer and Blood Disorders Center, Boston, MA, USA
e-mail: allison_oneill@dfci.harvard.edu

K. Watters
Boston Children's Hospital, Harvard Medical School, Otolaryngology and Communication Enhancement, Boston, MA, USA

R. Rahbar
Department of Otolaryngology, Boston Children's Hospital, Harvard Medical School, Boston, MA, USA

C. Rodriguez-Galindo
Department of Pediatric Oncology, Harvard Medical School; Dana-Farber/Boston Children's Hospital Cancer and Blood Disorders Center, Boston, MA, USA

R. Rahbar et al. (eds.), *Pediatric Head and Neck Tumors*,
DOI 10.1007/978-1-4614-8755-5_42, © Springer Science+Business Media New York 2014

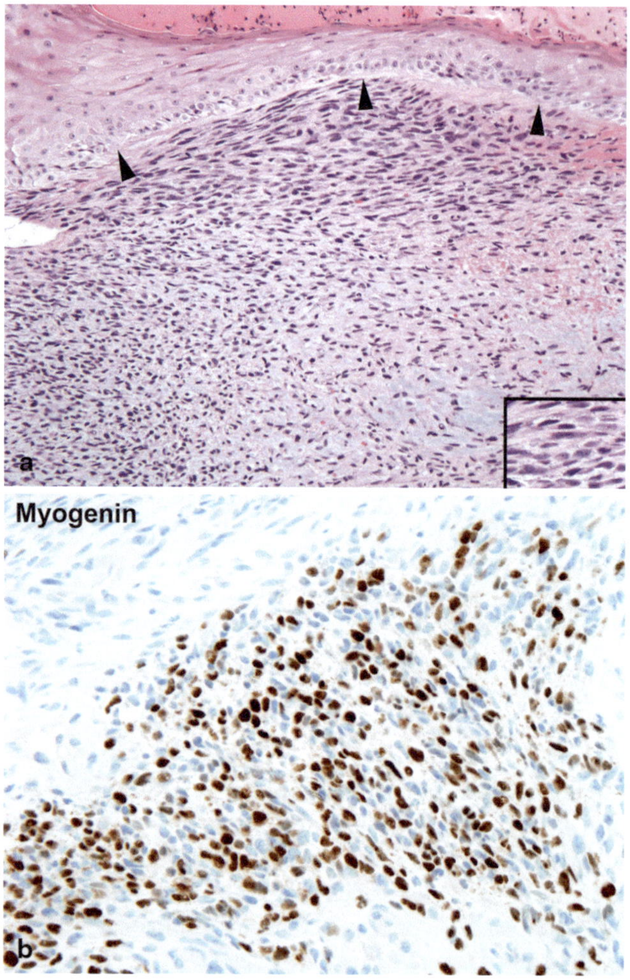

Fig. 42.1 Embryonal RMS of the right ear. **a** Cellular spindled cell proliferation of atypical cells with hyperchromatic nuclei and scant, elongated eosinophilic cytoplasm. The tumor is growing under the keratinizing squamous mucosa seen above the arrowheads. The neoplastic proliferation is more densely cellular under the epithelium and less cellular and myxoid in deeper locations. A densely cellular area at higher magnification is seen in the inset. **b** A large proportion of tumor cells show strong nuclear immunoreactivity for myogenin

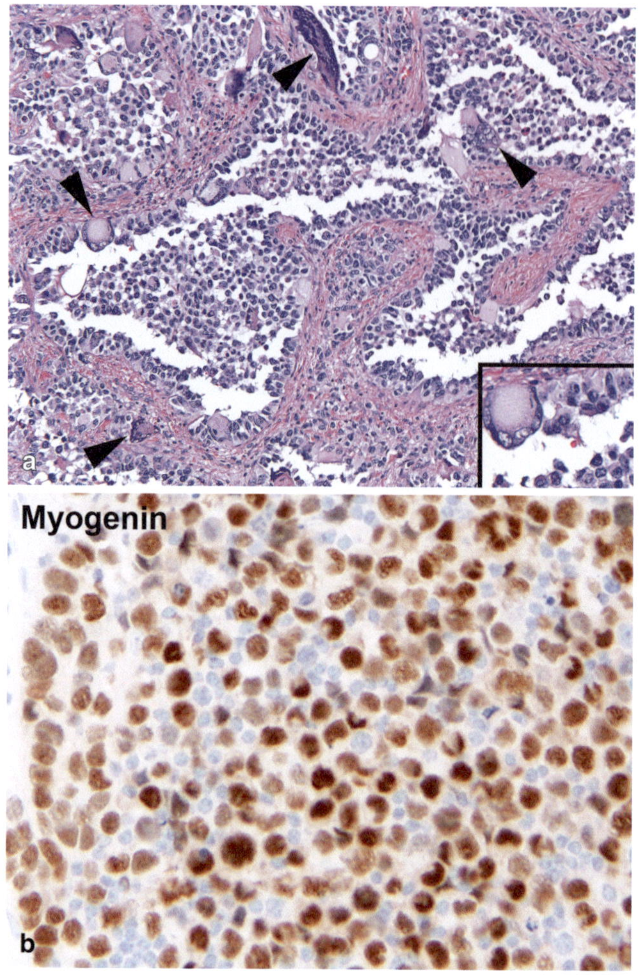

Fig. 42.2 Alveolar rhabdomyosarcoma. **a** Characteristic alveolar-like spaces delineated by connective tissue trabecules. Tumor cells are large and rounded, have uncohesive growth at the center, and appear to be attached to the connective tissue trabecules at the periphery. Occasional large pleomorphic giant tumor cells are also observed (*arrowheads*). Higher magnification of rounded tumor cells and of a giant multinucleated tumor cell is shown in the inset. **b** Most of the tumor cell nuclei are strongly immunoreactive to myogenin

croscopy. Distinct histologic groups with prognostic significance have been described:

- *Embryonal RMS* (55 %): Embryonal RMS is characterized histologically by both spindle and primitive round cells that are either tightly packed or loosely dispersed upon a myoid background (Fig. 42.1) [5]. The more differentiated cell, the rhabdomyoblast, can assume a variety of shapes (tadpole, racquet, strap cells), and reveal cross-striations [5]. The botryoid variant of embryonal RMS, which accounts for 5 % of cases, is characterized by polyploid masses and subepithelial aggregates of tumor cells microscopically. These tumors can arise in the mucosa-lined nasopharynx. Prognosis for embryonal RMS is generally good.
- *Alveolar RMS* (20 %): Alveolar RMS is characterized by the presence of fibrovascular septa forming spaces that contain freely floating round malignant cells with abundant eosinophilic cytoplasm (Fig. 42.2). This type is so named because of its distinct architecture resembling that of pulmonary alveoli. While the IRS Pathology Committee originally designated that more than 50 % of the tumor contain these elements to qualify as an alveolar RMS, it is now recognized that any degree of alveolar histology within a tumor specimen is diagnostic [7]. Tumors in the adolescent age group are typically of the alveolar type and have a poorer prognosis because of their aggressive and metastatic nature. Lymphatic and systemic metastases are more common. The prognosis of alveolar tumors is better if a child is less than 10 years of age.
- *Undifferentiated/Pleomorphic (25 %)*: Pleomorphic RMS can show features of both embryonal and alveolar his-

tologies [8] while undifferentiated, or RMS "not otherwise specified," are more difficult to categorize. The vast majority of RMS involving the head and neck, greater than 75 %, fall into the embryonal or alveolar subtypes [9].

Immunohistochemical expression of muscle-specific proteins including desmin, muscle-specific actin, and myogenin are the most important markers for establishing a pathologic diagnosis (Figs. 42.1 and 42.2) [10, 11].

Molecular/Genetic Pathology

RMS are associated with chromosomal abnormalities that can be used to confirm the diagnosis [12]. Some of these abnormalities have important prognostic and possibly therapeutic implications.

- Embryonal RMS have characteristically been linked to loss of heterozygosity at a specific site on the short arm of chromosome 11 (11p15). Loss of heterozygosity is associated with over-expression of insulin growth factor 2 and known to play a role in tumorigenesis. Embryonal type tumors have been found to have a DNA content between diploid and hyperdiploid. There have been varying reports as to the prognostic significance of ploidy in RMS, with hyperdiploidy associated with a better long-term survival than tetrapolidy. However, conflicting studies have likewise been published [13–15].
- Alveolar RMS has translocations involving the FKHR gene on the long arm of chromosome 13 with genes of the PAX family on either chromosome 2 (PAX3) or chromosome 1 (PAX7) [12]. PAX3 is a transcriptional regulatory protein expressed during embryogenesis and thought crucial for the development of mesenchymal precursors into myoblasts [16]. These translocations result in the fusion of the DNA-binding domain of the neuromuscular developmental transcription factors, encoded by PAX3, to the transcriptional activation domain FKHR (a relatively ubiquitous transcription factor)—the consequences of this fusion are not fully understood [17, 18]. However, the resultant hybrid molecule is a potent transcription activator thought to activate and repress other genes leading to abnormal cell growth.
- *TP53* mutations have been associated with both embryonal and alveolar histologic subtypes [19, 20]. Expression of this mutated tumor suppressor gene product is associated with decreased survival and anaplastic histology [21, 22].
- Elevated n-myc expression (10 % of patients with alveolar), and point mutations in N-ras and K-ras oncogenes (usually embryonal) have been described.
- Fluorescent in situ hybridization (FISH) can be used to determine if the above-mentioned translocations are present. It can also be used to assess for break-apart of the FKHR gene. Reverse transcription (i.e. reverse transcription) polymerase chain reaction (RT-PCR) can be helpful in assessing for characteristic translocations seen in alveolar RMS, especially when cytogenetic studies are not possible.

Incidence and Prevalence

- In the USA, there are approximately 850 cases of soft tissue sarcoma per year with approximately 40 %, or 350 cases, being RMS. More than 50 % of these cases occur in children younger than 10 years of age [6].
- About 35 % of all RMS cases arise in the head and neck region, with nearly 75 % of these tumors confined to the orbit or parameningeal regions [1].
- There has been a slight increase in head and neck RMS in the last 30 years with an overall incidence of 0.041 cases per 100,000 population and a statistically significant annual percentage increase of 1.16 % ($p<0.005$) [9].

Age Distribution

- In a retrospective review of 558 cases of RMS, roughly 2/3rds of head and neck RMS occurred in children 0–19 years of age, with a peak incidence between 0 and 9 years. The remainder occurred in adults aged 20–55 years [9]. The mean age of incidence is 5 years.
- Embryonal RMS comprises roughly 80 % of cases in children younger than 5 years of age, and 64 % among 15–19 year olds. The relative percentage of alveolar RMS increases from 15 % among children younger than 5 years of age to 30 % among 15–19 years [6]. This age differential between embryonal and alveolar RMS may partially reflect the higher incidence of head and neck cases in younger children, the majority of which are embryonal.

Sex Predilection

- While some studies note a slight male predilection for head and neck RMS, this finding is generally not statistically significant [9, 23].

Geographic Distribution

- Given that only small case series have been published regarding site-specific experiences with head and neck RMS, data on geographic distribution is not available.

Table 42.1 Genetic syndromes associated with pediatric and adolescent cases of rhabdomyosarcoma

1. Neurofibromatosis
2. Beckwith–Weidemann
3. Li Fraumeni syndrome
4. Rubinstein–Taybi syndrome
5. Costello syndrome
6. Gorlin basal cell nevus syndrome

Risk Factors

- There is limited evidence that the following environmental exposures are linked to RMS: paternal smoking, maternal use of recreational drugs, antibiotic use, low socioeconomic status, or ionizing radiation (in utero) [24–26]. There is no data linking any of the risks to head and neck RMS in particular.

Relationships to Other Disease States, Syndromes

- Most cases of RMS are sporadic; 9% of cases are syndrome-related. A number of genetic syndromes are thought to be associated with the development of early RMS [27]. (Table 42.1)
- There is some concordance with the location of RMS and major birth defects. One autopsy study showed 32% of 115 children with RMS to have at least one congenital anomaly [6, 28].

Presentation

Symptoms are dependent upon the tumor's location at diagnosis. Head and neck RMS is divided into three subtypes: orbital, parameningeal, and non-orbital non-parameningeal [9].

Orbital

- Eyelid: this is included in the "orbital category." Tumors of true eye origin can occur but are rare and arise from the conjunctiva.
- Orbit: this region refers to the bony cavity which contains the globe, nerve and vessels, and extraocular muscles. Tumors can occasionally invade the bony walls and extend into the sinuses.
- Orbital RMS is most typically associated with the insidious or rapid onset of unilateral proptosis and inferior or inferiotemporal displacement of the globe. Patients can likewise present with worsening eyelid or conjunctival edema and erythema, a palpable mass, ophthalmoplegia (inability to adduct the affected eye), or blepharoptosis (drooping of the upper eyelid). A review by Gandhi et al. reported that approximately 11% of patients presented after incidental trauma. Only 10–20% of patients note ocular or orbital pain [29].

Parameningeal (approximately 40% of head and neck RMS cases)

- Middle ear: patients may present with a mass in front or under the ear suggesting a parotid origin. The mass may also extend through the tympanic membrane and appear to be arising from the ear canal. This tumor is often advanced at presentation. Tumors of this type may be associated with otalgia, bloody otorrhea, and hearing loss [30, 31]. They may also be associated with a facial nerve paralysis (VII).
- Nasal cavity and paranasal sinuses: patients may present with tumor in any one of the three paranasal sinuses (maxillary, ethmoid, and sphenoid) which surround the nasal cavity. Tumor originating in one sinus will often spread to the others. Tumors arising in the maxillary or ethmoid sinuses may invade the orbit. Patients may have associated rhinosinusitis including nasal obstruction and bloody or mucopurulent rhinorrhea. Occasionally, proptosis can also be present (Fig 42.3).
- Nasopharynx: patients present with tumors in the region defined by the back of the nasal septum anteriorly, the sphenoid sinus superiorly, the soft palate inferiorly, and the pharyngeal walls laterally and posteriorly. Tumors of this type may be associated with upper airway obstruction, new onset sleep apnea, or an abducens (VI) nerve palsy.
- Infratemporal fossa/pterygopalatine and parapharyngeal areas: patients present with tumors in the region bounded laterally by the medial lobe of the parotid gland and medially by the pharynx.
- Approximately 65–80% of patients with parameningeal disease have high-risk features including intracranial extension, skull base erosion, and cranial nerve paresis at presentation: diplopia caused by involvement of the oculomotor (III), trochlear (IV), and abducens (VI) nerves. A Horner's syndrome may be the only clinical finding in some instances. Headache and papilledema may be present if there is intracranial involvement. Lymph node involvement is present in 7% of patients at the time of presentation [10].
- A retrospective review by Zorzi et al. of 35 children with parameningeal RMS showed that 54% presented with a cranial nerve palsy, with the facial nerve being the most commonly involved [32]. In large studies performed by the IRS (Intergroup Rhabdomyosarcoma Study) and European study groups, the nasopharynx and paranasal

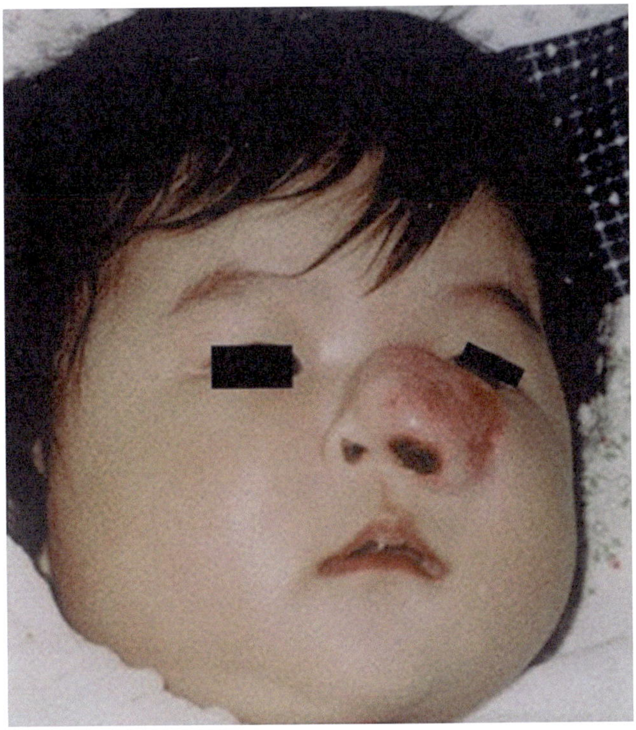

Fig. 42.3 A 4-month old female infant with a rapidly growing lesion in the region of her left nose and maxillary sinus. This lesion was mistakenly diagnosed as an infantile hemangioma, but failed to response to conventional treatment. A biopsy confirmed embryonal rhabdomyosarcoma

sinuses are the most commonly reported location of parameningeal tumors [33].

Non-orbital/Non-parameningeal

- These tumors arise from both superficial locations (cheek, external ear, scalp), and deep locations (parotid, oropharynx, palate, larynx, and neck).
- Superficial tumors may present as a painless mass lesion, while those in deeper locations, such as the oropharynx and larynx, may present with dysphagia, dysphonia, and/or obstructive airway symptoms. Facial nerve paralysis (VII) may be present with tumors of the parotid gland. The majority of non-parameningeal tumors are of the embryonal type, except those occurring in the cheek and scalp which have a tendency to be of the alveolar subtype.
- Tumors can occur in the thyroid and parathyroid but are rare.

Patterns of Evolution

- Parameningeal lesions carry a poorer prognosis given that their deep location renders them clinically silent. They must grow to considerable size before they are visualized from the outside.
- The most common sites of metastases for RMS are lung, bone, and bone marrow. Lung metastases are often asymptomatic unless large or progressive whereas bone metastases typically cause pain at the site of the lesion. Bone marrow disease may lead to diminished peripheral blood counts.

Evaluation at Presentation

Physical Exam

- Thorough history and physical exam of the head and neck region are recommended to determine the location and size of the mass, and examine for lymphadenopathy. Cranial nerves should be assessed. Flexible nasal endoscopy and laryngoscopy should be routinely performed. Referral to an ophthalmologist, audiologist and ear, nose, and throat (ENT) surgeon are imperative.

Initial Imaging

- RMS of the head and neck are best depicted with magnetic resonance imaging (MRI) due to superior soft-tissue contrast, excellent spatial resolution, multiplanar imaging, and absence of ionizing radiation. With these benefits, come the downside of a 30–45 min exam requiring anesthesia for younger children [34].
- Routine spin-echo (SE) T1- and T2-weighted sequences before and after intravenous contrast administration are routine. RMS appears relatively hypointense to brain on T2-weighted images. Coronal contrast-enhanced fat-suppressed T1-weighted images are useful for the detection of parameningeal tumors (Fig. 42.4). Volumetric interpolated breath-hold examination (or VIBE) can acquire images rapidly and allow for 3D reconstructions, which can detect subtle skull base abnormalities and perineural tumor spread. Dynamic contrast-enhanced MRI is useful in assessing tumor vascularity in vivo and may be relevant in assessing the nature of a residual mass post-treatment.
- CT scan of the primary site is often performed at diagnosis, but MRI is the preferred imaging modality for follow-up. On CT, RMS appears as a heterogeneous mass, often with necrosis. A CT scan can more readily identify bony erosion [35]. (Fig. 42.5)
- Imaging must assess the origin and local extent of the primary tumor, its size in centimeters, extension of tumor beyond the skull base, invasion into the anterior, middle or posterior cranial fossas, dural enhancement, and perineural enhancement [29].

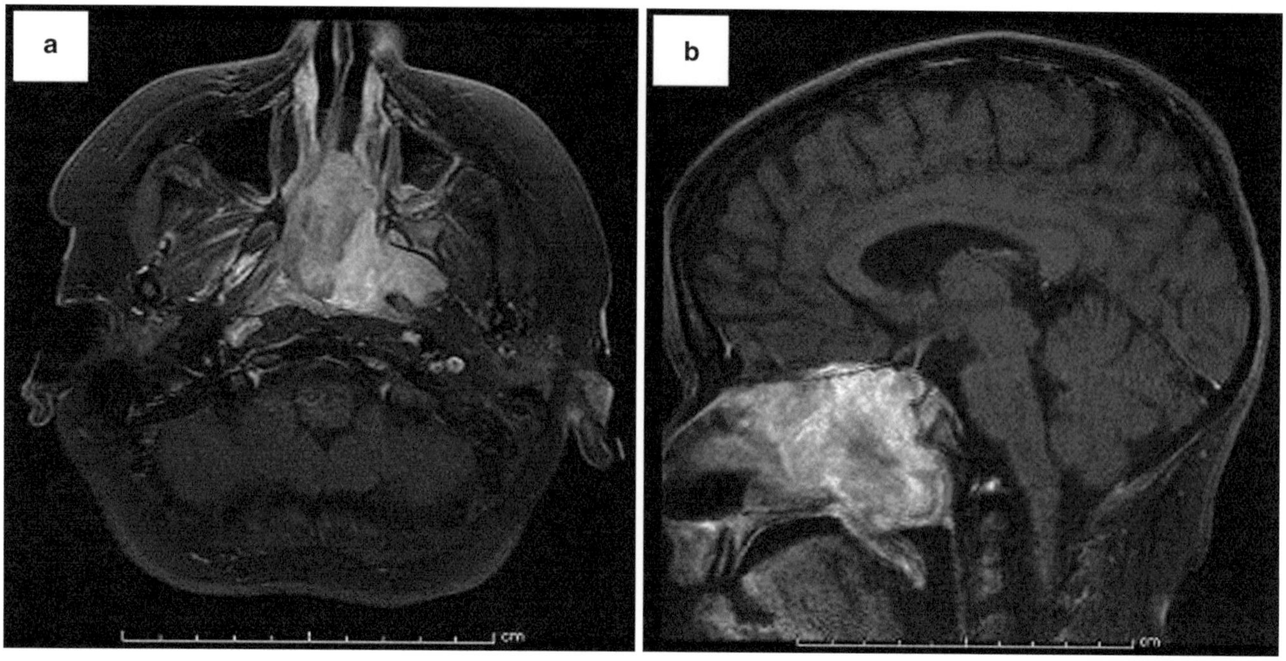

Fig. 42.4 Axial (**a**) and sagittal (**b**) T1 weighted high-resolution MR images of the paranasal sinuses of the patient in Fig. 42.3. A large lobulated relatively well-circumscribed heterogeneously enhancing hypercellular mass lesion is present. This lesion is centered within the nasopharyngeal cavity extending into the *left* inferior orbital fissure, the *left* masticator space and *left* pterygopalatine fossa laterally, to the posterior aspect of the nasal air cavity anteriorly, and extends superiorly with invasion of the anterior skull base at the level of the planum sphenoidale and anterior aspect of the pituitary fossa as well as involving the *left* cavernous sinus with extension superiorly through the left foramen of ovale along V3. Abnormal dural enhancement along the floor of the anterior cranial fossa, *left* middle cranial fossa, and along the dorsal aspect of the dorsum sella and clivus is also present, suggestive of intracranial extension of the mass lesion

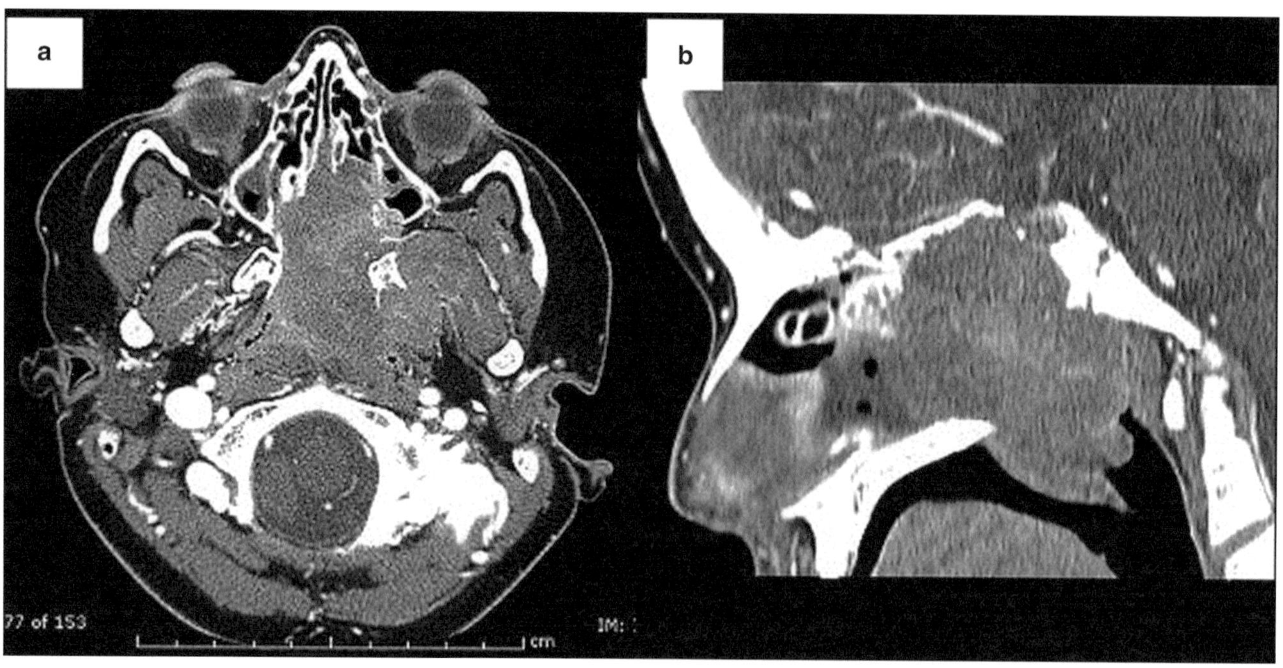

Fig. 42.5 Axial (**a**) and sagittal (**b**) CT images of the paranasal sinuses of a 10-year old male who presented with a 6-week history of increasing *left* nasal obstruction, *left* otalgia, a hyponasal voice and a 6th cranial nerve palsy. A large nasopharyngeal mass extending into the nasal cavity is present. There is complete destruction of the bony nasal septum and also the anterior wall and floor of the sphenoid sinuses. There is also dehiscence of the bony skull base. Intranasal biopsy confirmed an embryonal rhabdomyosarcoma

Table 42.2 Differential diagnosis for RMS

Oncologic	Benign
1. Non-Hodgkin's Lymphoma	Hemangioma/ Lymphangioma
2. Nasopharyngeal carcinoma	Nasal polyp
3. Osteosarcoma	Schwannoma
4. Ewing sarcoma and PNET	Plexiform neurofibroma
5. Juvenile angiofibroma	Giant cell granuloma
6. Neuroblastoma	Parotid tumor
7. Fibro-, chondro-, synovial sarcomas	Ossifying fibroma
8. Lymphadenopathy	Neck cyst
9. Lymphoproliferative disorders, LCH	Vascular malformation
10. Optic nerve glioma	Fibrous dysplasia

Biopsy

- Tissue sampling can occur either via open or needle biopsy. If possible, an open biopsy under anesthesia is preferred. Closed techniques such as fine needle aspiration and tru-cut biopsy are reserved for inaccessible lesions. They obtain smaller volumes of tissue, increase sampling error and inconclusive findings, and often preclude molecular studies [36]. Endoscopic techniques play an important role in exploring and biopsying sinonasal and nasopharyngeal tumors. A frozen section should be obtained at the time of open biopsy to ensure that the specimen is adequate. If it is suggestive of RMS, bone marrow aspiration for cytogenetic analysis can be performed under the same anesthesia.
- In the Children's Oncology Group protocols for RMS, lymph nodes >15 mm in short axis when assessed by CT scan (slice thickness less than 5 mm) or > 10 mm when palpated clinically, are considered concerning for malignancy. Imaging literature cites that a hypoechoic, rounded lymph node with obliteration of the fat center is likewise concerning [34]. Sampling of concerning lymph nodes by upfront neck dissection is recommended [37].

Stabilization

- In most cases, children presenting with head and neck RMS are stable. For patients with orbital RMS who are experiencing vision decline, immediate initiation of chemotherapy is recommended. Steroids to diminish inflammation and topical agents for proptosis are indicated to preserve vision.

Differential Diagnosis

The differential diagnosis of head and neck RMS includes both benign and malignant conditions. The greatest diagnostic challenge in RMS is the distinction from other poorly differentiated small round bluecell tumors (Table 42.2).

Additional Workup/Staging

Laboratory Data

- Complete blood count with differential, liver function tests, electrolytes.
- May consider LDH, ESR/CRP if considering other etiologies on the differential diagnosis.
- Lumbar puncture should be performed for children with orbital or parameningeal tumors with skull base erosion or intracranial extension.
- Bilateral bone marrow aspirates and biopsies.

Imaging Evaluation

- In addition to imaging of the primary site of disease, diagnostic biopsy, and nodal assessment (as above), a metastatic work-up should be performed as follows:
  - CT scan of the chest: recommended to assess for pulmonary nodules. This modality is limited by its inability to distinguish benign from malignant lesions [38].
  - Nuclear medicine bone scan: recommended in European and Children's Oncology Group protocols, however debate exists as to its yield for osteolytic lesions [39].
  - Positron Emission Tomography (PET): has been shown to be of equal accuracy in staging the primary tumor, regional lymph nodes and bony metastases [40, 41]. Distant metastases and lymph node metastases have been reported to be superiorly detected by PET/CT over conventional imaging studies [42]. The use of PET in pediatric patients with head and neck RMS is not yet routine, but will likely approach the standard of care.

In order to discuss treatment of head and neck RMS, we must first discuss staging and grouping classifications. The current staging system for treatment protocols was developed by the Soft Tissue Sarcoma Committee of the Children's Oncology Group (COG-STS) [43].

Staging

Staging is based on the site and size of the tumor and the presence or absence of metastases (Table 42.3). Most tumors of the head and neck present as stage III disease. The 3-year failure-free survival (FFS) rates are reported as 86, 80, 68, and 25% for Stages I, II, III, and IV in IRS-IV, respectively [43].

Tumor:

T1—confined to anatomic site of origin

T2—extension and/or fixation to surrounding tissues

a. ≤5 cm in diameter

b. >5 cm in diameter

Table 42.3 Disease staging dependent on tumor site, size, and the presence or absence of metastases

Stage	Sites	T	Size	N	M
I	Orbit, head and neck (excluding parameningeal)	T1 or T2	a or b	N0 or N1 or Nx	M0
II	Parameningeal	T1 or T2	a	N0 or Nx	M0
III	Parameningeal	T1 or T2	a	N1	M0
			b	N0 or N1 or Nx	M0
IV	All	T1 or T2	a or b	N0 or N1	M1

Regional Nodes:

N0—regional nodes not clinically involved

N1—regional nodes clinically involved by neoplasm

Nx—clinical status of regional nodes unknown

Metastases:

M0—No distant metastases

M1—metastases present

Grouping

Grouping is based on tumor status postsurgical resection, including assessment of the tumor margins (Table 42.4).

Caveats

Tumors arising in the orbit but invading the bony wall into the sinuses should be considered parameningeal.

Tumors arising in the infratemporal fossa and growing through the parotid should still be treated as parameningeal.

Risk Groups

Risk groups are determined by stage, surgical grouping, and histology (Table 42.5). Low-risk, intermediate-risk, and high-risk patients have a reported 3-year FFS rate of 88, 55–75, and <30 % respectively [43].

Treatment

Two important considerations must be taken into account before commencing treatment:

- Expected cure rate with the specific treatment approach.
- Acute and long-term toxicities associated with the treatment type.

Table 42.4 Disease grouping dependent upon extent of surgical resection

Group I	Localized disease, completely resected
	Confined to muscle/organ or origin
	Contiguous involvement-infiltration outside the muscle or organ of origin, as through fascial planes
Group II	Total gross resection with evidence of regional spread
	Microscopic residual disease
	Regional disease with involved nodes, completely resected with no microscopic residual
	Regional disease with involved nodes, grossly resected, but with evidence of microscopic residual and/or histologic involvement of the most distal regional node (from the primary site) in the dissection
Group III	Incomplete resection with gross residual disease
	After biopsy only
	After gross major resection of the primary (>50 %)
Group IV	Distant metastatic disease present at onset
	Lung, liver, bones, bone marrow, brain, distant muscle/nodes
	The presence of positive cytology in CSF, pleural or abdominal fluid, as well as implants on pleural or peritoneal surfaces

Table 42.5 Disease risk grouping dependent upon histology, stage, and surgical group

COG-STS risk group classification			
Risk group	Histology	Stage	Group
Low (35 %)[a]	Embryonal	I	I, II, III
	Embryonal	II, III	II, III
Intermediate (50 %)	Embryonal	II, III	III, IV[b]
	Alveolar	I, II, III	I, II, III
High (15 %)	Embryonal or alveolar	IV	IV[c]

[a] Two subsets of low risk: Subset 1 (lowest risk): Stage 1 or 2, Group I, II OR Stage 1, Group III (orbit only). Subset 2: Stage I, Group III OR Stage 3, Group I, II

[b] Intermediate risk includes: metastatic embryonal RMS <10 years of age

[c] High risk includes: metastatic embryonal RMS >10 years of age

Multidisciplinary Approach

Treatment should be coordinated by a multidisciplinary pediatric oncology team comprised of medical and radiation oncologists, head and neck surgeons, plastic surgeons, and neurosurgeons, in addition to a nutritionist, psychologist, and physiotherapist.

Treatment of RMS has evolved systematically through clinical trials. Commonly, children with RMS are treated within interdisciplinary study protocols: the IRSG (North America), SIOP (Europe), CWS (Germany) and ICS protocols (Italy). Current treatment for RMS relies on chemotherapy, with surgery and radiation as adjunct therapies. Treatment should focus on achieving both local control and eradication of metastases, without compromising functional or cosmetic outcome. Effective risk-adapted multimodality therapy has improved the prognosis for RMS patients. Current survival rates have increased from approximately 25% in the 1970s to over 70% in non-metastatic disease.

Chemotherapy

Chemotherapy is the backbone of treatment for RMS regardless of resectability, as all patients are presumed to have micrometastases at the time of diagnosis. Data from the IRS group shows remarkable improvement in progression-free and overall survival with the use of multi-agent chemotherapy [44, 45].

A combination of vincristine, actinomycin D, and cyclophosphamide (VAC) or ifosfamide (VAI) has been the gold standard for combination chemotherapy in the United States and Europe. Actinomycin D potentiates the action of radiation therapy. Consecutive large randomized trials have allowed for modifications of this combination, tailored to specific subgroups, according to clinical group and site of disease. For patients with low risk disease, outcomes are excellent (survival rates in excess of 90%) with standard VAC therapy. A subset of these patients (subset 1, including all localized orbital tumors of embryonal histology) can be treated without alkylators [46]. For patients of the intermediate-risk category, where the majority of head and neck primaries fall, treatment requires aggressive alkylator therapy, with either VAC or VAI [47]. In conjunction with radiation therapy, survival rates for this group of patients approach 60–70% [48]. Patients with metastatic disease have a poor prognosis, and a more intensive treatment is required. However, outcomes for children < 10 years of age with tumors of embryonal histology may be closer to the intermediate-risk category [49].

Surgical Therapy

- There has been critical discussion in the literature concerning the role of surgery as a primary treatment modality [50]. Because 50% of failures occur at the primary tumor site, there has been renewed interest in surgical excision as the primary mode of control. In addition, avoidance of complications such as arrest in facial growth and development of secondary malignancies following radiation therapy has become a consideration in the management of these patients.
- Approximately 10% of newly diagnosed patients have tumors that can be completely removed [44, 45].
- Tumors in non-parameningeal regions are more amenable to complete surgical excision; such locations include the ear, zygoma, soft palate, tongue, and supraglottic larynx.
- Parameningeal tumors present a surgical challenge; complete resection is not feasible in most patients, and even if possible, is unlikely to be achieved without major functional or cosmetic consequences.
- In selected cases, newer surgical approaches including craniofacial and skull base surgery, microvascular techniques, and nerve grafting procedures, allow surgery to be considered for eradicating both the primary tumor and residual disease. A combined intracranial/extracranial approach with en-bloc tumor removal is sometimes possible (Figs. 42.6, 42.7). If margins are narrow, biopsy specimens from the surrounding tissue are obtained to assess for residual local disease. Immediate reconstruction with free tissue transfer using microvascular techniques is useful to minimize functional and cosmetic deformities. The infratemporal approach for lateral skull base lesions allows surgical control of major neurovascular structures. It also permits removal of the contents of the infratemporal fossa and resection of the skull base, meninges, and if necessary, brain (Fig. 42.7).
- Complete surgical resection with negative margins offers the best chance of survival and can preclude use of radiotherapy [51–54]. However, primary surgery of head and neck RMS is discouraged if it leads to unacceptable morbidity.
- As with RMS primaries of other sites, there is no role for distant metastatectomy in head and neck RMS [55].

Radiation Therapy

A review of the COG literature for pediatric patients with rhabdomyosarcoma and microscopic residual disease indicates that failure to comply with radiation guidelines is associated with a high risk of local-regional disease recurrence [56]. Radiation therapy is an essential part of all treatment protocols except for low risk tumors that are completely resected.

Intermediate-Risk Patients (Per COG ARST0531)

- Group I, alveolar (stage 1–3): complete excision with negative margins, week 1–3 chemotherapy, radiotherapy at week 4:3,600 cGy [57]
- Group II, alveolar (stage 1–3): complete excision with positive margins and/or regional nodal disease prior to chemotherapy, week 1–3 chemotherapy, radiotherapy at week 4: node negative (3,600 cGy), node positive (4,140 cGy)
- Group III embryonal (stage 1 or 2) or alveolar (stage 1–3): incomplete excision prior to chemotherapy, week 1–3 chemotherapy, radiotherapy at week 4: orbital (4,500 cGy), non-orbital (5,040 cGy)

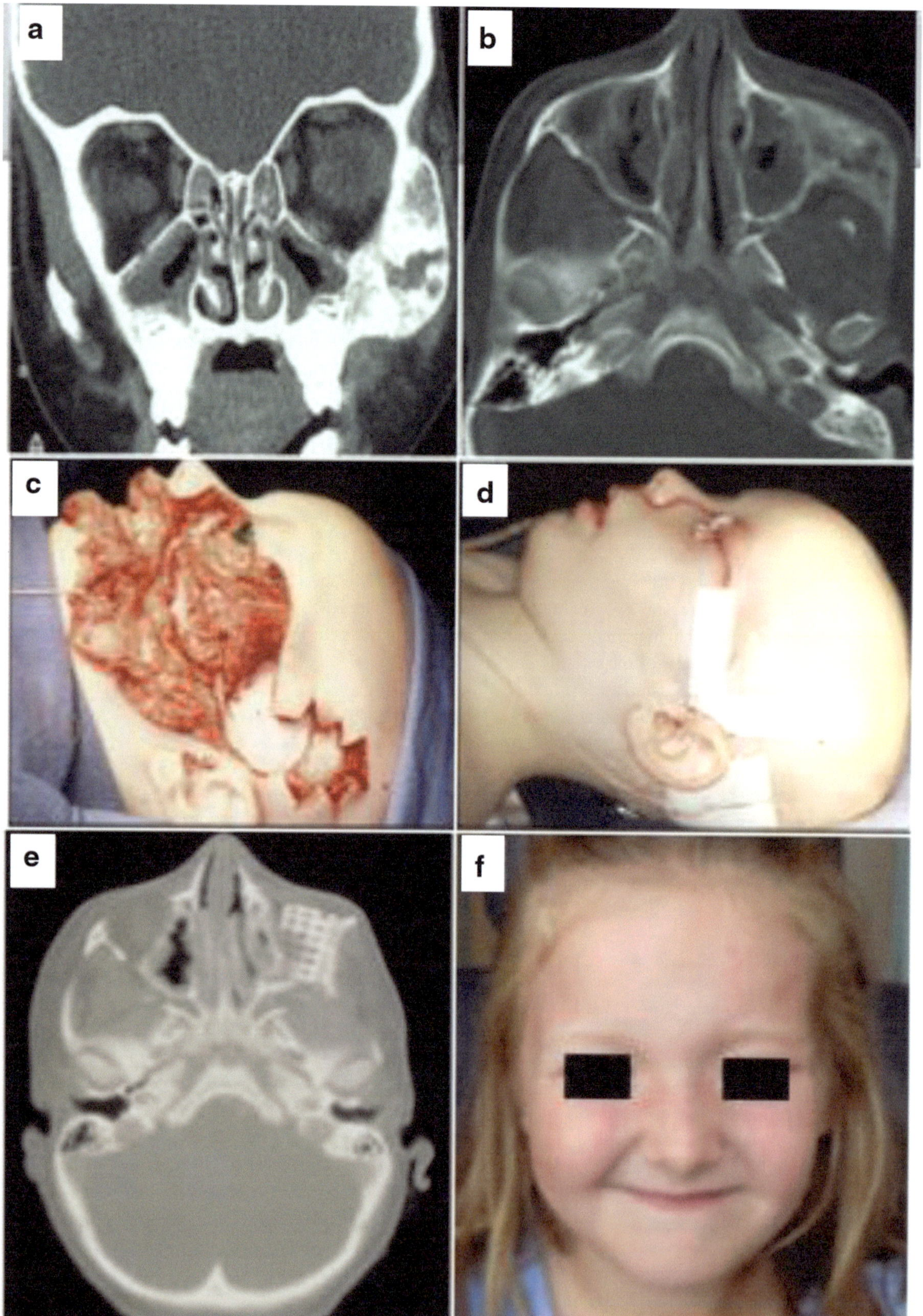

Fig. 42.6 Axial (**a**) and sagittal (**b**) CT images of the paranasal sinuses of a 4-year-old female who is status-post chemotherapy for an embryonal rhabdomyosarcoma of the *left* maxilla and lateral wall of the *left* orbit. Using a modified Weber–Ferguson incision, the tumor was removed en-bloc with preservation of the *left* facial nerve (**c**). The closed incision at the end of the procedure is shown in (**d**). Bone and temporalis muscle was used to reconstruct the defect, and titanium plates were used to reconstruct the lateral orbital wall. The orbital floor plates are seen on an axial CT scan 1-year later (**e**). The patient is shown 1-year postoperatively in (**f**). Facial nerve movement is nearly symmetric bilaterally

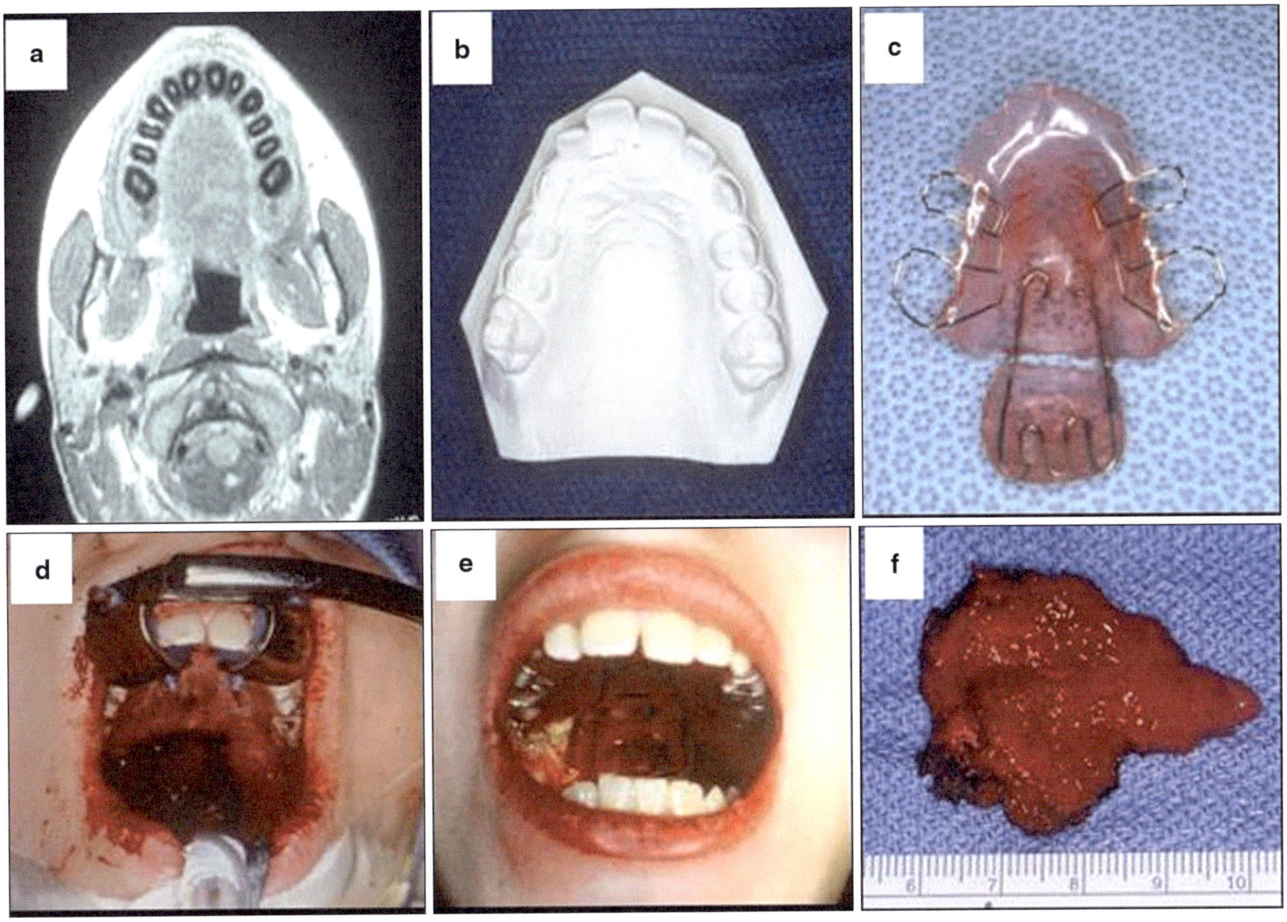

Fig. 42.7 Axial CT image (**a**) of a 14-year old with an alveolar rhabdomyosarcoma of her soft palate. An obturator prosthesis was made for the defect following surgery. The prosthesis mold was taken preoperatively (**b**). The obturator plate is seen in (**c**). A partial maxillectomy, including removal of the soft palate was performed. Intraoperative images are shown—the plate defect is seen in (**d**) and the obturator prosthesis is in situ in (**e**). The resected specimen was 4 × 3 cm in size (**f**)

Low Risk Patients (Per COG ARST0331)

- Orbital (stage 1): Chemotherapy is given for 13 weeks. Radiotherapy is given post-operatively in the following scenarios:
  - Group II: nodes not involved—3,600 cGy
    - nodes involved—4,140 cGy
  - Group III: any nodal status—4,500 cGy
- Non-orbital, Non-parameningeal: Chemotherapy is given for 13 weeks, radiation is then given at the following doses:
  - Group II: nodes not involved (3,600 cGy), nodes involved (4,140 cGy)
  - Group III: superficial site, nodes not involved, candidate for complete resection

Post-surgical resection:

  - Completely resected: nodes not involved (3,600 cGy)
  - Microscopic residual: nodes not nodes not involved (3,600 cGy), nodes involved (4,140 cGy)
  - Gross residual: any nodal status (5,040 cGy)

- Parameningeal, Non-orbital: Chemotherapy is given for 13 weeks. Radiation is then given for the following scenarios:
  - Stage 2, Group II: 3,600 cGy
  - Stage 3, Group II: nodes not involved (3,600 cGy), nodes involved (4,140 cGy)

Data reviewed from the Intergroup Rhabdomyosarcoma Study for Groups II through IV suggests that for children with evidence of meningeal impingement, earlier start to radiation therapy (within 2 weeks) is associated with lower rates of local failure [58].

Hyper-fractionated accelerated radiotherapy (HART) and intensity-modulated radiotherapy (IMRT) are two modalities of radiation that can deliver high doses of radiation to a defined target volume while sparing surrounding organs at risk. These techniques, along with proton beam radiotherapy, are being used with increasing frequency for pediatric patients with head and neck RMS [59, 60].

Table 42.6 Unfavorable prognostic factors in pediatric patients with rhabdomyosarcoma

1. Age > 10 years and < 1 year at diagnosis
2. Alveolar subtype
3. Parameningeal site
4. Direct intracranial tumor extension
5. Large tumor size (> 5 cm)
6. Skull base erosion
7. Cranial nerve palsy

Complications

Facial growth, neuroendocrine dysfunction, visual/orbital problems, dental abnormalities, asymmetry of the tissues at the primary tumor site, hypothyroidism, secondary malignancy, and intellectual and academic delays are all found to be associated with receipt of head and neck radiotherapy. Hearing abnormalities have been more frequently attributed to tumor location or cisplatin therapy than radiotherapy [61, 62].

Prognosis

- The treatment outcome for pediatric RMS depends on anatomic site, patient age, stage, and histology (the basis for risk stratification).
- Unfavorable prognostic factors include older age, metastatic disease, large tumor, alveolar histology, and parameningeal location [63]. (Table 42.6)
- Low-risk, intermediate-risk and high-risk patients have a 3-year failure free survival rate of 88, 55–75, and <30% respectively.
- The most unfavorable prognostic factor appears to be the presence of distant metastases at diagnosis: even with aggressive treatment, patients with metastases have only a 20% chance of long-term survival [9].

Recurrence

- Up to one-third of patients experience a local or metastatic recurrence yielding poor survival despite aggressive therapy; 50–95% of these patients die of progressive disease despite surgery and radiotherapy.
- Raney et al. reported that complete excision of the recurrent tumor was associated with better outcome [64]. Patients who underwent surgery had a better outcome (5 year survival of 54% vs. 24.7% in the non-surgical group), and it was observed that the overall survival increased to 61.4% for patients that also received radiotherapy [65].

Follow-up

Frequency of office visits

- Imaging studies should be performed no sooner than 6 weeks post-treatment to avoid confusion between residual disease and post-treatment changes. Enhancement of the tumor bed that remains stable for at least 3 months after treatment is suspicious for residual tumor.
- After completion of therapy, office visits with laboratory work (CBC, chemistry) should be performed q3 months × 1 year, q4 months for years 2–3, q6 months for year 4, and annually thereafter.

Frequency of imaging

- At each of the above-mentioned clinical visits, chest x-ray (CXR) should be performed along with imaging of the primary site of disease (preferably with MRI).

References

1. Pappo AS, Shapiro DN, Crist WM, Maurer HM. Biology and therapy of pediatric rhabdomyosarcoma. J Clin Oncol. 1995;13:2123–39.
2. Simon JH, Paulino AC, Smith RB, Buatti JM. Prognostic factors in head and neck rhabdomyosarcoma. Head Neck. 2002;24:468–73.
3. Horn RC Jr, Enterline HT. Rhabdomyosarcoma: a clinicopathological study and classification of 39 cases. Cancer. 1958;11:181–99.
4. Newton WA Jr, Soule EH, Hamoudi AB, et al. Histopathology of childhood sarcomas, intergroup rhabdomyosarcoma studies I and II: clinicopathologic correlation. J Clin Oncol. 1988;6:67–75.
5. Agamanolis DP, Dasu S, Krill CE Jr. Tumors of skeletal muscle. Hum Pathol. 1986;17:778–95.
6. Gurney JG, Young JL Jr, Roffers SD, Smith MA, Bunin GR. Soft tissue sarcomas SEER data pediatrics. National Cancer Institute; 1975–1995; 111–124.
7. Tsokos M, Webber BL, Parham DM, et al. Rhabdomyosarcoma. A new classification scheme related to prognosis. Arch Pathol Lab Med. 1992;116:847–55.
8. Kodet R, Newton WA Jr, Hamoudi AB, Asmar L, Jacobs DL, Maurer HM. Childhood rhabdomyosarcoma with anaplastic (pleomorphic) features. A report of the intergroup rhabdomyosarcoma study. Am J Surg Pathol. 1993;17:443–53.
9. Turner JH, Richmon JD. Head and neck rhabdomyosarcoma: a critical analysis of population-based incidence and survival data. Otolaryngol Head Neck Surg. 2011;145:967–73.
10. Dias P, Parham DM, Shapiro DN, Webber BL, Houghton PJ. Myogenic regulatory protein (MyoD1) expression in childhood solid tumors: diagnostic utility in rhabdomyosarcoma. Am J Pathol. 1990;137:1283–91.
11. Parham DM, Webber B, Holt H, Williams WK, Maurer H. Immunohistochemical study of childhood rhabdomyosarcomas 2 related neoplasms. Results of an intergroup rhabdomyosarcoma study project. Cancer. 1991;67:3072–80.
12. Barr FG. Molecular genetics and pathogenesis of rhabdomyosarcoma. J Pediatr Hematol Oncol. 1997;19:483–91.
13. Shapiro DN, Parham DM, Douglass EC, et al. Relationship of tumor-cell ploidy to histologic subtype and treatment outcome in

children and adolescents with unresectable rhabdomyosarcoma. J Clin Oncol. 1991;9:159–66.

14. San Miguel-Fraile P, Carrillo-Gijon R, Rodriguez-Peralto JL, Badiola IA. Prognostic significance of DNA ploidy and proliferative index (MIB-1 index) in childhood rhabdomyosarcoma. Am J Clin Pathol. 2004;121:358–65.
15. Kilpatrick SE, Teot LA, Geisinger KR, et al. Relationship of DNA ploidy to histology and prognosis in rhabdomyosarcoma. Comparison of flow cytometry and image analysis. Cancer. 1994;74:3227–33.
16. Goulding MD, Chalepakis G, Deutsch U, Erselius JR, Gruss P. Pax-3, a novel murine DNA binding protein expressed during early neurogenesis. EMBO J. 1991;10:1135–47.
17. Sorensen PH, Lynch JC, Qualman SJ, et al. PAX3-FKHR and PAX7-FKHR gene fusions are prognostic indicators in alveolar rhabdomyosarcoma: a report from the children's oncology group. J Clin Oncol. 2002;20:2672–9.
18. Barr FG, Galili N, Holick J, Biegel JA, Rovera G, Emanuel BS. Rearrangement of the PAX3 paired box gene in the paediatric solid tumour alveolar rhabdomyosarcoma. Nat Genet. 1993;3:113–7.
19. Felix CA, Kappel CC, Mitsudomi T, et al. Frequency and diversity of p53 mutations in childhood rhabdomyosarcoma. Cancer Res. 1992;52:2243–7.
20. Taylor AC, Shu L, Danks MK, et al. P53 mutation and MDM2 amplification frequency in pediatric rhabdomyosarcoma tumors and cell lines. Med Pediatr Oncol. 2000;35:96–103.
21. Qualman SJ, Coffin CM, Newton WA, et al. Intergroup rhabdomyosarcoma study: update for pathologists. Pediatr Dev Pathol. 1998;1:550–61.
22. Parham DM. Pathologic classification of rhabdomyosarcomas and correlations with molecular studies. Mod Pathol. 2001;14:506–14.
23. Hicks J, Flaitz C. Rhabdomyosarcoma of the head and neck in children. Oral Oncol. 2002;38:450–9.
24. Grufferman S, Wang HH, DeLong ER, Kimm SY, Delzell ES, Falletta JM. Environmental factors in the etiology of rhabdomyosarcoma in childhood. J Natl Cancer Inst. 1982;68:107–13.
25. Hartley AL, Birch JM, McKinney PA, et al. The inter-regional epidemiological study of childhood cancer (IRESCC): case control study of children with bone and soft tissue sarcomas. Br J Cancer. 1988;58:838–42.
26. Grufferman S, Schwartz AG, Ruymann FB, Maurer HM. Parents' use of cocaine and marijuana and increased risk of rhabdomyosarcoma in their children. Cancer Causes Control. 1993;4:217–24.
27. Ruymann FB, Maddux HR, Ragab A, et al. Congenital anomalies associated with rhabdomyosarcoma: an autopsy study of 115 cases. A report from the Intergroup Rhabdomyosarcoma Study Committee (representing the Children's Cancer Study Group, the Pediatric Oncology Group, the United Kingdom Children's Cancer Study Group, and the Pediatric Intergroup Statistical Center). Med Pediatr Oncol. 1988;16:33–9.
28. Yang P, Grufferman S, Khoury MJ, et al. Association of childhood rhabdomyosarcoma with neurofibromatosis type I and birth defects. Genet Epidemiol. 1995;12:467–74.
29. Gandhi PD, Fleming JC, Haik BG, Wilson MW. Ophthalmic complications following treatment of paranasal sinus rhabdomyosarcoma in comparison to orbital disease. Ophthal Plast Reconstr Surg. 2011;27:241–6.
30. Dehner LP, Chen KT. Primary tumors of the external and middle ear. III. A clinicopathologic study of embryonal rhabdomyosarcoma. Arch Otolaryngol. 1978;104:399–403.
31. Wiatrak BJ, Pensak ML. Rhabdomyosarcoma of the ear and temporal bone. Laryngoscope. 1989;99:1188–92.
32. Zorzi AP, Grant R, Gupta AA, Hodgson DC, Nathan PC. Cranial nerve palsies in childhood parameningeal rhabdomyosarcoma. Pediatr Blood Cancer. 2012;59:1211–4.
33. Bisogno G, Compostella A, Ferrari A, et al. Rhabdomyosarcoma in adolescents: a report from the AIEOP Soft Tissue Sarcoma Committee. Cancer. 2012;118:821–7.
34. Freling NJ, Merks JH, Saeed P, et al. Imaging findings in craniofacial childhood rhabdomyosarcoma. Pediatr Radiol. 2010;40:1723–38; quiz 855.
35. Scotti G, Harwood-Nash DC. Computed tomography of rhabdomyosarcomas of the skull base in children. J Comput Assist Tomogr. 1982;6:33–9.
36. Bisogno G, De Rossi C, Gamboa Y, et al. Improved survival for children with parameningeal rhabdomyosarcoma: results from the AIEOP soft tissue sarcoma committee. Pediatr Blood Cancer. 2008;50:1154–8.
37. Newman AN, Rice DH. Rhabdomyosarcoma of the head and neck. Laryngoscope. 1984;94:234–9.
38. Van Rijn RR, Wilde JC, Bras J, Oldenburger F, McHugh KM, Merks JH. Imaging findings in noncraniofacial childhood rhabdomyosarcoma. Pediatr Radiol. 2008;38:617–34.
39. Daldrup-Link HE, Franzius C, Link TM, et al. Whole-body MR imaging for detection of bone metastases in children and young adults: comparison with skeletal scintigraphy and FDG PET. AJR Am J Roentgenol. 2001;177:229–36.
40. Tateishi U, Hosono A, Makimoto A, et al. Comparative study of FDG PET/CT and conventional imaging in the staging of rhabdomyosarcoma. Ann Nucl Med. 2009;23:155–61.
41. Klem ML, Grewal RK, Wexler LH, Schoder H, Meyers PA, Wolden SL. PET for staging in rhabdomyosarcoma: an evaluation of PET as an adjunct to current staging tools. J Pediatr Hematol Oncol. 2007;29:9–14.
42. Volker T, Denecke T, Steffen I, et al. Positron emission tomography for staging of pediatric sarcoma patients: results of a prospective multicenter trial. J Clin Oncol. 2007;25:5435–41.
43. Breneman JC, Lyden E, Pappo AS, et al. Prognostic factors and clinical outcomes in children and adolescents with metastatic rhabdomyosarcoma—a report from the Intergroup Rhabdomyosarcoma Study IV. J Clin Oncol. 2003;21:78–84.
44. Crist W, Gehan EA, Ragab AH, et al. The third intergroup Rhabdomyosarcoma Study. J Clin Oncol. 1995;13:610–30.
45. Crist WM, Anderson JR, Meza JL, et al. Intergroup rhabdomyosarcoma study-IV: results for patients with nonmetastatic disease. J Clin Oncol. 2001;19:3091–102.
46. Raney RB, Walterhouse DO, Meza JL, et al. Results of the Intergroup Rhabdomyosarcoma Study Group D9602 protocol, using vincristine and dactinomycin with or without cyclophosphamide and radiation therapy, for newly diagnosed patients with low-risk embryonal rhabdomyosarcoma: a report from the Soft Tissue Sarcoma Committee of the Children's Oncology Group. J Clin Oncol. 2011;29:1312–8.
47. Spunt SL, Smith LM, Ruymann FB, et al. Cyclophosphamide dose intensification during induction therapy for intermediate-risk pediatric rhabdomyosarcoma is feasible but does not improve outcome: a report from the soft tissue sarcoma committee of the children's oncology group. Clin Cancer Res. 2004;10:6072–9.
48. Arndt CA, Stoner JA, Hawkins DS, et al. Vincristine, actinomycin, and cyclophosphamide compared with vincristine, actinomycin, and cyclophosphamide alternating with vincristine, topotecan, and cyclophosphamide for intermediate-risk rhabdomyosarcoma: children's oncology group study D9803. J Clin Oncol. 2009;27:5182–8.
49. Weigel BLE, Anderson JR, Galster A, Arndt CA, Michalski J, Hawkins DS, Meyer WH. Early results from Children's Oncology Group (COG) ARST0431: Intensive multidrug therapy for patients with metastatic rhabdomyosarcoma (RMS). J Clin Oncol. 2010. ASCO Annual Meeting Proceedings (Post-Meeting Edition).

50. Gradoni P, Giordano D, Oretti G, Fantoni M, Ferri T. The role of surgery in children with head and neck rhabdomyosarcoma and Ewing's sarcoma. Surg Oncol. 2010;19:e103–9.
51. Daya H, Chan HS, Sirkin W, Forte V. Pediatric rhabdomyosarcoma of the head and neck: is there a place for surgical management? Arch Otolaryngol Head Neck Surg. 2000;126:468–72.
52. Maurer HM, Gehan EA, Beltangady M, et al. The Intergroup Rhabdomyosarcoma Study-II. Cancer. 1993;71:1904–22.
53. Wharam MD, Beltangady MS, Heyn RM, et al. Pediatric orofacial and laryngopharyngeal rhabdomyosarcoma. An Intergroup Rhabdomyosarcoma Study report. Arch Otolaryngol Head Neck Surg. 1987;113:1225–7.
54. Stevens MC. Treatment for childhood rhabdomyosarcoma: the cost of cure. Lancet Oncol. 2005;6:77–84.
55. Temeck BK, Wexler LH, Steinberg SM, McClure LL, Horowitz M, Pass HI. Metastasectomy for sarcomatous pediatric histologies: results and prognostic factors. Ann Thorac Surg. 1995;59:1385–9; discussion 90.
56. Million L, Anderson J, Breneman J, et al. Influence of noncompliance with radiation therapy protocol guidelines and operative bed recurrences for children with rhabdomyosarcoma and microscopic residual disease: a report from the Children's Oncology Group. Int J Radiat Oncol Biol Phys. 2011;80:333–8.
57. Breneman J, Meza J, Donaldson SS, et al. Local control with reduced-dose radiotherapy for low-risk rhabdomyosarcoma: a report from the Children's Oncology Group D9602 study. Int J Radiat Oncol Biol Phys. 2012;83:720–6.
58. Michalski JM, Meza J, Breneman JC, et al. Influence of radiation therapy parameters on outcome in children treated with radiation therapy for localized parameningeal rhabdomyosarcoma in Intergroup Rhabdomyosarcoma Study Group trials II through IV. Int J Radiat Oncol Biol Phys. 2004;59:1027–38.
59. Curtis AE, Okcu MF, Chintagumpala M, Teh BS, Paulino AC. Local control after intensity-modulated radiotherapy for head-and-neck rhabdomyosarcoma. Int J Radiat Oncol Biol Phys. 2009;73:173–7.
60. Yock T, Schneider R, Friedmann A, Adams J, Fullerton B, Tarbell N. Proton radiotherapy for orbital rhabdomyosarcoma: clinical outcome and a dosimetric comparison with photons. Int J Radiat Oncol Biol Phys. 2005;63:1161–8.
61. Paulino AC, Simon JH, Zhen W, Wen BC. Long-term effects in children treated with radiotherapy for head and neck rhabdomyosarcoma. Int J Radiat Oncol Biol Phys. 2000;48:1489–95.
62. Raney RB, Asmar L, Vassilopoulou-Sellin R, et al. Late complications of therapy in 213 children with localized, nonorbital soft-tissue sarcoma of the head and neck: A descriptive report from the Intergroup Rhabdomyosarcoma Studies (IRS)-II and—III. IRS Group of the Children's Cancer Group and the Pediatric Oncology Group. Med Pediatr Oncol. 1999;33:362–71.
63. Mazzoleni S, Bisogno G, Garaventa A, et al. Outcomes and prognostic factors after recurrence in children and adolescents with nonmetastatic rhabdomyosarcoma. Cancer. 2005;104:183–90.
64. Raney RB Jr, Crist WM, Maurer HM, Foulkes MA. Prognosis of children with soft tissue sarcoma who relapse after achieving a complete response. A report from the Intergroup Rhabdomyosarcoma Study I. Cancer. 1983;52:44–50.
65. Klingebiel T, Pertl U, Hess CF, et al. Treatment of children with relapsed soft tissue sarcoma: report of the German CESS/CWS REZ 91 trial. Med Pediatr Oncol. 1998;30:269–75.

Thyroglossal Duct Cysts

43

Joel W. Jones and Dwight T. Jones

Introduction

Thyroglossal duct cysts (TGDC) do not present to the otolaryngologist every day, but they are abnormalities that most busy practitioners will see two to six times a year. After lymph nodes, they are the most common neck mass in children [1]. Their workup and proper management are important since they can enlarge and be unsightly, become chronically infected, and rarely degenerate to carcinoma. Other midline neck masses can present as TGDC anomalies, thus, mandating proper evaluation for all neck masses in children.

Biology and Epidemiology

The embryology of the thyroid gland is crucial for understanding the pathology of thyroglossal lesions, their clinical presentation, and the rationale for surgical treatment. During the 4th week of life, the thyroid gland begins as a cluster of cells in the base of the developing tongue [2]. The thyroid's origin is located at the midpoint of the region where the anterior ectodermal and posterior endodermal structures of the tongue meet. In the adult, this marks the location of the foramen cecum. This primitive thyroid tissue becomes a ventral diverticulum and proceeds caudally through the floor of the assembling pharynx and within the mesoderm of the neck until it reaches its final location at the upper tracheal rings. This journey is completed in the 7th week of life. At this time the thyroid tissue is mainly composed of follicular cells, which will produce thyroxin and store colloid. The mature gland has a dual embryological origin. The ultimobranchial body will unite with the thyroid primordium and eventually develop into parafollicular cells that produce calcitonin.

During decent, the thyroid gland remains connected to the tongue by a patent epithelial tract known as the thyroglossal duct. The duct serves as a marker for the thyroid gland's movement. Embryological studies of the tract have revealed that the thyroid gland takes a predictable yet indirect path and has a close relationship with the developing hyoid bone [3]. The tract initially courses ventral to the developing hyoid bone, but its path is altered as the hyoid assumes its anatomical position. The hyoid pulls the tract underneath and around the inferior surface of its body. The tract then arches back and follows a downward descent ventral to the thyrohyoid membrane and tracheal rings. Multiple abnormalities in thyroid development can occur at any point along this embryological pathway. Small deposits of thyroid tissue may be left behind during the gland's descent. These ectopic rests can enlarge and function as a thyroid nodule. Migration of the gland can also completely arrest anywhere along the tract and result in a functioning ectopic thyroid gland [4].

After decent, the thyroglossal duct will normally detach from the thyroid and atrophy by the 10th week of life [5]. A vestigial portion of the duct at the thyroid's origin will form the foramen cecum. The thyroglossal duct may fail to atrophy at any point along the path of decent and persist as a remnant. The true prevalence of thyroglossal duct remnants is approximately 7%, but only a fraction of these will become symptomatic and require medical treatment [3]. The remnants consist of ductal epithelium and can maintain secretory activity [6, 7]. A thyroglossal duct cyst can form as the opening of the tract becomes blocked and secretory fluid accumulates. The cyst reveals itself as a varying size mass classically in the midline neck. This most commonly occurs anywhere just below the level of the hyoid bone to the normal level of the thyroid gland [5, 8].

D. T. Jones (✉)
Department of Otolaryngology - Head and Neck Surgery,
University of Nebraska College of Medicine, Omaha, NE, USA
e-mail: dwight.jones@unmc.edu

J. W. Jones
Department of Otolaryngology - Head and Neck Surgery,
University of Kansas College of Medicine, Kansas City, KS, USA

R. Rahbar et al. (eds.), *Pediatric Head and Neck Tumors*,
DOI 10.1007/978-1-4614-8755-5_43, © Springer Science+Business Media New York 2014

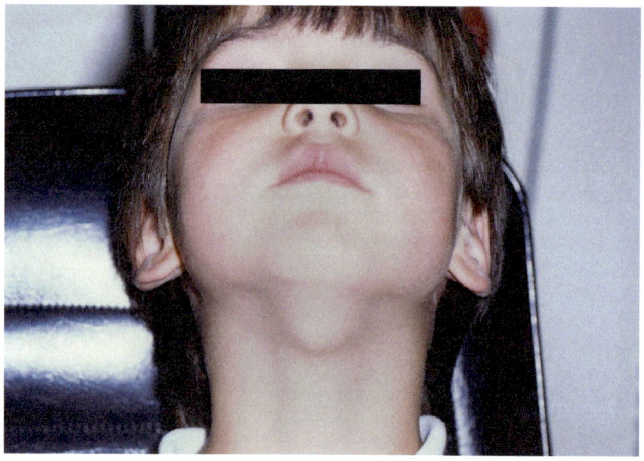

Fig. 43.1 A midline neck mass illustrating the typical presentation and position for a thyroglossal duct cyst

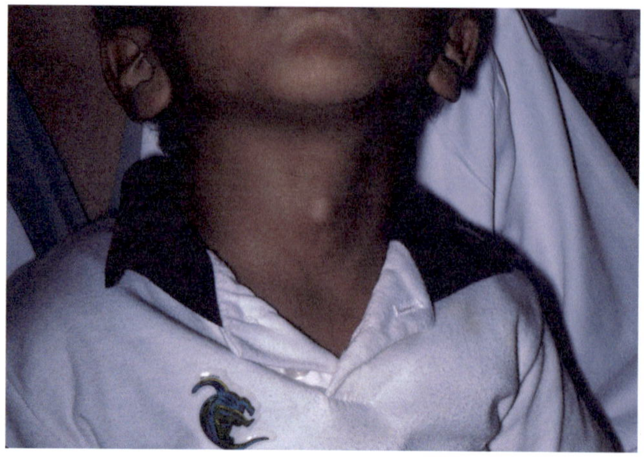

Fig. 43.2 Any midline neck mass should raise suspicion for a thyroglossal duct cyst

After lymph nodes, TGDC are the most common mass in the pediatric neck. They most often present during childhood, usually in the first decade of life and before the age of five [9]. About 35 % of cases will present after 30 years of age [5]. There is minimal gender difference, occurring equally in male and female populations [5, 9]. TGDC occur sporadically within the population and despite reports of occurrence in multiple members of some families, they do not appear to have any genetic pattern of inheritance [10].

Presentation

TGDC classically present in the midline of the neck at or below the level of the hyoid bone and above the thyroid gland (Fig. 43.1). Most patients will present with a firm midline neck mass and no other symptoms. If symptoms are present, they vary depending on the exact location, size of the mass, and age of the patient. Usually there is no pain [8, 11]. Tenderness or redness may occur if the cyst has been inflamed or infected. This usually happens with upper respiratory tract infections. Other symptoms, which are unusual, include: difficulty swallowing, choking, coughing, or globus sensation. Although rare, sudden death from airway compromise has been reported in infants [12].

A TGDC can enlarge several centimeters in size but on presentation they are typically pea size to 2 cm. They are commonly firm but not solid or soft on palpation. They may be freely mobile under the skin and classically elevate on swallowing. TGDC can develop a variety of secondary features. The thyroid's embryological relationship with the tongue makes a cyst susceptible to infection from microbes that enter the tract from the oral cavity. Infection has been reported in up to 50 % of cases [13]. Infected cysts may present as an abscess with inflammation and tenderness. TGDC do not typically communicate with the skin, but infection can lead to the development of a draining fistula [14].

Differential Diagnosis

The majority of neck masses in the pediatric population have a congenital or infectious etiology. Despite being a common cause for a midline neck mass in the child, TGDC have a broad differential diagnosis. Even after proper clinical evaluation, other masses such as lymph nodes and thyroglossal carcinomas have been misdiagnosed as TGDC [9, 15]. The wary physician must always consider the full range of diagnostic possibilities when accessing any neck mass in a child. The most important lesion to distinguish from a TGDC is a median ectopic thyroid gland. Most patients with an ectopic thyroid gland will have their entire functioning tissue located in an aberrant midline location [4]. Removal will result in lifelong hypothyroidism so care must be taken during the evaluation to rule out this possibility.

Dermoid cysts can also be readily mistaken for TGDC [5, 9]. They can present midline in the same locations as a TGDC and may also have the same consistency on palpation. Unlike TGDC, dermoid cysts do not move with swallowing. Other midline considerations include lymph nodes, branchial anomalies, lipomas, lymphatic malformations, and ranulas [5, 9, 16].

Diagnosis and Evaluation

Physical Examination

The classical TGDC is not soft or hard, but is firm and usually midline (Fig. 43.2). A complete head and neck examination should be performed on all patients. The clinician should inspect the base of the tongue and floor of mouth with visual and bimanual palpation. Ranulas and lingual thyroids can often be ruled out in this manner. Next the neck should be palpated on both sides. This is classically done from the rear of the patient using a hand on each side of the neck and systematically checking each neck level, including the midline. In a very young patient, the behind the neck approach may not be feasible. Care should be taken to check for masses in the submandibular spaces and along the jugular digastric chain. Midline masses should be palpated with both hands and the patient should be asked to swallow to see if the mass elevates and descends with deglutition. This finding may be difficult to observe in some pediatric patients. Although not always possible, it is advisable to try and palpate the thyroid gland to determine if it is in its normal location. If the mass is small or changing in size, it may be difficult to locate on the first evaluation. If the mass cannot be located, it is important to have the patient or their guardian/parent show the physician where the area of concern is after the examination is complete. TGDC do not commonly reduce in size or disappear. If this occurs with a suspected TGDC, the diagnosis should be in question. Unless the cyst has been infected and drained spontaneously, there is usually not a fistulous opening to the skin.

Laboratory Data

Most midline neck masses, including TGDC, do not require any laboratory data prior to removal. Most patients will be euthyroid and rarely will the TSH or other thyroid function tests (TFT) show any abnormalities. TFT should be ordered in cases where the presumed TGDC is an ectopic thyroid gland or if the patient appears clinically hypothyroid [9, 16]. In the healthy child without other comorbidities, other laboratory testing will typically be normal and not necessary prior to treatment.

Imaging Evaluation

The presence of a TGDC implies that normal thyroid decent has occurred. The main goal and advantage of any imaging is to document that the thyroid gland is indeed located in its usual location and not ectopic. While many ectopic thyroid glands will eventually require removal, it serves the surgeon well to advise the patient or their guardians of this possibility prior to surgery [14].

In the past many practitioners relied on thyroid scans to document the actual location of the thyroid gland and any ectopic functioning thyroid tissue [17]. Thyroid scans are accurate, but require intravenous access, time, and patience

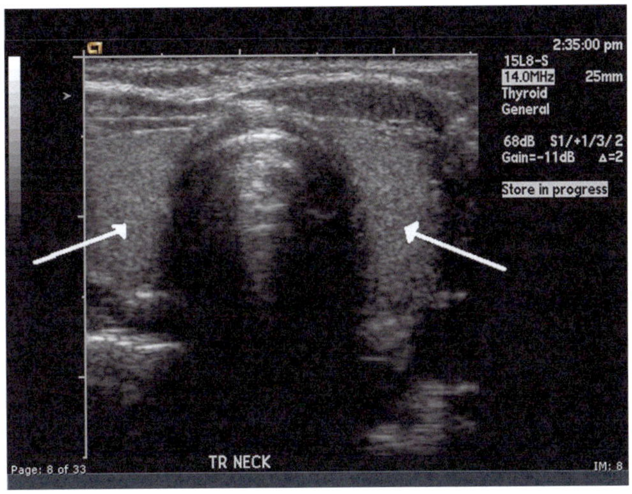

Fig. 43.3 U/S imaging documenting the location of the thyroid gland (*arrows*)

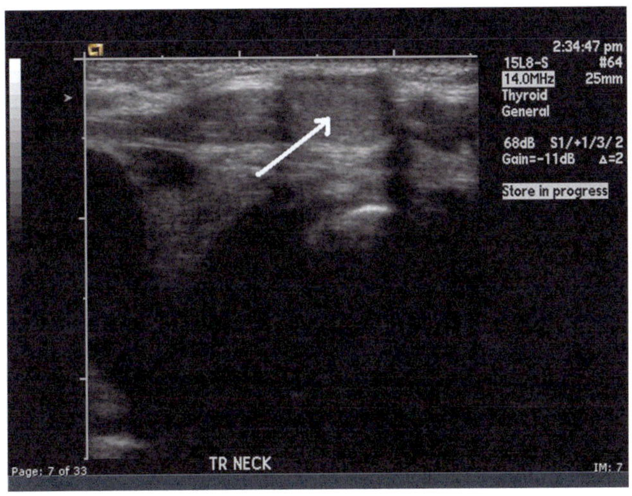

Fig. 43.4 U/S showing the typical location of a thyroglossal duct cyst (*arrow*)

on the part of the patient. They may involve separate evaluations and appointments. Sedation may also be necessary in young children. In recent years, ultrasound (U/S) has replaced thyroid scans in many institutions [8, 14, 18]. U/S has the benefit of documenting the presence of a normal thyroid gland as well as locating the TGDC (Figs. 43.3, 43.4). It is not time consuming and does not expose the patient to radiation. It usually can be scheduled quickly, sometimes on the day of the primary evaluation. Although other midline anomalies can be discerned with U/S, at times it can be misleading. For example, in young infants a large thymus gland can protrude up into the neck and masquerade as a normal thyroid gland on U/S. The senior author has had this occur twice in 25 years of practice.

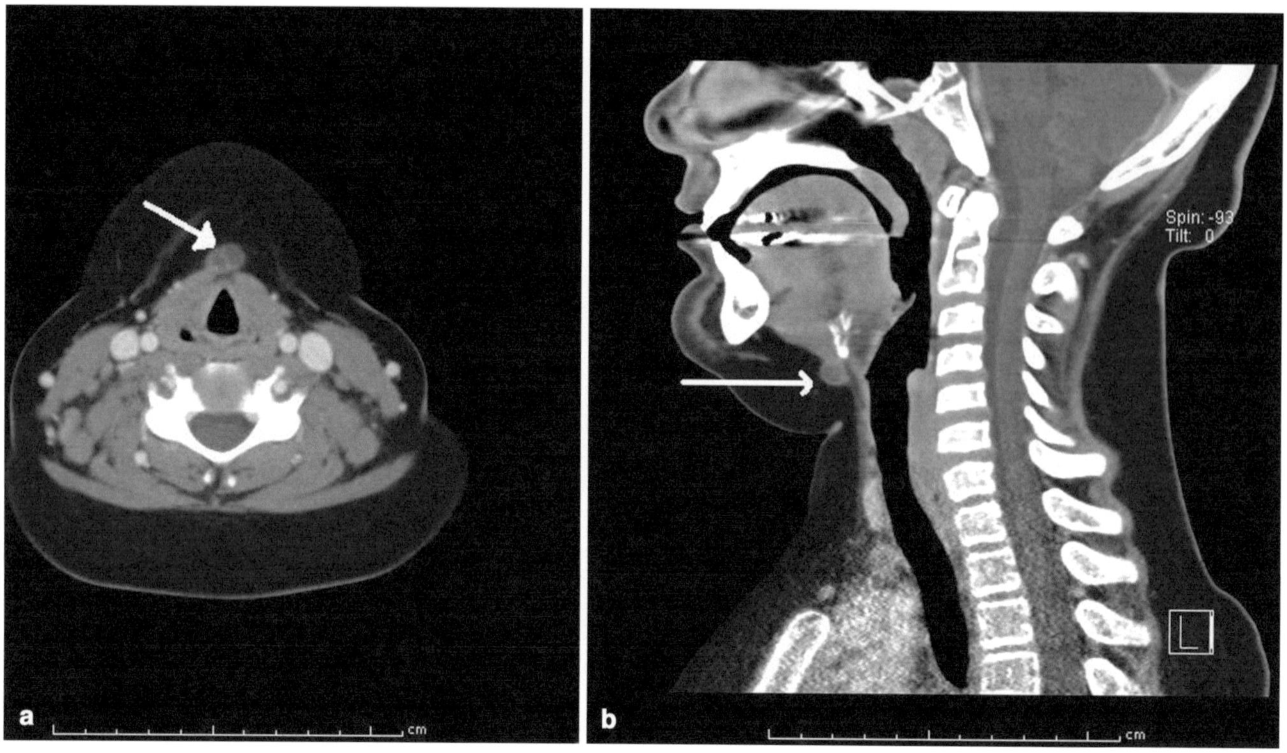

Fig. 43.5 a, b CT scan with *arrows* indicating the location of a thyroglossal duct cyst

Some have used computed tomography (CT) scanning with contrast to evaluate a TGDC (Fig. 43.5a, b). This is typically not necessary unless the physician senses some other pathological process that U/S could not properly evaluate. CT scanning with contrast may be of help when accessing a reoccurring TGDC [18]. Extra tracts or other diagnostic possibilities can at times be better delineated on CT scans. Like thyroid scans, sedation or general anesthesia might be necessary in select patients.

Pathology

The pathology of a TGDC is straightforward. The cystic tract is lined by either squamous or pseudostratified ciliated columnar epithelium (Fig. 43.6) [19]. Inflammatory cells and thyroid follicles may also be present [20]. Confirmation of the correct diagnosis is mandatory to avoid postoperative complications. If there is any question of a possible ectopic thyroid gland during surgery, an intraoperative frozen section should be obtained. If the frozen section reveals thyroid glandular tissue or colloid follicles without any cystic components, it is imperative to obtain a thyroid scan in the postoperative period to document that an actual functioning thyroid gland exists. The surgeon may also opt to explore the area where the thyroid gland should be located to see if a gland is present.

The most common midline mass mistaken for a TGDC is a dermoid cyst. If opened in the operating room after excision, dermoid cysts will classically be filled with cheesy white sebaceous material. In contrast, a TGDC will typically reveal dishwater colored material. No ascending tract is usually seen with a dermoid cyst.

Treatment

Medical

TGDC are usually not treated medically. Some have advocated following these lesions conservatively unless there is some specific indication for removal. It is important to keep in mind that many TGDC will become infected and some will abscess to the point that they must be incised and drained. Often cysts will only continue to enlarge until they are cosmetically unsightly and thus necessitate removal. Patients who present with infected cysts should be treated with oral antibiotics until the infection subsides. If antibiotics fail to eliminate the infection, simple incision and drainage may be necessary. All patients who choose conservative management without resection should be advised that over time there is a 1 % occurrence of thyroglossal cancer within the cyst or its tract [21]. It is important that patients opting

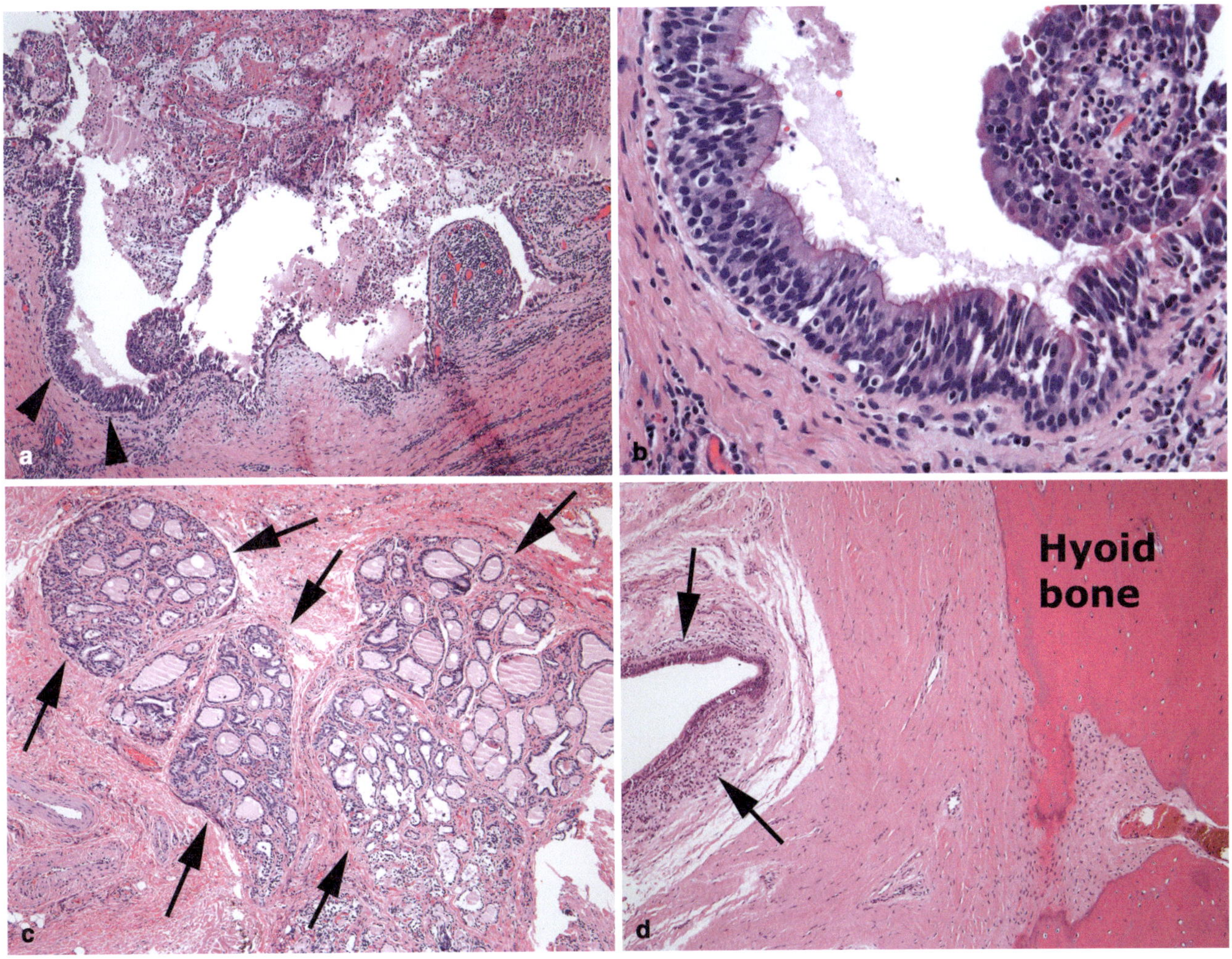

Fig. 43.6 Thyroglossal duct cyst, midline neck. **a** Large soft tissue cyst lined by well-formed respiratory ciliated epithelium (*arrowheads*) containing sloughed surface epithelial cells, cellular debris, inflammatory cells, and mucus. **b** Higher magnification of ciliated respiratory epithelium (*detail from area indicated by arrowheads in* **a**). **c** Ectopic islands of thyroid tissue with well-formed follicles (*between arrows*). **d** Thyroglossal duct remnant (*between arrows*) adjacent to *hyoid bone*

for nonsurgical treatment be followed closely every 6–12 months, checking on TGDC size and neck adenopathy. If the midline neck mass is thought to be a reactive lymph node, then a 10–20 day course of oral antibiotics is indicated to see if any decrease in size occurs. TGDC typically decrease in size with oral antibiotics if they have enlarged secondary to infection.

Surgical

The standard treatment for a TGDC is complete resection using the Sistrunk method, which mandates resection of the midportion of the hyoid bone and proximal tract [22]. This entails dissection of the cyst in the neck from surrounding tissue and then carefully following the attached tract up to the hyoid bone. The cysts are usually located anterior to the hyoid, but there have been scattered reports of intrahyoid involvement [23, 24]. It is important that the midportion of the hyoid bone be resected in toto with the rest of the specimen and that after midhyoid resection, the dissection continues up as far as possible to the base of the tongue. The cyst may appear as a poorly defined mass that is difficult to dissect from the adjoining tissue, especially if inflammation and infection has occurred. It is important during dissection that a tissue core of approximately 3 mm be resected with the cyst and adjoining tract (Fig. 43.7). On microscopic sections thyroglossal duct remnants frequently have branching tracts, thus aggressive dissection of the cyst and tract from surrounding tissue should be avoided for fear of leaving small accessory tracts, which can lead to recurrence and further surgery [6].

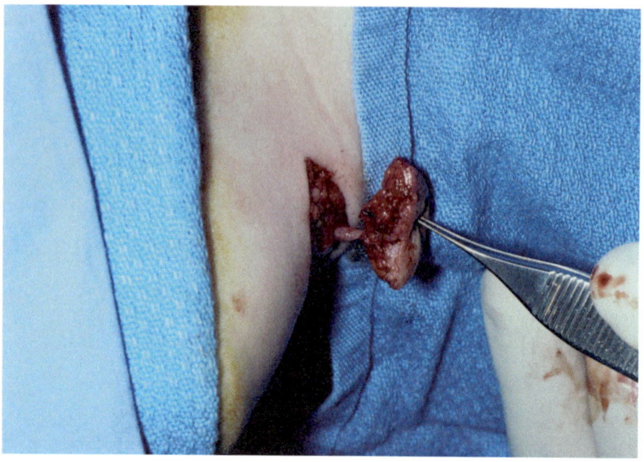

Fig. 43.7 The Sistrunk procedure showing excision of the cyst with the accompanying thyroglossal tract

During cyst removal, no part of the airway should be entered since TGDC are confined to the neck and lie anterior to the larynx and trachea. Entering the airway during resection may cause severe injury to the true vocal cords, trachea, supraglottic structures, and esophagus. If the airway is entered and air bubbles are seen in the neck, a laryngoscopy and bronchoscopy should be preformed to assure that no damage to these structures has taken place. Any noted injury should be immediately repaired, especially if damage has occurred to the glottis. Delay in repair of laryngeal trauma only hampers a successful outcome.

The recurrence rate following a Sistrunk procedure is 3 % [25, 26]. Reoperation should focus on wider and deeper removal of midline fascial tissue involving the area of recurrence [27]. This will help to ensure that any previously missed tracts have been resected. If the midportion of the hyoid bone was not previously resected, it is imperative to remove it during reoperation.

TGDC that present with abscess formation should be treated with simple incision and drainage in the operating room. Cultures should be taken. The wound should be rigorously irrigated and packed with gauze that can be advanced and removed over 3 or 4 days. Twenty-four to forty-eight hours of IV antibiotics postoperatively are helpful in rapid resolution of the infection after the area has been opened and drained. Once the area has healed, the patient should be scheduled in a timely manner for complete resection since TGDC have a propensity to become repeatedly infected. It is not wise to attempt resection of an infected TGDC. The cyst and accompanying tract can be hard if not impossible to locate due to the intensity of the inflammation. The patient is also at increased risk of injury to surrounding structures from a loss of tissue plains. Infected and abscessed cysts usually defervesce quickly if treated properly.

If the cyst cannot be located preoperatively on the day of surgery, consideration should be given to postponing the surgery and the patient be advised to return for examination when the mass returns. Neck exploration in patients without a palpable lesion preoperatively can be frustrating and fruitless since many times no mass or tract can be located. If a suspected TGDC is changing in size, observation with or without a contrast-enhanced CT scan might be indicated to confirm the exact diagnosis. Patience and time will allow suspected lesions to declare themselves.

References

1. Enepekides DJ. Management of congenital anomalies of the neck. Facial Plast Surg Clin North Am. 2001;9(1):131–45.
2. Sadler TW. Langman's medical embryology. 11th ed. Philadelphia: Lippincott Williams and Wilkins; 2010. S. 277–9.
3. Ellis PD, van Nostrand AW. The applied anatomy of thyroglossal tract remnants. Laryngoscope. 1977;87(5):765–70.
4. Mussak EN, Kacker A. Surgical and medical management of midline ectopic thyroid. Otolaryngol Head Neck Surg. 2007;136(6):870–2.
5. Allard RH. The thyroglossal cyst. Head Neck Surg. 1982;5(2):134–46.
6. Soucy P, Penning J. The clinical relevance of certain observations on the histology of the thyroglossal tract. J Pediatric Surg. 1984;19(5):506–9.
7. Todd NW. Common congenital anomalies of the neck. Embryology and surgical anatomy. Surg Clin North Am. 1993;73(4):599–610.
8. Brousseau VJ, Solares CA, Xu M, et al. Thyroglossal duct cysts: presentation and management in children versus adults. Int J Pediatr Otorhinolaryngol. 2003;67(12):1285–90.
9. Radkowski D, Arnold J, Healy GB, et al. Thyroglossal duct remnants. Preoperative evaluation and management. Arch Otolaryngol Head Neck Surg. 1991;117(12):1378–81.
10. Greinwald JH Jr, Leichtman LG, Simko EJ. Hereditary thyroglossal duct cysts. Arch Otolaryngol Head Neck Surg. 1996;122(10):1094–6.
11. Josephson GD, Spencer WR, Josephson JS. Thyroglossal duct cyst: the New York Eye and Ear Infirmary experience and a literature review. Ear Nose Throat J. 1998;77(8):642–4, 646–7, 651.
12. Byard RW, Bourne AJ, Silver MM. The association of lingual thyroglossal duct remnants with sudden death in infancy. Int J Pediatr Otorhinolaryngol. 1990;20(2):107–12.
13. Solomon JR, Rangecroft L. Thyroglossal-duct lesions in childhood. J Pediatr Surg. 1984;19(5):555–61.
14. Foley DS, Fallat ME. Thyroglossal duct and other congenital midline cervical anomalies. Semin Pediatr Surg. 2006;15(2):70–5.
15. Peretz A, Leiberman E, Kapelushnik J, et al. Thyroglossal duct carcinoma in children: case presentation and review of the literature. Thyroid. 2004;14(9):777–85.
16. Tracy TF Jr, Muratore CS. Management of common head and neck masses. Semin Pediatr Surg. 2007;16(1):3–13.
17. Pinczower E, Crockett DM, Atkinson JB, et al. Preoperative thyroid scanning in presumed thyroglossal duct cysts. Arch Otolaryngol Head Neck Surg. 1992;118(9):985–8.
18. Gupta P, Maddalozzo J. Preoperative sonography in presumed thyroglossal duct cysts. Arch Otolaryngol Head Neck Surg. 2001;127(2):200–2.
19. Chandra RK, Maddalozzo J, Kovarik P. Histological characterization of the thyroglossal tract: implications for surgical management. Laryngoscope. 2001;111(6):1002–5.

20. Hirshoren N, Neuman T, Udassin R, et al. The imperative of the Sistrunk operation: review of 160 thyroglossal tract remnant operations. Otolaryngol Head Neck Surg. 2009;140(3):338–42.
21. Heshmati HM, Fatourechi V, van Heerden JA, et al. Thyroglossal duct carcinoma: report of 12 cases. Mayo Clin Proc. 1997;72(4):315–9.
22. Sistrunk WE. The surgical treatment of cysts of the thyroglossal tract. Ann Surg. 1920;71(2):121–2.
23. Bourjat P, Cartier J, Woether JP. Thyroglossal duct cyst in hyoid bone: CT confirmation. J Comput Assist Tomogr. 1988;12(5):871–3.
24. Podoshin L, Fradis M, Goldstein J, et al. Intrahyoid thyroglossal cyst. J Laryngol Otol. 1989;103(5):539–42.
25. Pelausa ME, Forte V. Sistrunk revisited: a 10-year review of revision thyroglossal duct surgery at Toronto's Hospital for Sick Children. J Otolaryngol. 1989;18(7):325–33.
26. Bennett KG, Organ C, Willliams R. Is the treatment for thryroglossal duct cysts too extensive? Am J Surg. 1986;152(6):602–5.
27. Patel NN, Hartley BE, Howard DJ. Management of thyroglossal tract disease after failed Sistrunk's procedure. J Laryngol Otol. 2003;117(9):710–2.

44 Thyroid Tumors

Biren P. Modi and Robert C. Shamberger

Introduction

Thyroid tumors include global thyroid enlargement (goiter), typically as a result of Graves' disease or Hashimoto's thyroiditis, and focal nodule formation, with or without background thyroiditis. The majority of this chapter will be spent discussing the pathophysiology and clinical care of the child with thyroid nodule disease. Other thyroid related lesions, such as thyroglossal duct cysts and parathyroid tumors, are discussed elsewhere in this book.

Though uncommon, thyroid nodules in children are much more likely to be malignant than in adults. Appropriate diagnostic investigation requires fine-needle aspiration (FNA) of all nodules >1 cm, with subsequent surgical management dependent on cytologic results. Surgical intervention for thyroid malignancies in children should be undertaken by experienced surgeons with adequate clinical volume to limit complications. In addition, surgery for thyroid malignancies is part of a multimodal treatment regimen which includes suppressive thyroid hormone therapy, radioactive iodine (RAI) ablation, and both laboratory and imaging surveillance. Syndromes which include thyroid malignancies, such as the phosphatase and tensin homolog (PTEN) hamartoma tumor syndrome and the multiple endocrine neoplasia (MEN) syndromes, must be given special consideration.

Key Points

- Although thyroid nodules in the pediatric population are more likely to be malignant and more likely to present with metastatic disease, outcomes for differentiated thyroid cancer in children are excellent.
- Ultrasound (US) identification and characterization of thyroid nodules and US-guided fine-needle aspiration are the mainstays of diagnostic testing for malignancy in thyroid nodule disease.
- Surgical intervention for thyroid nodules is guided by cytologic interpretation of fine-needle aspiration biopsies as specified by the Bethesda criteria. In general, near-total thyroidectomy with selective lymph node dissection is the surgical treatment of choice for local control of thyroid cancer, facilitating the use of RAI and monitoring for recurrence with measurement of serum thyroglobulin.
- Overall, differentiated thyroid cancer is treated using multimodal therapy including surgical resection, RAI, and suppressive thyroid hormone therapy.

Biology and Epidemiology

The thyroid gland is composed primarily of follicles of cuboidal thyroid cells. These cells are responsible for the production of triiodothyronine (T3) and thyroxine (T4). The central portion of the follicle is composed of colloid, containing thyroglobulin and stored thyroid hormone. Intermittently dispersed between the follicles are parafollicular C-cells, which are derived from the fourth branchial pouch and secrete calcitonin. These distinctions are key in understanding the cells of origin for the various types of thyroid cancer and the laboratory detection and surveillance of these tumors.

The hypothalamic-pituitary-thyroid axis is comprised of thyrotropin-releasing hormone secretion by the hypothalamus, thyrotropin or thyroid-stimulating hormone (TSH) secretion by the anterior pituitary, and thyroid hormone secretion by the thyroid gland. Thyroid hormones, T3 and T4, are formed by the iodination of tyrosine from thyroglobulin followed by coupling of the iodinated tyrosine. The active form of the hormone, T3, binds a nuclear receptor in target cells, thus allowing it to bind DNA and regulate genetic transcription. The end result is modulation of metabolism via effects

B. P. Modi (✉) · R. C. Shamberger
Department of Surgery, Boston Children's Hospital, Harvard Medical School, Boston, MA, USA
e-mail: biren.modi@childrens.harvard.edu

R. Rahbar et al. (eds.), *Pediatric Head and Neck Tumors*,
DOI 10.1007/978-1-4614-8755-5_44, © Springer Science+Business Media New York 2014

on cellular oxygen consumption, basal metabolic rate, and lipid, protein, and carbohydrate management [1].

Pathophysiology

- Goiters are diffusely enlarged thyroid glands. In children living in developed countries without concern for iodine provision, these are typically the result of autoimmune disease. Graves' disease, or diffuse toxic goiter, is a hyperthyroid state resulting from stimulating antibodies directed against the thyroid plasma membrane. Hashimoto's disease, or chronic lymphocytic thyroiditis, is also of autoimmune etiology and typically results in a hypothyroid state, though hyper-, eu-, and hypothyroid states are possible [2].
- Thyroid nodules are described by composition, size, and function. Though functional autonomous nodules (hot nodules) can harbor malignancy, this is felt to be extremely rare. Both benign and malignant nodules can be cystic or solid or mixed.
- Features which increase the likelihood of a nodule being malignant include:
  - Young age of patient
  - History of radiation exposure
  - Larger size of nodule
  - Cold nodule
  - Evidence of cervical adenopathy
  - History of prior malignancy
  - Family history of thyroid cancer or cancer syndromes
  - Likely, background thyroiditis, though this point is debated [3]

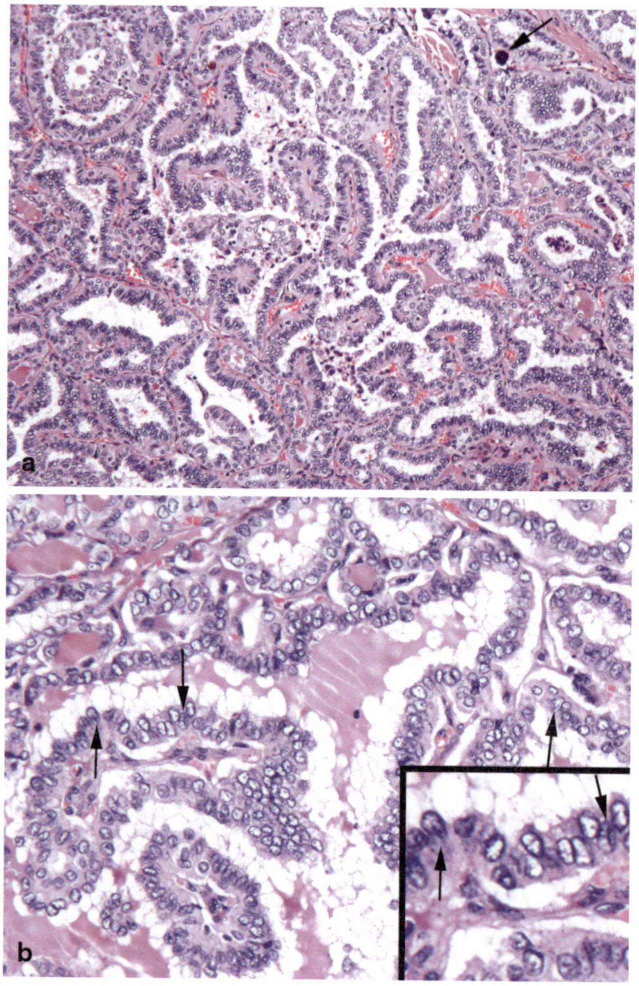

Fig. 44.1 Histopathology of papillary carcinoma. **a** Distinct branching papillae with delicate fibrovascular cores and occasional psammoma bodies (*arrow*). **b** Nuclei are typically large, crowded (*on top of each other*), ovoid, clear ("Orphan Annie eye"), and occasionally grooved (*arrows*). In the *inset*, nuclear grooves at higher magnification are indicated by *arrows*

Molecular/Genetic Pathology

- In Graves' disease, TSH-receptor antibodies are present in more than 95 % of patients. Hashimoto's disease results from antithyroid microsomal antibodies or antithyroid peroxidase antibodies in 95 % of patients [2].
- Three histologic types of primary differentiated thyroid cancer are predominant [2, 4, 5]:
  - Papillary carcinoma is the most common in children and adults and is characterized pathologically by psammoma bodies, a prominent follicular pattern, and nuclear grooving (Fig. 44.1). Subtypes include classical, follicular, and diffuse sclerosing variants.
  - Follicular adenocarcinoma is less common and is difficult pathologically to differentiate from normal thyroid tissue or follicular adenoma.
  - Medullary carcinoma differs from the other two in that the cell of origin is the parafollicular C-cell (Fig. 44.2). This subtype accounts for 2–5 % of thyroid tumors and arises spontaneously or in association with described cancer syndromes (MEN 2a and 2b, familial medullary thyroid carcinoma (FMTC)) [2, 6].
- Rat sarcoma (RAS) proto-oncogene mutations are found in 20 % of papillary cancers and 80 % of follicular cancers [2, 7].
- Specific rearranged during transfection (RET) proto-oncogene mutations are associated with the MEN and FMTC syndromes. In addition, mutations in rearranged during transfection (RET) are associated with 40 % of sporadic medullary cancer and 35 % of papillary cancers [7, 8].
- Additional genetic mutations in the v-Raf (Virus-induced rapidly accelerated fibrosarcoma) murine sarcoma viral oncogene homolog B1 (BRAF) oncogene are also associated with papillary cancer, with more recent data suggesting that particular BRAF mutations may be predictive of a more aggressive malignancy.

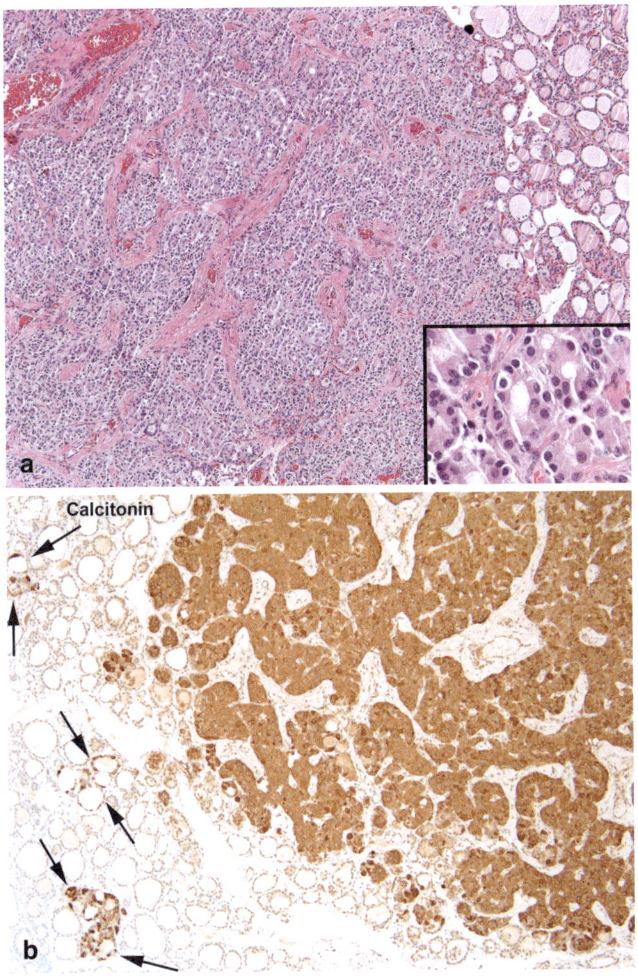

Fig. 44.2 Histopathology of medullary thyroid carcinoma. **a** Well demarcated nodule of medullary carcinoma composed of large sheets of tumor cells outlined by dense fibrovascular septae. Tumor cells have regular round nuclei with fine chromatin and abundant eosinophilic cytoplasm (*inset*). **b** Strong cytoplasmic immunoreactivity for *calcitonin* in the nodule of medullary carcinoma, in adjacent tumorlets and in foci of C-cell hyperplasia (*between arrows*)

- Other types of primary thyroid neoplasms (e.g., lymphoma) are not discussed here due to their extreme rarity [4].

Incidence and Prevalence

- The reported incidence of thyroid nodules in children is approximately 1 % [9].
- The incidence of malignancy within thyroid nodules in children is relatively high, ranging from 12 to 36 % in recent reports [9–11].
- Overall, thyroid carcinoma accounts for 3 % of pediatric malignancies. Evaluated in the opposite fashion, approximately 10 % of thyroid cancers occur in children [2].
- The pediatric population accounts for approximately 2 % of all newly diagnosed thyroid cancers [6].

Age Distribution

- Graves' disease typically occurs in adolescence to early adulthood, though neonatal Graves' disease in infants of affected mothers is well described.
- Hashimoto's disease incidence peaks during puberty and adolescence.
- In children, the peak incidence of thyroid cancer, like that of thyroid nodules, occurs in early adolescence (Fig. 44.3) [2, 11].

Sex Predilection

- Graves' disease carries a 5:1 predilection for female patients [2].
- Hashimoto's disease is more prevalent in female patients.
- Thyroid nodules in children have a 3.6:1 predilection for female patients [11].
- Thyroid cancer in children has a 2:1 to 3.3:1 predilection for female patients [2, 11].

Geographic/Ethnic Distribution

- Higher rates of thyroid cancer are found in adolescent female patients of white and Hispanic backgrounds than black female patients or male patients of any race [6].

Risk Factors

- Previous radiation, in the form of directed neck radiation, environmental disasters such as Chernobyl, or previous radiotherapy for other malignancy is related to a higher incidence of thyroid cancer in a dose-dependent manner [6]. The time from radiation exposure to development of thyroid carcinoma is 4–6 years, though the identification of the thyroid malignancy may take longer [2, 12].
- Prior malignancy is also related to an increased incidence of thyroid cancer. Thyroid cancer accounts for 9 % of secondary malignancies and is the most common secondary malignancy in survivors of childhood Hodgkin's and non-Hodgkin's lymphoma [6]. Conversely, Hodgkin's disease is the most common primary cancer in patients with secondary thyroid cancer [2, 12].
- Age is an independent risk factor predicting malignancy in thyroid nodules. In general, 20 % of nodules in children compared to only 5 % of nodules in adults are malignant. This rate is higher in children younger than 10 years of age [6, 13].

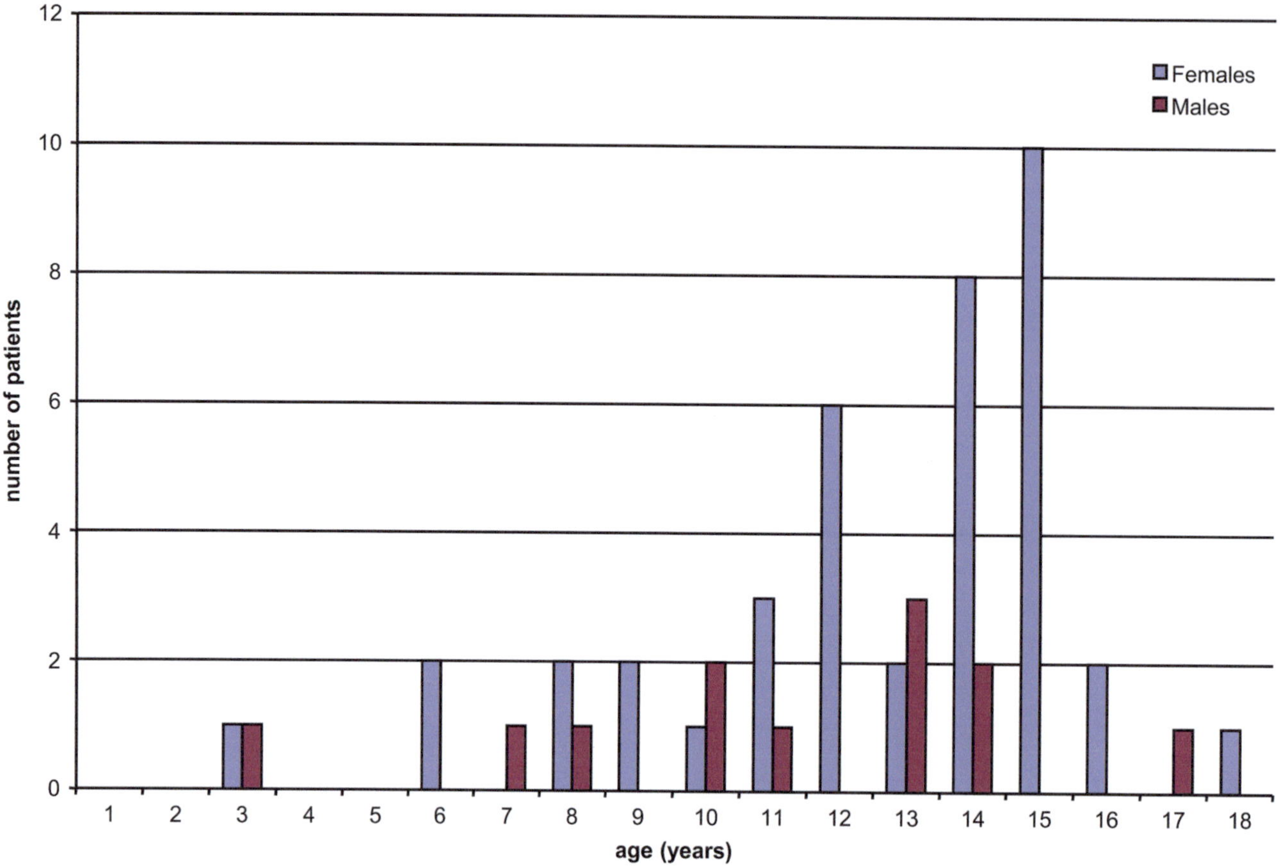

Fig. 44.3 Age distribution of thyroid nodules operated upon at our institution. A similar age distribution exists for pediatric thyroid cancer. (Reprinted from S. Scholz et al. [11], with permission from Elsevier)

Relationships to Other Disease States, Syndromes

- Medullary carcinoma is the thyroid malignancy associated with FMTC, MEN 2a, and MEN 2b. FMTC is self-explanatory. MEN 2a is comprised of hyperparathyroidism, pheochromocytoma, and medullary carcinoma of the thyroid. MEN 2b is also comprised of pheochromocytoma and medullary thyroid cancer (MTC, without hyperparathyroidism), but also manifests with a marfanoid habitus and cutaneous neuromas.
- In the MEN syndromes, medullary carcinoma of the thyroid has nearly 100% penetrance, is typically the first malignancy to present, and is invariably the most common cause of death. Treatment guidelines are derived from this principle and the genotypic variations that have now been delineated [8].
- The PTEN hamartoma tumor syndrome follows a germline mutation in the tumor suppressor PTEN gene. Patients with this syndrome develop benign and malignant growths of multiple tissues, most notably the breast, thyroid, bowel, and skin. The thyroid component can present as either follicular or papillary or both histologic subtypes of thyroid cancer. Recent data suggest that this presentation can occur early, in preteenage to teenage children, rather than adulthood as previously suspected. Patients suspected to have this syndrome should undergo an annual US surveillance from the time of diagnosis [14].
- Gardner syndrome, one of the familial adenomatous polyposis (FAP) syndromes, is caused by a defect in the adenomatous polyposis coli (APC) gene. It is characterized by multiple colonic polyps, osteomas and other soft tissue tumors, desmoid tumors, retinal pigmentation, and an increased risk of thyroid cancer. In one series, the average age at which thyroid cancer was diagnosed in patients with Gardner syndrome was 23 years, with many of the patients diagnosed in their adolescent years [4, 15].

Presentation

Symptoms

- Most pediatric patients with differentiated thyroid cancer present with an asymptomatic, incidentally noted solitary neck mass due to a thyroid nodule [4].

- Recently, as imaging studies become more sensitive, many patients present with thyroid nodules noted incidentally on imaging for trauma or other indications. In addition, nodules are often detected early and incidentally in patients followed for the development of secondary cancers after therapy for a childhood malignancy (e.g., Hodgkin's lymphoma).
- Children present with malignant involvement of the cervical lymph nodes more frequently than adults. Lymph node involvement at diagnosis is present in 40–80% of children with differentiated thyroid cancer, compared with a 20–50% incidence in adults. Distant metastases are likewise more common in children, with 7–25% of children presenting with metastatic disease outside the neck [5–7, 16].
- Rarely, patients present with symptoms other than a simple neck mass.
  - Hoarse voice suggestive of recurrent laryngeal nerve involvement with paralysis of the ipsilateral vocal cord. This is strongly suggestive of malignancy [13].
  - Swallowing difficulty due to mass effect.
  - Shortness of breath or dyspnea due to mass effect, especially while recumbent, or due to diffuse pulmonary metastatic involvement. Similar to lymph node involvement, children are more likely than adults to present with pulmonary metastases, in the 20–30% range [6].

Patterns of Evolution

- As mentioned above, the majority of thyroid cancers are detected as solitary nodules. If left untreated, the presentation will evolve to larger primary tumors, potentially with compressive symptoms, cervical lymphadenopathy, and ultimately, possible pulmonary compromise.

Evaluation at Presentation

- Evaluation of the child with a neck nodule should include a thorough history geared toward the differential diagnosis, a focused physical examination and appropriate imaging and laboratory studies as indicated below. Emergent presentations are rare.

Differential Diagnosis

Most patients are asymptomatic or have a simple chief complaint of a lump in the neck. Though the differential for this is broad, a more concise differential exists once the lesion is determined to be within the thyroid on US examination. The major diagnoses in this group include:

- Benign cyst
- Adenoma
- Colloid nodule
- Hyperplastic nodule
- Infectious nodule
- Lymphocytic nodule
- Differentiated thyroid cancer

Diagnosis and Evaluation

Physical Examination

- Physical exam should be focused to evaluate the location of the primary nodule, including mobility with swallowing and freedom from adjacent structures. In addition, assessment for additional nodules, the size of the thyroid gland, and enlarged cervical lymph nodes should be performed. The voice is immediately evident on evaluation of the patient [4].
- Findings concerning for malignancy include solitary nodule, evidence of cervical adenopathy in conjunction with a thyroid nodule, fixed lesions, and hoarseness. Compressive symptoms associated with goiter are rarely associated with malignant thyroid nodules.

Laboratory Data

- Initial laboratory studies should include TSH. In addition, measurement of serum calcitonin level can help in the identification of medullary cancer if this is suspected based on family history [4, 6].

Imaging Evaluation

- In children, any neck nodule should prompt a neck and thyroid US, which will localize the nodule. In addition, US characteristics of the nodule can assist in determining the possibility of malignancy. Concerning features include vague margins, calcifications, hypoechoic solid nodules or heterogenous appearance, intranodular vascularity, invasive growth, and suspicious regional lymph nodes [6, 13, 17].
- If the TSH is suppressed, an independently active nodule should be suspected and can be confirmed with radionuclide thyroid scintigraphy. Although possible, "hot" active nodules are very rarely malignant and are generally managed with medical therapy targeting the hyperthyroid state [17].

Table 44.1 FNA categories under the Bethesda classification scheme and the typical surgical management associated with each category. (Adapted from E. S. Cibas [17], with permission from Elsevier)

Diagnostic category	Risk of malignancy	Typical management
Nondiagnostic or unsatisfactory	N/A	Repeat US-guided FNA
Benign	0–3 %	Routine surveillance
Atypia	5–15 %	Repeat FNA
Follicular neoplasm or suspicious for follicular neoplasm	15–30 %	Thyroid lobectomy
Suspicious for malignancy	60–75 %	Near-total thyroidectomy or thyroid lobectomy followed by completion thyroidectomy if indicated
Malignant	97–99 %	Near-total thyroidectomy

Pathology

- Although no consensus pediatric guidelines exist, in general any solid nodule greater than 1 cm in diameter, any nodule with concerning sonographic features regardless of size, and any nodule in a patient with significant risk factors (age, radiation, family history, associated syndrome history) should undergo fine-needle aspiration (FNA) for cytologic evaluation of the nodule. Lesions of borderline size or complex nodules with a significant cystic component may either undergo FNA or be monitored with serial US [17, 18]. If cystic lesions recur after initial aspiration, they should be monitored more closely, sampled with FNA, or be surgically resected for diagnostic purposes [2, 4].
- Despite the relatively high risk of malignancy in pediatric thyroid nodules, recent data suggest that the use of FNA, especially US-guided FNA, can beneficially impact the management of pediatric thyroid nodules. Specifically, FNA may preclude the need for surgery in lesions with clearly benign cytology and has been shown to decrease the rate of surgery for benign lesions [6, 9, 17]. Without definite demonstration of efficacy in pediatric patients, however, some authors still recommend immediate surgery for younger patients, whose risk of malignancy is high [2].
- FNA is considered cost-effective and highly accurate, in both adult and pediatric patients [4]. This has been demonstrated in multiple single-institution series [6, 9, 11]. A dedicated pediatric meta-analysis found the sensitivity and specificity of FNA for thyroid malignancy to be 94 % and 81 %, with a negative predictive value of over 98 % [19].
- The technique for FNA has been evaluated for maximal yield of cellularity without dilution of the sample or excessive blood. In general, US guidance offers the ability to guide biopsy to specific portions of a nodule. This includes the wall, specific solid components of mixed solid and cystic lesions, and areas involved with microcalcifications. Small, generally 25–27 gauge needles are used, with standard syringes to apply suction and collect the specimen. Three back and forth oscillations per second, for 3–5 s per pass, will provide good cellularity without excessive blood. Typically, 2–5 passes per nodule are performed, as tolerated, and each pass should yield 1–2 slides [17]. FNA is generally well tolerated, even by children, but can be made more tolerable with the application of topical anesthetic cream prior to planned biopsy. A variety of slide preparation techniques and processes exist, with prompt slide preparation being the most important factor to ensure adequate assessment and limit unsatisfactory specimens.
- Guidelines for the interpretation of FNA cytology (the Bethesda classification) have been set forth in the adult population and have been applied to pediatric patients [17]. Based on the results of cytology, an estimate of the likelihood of malignancy can help guide surgical decision making (Table 44.1).
  - Nondiagnostic/unsatisfactory: This category comprises approximately 10 % of thyroid FNA samples. This result can occur because the sample contains cyst fluid only or is virtually acellular.
  - Benign: This category comprises approximately 60–70 % of thyroid FNA samples and is the source of greatest benefit of performing FNA, as samples with this diagnosis obviate the need for surgical excision of a benign thyroid nodule. This result can be subclassified into benign follicular nodules or various forms of thyroiditis. The false negative rate is only 0–3 %, but nodules should be followed clinically nonetheless, with repeat FNA performed for nodules which demonstrate significant growth or new suspicious sonographic changes.
  - Atypia: This category is reserved for specimens that are not easily identified as benign, suspicious, or malignant. Approximately 3–6 % of FNA samples fall into this category, and this reading conveys a malignancy rate of 5–15 %. In general, these lesions undergo repeat biopsy, resulting in a more definitive diagnosis 80 % of the time. However, the specific clinical scenario, including physical findings or sonographic features, may persuade the physician to elect to monitor the lesion or proceed with resection for definitive diagnosis.

  - Follicular neoplasm or suspicious for follicular neoplasm: This category defines samples with hypercellularity and follicular cells with atypical cellular architecture, but without the nuclear and cellular features that would describe papillary carcinoma. Despite these abnormal features, however, only 15–30% of these samples will prove to be malignant, either as follicular carcinoma or the follicular variant of papillary carcinoma. The remaining lesions prove to be follicular adenomas or adenomatoid nodules of multinodular goiter. A special subset of this category may be further described in the FNA result as Hürthle cell or suspicious for Hürthle cell neoplasm, characterized by the oncocytic cells of Hürthle cell carcinoma.
  - Suspicious for malignancy: This category describes specimens with cells which clearly have signs of nuclear and architectural features of carcinoma but which have low cellularity or only focal populations of cells that have these features. The lesions are truly malignant in 60–75% of cases. The nonmalignant lesions are typically follicular adenomas.
  - Malignant: This category is used when the cytologic features of the FNA specimen are conclusively malignant (Fig. 44.4). This category accounts for 3–7% of thyroid FNA specimens and carries a likelihood of malignancy of 97–99%.
- In addition to traditional cytopathologic features, recently available commercial molecular diagnostic assays targeting known genetic mutations in the RET, RAS, and BRAF proto-oncogenes may add to the predictive value of FNA. Although no pediatric studies exist regarding these assays, emerging studies in adults may shed light on their utility. Immunohistochemical testing has not been shown to have a significant impact on the predictive value of FNA [20].
- In patients with large nodules, usually defined as >4 cm, the diagnostic sensitivity of FNA drops significantly due to sampling error. For this reason, nodules that grow to this size should be treated with surgical lobectomy for diagnostic and therapeutic purposes.

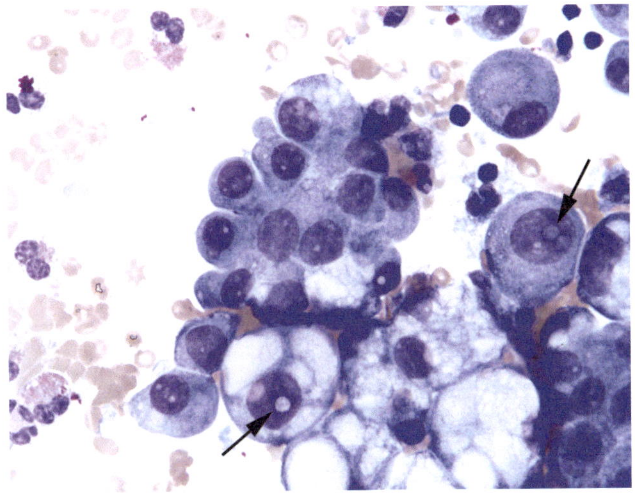

Fig. 44.4 FNA cytology of papillary carcinoma. Cellular specimen with rounded clusters of closely apposed tumor cells with abundant granular cytoplasm and round nuclei with powdery chromatin, single distinct nucleolus and characteristic pseudoinclusions (*arrows*)

Treatment

Goal Complete resection and eradication of malignant-differentiated thyroid cancer without treatment-related morbidity.

- The goal of therapy for differentiated thyroid cancer is eradication of the malignancy without undue operative or treatment-related morbidity. Since these malignancies are indolent and outcomes are excellent, aggressive therapy, which may result in significant complications, is discouraged [6].
- In most cases, treatment of differentiated thyroid cancer is multi-modal, with surgery playing a prime role for eradication of the primary tumor and associated cervical adenopathy. RAI ablation plays an adjuvant role for the control of residual and metastatic disease. Thyroid suppression via thyroid hormone replacement therapy essentially plays the role of chemotherapy, functioning to treat residual disease systemically by suppressing the growth and spread of any residual thyroid tissue.

Surgical Therapy

Choice of Operation Cytologic results of FNA typically guide appropriate surgical therapy as do radiographic abnormalities of the cervical lymph nodes (Table 44.1). In the intermediate range cytologic categories, such as atypia, follicular neoplasm, and suspicious for malignancy, individual patient characteristics may play a factor in determining a variation from the typical surgical therapy. In general, higher suspicion for malignancy will guide the surgeon to perform a near-total thyroidectomy, while intermediate-risk cytology results typically guide the surgeon toward a partial thyroid resection, with plan for completion thyroidectomy if the nodule returns as a true malignancy. Nodulectomy is a consideration of the past, and is no longer considered an appropriate surgical intervention [2, 5–7].

- For papillary carcinoma, near-total thyroidectomy is an accepted surgical option to limit injury to the parathyroid glands and recurrent laryngeal nerves. Residual disease left behind on these vital structures limits morbidity without affecting survival [2]. The surgical resection in medullary carcinoma is typically more extensive, due to the relatively aggressive nature of this tumor. In general, these patients undergo total thyroidectomy with central lymph node dissection. Ideally, this surgery is performed in a prophylactic manner obviating the need for lymph node dissection in patients with familial syndromes (see below).

- Although thyroid lobectomy can often be used to completely resect thyroid malignancy, this more conservative procedure is most often utilized only for small lesions (less than 1 cm). No survival benefit has been demonstrated for more extensive resection, as long as complete resection is achieved, although most multi-institutional series that have examined this are retrospective, confounded by lack of homogeneity, and demonstrated a treatment bias whereby larger lesions or lesions with more concerning preoperative findings were treated by more aggressive therapy, thus making true comparison difficult [16, 21].
- The benefit of more extensive resection, despite a slightly higher risk profile, is that removal of the entire thyroid facilitates adjuvant therapy. Complete thyroid resection allows for more efficacious therapy with RAI, such that native thyroid tissue does not compete with any potential residual malignant disease. It also allows for surveillance with serum thyroglobulin levels, which should be close to zero in a patient with a surgically absent thyroid and complete eradication of malignant thyroid cancer cells. Likewise, in MTC patients, serum calcitonin levels can be followed for early detection of recurrence [2, 6, 22]. Finally, since approximately 40% of pediatric thyroid cancers are multifocal, based on pathology specimens, a more complete resection can be achieved by the near-total thyroidectomy [23].
- Formal neck dissections are not performed, as there does not appear to be a survival benefit. There is, however, a clear increase in operative complications in patients undergoing more aggressive neck dissections. Thus, most surgeons perform selective node dissections for patients with evidence of lymph node metastases by exam or US. While minimizing operative morbidity, and not reducing survival, this strategy does increase the likelihood of the need for additional surgery to remove recurrent or additional lymph node metastases [2, 6, 7]. When excision of lymph node disease requires dissection high in the neck (level 2 submandibular nodes), we prefer a second transverse counter-incision fashioned in an upper skin crease rather than extension of the standard collar incision into a "hockey stick," as this provides a better cosmetic outcome. Finally, the use of intraoperative US to guide complete node dissection can be beneficial to ensure complete removal of all involved or radiographically "concerning" lymph nodes.

Timing Because of its indolent nature, surgical resection of papillary thyroid cancer occurs on an elective basis once the diagnosis has been made. Exceptions to this rule include patients with evidence of locally advanced disease (fixed lesion, evidence of nerve involvement) and patients with nonpapillary cancer.

- In the MEN syndromes, timing of thyroid resection is determined by the specific syndrome, and in many cases, the specific genetic mutation identified. As mentioned, MTC is the first presenting tumor in these patients and is the most common cause of death. In addition, some genetic mutations have been linked to early onset of disease and more aggressive disease. These discoveries have recently been used to help determine optimal timing for surgical resection of the thyroid, to facilitate surgery by allowing the patient to be as old as possible while limiting the possibility of early aggressive tumors forming prior to surgical resection.
- The current recommendations for patients with familial MTC or MEN 2a are for total thyroidectomy by 5 years of age for the majority of mutations, or between 5 and 8 years of age for some less high-risk mutations. This is an area of ongoing active evaluation, and complete consensus recommendations do not exist. For patients with one of these familial MTC syndromes, central neck lymph node dissection, between the carotids and from hyoid to sternal notch, is recommended at the time of thyroidectomy. Using these criteria, 80% of children undergoing prophylactic thyroidectomy will already have foci of MTC within their thyroid specimen [2, 8, 22].
- Patients with MEN 2b, especially those with RET mutations in codon 918, have a more aggressive form of disease, with very early development of MTC. As such, these patients should undergo total thyroidectomy and central neck dissection at diagnosis, preferably by 6 months to 1 year of age [2, 22].

Complications In the hands of experienced thyroid surgeons, operative morbidity is quite low. The extent of surgical resection, including both extent of thyroid resection and extent of lymph node dissection, correlates with the risk of complications [11].

- Permanent hypocalcemia as a result of hypoparathyroidism has been reported with an incidence of 1–17%, with most reports in the 10% range. More recent reports, with a trend toward less aggressive surgical therapy, report the lowest rates [7, 11, 16, 21].
- Transient postoperative hypocalcemia varies greatly in reported incidence, from 5 to 50%, with a clear correlation between more extensive resection (lobectomy vs. near-total thyroidectomy) and higher incidence [7, 11, 16].
- Permanent recurrent laryngeal nerve injury is an exceptionally rare event in most recent series, with an incidence of 1–4% [11, 16, 21].

- Transient recurrent laryngeal nerve injury, with hoarseness that resolves over several weeks to months, occurs in 1–10 % of patients [11, 16].
- The risk of significant postoperative neck hematoma requiring reoperation is not well reported, though always a concern following any neck surgery. Reported incidence of major wound complications, which includes hematoma as well as pneumothorax or infection, ranges from 5 to 10 %. The majority of these were related to significant lymph node dissections such as radical neck dissections, which are no longer routinely performed [16, 21]. The true incidence of neck hematoma requiring reoperation is more likely in the 1 % range.

Radioactive Iodine Therapy (RAI)

- RAI is used in cases of follicular or papillary cancer for the purpose of both surveillance for occult metastatic or residual disease (I^{123}) and ablation of this residual disease (I^{131}). RAI is most sensitive for the identification and ablation of residual disease when there is minimal normal thyroid tissue remaining; hence near-total thyroidectomy is the surgical procedure of choice when this modality is anticipated. In addition to the possibility of multi-focal disease, this is one of the underlying indications for completion thyroidectomy in patients who have undergone thyroid lobectomy and are found to have malignant disease. When residual thyroid is left, RAI can be effective in larger doses, though this increases the risks of secondary pulmonary fibrosis [7].
- RAI is usually performed 4–6 weeks after surgery following withdrawal of thyroid hormone therapy; the goal of withdrawal is to raise TSH above 30 mIU/mL, thus driving iodine uptake by residual thyroid (normal and malignant) cells. Withdrawal occurs 2 weeks prior to scanning, with confirmation of elevated TSH prior to the scan. Typically, a diagnostic test will be performed first, with I^{123} or low-dose I^{131}, which will then allow for determination of burden of disease and dosing of I^{131} for the ablative scan. Some centers obtain posttherapy scans to verify adequate uptake of RAI within the lesions.
- In retrospective studies of pediatric patients with differentiated thyroid cancer, lack of RAI therapy postoperatively increased the risk of both thyroid bed and lymph node recurrence [6, 24].
- Although RAI and even the withdrawal of hormone replacement preceding it are usually well tolerated, pulmonary fibrosis can be a complication of RAI at high doses [7]. In addition, transiently decreased sperm count and testosterone levels have been demonstrated in boys and young men [5].

Thyroid Hormone Suppression Therapy

- Following thyroid resection, thyroid hormone replacement is provided with a goal of suppressing TSH below normal levels (typical goal is 0.1–0.4 μU/mL) while avoiding symptoms of hyperthyroidism. The use of TSH suppressive doses of hormone replacement can limit both normal and malignant cell proliferation and, therefore, plays a significant role in the prevention of progression and recurrence [7].

Outcomes

- Despite frequently presenting with lymph node and distant metastatic disease, children afflicted with differentiated thyroid cancer have excellent outcomes.
- One multi-institutional study of nonmedullary thyroid cancer demonstrated an overall progression-free survival of 67 % with a median follow-up of over 11 years. The factors associated with progression of disease included younger age and residual cervical disease after surgical therapy. Of note, tumor size and choice of operation were not correlated with risk of progression, though bias based on features of the primary lesion could have affected which operation was chosen by the surgeon. In this study, only 2 disease-related deaths and 8 overall deaths occurred during the follow-up period (overall survival 98 %) [16].
- In one multi-institutional retrospective study of patients with nonmedullary thyroid cancer who presented with distant metastases, overall survival at 10 years was 100 %. Progression-free survival was 76 % at 5 years and 66 % at 10 years from diagnosis [21].

Follow-up

Frequency of Office Visits

- Patients are typically seen at 1 month, 3 months, 6 months, and 1 year following surgery, after which they are followed annually. The visits are geared toward physical examination of the thyroid bed and lymph nodes, evaluation of the efficacy of thyroid hormone suppressive therapy, and for preparation and follow-up of RAI scanning and ablation.
- In general, titration of thyroid hormone suppressive therapy can be performed over the phone with local laboratory value measurements to ensure TSH suppression and phone conversations to determine symptoms of hypothyroidism or hyperthyroidism.

Frequency of Imaging

- Annual surveillance with dedicated neck and thyroid bed US is performed, to assess for growth of recurrence within the thyroid bed and development of cervical nodal disease.
- RAI scanning and ablation typically occur 6 weeks to 3 months postoperatively and can be scheduled electively at the convenience of the patient. Consideration should be given to the potential symptoms the patient may experience during thyroid hormone withdrawal.

References

1. Brent GA. The molecular basis of thyroid hormone action. N Engl J Med. 1994;331:847–53.
2. Safford SD, Skinner MA. Thyroid and parathyroid disease in children. Semin Pediatr Surg. 2006;15:85–91.
3. Koo JS, Hong S, Park CS. Diffuse sclerosing variant is a major subtype of papillary thyroid carcinoma in the young. Thyroid. 2009;19:1225–31.
4. Bentley AA, Gillespie C, Malis D. Evaluation and management of a solitary thyroid nodule in a child. Otolaryngol Clin North Am. 2003;36:117–28.
5. Thompson GB, Hay ID. Current strategies for surgical management and adjuvant treatment of childhood papillary thyroid carcinoma. World J Surg. 2004;28:1187–98.
6. Dinauer CA, Breuer C, Rivkees SA. Differentiated thyroid cancer in children: diagnosis and management. Curr Opin Oncol. 2008;20:59–65.
7. Gingalewski CA, Newman KD. Seminars: controversies in the management of pediatric thyroid malignancy. J Surg Oncol. 2006;94:748–52.
8. Danko ME, Skinner MA. Surgical intervention in children with multiple endocrine neoplasia type 2. Curr Opin Pediatr. 2006;18:312–5.
9. Izquierdo R, Shankar R, Kort K, Khurana K. Ultrasound-guided fine-needle aspiration in the management of thyroid nodules in children and adolescents. Thyroid. 2009;19:703–5.
10. Al-Shaikh A, Ngan B, Daneman A, Daneman D. Fine-needle aspiration biopsy in the management of thyroid nodules in children and adolescents. J Pediatr. 2001;138:140–2.
11. Scholz S, Smith JR, Chaignaud B, Shamberger RC, Huang SA. Thyroid surgery at Children's Hospital Boston: a 35-year single-institution experience. J Pediatr Surg. 2011;46:437–42.
12. Green DM. Late effects of treatment for cancer during childhood and adolescence. Curr Probl Cancer. 2003;27:127–42.
13. Niedziela M. Pathogenesis, diagnosis and management of thyroid nodules in children. Endocr Relat Cancer. 2006;13:427–53.
14. Smith JR, Marqusee E, Webb S, et al. Thyroid nodules and cancer in children with PTEN hamartoma tumor syndrome. J Clin Endocrinol Metab. 2011;96:34–7.
15. Bell B, Mazzaferri EL. Familial adenomatous polyposis (Gardner's syndrome) and thyroid carcinoma. A case report and review of the literature. Dig Dis Sci. 1993;38:185–90.
16. Newman KD, Black T, Heller G, et al. Differentiated thyroid cancer: determinants of disease progression in patients <21 years of age at diagnosis: a report from the Surgical Discipline Committee of the Children's Cancer Group. Ann Surg. 1998;227:533–41.
17. Cibas ES. Fine-needle aspiration in the work-up of thyroid nodules. Otolaryngol Clin North Am. 2010;43:257–71, vii–viii.
18. Cooper DS, Doherty GM, Haugen BR, et al. Revised American Thyroid Association management guidelines for patients with thyroid nodules and differentiated thyroid cancer. Thyroid. 2009;19:1167–214.
19. Stevens C, Lee JK, Sadatsafavi M, Blair GK. Pediatric thyroid fine-needle aspiration cytology: a meta-analysis. J Pediatr Surg. 2009;44:2184–91.
20. Ferraz C, Eszlinger M, Paschke R. Current state and future perspective of molecular diagnosis of fine-needle aspiration biopsy of thyroid nodules. J Clin Endocrinol Metab. 2011;96:2016–26.
21. La Quaglia MP, Black T, Holcomb GW 3rd, et al. Differentiated thyroid cancer: clinical characteristics, treatment, and outcome in patients under 21 years of age who present with distant metastases. A report from the Surgical Discipline Committee of the Children's Cancer Group. J Pediatr Surg. 2000;35:955–9; discussion 60.
22. Akerstrom G, Stalberg P. Surgical management of MEN-1 and -2: state of the art. Surg Clin North Am. 2009;89:1047–68.
23. Chadha NK, Forte V. Pediatric head and neck malignancies. Curr Opin Otolaryngol Head Neck Surg. 2009;17:471–6.
24. Handkiewicz-Junak D, Wloch J, Roskosz J, et al. Total thyroidectomy and adjuvant radioiodine treatment independently decrease locoregional recurrence risk in childhood and adolescent differentiated thyroid cancer. J Nucl Med. 2007;48:879–88.

45 Venous Malformations

Rafael A. Couto and Arin K. Greene

Introduction

Venous malformation (VM) is a slow-flow vascular anomaly characterized by dilated, thin-walled veins with abnormal smooth muscle (see Figs. 45.1 and 45.2) [1]. Consequently, lesions expand, flow stagnates, and clotting occurs. Although present at birth, VM may not be clinically evident until it has enlarged or become symptomatic [2]. VMs are typically sporadic; however, they also may be familial (cerebral cavernous malformation (CCM), cutaneomucosal-venous malformation (CMVM), glomuvenous malformation (GVM)) [3–5]. VMs can range from small, localized skin lesions to diffuse malformations involving multiple tissue planes. VMs can cause bleeding, pain, thrombosis, and distortion/obstruction of anatomic structures [6]. Treatment consists of sclerotherapy and/or resection.

Key Points

- VM is particularly problematic because it can expand, especially during adolescence, and often recurs after treatment.
- The majority of patients who present with asymptomatic lesions ultimately will require intervention.
- VMs should be treated in a vascular anomalies center by a multidisciplinary team.

A. K. Greene (✉)
Department of Plastic and Oral Surgery, Boston Children's Hospital, Harvard Medical School, Boston, MA, USA
e-mail: arin.greene@childrens.harvard.edu

R. A. Couto
Department of Plastic and Oral Surgery, Boston Children's Hospital, Harvard Medical School, Boston, MA, USA

Biology and Epidemiology

VMs arise from an error in vascular morphogenesis, which results in dilated, thin walled channels of variable size and mural thickness [1]. VM is sporadic and solitary in 90% of patients; 10% have multifocal, familial lesions (GVM: 8.0% or CMVM: 2.0%) [4, 5].

Pathophysiology

- The mechanism for VM enlargement is unknown. Atypical structural characteristics of the vein may predispose the lesion to distention causing stagnation, thrombus, pain, deformation, and/or obstruction [2].
- Neovascularization may be involved in VM progression. Hypoxia-inducible factor (HIF), matrix metalloproteinases (MMPs), vascular endothelial growth factor (VEGF), and endothelial proliferation are upregulated in cerebral VMs [7–9].
- Lesions progress 2.6 times more often in adolescence compared to childhood, indicating that pubertal hormones may be involved in the pathogenesis of VM [2].

Molecular/Genetic Pathology

- Sporadic VMs arise from abnormal vasculogenesis; approximately one-half of lesions have a somatic mutation in the endothelial tyrosine kinase receptor *TIE2* [4, 5]. Angiopoetins, the ligands for *TIE2*, are involved with vascular stabilization; the mutation alters endothelial–pericyte contact affecting venous development [5, 10].
- GVM is an autosomal dominant condition with abnormal smooth muscle-like glomus cells along the ectatic veins; it is caused by a mutation in the *glomulin* gene [11, 12].
- CMVM is an autosomal dominant disorder produced by a mutation in the *TIE2* receptor [10].

R. Rahbar et al. (eds.), *Pediatric Head and Neck Tumors*,
DOI 10.1007/978-1-4614-8755-5_45, © Springer Science+Business Media New York 2014

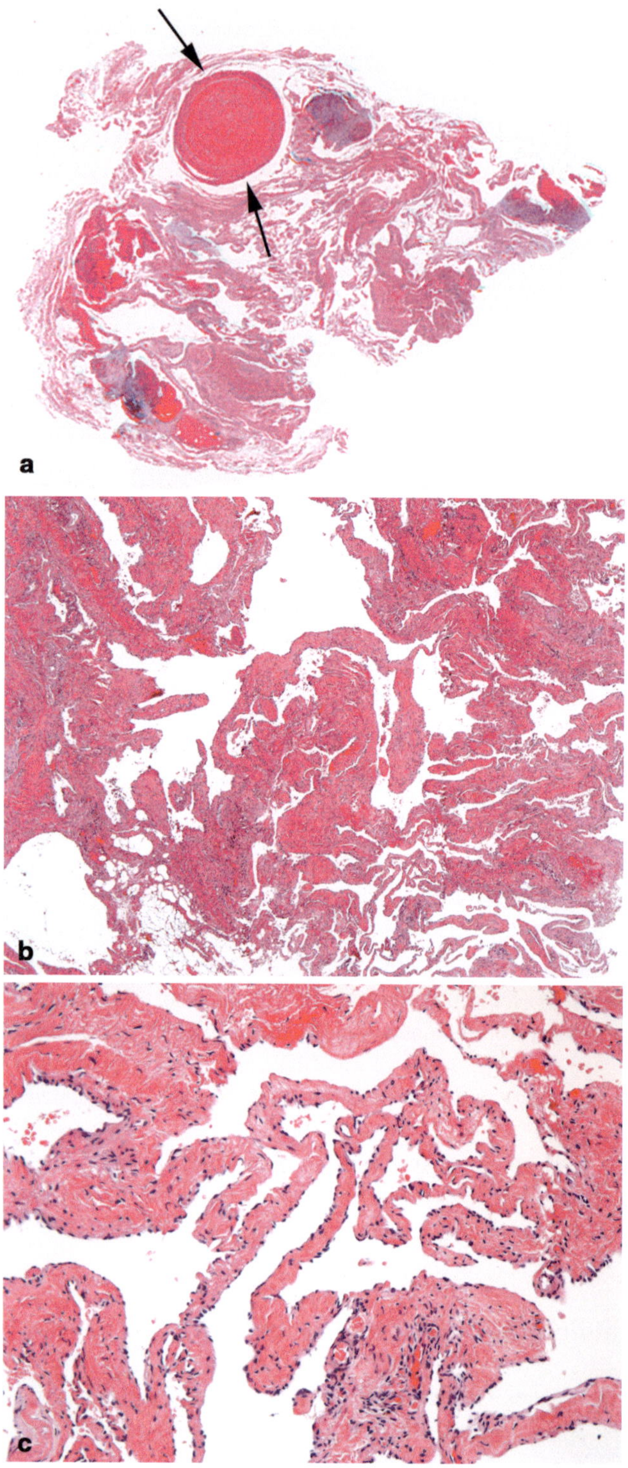

Fig. 45.1 Venous malformation, neck. **a** Intramuscular VM composed of large, irregular, thin-walled channels. A phlebolith is indicated by *arrows*. **b** The channels vary in size and are arranged back to back with scant intervening stroma. **c** Abnormal venous channels with flat endothelium and thin, variably muscular walls

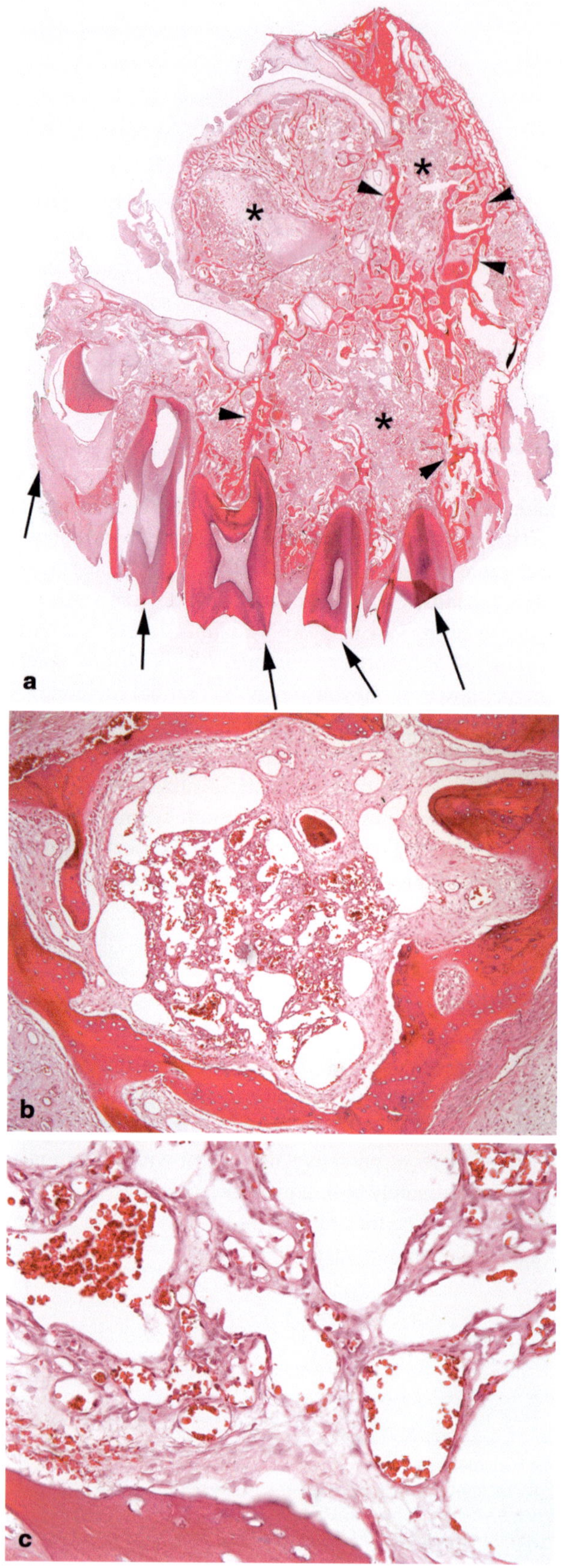

Fig. 45.2 Venous malformation, maxillary bone. **a** Portion of maxillary bone with intraosseous VM associated with osteolysis (*asterisks*). *Arrows* indicate teeth and *arrowheads* indicate residual trabeculae of bone. **b** Cluster of intramedullary, thin-walled venous channels of variable size. **c** Back to back, thin-walled venous channels with flat endothelium and luminal red blood cells

- CCM is an autosomal dominant condition that results from mutations in *CCM1/KRIT1*, *CCM2*, and *CCM3* genes [13–15].

Incidence and Prevalence

- VMs are the most common vascular malformation treated in a vascular anomalies center, comprising 36.8% of referrals [16].

Age Distribution

- VM is present at birth, but may not become obvious until childhood or adolescence [2].

Sex Predilection

- Men and women are affected equally.

Risk Factors

- The offspring of patients with GVM, CMVM, or CCM have a 50% risk of inheriting the condition [11–15].
- Progesterone-only oral contraceptives are recommended because estrogen has more potent proangiogenic activity than progesterone [6, 17–20].
- Pregnant women do not have an increased risk of VM expansion and thus pregnancy is not contraindicated [2]. Nevertheless, women with significant lesions should be cautioned about possible worsening of symptoms during pregnancy.

Relationships to Other Disease States, Syndromes

- Blue rubber bleb nevus syndrome (BRBNS) is a rare condition with multiple VMs in the skin, soft tissue, and gastrointestinal tract [21].
- Diffuse phlebectasia of Bockenheimer is an extensive extremity VM that affects the skin, subcutaneous tissue, muscle, and bone [22].
- Kippel-Trénaunay syndrome (KTS) is an eponym used to describe capillary-lymphatic-venous malformation (CLVM) of an overgrown extremity.
- Sinus pericranii is a soft tissue/cutaneous VM of the scalp or face that has a transcranial communication with the dural venous system.

Presentation

Symptoms

- Bleeding
  - Head/neck VM may present with mucosal bleeding.
  - BRBNS can cause gastrointestinal bleeding and chronic anemia.
- Distortion/obstruction of anatomical structures
  - Head/neck VM may compromise airway or orbital function.
- Pain
  - Caused by thrombosis and phlebolith formation.
  - VM of muscle may result in fibrosis and contractures.
  - GVMs are typically more painful than sporadic VM.
- Thrombosis
  - Large VMs are likely to have venous pooling and are predisposed to localized intravascular coagulopathy (LIC) causing thrombosis and pain [23].
  - Phlebectasia that communicates with the deep venous system is at risk of thrombosis and pulmonary embolism [6].

Differential Diagnosis

Arteriovenous malformation (AVM)
Capillary malformation (CM)
Congenital hemangioma (CH)
Infantile hemangioma (IH)
Kaposiform hemangioendothelioma (KHE)
Lymphatic malformation (LM)

Diagnosis and Evaluation

Physical Examination

Venous Malformation

Approximately 90% of VMs are diagnosed by history and physical examination [24, 25]. VMs can be small and well localized, or involve multiple tissue planes and important structures. Almost all lesions involve the mucosa, skin, and/or subcutaneous tissue; 50% also affect deeper structures (e.g., muscle, bone, joints, viscera) [4]. The primary differential diagnosis is LM.

- Findings:
  - VMs are blue, soft, and compressible; dependent positioning may enlarge the lesion.
  - VMs are usually >5 cm (56%) and solitary (99%), they are located on the extremities (48.3%), head/neck (30.3%), trunk (16.6%), or viscera (4.8%) [16].

- VMs are slow-flow lesions; hand-held Doppler excludes fast-flow vascular anomalies (e.g., AVM, hemangioma) [6].

Glomuvenous Malformation

Patients with a family history of VM should be evaluated for GVM. This condition is autosomal dominant, and individuals are counseled about the risk of transmitting the gene to their offspring [6]. Patients are also predisposed to develop new lesions [4, 12].

- Findings:
  - Confined to the skin and subcutaneous tissue. Lesions are usually <5 cm, and multiple (70%) [4].
  - Involve the extremities (76%), trunk (14%), or head/neck (10%) [4].
  - More painful than VM, especially on palpation [12].

Cutaneomucosal-Venous Malformation

Patients with a family history of similar lesions should be examined for CMVM. Individuals are counseled about the autosomal dominant inheritance pattern of this condition.

- Findings:
  - Lesions are small (76% <5 cm), multiple (73%), and located on the head/neck (50%), extremity (37%), or trunk (13%) [4].
  - Unlike GVM, CMVM is not painful on palpation [4].

Laboratory Data

- Large VMs are at risk for blood stagnation and subsequent coagulation.
  - Plasma D-dimers and fibrin split products may be elevated [26].
  - Antithrombin, fibrinogen, and factors V, VIII, and XIII can be low [26].
  - Prothrombin and partial thromboplastin time are normal [26].

Imaging Evaluation

Imaging is usually performed for large or deep VMs. Small, superficial lesions typically do not require radiographical work-up.

Ultrasonography (US)

US can be performed without sedation and demonstrates compressible, anechoic-hypoechoic spaces with septations [27]. Phleboliths are hyperchoic and cause acoustic shadowing [28].

Computed Tomography (CT)

CT may be indicated if there is bony involvement [6].

Magnetic Resonance Imaging (MRI)

MRI is usually obtained for large, deep, or problematic lesions to (1) confirm the diagnosis, (2) define the extent of the malformation, and (3) plan treatment [6]. VMs are hyperintense on T2-weighted images; phleboliths are hypointense [6]. VMs enhance following gadolinium administration [29].

Venography

Venography is not required for diagnostic confirmation, but is often performed during sclerotherapy.

Pathology

Histopathological diagnosis of VM is rarely necessary, but may be indicated if imaging is equivocal. Histopathologically, VMs show abnormal, thin-walled venous channels with irregular layers of smooth muscle (see Figs. 45.1 and 45.2) [1]. Vessels frequently have thrombi or phleboliths in their lumens (see Fig. 45.1a) [1]. GVMs are characterized by abnormal venous channels surrounded by characteristic cuboidal myoid “glomus” cells (see Fig. 45.3) [1].

Treatment

Nonoperative Management

Drug therapy for VMs is not available. Patients with a large extremity VM are prescribed custom-fitted garments to reduce blood stagnation which minimizes expansion, LIC, phlebolith formation, and pain [23, 26, 30]. Prophylactic daily aspirin (81 mg) may be given to patients with recurrent pain from phlebothrombosis [6]. Anticoagulation with low-molecular-weight heparin (LMWH) or warfarin is considered for patients with significant LIC or those at risk for disseminated intravascular coagulation (DIC) [26, 31]. An inferior or superior vena cava filter may be indicated if anticoagulantion is contraindicated or ineffective [26].

Operative Management

Indications

VM is a benign condition, and thus nonproblematic lesions do not require intervention. Treatment usually is reserved for symptomatic VMs that cause pain, deformity, or threaten vital structures. Lesions are managed with sclerotherapy and/or resection. VM involving an anatomically sensitive area or causing gross deformity may require management as early as infancy. If possible, intervention should be postponed until after 12 months of age when the risk of anesthesia is lowest [6]. Long-term memory and self-esteem begin to form around 3.5 years; thus, it is ideal to treat a lesion

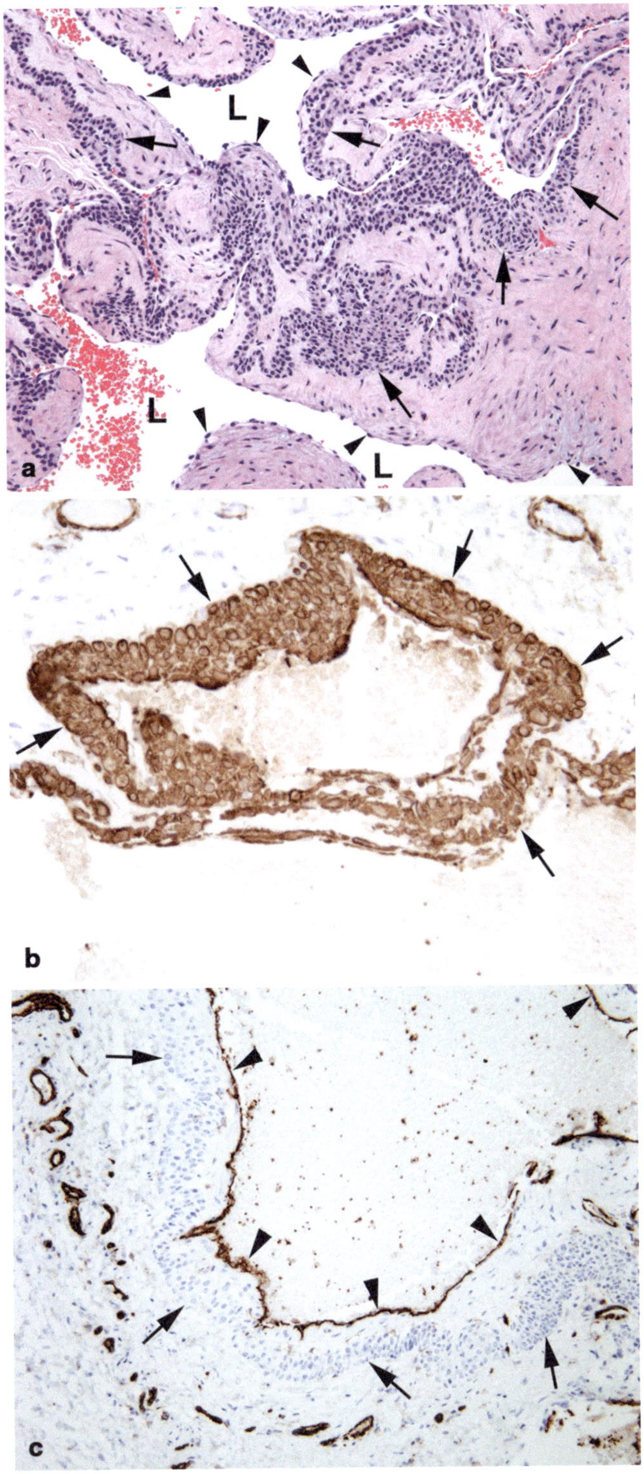

Fig. 45.3 Glomovenous malformation, soft tissue. **a** Large tortuous venous channels surrounded by layers of uniform glomus cells (*arrows*). Venous channels are lined by flattened endothelium (*arrowheads*) and their lumens (*L*) have irregular shapes. **b** Glomus cells (*arrows*) are strongly and diffusely immunoreactive for smooth muscle actin. **c** Endothelium shows strong immunoreactivity for CD31 (*arrowheads*) while surrounding glomus cells are negative (*arrows*)

causing a deformity before this age to limit psychological morbidity [6]. Some parents, however, elect to wait until the child is older and able to make the decision to proceed with operative intervention, especially if the deformity is minor. However, if a lesion enlarges over time, it may become more difficult to treat.

Sclerotherapy

Sclerotherapy is the first-line intervention for problematic VM because it is safer and more effective than resection (see Fig. 45.4) [6, 28, 32]. It involves the injection of a sclerosant into the lesion which causes inflammation, cellular destruction, thrombosis, and shrinkage. Diffuse malformations are treated by targeting specific symptomatic regions [6, 28]. Sclerotherapy is continued until symptoms are alleviated or when there are no further vascular spaces to inject. Although sclerotherapy reduces the size of the lesion and improves symptoms, it does not cure the condition. Consequently, patients may still have a deformity after treatment, which can be improved by a surgical procedure [6].

Sodium tetradecyl sulfate (STS), absolute ethanol (95–98 %), and bleomycin are the preferred sclerosants at our institution [6, 28]. Ethanol is more toxic to the VM than STS, but it has to be carefully used due to potential local and systemic complications [6, 28]. Small lesions may be treated in the office without image guidance; 3 % STS is diluted in saline to inject a 1 % solution [6].

Ulceration is the most common local complication following sclerotherapy, and is more likely if the VM involves the dermis or if ethanol is used [6, 28, 32, 33]. Wounds are allowed to heal secondarily, and depending on the depth of the wound, topical antibiotics or dressing changes are used [6]. Transient or permanent nerve injury can result from extravasation of scleroscent, especially when ethanol is used [6, 28, 32, 33]. Extravasation of scleroscent into muscle can cause atrophy and contracture [6, 28, 32, 33]. Post-treatment swelling in certain anatomic areas may require close monitoring. Since orbital injections can cause orbital compartment syndrome, patients are examined by an ophthalmologist immediately after the procedure [6, 28].

Systemic complications from sclerotherapy, including hemolysis, hemoglobinuria, and oliguria are more common when large lesions are managed with a significant volume of sclerosant [6, 28]. To prevent renal injury, patients receive intravenous fluid to alkalinize the urine [6, 28]. Patients who are at risk of thromboembolism may be given LMWH 14 days before and after the procedure [6, 28].

Resection

Excision of a VM can cause major blood loss, iatrogenic injury, and/or disfigurement. Resection usually is not first-line treatment because (1) complete removal of the lesion is rarely accomplished, (2) the recurrence rate is high, (3) the risk of bleeding and iatrogenic injury is significant, and (4)

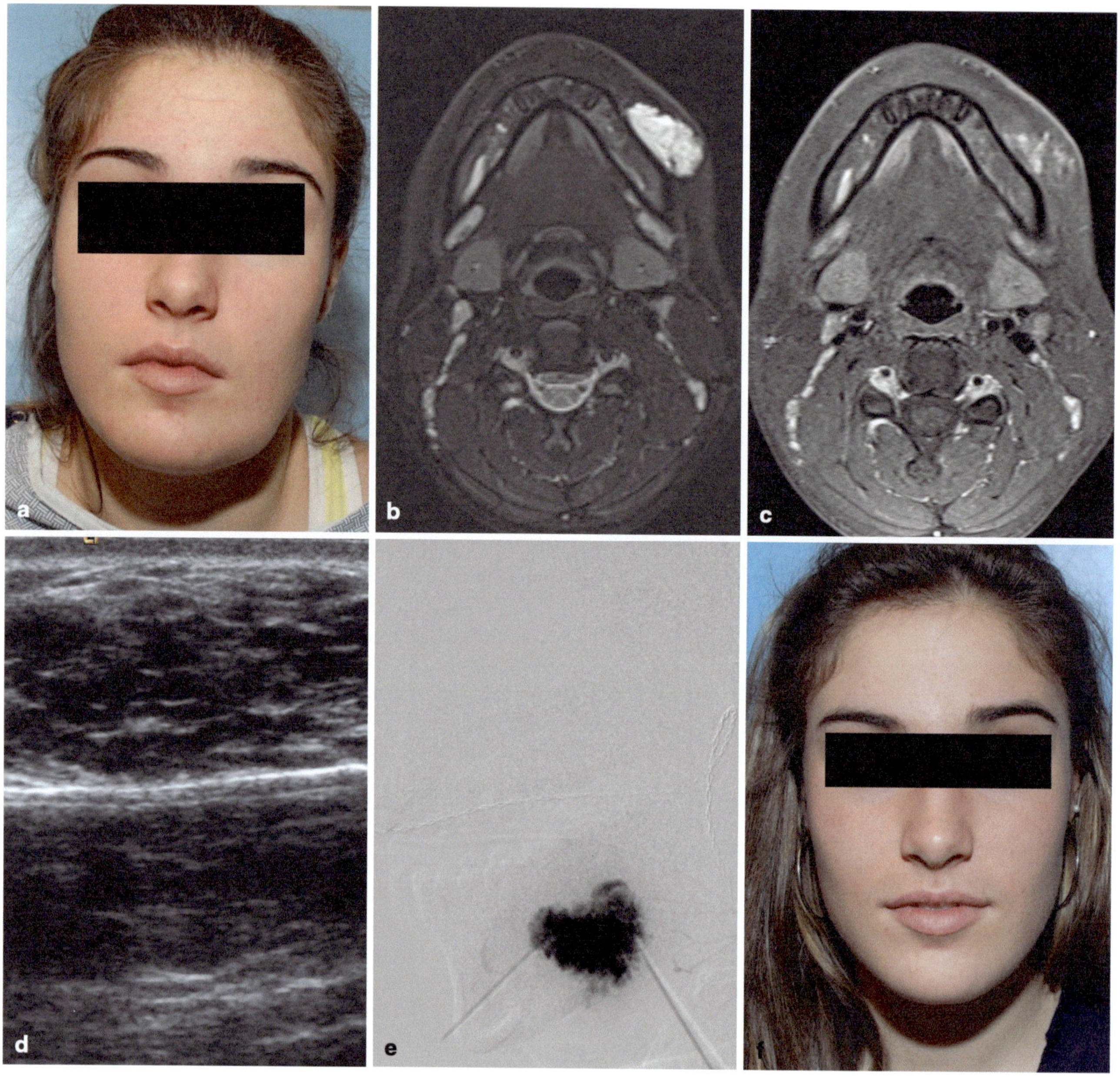

Fig. 45.4 Management of VM with sclerotherapy. **a** 15-year-old girl with an enlarging lesion of the left cheek. **b** T2-weighted axial magnetic resonance with fat suppression illustrates a localized VM involving the cheek. **c** Axial T1 image exhibits heterogeneous enhancement of the lesion with contrast. **d** Ultrasound exhibits compressible hypoechoic venous spaces with echogenic walls. **e** Venogram of a spongiform VM with minor draining vein. **f** Resolution of facial asymmetry 2 months following sclerotherapy with sodium tetradecyl sulfate. Reprinted from Clinics in Plastic Surgery, 38/1, Greene AK, Alomari AI, Management of Venous Malformations, 87, 2011, with permission from Elsevier

extirpation may cause a worse deformity than the appearance of the VM. An operation should be considered for small, well-localized lesions that can be completely removed, or for malformations that continue to be symptomatic after sclerotherapy.

Generally, VMs should undergo sclerotherapy several months prior to excision to (1) facilitate the resection, (2) improve the outcome, and (3) reduce the recurrence rate (see Fig. 45.5) [6]. Sclerotherapy converts the VM into scar tissue, which reduces the risk of blood loss, iatrogenic injury, and recurrence. Patients receiving chronic anticoagulation, should have the anticoagulant held 12 h before and after the procedure to prevent bleeding complications [26, 28]. Cryoprecipitate may be administered if the fibrinogen levels are low on the day of the operation [32]. Because GVMs are small, localized, and less amenable to sclerotherapy, resection usually is first-line therapy for symptomatic areas [6].

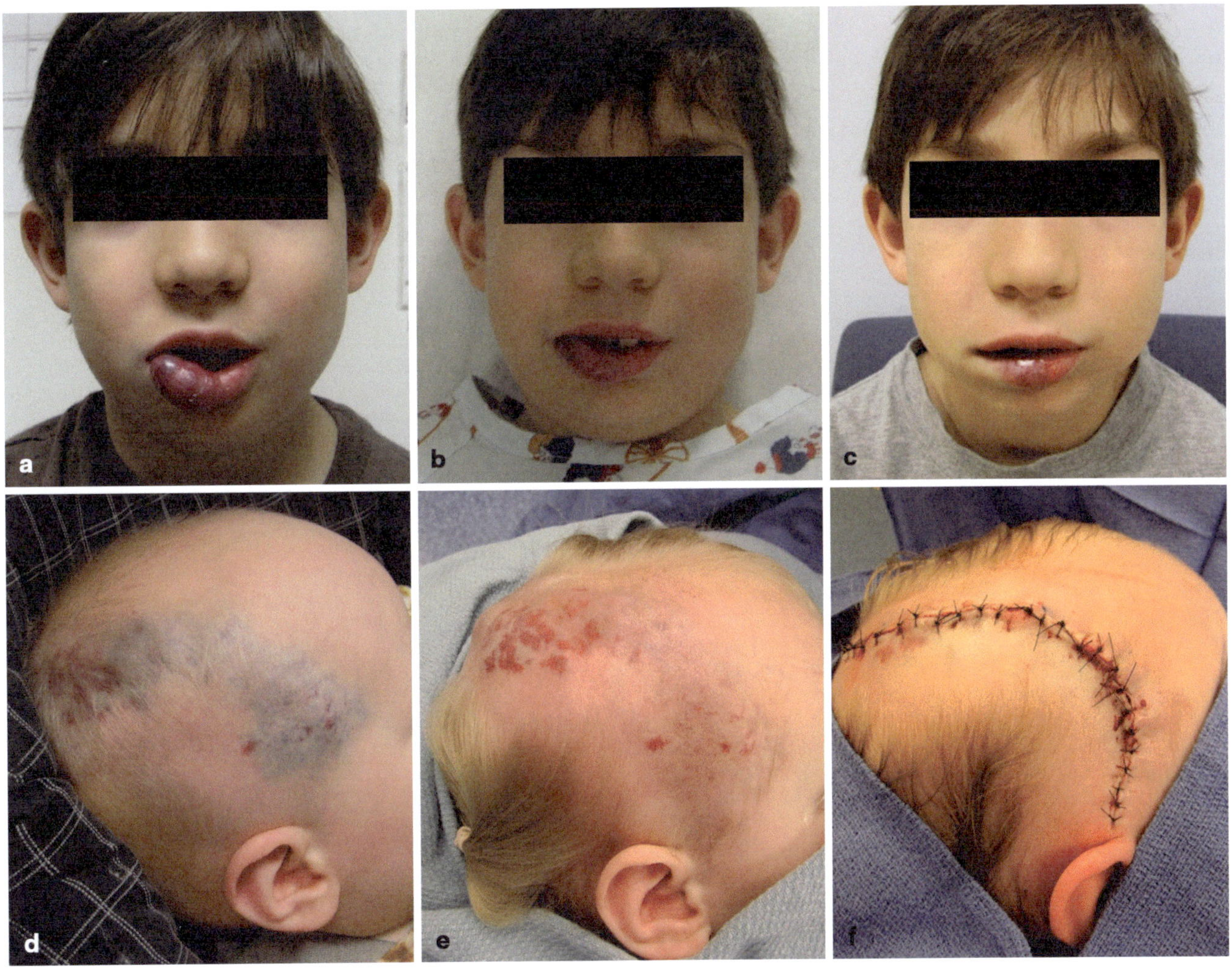

Fig. 45.5. Management of VM with sclerotherapy followed by resection. **a** 5-year-old boy with an enlarging VM of the lower lip. **b** Reduction of VM after three sclerotherapy treatments with STS. Sclerotherapy could not be continued due to the replacement of venous spaces by fibrotic tissue. **c** Improved contour 6 weeks following excision of residual VM and scar tissue using a transverse mucosal incision. **d** 7-month-old girl with a VM of the scalp. **e** Reduction of lesion following three STS treatments. Additional sclerotherapy was not possible because accessible venous spaces had been obliterated. **f** Following resection of residual VM and scar tissue. Reprinted from Clinics in Plastic Surgery, 38/1, Greene AK, Alomari AI, Management of Venous Malformations, 89, 2011, with permission from Elsevier

Head and neck lesions are removed through a coronal (forehead, orbit), tarsal (eyelid), preauricular-melolabial-transoral (cheek), or transverse mucosal (lip) incision. In order to reduce blood loss, local anesthetic with epinephrine should be administered. Subtotal resections of problematic areas (e.g., overgrown lip) should be performed rather than attempting total excision which would result in a worse deformity than the malformation (see Fig. 45.5) [6]. Staged resection of defined regions is recommended for diffuse VMs. Patients and families are counseled that VM can reexpand, and thus additional intervention may be required in the future.

Outcome

Operative Management

Sclerotherapy

Seventy to ninety percent of patients experience a reduction in the size of the VM, and have improved symptoms (see Fig. 45.4) [6, 28, 32, 33]. However, VMs can reexpand after sclerotherapy [6]. For example, 6 months following treatment with STS, 45 % of patients have partial recannalization [34]. Patients often require additional interventions over the course of their lifetime.

Resection

Recurrence following resection is common. Excision is usually subtotal because the lesion often involves important anatomical structures, and it is difficult to appreciate the extent of the malformation.

References

1. Gupta A, Kozakewich H. Histopathological of vascular anomalies. Clin Plast Surg. 2011;38(1):31–44.
2. Hassanein AH, Mulliken JB, Fishman SJ, et al. Venous malformation: risk of progression during childhood and adolescence. Ann Plast Surg. 2012;68(2):198–201.
3. Labauge P, Enjolras O, Bonerandi JJ, et al. An association between autosomal dominant cerebral cavernous and a distinctive hyperkeratotic cutaneous vascular malformations in 4 families. Ann Neurol. 1999;45:250–4.
4. Boon LM, Mulliken JB, Enjolras O, et al. Glomuvenous malformation (glomangioma) and venous malformation: distinct clinicopathologic and genetic entities. Arch Dermatol. 2004;140:971–6.
5. Limaye N, Wouters V, Uebelhoer M, et al. Somatic mutations in angiopoietin receptor gene TEK cause solitary and multiple sporadic venous malformations. Nat Gen. 2009;41:118–24.
6. Greene AK, Alomari AI. Management of venous malformation. Clin Plast Surg. 2011;38(1):83–93.
7. Notelet L, Houtteville JP, Khour S, et al. Proliferating cell nuclear antigen (PCNA) in cerebral cavernomas: an immunohistochemical study in 42 cases. Surg Neurol. 1997;47:364–70.
8. Sure U, Freman S, Bozinov O, et al. Biological activity of adult cavernous malformations: a study of 56 patients. J Neurosurg. 2005;102(2):342–7.
9. Bicer A, Gucu B, Ozkan A, et al. Expressions of angiogenesis associated matrix metalloproteinases and extracellular matrix proteins in cerebral vascular malformations. J Clin Neurosci. 2010;17:232–6.
10. Vikkula M, Boon LM, Carraway KL, et al. Vascular dysmorphogenesis caused by an activating mutation in the receptor tyrosine kinase TIE2. Cell. 1996;87:1181–90.
11. Brouillard P, Boon LM, Mulliken JB, et al. Mutations in a novel factor, glomulin, are responsible for glomuvenous malformations ("glomangiomas"). Am J Hum Genet. 2002;70:866–74.
12. Brouillard P, Ghassibe M, Pennington A, et al. Four common glomulin mutations cause two thirds of glomuvenous malformations ("familial glomangiomas"): evidence for a founder effect. J Med Genet. 2005;42:e13.
13. Labergele-Couteulx S, Jung HH, Labauge P, et al. Truncated mutations in CCM1, encoding KRIT1, cause cavernous angiomas. Nat Genet. 1999;23:189–93.
14. Labauge P, Brunereau L, Levy C, et al. The natural history of familial cerebral cavernomas: a retrospective MRI study of 40 patients. Neuroradiology. 2000;42:327–32.
15. Pagenstecher A, Stahl S, Sure U, et al. A two-hit mechanism causes cerebral cavernous malformations: complete inactivation of CCM1, CCM2 or CCM3 in affected endothelial cells. Hum Mol Genet. 2009;18:911–8.
16. Greene AK, Liu AS, Mulliken JB, et al. Vascular anomalies in 5621 patients: guidelines for referral. J Peditr Surg. 2011;46(9):1784–9.
17. Johanisson E, Oberholzer M, Swahn ML, et al. Vascular changes in the human endometrium following the administration of the progesterone antagonist RU 486. Contraception. 1989;39:103–17.
18. Hyder SM, Huang JC, Nawaz Z, et al. Regulation of vascular endothelial growth factor expression by estrogens and progestins. Environ Health Perspect. 2000;108(Suppl 5):785–90.
19. Heryanto B, Rogers PA. Regulation of endometrial endothelial cell proliferation by oestrogen and progesterone in the ovariectomized mouse. Reproduction. 2002;123:107–13.
20. Kayisli UA, Luk J, Guzeloglu-Kayisili O, et al. Regulation of angiogenic activity of human endometrial endothelial cells in culture by ovarian steroids. J Clin Endocrinol Metab. 2004;89:5794–802.
21. Fishman SJ, Smithers CJ, Folkman J, et al. Blue rubber bleb nevus syndrome: surgical eradication of gastrointestinal bleeding. Ann Surg. 2005;241:523–8.
22. Kubiena HF, Liang MG, Mulliken JB. Genuine diffuse phlebectasia of Bockenheimer: dissection of an eponym. Pediatr Derm. 2006;23:294–7.
23. Mazoyer E, Enjolras O, Laurian C, et al. Coagulation abnormalities associated with extensive venous malformations of the limbs: differentiation from Kasabach-Merritt syndrome. Clin Lab Haematol. 2002;24:243–51.
24. Mulliken JB, Glowacki J. Hemangiomas and vascular malformations in infants and children: a classification based on endothelial characteristics. Plast Reconstr Surg. 1982;69:412–22.
25. Finn MC, Glowacki J, Mulliken JB. Congenital vascular lesions: clinical application of a new classification. J Pediatr Surg. 1983;18:894–900.
26. Adams DM, Wentzel MS. The role of the hematologist/oncologist in the care of patients with vascular anomalies. Pediatr Clin N Am. 2008;55:339–55.
27. Paltiel H, Burrows PE, Kozakewich HP, et al. Soft-tissue vascular anomalies: utility of US for diagnosis. Radiology. 2000;214:747–54.
28. Choi DJ, Alomari AI, Chaudry G, et al. Neurointerventional management of low-flow vascular malformations of the head and neck. Neuroimag Clin N Am. 2009;19:199–218.
29. Burrows RE, Laor T, Paltiel H, et al. Diagnostic imaging in the evaluation of vascular birthmarks. Dermatol Clin. 1998;16:455–88.
30. Enjolras O, Ciabrini D, Mazoyer E, et al. Extensive pure venous malformations in the upper or lower limb: a review of 27 cases. J Am Acad Dermatol. 1997;36:219–25.
31. Dompmartin A, Acher A, Thibon P, et al. Association of localized intravascular coagulopathy with venous malformations. Arch Dermatol. 2008;144:873–7.
32. Berenguer B, Burrows PE, Zurakowski D, et al. Sclerotherapy of craniofacial venous malformations: complications and results. Plast Reconstr Surg. 1999;104:1–11.
33. Burrows PE, Mason KP. Percutaneous treatment of low flow vascular malformations. J Vasc Interv Radiol. 2004;15:431–45.
34. Yamaki T, Nozaki M, Sakurai H, et al. Prospective randomized efficacy of ultrasound-guided foam sclerotherapy with ultrasound-guided liquid sclerotherapy in the treatment of symptomatic venous malformations. J Vasc Surg. 2008;47:4578–84.

Index

R. Rahbar et al. (eds.), *Pediatric Head and Neck Tumors*,
DOI 10.1007/978-1-4614-8755-5, © Springer Science+Business Media New York 2014

MIX
Papier aus verantwortungsvollen Quellen
Paper from responsible sources
FSC® C105338

If you have any concerns about our products,
you can contact us on
ProductSafety@springernature.com

In case Publisher is established outside the EU,
the EU authorized representative is:
Springer Nature Customer Service Center GmbH
Europaplatz 3, 69115 Heidelberg, Germany

Printed by Libri Plureos GmbH
in Hamburg, Germany